THE COMPLETE GUIDE TO FERTILITY AWARENESS

Fertility awareness is key to understanding and making decisions about sexual and reproductive health at all life-stages. It can be used to plan or avoid pregnancy. Fertility Awareness Methods (FAMs) are highly effective when motivated couples are taught by trained practitioners. These methods are in demand for ecological, medical, cultural, religious and moral reasons. The ability to control fertility naturally is a lifestyle choice.

The Complete Guide to Fertility Awareness provides the science and methodology suitable for health professionals and a general audience. It covers reproductive physiology and the fertility indicators: temperature, cervical secretions and cycle length calculations. It explores ways to optimise conception and to manage conception delays. Case studies and self-assessment exercises are included throughout. The book addresses the scientific credibility of new technologies including fertility apps, home test kits, monitors and devices.

The Complete Guide to Fertility Awareness offers:

- evidence-based information for general practitioners, practice nurses, school nurses, midwives, and sexual health doctors and nurses;
- a unique perspective on subfertility for gynaecologists and fertility nurses;
- an authoritative source of reference for medical, nursing and midwifery students;
- a balanced source of information for complementary therapists;
- a straightforward and practical reference for new and experienced FAM users;
- the core text for the FertilityUK Advanced Skills Course in Fertility Awareness.

Jane Knight is a fertility nurse specialist with over 30 years experience teaching fertility awareness in both NHS and private practice. She was the UK Principal Investigator for the European multi-centre study on the probability of conception on different days of the menstrual cycle. She trains health professionals in the UK and internationally.

THE COMPLETE GUIDE TO FERTILITY AWARENESS

JANE KNIGHT

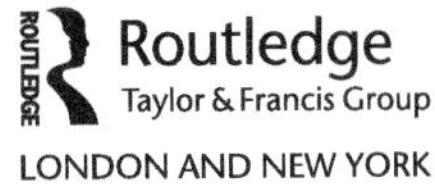

LONDON AND NEW YORK

First published 2017
by Routledge
2 Park Square, Milton Park, Abingdon, Oxon OX14 4RN

and by Routledge
711 Third Avenue, New York, NY 10017

Routledge is an imprint of the Taylor & Francis Group, an informa business

Cover design by Burnt Peach www.burntpeach.com

British Library Cataloguing in Publication Data
A catalogue record for this book is available from the British Library

Library of Congress Cataloging in Publication Data
A catalogue record has been requested for this book.

ISBN: 978-1-138-79009-4 (hbk)
ISBN: 978-1-138-79010-0 (pbk)
ISBN: 978-1-315-76441-2 (ebk)

Typeset in Sabon
by Apex CoVantage, LLC

Dedicated to the memory of Dr Elizabeth Clubb FRCGP, DSG

CONTENTS

PREFACE

My interest in fertility awareness was first sparked as a student midwife. Our *Maggie Myles* textbook sternly warned us that "the safe period is not safe" but an enlightened tutor gave us a review article by an American gynaecologist entitled "Fertility awareness as a method of conception control" – and finally the menstrual cycle made sense. My quest for more information led me to Oxford – to Dr Elizabeth Clubb, a general practitioner who had been teaching Catholic couples for many years. In the 1970s there was an increasing interest from the "Green Movement", so Elizabeth took me on to cope with the demand.

Elizabeth was Medical Director of Catholic Marriage Advisory Council (CMAC) and I became the first non-Catholic head of the Fertility Awareness Service. It was apparent that women expect to access family planning information not through CMAC centres but through mainstream health services, so attention was focussed on training health professionals to teach Fertility Awareness Methods (FAMs) alongside other contraceptive methods. We developed audio-visual aids to reduce teaching time and conducted a pilot study which showed that group teaching is both effective and cost-effective in primary care. The multi-disciplinary training achieved university accreditation in the late 1990s and FAMs were finally seen as credible methods which could be integrated into NHS services. We co-authored our first book for general readers in 1986.

Much has changed in the 30 years since the first edition of *Fertility*. At that time combining the indicators was definitely seen as the way forward, but we now have a much clearer picture of the actual fertile time, based on hormonal assays and ultrasound. Years of painstaking research have determined the optimum combination of indicators to identify the fertile time. Women now have real choice – from the simplest calendar-based methods, different combinations of indicators through to Lactational Amenorrhoea Method and beyond. The way forward is undoubtedly gadgets and apps, but the research evidence is lacking. Without it we run the risk of going full circle back to the unreliability of the Calendar/Rhythm Method.

ACKNOWLEDGEMENTS

I would like to thank my colleagues who have provided comments on specific chapters: Dr Allan Pacey, Dr Victoria Jennings, Dr Cecilia Pyper, Dr Jill Shawe, Dr Christian Gnoth, Judy Sotudeh, Anita O'Neill, Terri Morgan-Collins, Dr Sheryl Homa, Melanie Brown and Zita West. I owe an enormous debt to Toni Belfield who tackled the whole book, provided much-needed encouragement and made a major contribution to the finished product. And finally to my family: to my husband Peter, to Kyle who supported the IT and to Pia for her tireless work on the images.

ABBREVIATIONS

AFC	Antral follicle count
AMH	Anti-mullerian hormone
ASRM	American Society for Reproductive Medicine
BBT	Basal body temperature
BIP	Basic infertile pattern
BMI	Body mass index
COC	Combined oral contraceptive
CPR	Cumulative pregnancy rate
E3G	Estrone 3–glucuronide
ESHRE	European Society of Human Reproduction and Embryology
FA	Fertility awareness
FAM(s)	Fertility Awareness Method(s)
FFD	First fertile day
FIGO	International Federation of Gynecology and Obstetrics
FPA	Family Planning Association
FSH	Follicle-stimulating hormone
FSRH	Faculty of Sexual and Reproductive Health Care
GnRH	Gonadotrophin-releasing hormone
hCG	Human chorionic gonadotrophin
HFEA	Human Fertilisation and Embryology Authority
HPV	Human papilloma virus
HRT	Hormonal replacement therapy
IPPF	International Planned Parenthood Federation
IRH	Institute for Reproductive Health (Georgetown University, Washington DC)
IUC	Intrauterine contraception
IUD	Intrauterine device
IVF	In-vitro fertilisation
LAM	Lactational Amenorrhoea Method
LARC	Long-acting reversible contraceptive
LFD	Last fertile day
LH	Luteinising hormone
LNG-IUS	Levonorgestrel-releasing intrauterine systems
LPD	Luteal phase deficiency
LUF	Luteinised unruptured follicle
NFP	Natural Family Planning
NICE	National Institute for Health and Clinical Excellence

NSAID	Non-steroidal anti-inflammatory drug
OC	Oral contraceptive
OPK	Ovulation predictor kit
PCOS	Polycystic ovary syndrome
PMS	Premenstrual syndrome
POI	Premature ovarian insufficiency
POP	Progestogen-only pill
PSA	Prostate specific antigen
PSHE	Personal social, health and economic education
RCOG	Royal College of Obstetricians and Gynaecologists
RHA	Reproductive health awareness
SDM	Standard Days Method
STI	Sexually transmissible infection
TDM	TwoDay Method
TSH	Thyroid stimulating hormone
USAID	US Agency for International Development
WHO	World Health Organisation

FIGURES

TABLES

IMAGES AND PERMISSIONS

Artwork by Burnt Peach www.burntpeach.com

Figures 2.1, 2.3, 2.4, 3.1, 3.4, 3.5, 3.6, 4.15, 5.2, 7.1, 12.1, 13.1, 14.1, 18.6, 18.7 and appendices A–E adapted from Clubb and Knight, Fertility, David and Charles 1996 and FertilityUK training materials.

Figures 3.2, 3.7, 3.9, 3.12, 3.13, 4.1, 5.1, 6.1 copyright © Dr Cecilia Pyper and Jane Knight 2016. Produced in collaboration with FertilityUK and the Institute for Reproductive Health, Georgetown University.

Figures 4.2, 4.3, 4.4, 4.5, 4.6, 4.7, 4.8, 4.10, 4.11, 4.12, 5.3, 5.4, 5.5, 5.6, 6.2, 7.2, 8.1, 9.1, 10.3, 12.2, 12.3, 12.4, 12.5, 15.1, 15.2, 15.3, 16.4, 16.5, 17.2, 17.3, 18.2, 18.3, 18.4, 19.1 and 19.2 copyright © Jane Knight, FertilityUK 2016.

Figure 3.8 Copyright © Prof. Erik Odeblad. Verbal permission for reproduction from Odeblad 18.02.15.

PART I

Scientific background and methodology

OVERVIEW OF FERTILITY AWARENESS

1

The term **fertility awareness (FA)** is used in different ways. It is essentially an educational process which provides individuals with a better understanding about fertility so that they are in a stronger position to make informed decisions about how they wish to both manage their reproductive health and take control of their fertility.

In the 1990s the Institute for International Studies in Natural Family Planning (Georgetown University) defined FA as:

> Basic information and education on male and female reproductive physiology as it relates to fertility. For a woman this includes the ability to identify and interpret the signs, symptoms and patterns of fertility throughout her menstrual cycle. For a man it includes understanding his own reproductive potential. For both women and men, it contributes to their knowledge about their combined fertility at different stages throughout their lives and to their ability to communicate about fertility issues with health professionals and one another. [300]

The Institute for Reproductive Health (IRH), formerly the Institute for International Studies in NFP, now proposes a much broader definition of FA and one which more appropriately defines the ongoing educational process:

> Fertility awareness is actionable information about fertility throughout the life-course and the ability to apply this knowledge to one's own circumstances and needs. Specifically it includes basic information about the menstrual cycle, when and how pregnancy occurs, the likelihood of pregnancy from unprotected intercourse at different times during the cycle and at different life stages, and the role of male fertility. FA also can include information on how specific family planning methods work, how they affect fertility, and how to use them; and it can create the basis for understanding, communicating and correctly using family planning. [301]

FERTILITY AWARENESS: EDUCATION THROUGH REPRODUCTIVE LIFE

Men and women have a right to understand their differences in reproductive physiology and their combined fertility potential. A man needs to understand that he is always potentially fertile, producing sperm continuously from puberty until well into old age; but the reproductive lifespan of a woman is much shorter by comparison: from menarche (first period) to menopause (final period), and her fertility is cyclical.

A woman's reproductive lifetime can be roughly divided into four ages:

- teenage years with the menarche and emerging fertility (12–18 years);
- most fertile years (18–35);
- mature years with declining fertility (35–45); and
- peri-menopausal years with cessation of fertility at the menopause (45–55).

Family planning needs and intentions are likely to change throughout reproductive life, starting with a very strong need to avoid pregnancy, to a more relaxed approach when contemplating pregnancy, a time of actively trying to conceive, postnatal recovery and breastfeeding, family spacing, followed by a strong need to avoid pregnancy again when limiting the family.

A key insight from the 2013 National Survey of Sexual Attitudes and Lifestyles (Natsal3): a poll of 15,000 Britons (aged 16–44) revealed that people are having sex earlier and having children later, which means that, on average, women in Britain spend about 30 years of their life needing to avert an unplanned pregnancy, yet many are not being informed about or offered the full range of services. [401]

FA education provides fundamental knowledge at all stages of reproductive life:

- FA helps young people to understand bodily changes associated with puberty and emerging fertility. It explains reproductive physiology and normal variations in the menstrual cycle, helping to distinguish between normal physiological vaginal secretions and pathological discharges including sexually transmissible infections (STIs). FA improves understanding about the vulnerability of the reproductive organs, the potentially damaging effects of STIs and the importance of protecting future fertility. This is sometimes referred to as **reproductive health awareness (RHA)**.
- FA information helps people to understand **family planning choice**, how different methods work, how a method interrupts fertility, how it fails if not used correctly and how fertility returns after the method is discontinued. Fertility awareness–based methods of family planning should be offered alongside other methods as part of a comprehensive sexual and reproductive health service.
- **FA-based methods** of family planning are sometimes referred to as FAB methods, but referred to here as Fertility Awareness Methods (FAMs). They include all methods based on identifying the woman's fertile time. It is essential to understand the length and variability of the menstrual cycle, the timing of ovulation during the cycle, changes in cervical secretions, changes in waking temperature and the effect of intercourse timing on the probability of conception. FAMs can be used to avoid pregnancy through **natural family planning (NFP)** requiring abstinence during the fertile time. They can also be used in combination with barrier methods or withdrawal. FAMs can provide effective family planning at all stages of reproductive life.
- FA information helps couples to **plan pregnancies** and optimise preconception health; this can be particularly beneficial if they are having difficulty conceiving. Fertility-focussed intercourse may reduce time to pregnancy and avoid unnecessary fertility investigations and treatments. FA knowledge also helps to accurately time fertility tests and investigations. FA education should be a fundamental part of primary care preconception advice when couples first report difficulties conceiving.
- FA information helps people to a better understanding of the woman's reproductive lifespan, to consider the "right time" to have a baby and the risks of delaying childbearing, recognising that assisted fertility such as in-vitro fertilisation (IVF) cannot compensate for lost years.
- In the first six months after childbirth, women who are fully breastfeeding and amenorrhoeic can make use of the natural time of infertility or **Lactational Amenorrhoea Method (LAM)** to space their families.

- FA information can help women to understand cyclic changes associated with declining fertility approaching the menopause, the onset of permanent infertility and post-menopausal changes which may be pathological.

FAMs fulfil the broader definition of **family planning** which encompasses reproductive health, planning a family as well as avoiding pregnancy. Family planning is about deciding if and when to start a family, and determining the number and spacing of children. Family planning needs change with age and social circumstances, and although practical instruction in FAMs may be requested only by a small percentage of women, there are many more who can benefit from general FA information. [475]

Health professionals need to improve women's knowledge about fertility at all ages and stages: from young people's contraception and sexual health services, through primary care to specialist preconception and fertility clinics, maternity services and menopause clinics. This life-course approach fits with the 2011 Royal College of Obstetricians and Gynaecologists (RCOG) report *Women's health care: A proposal for change*, which states that

> The women's health network concept is about a woman-centred life-course approach based on the principle of the right care, at the right time, in the right place and provided by the right person. . . . The life-course approach sets out to maximise every opportunity that the health service has with a woman to improve her lifestyle and her general health, ultimately to improve her outcomes irrespective of her situation in society. Adopting such an approach to delivering health care will provide women with consistent information from a young age, enabling them to make better decisions about their health. . . . Reproductive and sexual health are relevant to almost all women and unfold across the life course; by default, health care needs are more predictable over a woman's life compared with, for example, sporadic disease episodes. [494]

WOMEN'S KNOWLEDGE OF FERTILITY

Despite our sexually enlightened age, knowledge about fertility generally remains poor. A UK survey of fertility and reproductive health knowledge, conducted in 2007 by the Family Planning Association (FPA) and National Opinion Polls, reported that 29% of respondents thought short bursts of vigorous exercise, douching or urinating would stop a woman from getting pregnant after sex; 50% gave the wrong answer or did not know when the most fertile time is in a woman's menstrual cycle; and 89% gave the wrong answer or did not know that sperm can live inside a woman's body for up to seven days [182]

Most women lack a clear understanding about the fertile time. In the late 1990s, nearly 1,500 postnatal women were surveyed in South America, revealing that almost 60% of pregnancies were unintended. A substantial proportion of the women could not identify the time during the menstrual cycle when conception was most likely to occur: 40% thought conception was most likely mid-cycle, 25% thought conception was most likely immediately after a period and 7% thought conception was most likely just before a period. Almost 30% gave miscellaneous answers, including identifying menstruation as the most likely time of conception. The younger women were less knowledgeable about the fertile time. [219]

One might anticipate that women who are trying to conceive and actively seeking fertility knowledge may be better informed about their fertile time, but this is not necessarily the case. In 1997, a fertility clinic in New Zealand assessed the fertility knowledge of 80 new patients. Only a quarter of the women were considered to have an adequate understanding of FA to optimise conception, supporting the study hypothesis of a generally poor level of fertility knowledge among women presenting for treatment. [54] Similar results were found in a 2006 clinic audit. Of 281 women who had been trying to conceive for an average of one year, 50%

were using ovulation predictor kits (OPKs), and 30% were using cervical secretions to optimise sex targeting, but less than half of the couples were estimated to be targeting the full width of the fertile time. [611]

In 2008, two fertility clinics in Australia conducted a questionnaire survey on the knowledge, attitudes and practices of 204 women, most of whom had been trying to conceive for more than a year:

- 87% had used books and the Internet to try and improve their FA knowledge;
- 68% believed they had timed intercourse to the fertile time, but
- only 13% could accurately identify their actual fertile time;
- 94% believed that a woman should receive FA education when she first goes to her doctor with difficulties conceiving. [260]

This lack of knowledge about the fertile time is reflected in both unintended pregnancies for the pregnancy avoiders and delayed conception for the pregnancy planners. The knowledge gap is costly in financial terms for public health services and, importantly, can have serious implications for women's physical and mental health. Men and women have a right to essential information about fertility.

An online survey of women aged 18–40 in the US found that around:

- 40% of women across all age groups expressed concerns about their ability to conceive; yet
- 30% of women were unaware of the adverse implications of STIs, obesity or irregular periods;
- 20% were unaware of the effects of reproductive ageing; and
- 40% were unfamiliar with the fertile time in the menstrual cycle.

As with the Gadow research in South America, younger women were less knowledgeable about fertility and older women were more likely to believe in common myths and misconceptions. The researchers concluded that fertility knowledge was limited and recommended that future initiatives should prioritise dissemination of accurate fertility information through Web-based sources and encourage contact with health professionals. [366]

FERTILITY KNOWLEDGE AND CONTRACEPTIVE RISK-TAKING

A lack of accurate fertility knowledge directly contributes to risk-taking behaviour. Sociologist Kristen Luker developed a theory of contraceptive risk-taking from studying 500 women seen at an abortion clinic in California. [363] Her theory proposes that a woman uses a cost-benefit analysis, although she may not perceive it as such, and essentially goes through a three-step decision-making process:

1 Weigh up the psycho-social costs of contraception vs. the benefits of pregnancy.
2 Make a subjective assessment of the risk of conception based on knowledge of fertility.
3 Consider the probability of reversing the pregnancy based on personal views on abortion.

Luker suggests that the more aware that women are of this complex process, the more effective they are likely to be in using contraception.

Costs of contraception vs. benefits of pregnancy

Luker describes a number of psycho-social costs in using contraception: the woman has to acknowledge that she is sexually active (this may be difficult for some women); contraception may affect the spontaneity of sex; contraception may require a medical appointment or embarrassment in a pharmacy; she may fear rejection or a negative reaction from her partner, especially if she asks him to use a condom; and she may have medical concerns (for example, about side effects of the pill).

Luker also describes anticipated benefits of pregnancy: proof of womanhood, proof of fertility (two-thirds of the women interviewed had been told by a gynaecologist that they may have difficulties conceiving), improved self-worth, rebellion against parents or a bid for independence, to force commitment from a partner, and finally the pure thrill of taking risks. These calculated costs and benefits are individually determined and vary from woman to woman and at different stages of life for each woman.

Chance of conceiving from unprotected sex

The next step in this decision-making process, and of most relevance to this discussion, is to make a subjective assessment of the probability of conceiving from unprotected sex. If a woman does not understand her fertility, she cannot accurately assess her actual risk of pregnancy on any given day of the cycle. Every time she takes a risk and does not conceive, this information is added to her decision-making as evidence of a correct assessment, that pregnancy was not possible at that time. The woman may therefore either believe she is infertile or that she has correctly identified an infertile day. So if she has unprotected sex and gets away with it, this actually encourages more risk-taking behaviour. If a woman assigns a low risk to the subjective probability of conception, she is likely to go to the final step.

Probability of reversing the pregnancy

The last step in Luker's theory involves assigning probabilities to the likelihood of reversing the pregnancy, and depends on the woman's knowledge of abortion services and her own personal views on abortion.

Freely and Pyper looked at some of the choices we face over family planning, pregnancy, abortion, genetic screening and infertility, and the complex decision-making processes involved. In *Pandora's Clock* [192], the men and women interviewed often had a narrow and patchy understanding of fertility. Whilst just about everyone welcomed the introduction of reproductive choice into their lives, very few had had an easy time with the problems and dilemmas that choice has actually created.

A number of studies highlight similar issues for women with unintended pregnancies – women generally perceive their risk of pregnancy as low, either because they thought they could not conceive on that particular day of the cycle or they believe themselves or their partner to be infertile or have low fertility. Women also over-estimate the actual chance of conceiving at the fertile time so, if a woman has successfully taken risks, this perpetuates risk-taking – until she takes one risk too many. Luker's theory of calculated risk-taking demonstrates the fundamental need for accurate knowledge about fertility to help couples take "intelligent risks".

FERTILE TIME IN HUMANS

Research using hormone metabolites clearly shows that conception occurs only during a six-day interval that ends on the estimated day of ovulation and falls to zero 24 hours after ovulation. [631] As ovulation is a hidden event in women we have to rely on observable signs which reflect hormonal changes: the indicators of fertility. Using observed indicators, the potential fertile time is slightly longer than six days.

A man is always potentially fertile, producing sperm capable of surviving in the female reproductive tract for an average of 72 hours and up to seven days in optimal conditions. A woman's fertility, however, works on a cyclical basis. Ovulation (release of the egg) occurs at a fixed interval of 10–16 days (average 14 days) before the *next* period. The egg is fertilisable for around 24 hours but there is always a possibility of a second ovulation within 24 hours (as with non-identical twins) giving a maximum of 48 hours for egg survival. The total fertile time therefore has a fairly constant number of days:

- seven days for maximum sperm survival, plus
- two days for maximum egg survival.

The challenge of FAMs is to accurately identify the start and end of the fertile time. The fertile time starts at the earliest opportunity that sperm could survive in the female reproductive tract (onset of estrogenised cervical secretions); the fertile time ends when the egg is no longer fertilisable (observable progesterone-related changes in cervical secretions and elevated waking temperature). The relative position of this nine-day fertile window will vary dependant on the day of ovulation, starting earlier in a short cycle and later in a longer cycle (see figure 3.13 in chapter 3). Intercourse at the fertile time does not, of course, guarantee conception. The probability of conception during a menstrual cycle (fecundability) is discussed on page 80; it is, however, apparent that some physiological aspects may encourage conception whilst others are not conducive.

ASPECTS WHICH ENCOURAGE CONCEPTION

The following aspects are favourable to conception:

- Physical attraction between a man and a woman often provides an irresistible urge for sexual intercourse.
- There are biological factors which promote intercourse during the fertile time. In the North Carolina study, intercourse frequency was shown to increase during the follicular phase, peak at ovulation and then decline abruptly. The six consecutive days with the most frequent intercourse coincided with the six fertile days of the cycle (assessed by hormone metabolites). The women in this study had intrauterine devices (IUDs) or tubal ligation, so were not trying to time sex to conceive. [628]
- Men are particularly attracted to women during their fertile time. One study found that lap dancers earned nearly $100 more per shift during their fertile time than in the luteal phase. The dancers on hormonal contraception showed no oestrus earnings peak. [405] [223]
- Many women report an increased libido at their most fertile time, with an abundance of estrogenic secretions favouring sperm survival. Research shows that women who are not using hormonal contraception are more likely to initiate sexual activity around ovulation. [3]
- Sexual arousal fluids increase the pH of the vagina, encouraging sperm survival.
- Prostatic fluid in semen contains prostaglandins, which stimulate the woman's vagina to contract, encouraging sperm to move towards the cervix.
- The cervix is in an optimal position for sperm penetration at the fertile time – centrally positioned, straight, soft and open.
- Negative pressure in the uterus at orgasm might promote physical aspiration of sperm – the "in-suck theory".
- Sperm are fast swimmers – they are found in the cervix within 90 seconds of ejaculation.

- A sperm-friendly environment extends from the cervix, through the uterine cavity to the Fallopian tubes. Cervical secretions assist sperm capacitation and provide the optimum environment for sperm transport through the reproductive tract.
- During intercourse approximately 250 million sperm are deposited in the anterior vagina – their sheer numbers facilitate conception.
- Sperm survival depends on the quality of the sperm, the seminal fluid and the cervical secretions. As Guillebaud reminds us: "one must be concerned not with the average sperm survival but the *lunatic fringe.*" Sperm survival may reach seven days, particularly if a woman is producing high-quality cervical secretions for an unusually long time. [256]
- When seminal fluid is first ejaculated it is highly viscous and sticks to the cervix. This temporary "gluing" effect has an obvious advantage in reproduction. Within a few minutes, seminal fluid liquefies, releasing the sperm to swim the shortest practicable distance through the cervix, giving the best swimmers a "head start".
- Although many women believe they have cycles of around 28 days, they are often very different and frequently shorter, 26 days or less. The unpredictable nature of the start of the fertile time makes conception more likely.

ASPECTS NOT CONDUCIVE TO CONCEPTION

There are two major physiological aspects which are not conducive to conception:

- The human egg has a very short lifespan (12–24 hours).
- Approximately 30–40% of fertilised eggs fail to implant, resulting in embryo wastage. This may be due to chromosomal abnormalities or to the receptivity of the endometrium.

External factors not conducive to conception:

- Less frequent sex: Natsal3 found that heterosexual couples, surveyed between 2010 and 2012, were having sex less than five times a month, a decrease from six times per month in the previous two decades. Modern living may be having an impact on libido. [401]
- Lifestyle: Negative lifestyle factors include smoking, alcohol, caffeine, illicit (recreational) drugs, sub-optimal weight and poor physical health.
- Stress and adaptation to stress: Physiologically, reproduction is a non-essential system and one of the first bodily systems to shut down during stress. In his book *Why Zebras Don't Get Ulcers*, Sapolsky explains how the human stress response inhibits reproduction. He vividly describes how stress "halts long-term expensive building projects;" and reminds us that reproduction is an expensive, optimistic thing to be doing, especially for women. [523]

CHANGES IN SEXUAL ATTITUDES AND LIFESTYLE

Demographic surveys such as Natsal3 reveal interesting changes in sexual attitudes and lifestyles. We need to question our assumptions about sex and what we mean by "sex" without assuming heterosexual intercourse. We also need to give clear and consistent messages when working with couples planning pregnancy. In 2013 the word "vaginal" was added to the National Institute for Health and Clinical Excellence (NICE) fertility guidelines on the frequency and timing of sexual intercourse: "People who are concerned about their fertility should be informed that *vaginal* sexual intercourse every 2 to 3 days optimises the chance of pregnancy." [428] For the purposes of this book, if the term "sex" is used loosely, it refers to vaginal sexual intercourse which could result in pregnancy.

Sexual pleasure is an area that women increasingly feel that they can discuss with a health professional. Some women are very open about their sexual needs, including their use of sex toys, but for others the whole area of sexual enjoyment may feel embarrassing, particularly in a clinical setting. Anxieties about sexual function and what is normal know no boundaries in terms of religion or culture, but when women (and men) feel safe they will share many of their most intimate moments, their pleasures and concerns.

TAKING CONTROL OF FERTILITY

The fact that FAMs can be used both to plan and avoid pregnancy is a bonus, but it also means that they are highly dependent on the motivation of the user and the moment of intercourse. A phrase often associated with FAMs is "unforgiving of imperfect use". When considering any method of family planning, it depends on how unforgiving of imperfect use the method is and how hard it is to use that method correctly. [589] If a woman misses a pill, depending on the time in her pill cycle, she is likely to get away with it; if a condom splits, there is a good chance that the accident will happen outside the fertile time. Unlike contraceptive methods which act by interrupting fertility in some way, with FAMs, a woman's physiology is not compromised – her body is primed to conceive. If a couple wish to avoid pregnancy, they need to modify their sexual behaviour.

Women often cite the control aspect as a distinct advantage of FAMs if they are using their knowledge to avoid pregnancy. Conversely for women who are planning pregnancy, particularly if they have a delay in conceiving, a lack of control over biological processes can be very challenging; women often describe it as the first time in their life that they have felt out of control. Essentially, FAMs offer couples an opportunity to control the elements of reproduction which are within human control.

REPRODUCTIVE HEALTH AWARENESS (RHA)

The term "reproductive health awareness" (RHA) describes an educational approach which empowers people to make responsible decisions about *all* aspects of their sexual and reproductive health. It is a broader term than FA. IRH conceptualized this approach based on its work in FAMs. It helps community, educational and health organisations to offer knowledge and skills development in body awareness and self-care, gender awareness, sexuality and interpersonal communication to their clients. IRH reminds us of the World Health Organisation (WHO) definition of health as "a state of complete physical, mental, and social well-being and not merely the absence of disease or infirmity" (WHO 1946). Increasingly, patients have moved from being passive recipients of care to clients or consumers who weigh alternatives, seeks second opinions, and assumes responsibility for their own health care. The training manual *RHA: A Wellness, Self-Care Approach* has been designed for providers to develop reproductive health training programmes. [386]

Although public health programmes in the UK may not use the term "RHA", they may be using similar participatory techniques when facilitating discussions about sexual or reproductive health. [472] These programmes are well-integrated into NHS services in the UK, so health professionals who gain a more in-depth understanding of FA will be in a better position to integrate this knowledge into existing contraception and sexual health services. Teachers and school nurses also have opportunities to integrate this approach into the science curriculum and personal social, health and economic education (PSHE) programmes (page 359).

A comprehensive literature review: "Fertility awareness across the life course" [301] explores what people know, what they don't know, and how it influences their attitudes and behaviours related to sexual and reproductive health. Sadly, not only do many women lack knowledge about their fertile time during each menstrual cycle, but many also lack a real understanding about age and the impact of delaying conception.

AGE AND FERTILITY

Pregnancy in women over 40 has become increasingly common due in part to advances in assisted conception, but largely to the increased use of egg donation. It may appear that older women are having babies using IVF, but many are either using eggs donated by a younger woman, or their own eggs or embryos which were frozen at a younger age.

Student knowledge about reproductive ageing

The average age of childbirth in the UK now stands at almost 30 years – higher than any other time in history. Twenty percent of women now reach 45 without having children – twice the proportion among the previous generation born in 1945. Some women will be childless by choice, some will have fertility problems, but others will have left it too late. [441] The issues are complex.

The Swedish FA Survey investigated fertility knowledge and attitudes to parenthood in 256 post-graduate students:

- Only 3% did not plan to have any children.
- Most childless respondents wanted at least two children.
- The majority wanted their first child at 29 and their last child around 35.
- Only 18% ranked having children before they got *too old* as very important.
- One in four over-estimated the chances of pregnancy at 35–40 years.
- One in two had overly optimistic estimates of IVF success rates.
- The most important circumstances for women's decision to have children were to be sufficiently mature, have a committed partner to share parenthood with, to have completed studies and to be financially secure. [591]

US researchers adapted the Swedish survey for online use studying the perceptions of female fertility in 246 undergraduate students. Nine out of ten students wanted children in the future, but they over-estimated the age at which a woman's fertility declines, the chances of pregnancy following unprotected intercourse and the chances of IVF success. The survey reached the same conclusion: individuals need accurate information about fertility to help make informed reproductive health decisions. [466] A New Zealand study similarly found that students over-estimated the chances of natural conception and IVF success in all age groups, and they had a poor understanding of the role of egg donation in older women. [362] [565]

What women need to know about delaying childbearing

Women need to fully comprehend the facts about age and fertility and the concerns about delaying any plans for conception.

- The optimal age for childbearing is between 20 and 35 years. [47] [46] [493]
- A woman continues to have "periods" for many years after her fertility stops.
- The probability of pregnancy is twice as high for women aged 19–26 compared with women aged 35–39 years. [145]
- Women need to consider what constitutes a family: one, two or more children; and allow time accordingly.
- Women need to be aware of any family history of premature menopause.
- A pregnancy in an older woman is more likely to miscarry or be affected by chromosomal abnormalities (for example, Down's or Edward's syndrome).

- Men are affected by reproductive ageing (although less so than women).
- IVF cannot compensate for lost years of fertility, and egg donation remains the only option for many older women. [375]
- There are currently no reliable predictors of fertility to guide women as to how long childbearing can safely be deferred. [371]
- Egg freezing may be a sensible option for women under 35 who are not in a position to start their families – provided that they are fully informed about the risks and success rates. [637]

Scientists at the university of Rotterdam used a computer-simulation model based on the natural fertility of 58,000 women spanning 200 years, updated with data from recent IVF statistics. They calculated that in order to have at least a 90% chance of achieving a one-child family, couples should start trying to conceive when the woman is 35 or younger. For two children, the latest starting age is 31; and for three children, 28 years. Without recourse to IVF, couples need to start earlier to achieve their desired family size. For a one-child family, couples need to start no later than 32, for two children at 27, and for three children no later than 23 years. [257]

The age conundrum

Public health messages about age as a leading cause of infertility are important; however, there have been legitimate concerns that this may encourage older women to abandon contraception too soon. [183] British Pregnancy Advisory Service (BPAS) statistics show that the majority of women believe it becomes very difficult to conceive after 35 and women in their late 30s and 40s were far less likely to use contraception than younger women. [60]

Educating women about age and declining fertility is challenging, but essential. Simple messages about menstrual cycles, contraception, the dangers of STIs and age-related risks should be reinforced through schools, family planning and sexual health clinics and in the media. [594] [565] Online fertility education may also have a role, but this should be paired with policies and practices that help individuals to make informed decisions about reproductive health and the timing of childbearing. [635]

FERTILITY AWARENESS TO PLAN PREGNANCY

Couples who are planning pregnancy are faced with conflicting advice. A few quotes from new clients in an Oxford FA clinic questionnaire survey highlight the confusion around targeting sex for conception:

- "We always *do it* on day 14 – the day I ovulate."
- "I know exactly when I ovulate – my temperature goes up, then we start having sex from about day 15 onwards."
- "I never let him near me until I am ready to ovulate – to save up his sperm."
- "We never do it after day 16 in case we dislodge it."

The NICE fertility guidelines [428] sensibly encourage regular sex throughout the cycle; however, this is often not practical due to busy lives and work commitments, and couples often seek more specific information. The best prospective marker of the fertile time is the cervical secretions which reflect rising estrogen levels during follicular development. Temperature changes are less relevant as the rise does not occur until after ovulation, which is too late for conception. The waking temperature does, however, have a diagnostic value, so may be of practical significance for some women. A fine line exists between encouraging a woman to develop an awareness of her fertility indicators, thus giving her a sense of control, and encouraging her to become obsessed by meticulous charting or home tests. The demands of scheduled intercourse can undoubtedly cause sexual and relationship difficulties.

FAMs TO AVOID PREGNANCY

Modern FAMs include family planning methods which are based on the identification of the woman's fertile time. [620] The effectiveness of these methods depends on two key variables: the accurate identification of the fertile time in a woman's menstrual cycle and the modification of sexual behaviour. [473]

A brief history of FAMs

Throughout history, men and women have been intrigued by fertility and ways to control it. Attempts to block, expel or divert the course of sperm date back to the Ancient Egyptians, whose concoctions for vaginal pastes included honey and crocodile dung. The Ancient Greeks were convinced that physical exertion was the answer, so there was a lot of prescribed jumping and sneezing after sex; and the Old Testament describes the "spilling of seed" (withdrawal).

Attempts to identify the fertile time date back to around 1000 BC with Hindu teachings describing the "natural season of woman". The Old Testament gives instructions regarding menstruation, the ritual bath and permitting sex from the 13th day. In the fourth century BC, Aristotle asserted that conception was most likely immediately before or after menstruation. It was not until the mid-19th century that Bischoff and Pouchet independently discovered that the ovaries released an egg about once a month – but unfortunately both scientists assumed the egg came down at the time of menstruation, comparable to the animal oestrus cycle. The image of the egg travelling down the tube and out during a period is still one held by some girls and the perpetuation of such myths is concerning.

The scientific background of the fertile time was first presented by Hartman in his classical work *Science and the Safe Period*. He reviewed the evidence for 11 different fertility indicators, including hormone assays, analysis of the corpus luteum, changes in vaginal smears, liquefaction of cervical secretions, endometrial biopsies, direct observation and recovery of oocytes, mittelschmerz (German for middle-pain) and temperature rise. [268] By 1977, Vollman published his classic volume *The Menstrual Cycle* analysing the characteristics of over 30,000 menstrual cycles – a significant contribution to current understanding of physiological methods. [601] See table 1.1 for the history and development of modern FAMs.

Identification of the fertile time

Ovulation is a cryptic event in humans. Compared with other primates where the female in oestrus provides surrounding males with clear visual advertisements of her sexual availability, ovulation in women is so well-concealed that the timing of ovulation was not discovered until around 1930. As Jared Diamond writes:

> A woman herself may learn to recognise sensations associated with ovulation, but it is tricky, even with the help of thermometers and ratings of vaginal mucus quality. Furthermore today's would-be-mother, who tries in such ways to achieve (or avoid) fertilisation, is responding by cold-blooded calculation to hard-won modern book knowledge. She has no other choice; she lacks the innate, hot-blooded sense of sexual receptivity that drives other female mammals. [121]

Table 1.1 History and development of Fertility Awareness Methods

Date	*Researcher*	*Description*
Circa 1000 BC	Laws of Manu Hindu teaching on married life	**Hindu scripture: the fertile time** The first known attempts at identifying the fertile time: "sixteen days and nights in each month, including four days which differ from the rest, are censured by the virtuous – the natural season of woman." The fertile cervix was described as "like the flowers of the water lily in the beams of the sun". [416]
Circa 1000 BC	Old Testament Genesis (38:3–10)	**Biblical reference to withdrawal method** After Onan's brother died, his father Judah told him to fulfil his duty as a brother-in-law to Tamar by giving her offspring (in a Levirate union, where the brother of the deceased provides offspring for the childless widow to preserve the family line). Onan withdrew before ejaculation and "spilled his seed on the ground" because the child would not be his legal heir. It was said that God struck him down for flouting Levirate marriage custom.
Circa 800 BC	Old Testament Leviticus (15:9).	**Jewish law** "When a woman has her menstrual flow, she will be in a state of impurity for seven days." A menstruating woman (*niddah*) was considered unclean for the first five days of menstruation and for the following seven days. The ritual bath (*mikvah*) was taken on the evening of the 12th day, after which she could be touched by her husband. The Torah prohibits sexual intercourse with a niddah. *Note:* this traditional Jewish law promotes conception.
Circa 400 BC	Hippocrates, Greek physician "Father of Medicine"	**Greek contraceptive advice** Hippocrates stated that: "After coitus if a woman does not wish to conceive, she makes it a custom for the semen to fall outside." He advised women to "jump so that the buttocks are touched by the feet". [416]
Circa 400 BC	Aristotle, Greek philosopher	**Greek anatomy** Aristotle asserted that the human embryo was produced by "the seed" of the male and merely nurtured by the "soil", or menstrual blood, believing that the woman made no material contribution. He thought that conception was most likely immediately before or after menstruation. One of Aristotle's anatomical drawings shows a duct connecting the uterus to the nipple. He assumed that breast milk was made from menstrual blood as he had observed that lactating women did not menstruate. (This was possibly the earliest description of lactational amenorrhoea.)

Date	*Researcher*	*Description*
Circa AD 100	Rabbi Eliezer ben Hurcanus	**Jewish withdrawal method** Rabbi Eliezer, a second-generation Tannaitic teacher of the Talmud approved the withdrawal method if pregnancy would affect a woman's health. Thereon he stated that a man was permitted to "thresh inside and winnow outside". [416]
Circa AD 120	Soranus of Ephesus, Greek physician	**Descriptions of the cervix in nulliparous and parous women** Soranus described the cervix as "soft and fleshy in virgins, like the sponginess of the lung and smoothness of the tongue, but in those who have born it becomes more callous like the head of a polypus" (polyp). [416] **Female orgasm and conception** Soranus made a link between orgasm and conception, observing that conception was more likely if the woman had an orgasm as this dilated the uterus. **Contraceptive sneezing** Soranus' gynaecology textbook advised that "the woman ought, in the moment during coitus when the man ejaculates his sperm, to hold her breath, draw her body back a little so that the semen cannot penetrate the os uteri. She should immediately crouch down with bent knees and provoke sneezes." [416]
12th century	Moses Maimonides, Jewish physician	**First observation of cervical secretions or pathological discharge?** Moses Maimonides noted that "lean women often have a white discharge." [416]
12th century	Chinese maintaining the stream of life	**Chinese myth** The Ancient Chinese wanted many sons, but fearing that sperm were in limited supply they developed coitus reservatus (withholding). The Yin essence (vaginal secretions) was believed to strengthen the Yang essence (semen). They advised gripping the testicles tightly or applying pressure to the perineum just before ejaculation, thus forcing semen into the bladder (retrograde ejaculation) and back through the spinal cord to the brain to maintain "the stream of life".
15th century	T.L.W. Bischoff, Germany; Felix Pouchet, French zoologist	**Ovulation during menstruation** Bischoff and Pouchet independently discovered that the ovaries release an egg about once a month. Both erroneously assumed that this occurred during menstruation so that women were fertile during a period (similar to animal oestrus).
1660s	Reinier de Graaf, Dutch physician and anatomist	**The egg theorised** De Graaf concluded that the follicle was not the egg itself but that it contained the much smaller egg (oocyte), although he never observed it. It would be 250 years until its discovery in 1928.

(*Continued*)

Table 1.1 (Continued)

Date	*Researcher*	*Description*
1678	Antonie van Leeuwenhoek, "Father of Microbiology"	**Semen discovered – the microscope** Leeuwenhoek used one of the first microscopes to study his own semen and discovered the sperm: "Animals in the semen moving forward with a snake-like motion of the tail". [416]
1827	Karl Ernest von Baer, German zoologist	**The mammalian egg discovered** Von Baer discovered the mammalian egg: "wherein lie the properties transmitting the physical and mental characteristics of the parent or grandparent or of even more remote ancestors". [416] (The human egg was not discovered until around 1928, by Edgar Allen.)
1842	Alexandre Brierre de Boismont, French physician	**Cervical secretions distinguished from pathological discharge** De Boismont used an early speculum to distinguish between normal physiological cervical secretions and pathological discharge, advising that "a white, opaque secretion, innocent in nature, should be distinguished from the inveterate white spotting or gonorrhoeal flows." [416]
1860	Edouard van Beneden, Belgian embryologist	**Fertilisation described** Beneden described the fusion of egg and sperm. **Meiosis discovered** Beneden discovered meiosis – the specialised cell division which halves the number of chromosomes to form the gametes.
1868	J. Marion Sims, American surgeon and founder of modern gynaecology	**Function of cervical secretions described** Sims (inventor of the Sims speculum) described the appearance of cervical secretions and their potential to encourage or impede sperm migration. He conducted the first post-coital test (for fertility assessment), observing that the test is positive when the secretions become clear and translucent with the consistency of raw egg white.
1869	W. Squire, London	**Biphasic temperature** Squire observed that a woman's waking temperature falls at menstruation, with a variable rise beforehand giving two distinct levels (biphasic), whereas a man's temperature remains on one level (monophasic).
1876	Mary Putnam Jacobi, Harvard student	**Harvard thesis: observational study of menstrual cycles** Jacobi observed six students for 12 cycles for her thesis *The Question of Rest for Women During Menstruation*. She measured pulse rate, blood pressure, grip-strength and total urea excretion in 24-hour urine samples. She also measured axillary, oral, vaginal and rectal temperatures. All findings showed some fluctuations over the menstrual cycle, but temperature was the most distinct.

Date	*Researcher*	*Description*
		Jacobi noted the raised temperature level premenstrually but did not link it to ovulation. She may also have overlooked a raised temperature for more than 22 consecutive days, possibly the first observation of temperature in early pregnancy. It is not known whether she realised that one of her students had conceived during the study.
1904	Theodor Hendrick van de Velde, Dutch gynaecologist, confirmed Jacobi's findings	**Temperature, corpus luteum and the ovulatory cycle** Van de Velde related the temperature rise to the activity of the corpus luteum. He showed that a woman ovulates only once per menstrual cycle, the length of the pre-ovulation phase varies and the rise in temperature is related to progesterone from the corpus luteum. He observed that the biphasic curve disappears at the menopause and is not dependent on a functional uterus. He noted four temperature phases during the menstrual cycle: • From the start of menstruation, the temperature remains low. • Around the 15th day before the following period, the temperature climbs over the course of a few days (temperature rise or shift). • The temperature remains at this higher level for about 10 days. • The temperature falls again just before or during menstruation.
1913	T.B. Hansen, German gynaecologist	**Temperature changes through reproductive life** Hansen noted that temperature patterns differ through reproductive life, observing monophasic charts in a girl before menarche, in a post-menopausal woman and in a woman after bilateral oophorectomy. He observed that: • The length of the luteal phase averages 10.7 days (range 5–16 days). • The temperature drops from as early as seven days before the start of a period, until the day after the period starts (day 2 of the cycle). • The temperature remains at the higher level following conception. • The temperature drops to the lower level following miscarriage.
1920s	Edgar Allen, American physiologist	**Discovery of estrogen** Allen's research on sex hormones led to the discovery of estrogen. **Discovery of the human egg** His studies focused on the ovarian follicles and led to the discovery of the human egg in 1928.

(*Continued*)

Table 1.1 (Continued)

Date	*Researcher*	*Description*
1929	Kyusaku Ogino, Japanese gynaecologist, and Hermann Knaus, Austrian physiologist	**Backwards thinking: ovulation in relation to the *next* period** Ogino and Knaus independently established that ovulation occurs at a fixed interval 12–16 days before the start of the *next* period. They used very different methods: • Ogino examined the ovaries of women during abdominal surgery (laparotomy) on different days of the menstrual cycle and found that none of them ovulated before the 16th day or after the 12th day before the *end* of the cycle. • Knaus used a small inflatable balloon linked to a recording system to observe the uterine response to oxytocin (pituitary extract). The contractile response of the uterus decreased sharply after ovulation, due to the action of progesterone on the myometrium. All previous attempts to relate ovulation to the preceding menstruation had been unsuccessful and had confused rather than clarified the problem, but Ogino and Knaus deduced the relationship between ovulation and the *next* period. They both concluded that: • There is only one ovulatory event in each menstrual cycle. It occurs at a fixed interval two weeks before the next period, irrespective of the length of the cycle. • Egg survival is limited to a few hours. • Conception occurs only when intercourse takes place on the days near ovulation. Ogino and Knaus reached slightly different conclusions on two aspects: • **Length of the luteal phase:** Knaus said categorically that the luteal phase was always 14 days, but Ogino gave a wider variation of 12–16 days. • **Sperm survival:** Knaus believed that sperm survival was limited to 48 hours, but Ogino believed that sperm could survive for 72 hours and exceptionally up to eight days. **Ogino's formula to achieve pregnancy** Ogino used his discovery to develop a formula for use in helping infertile women to time intercourse to achieve pregnancy.
1930	Jan Smulders, Dutch neurologist	**Calendar/Rhythm Method** Smulders saw the potential of the Ogino & Knaus discoveries to develop a method for avoiding pregnancy – the start of the Calendar/Rhythm Method. He based his calendar rules on two probabilities: • The next cycle has a high probability of fitting into the cycle length range of the preceding 12 cycles. • In a high proportion of cycles, ovulation takes place between the 16th day and 12th day before the next period.

Date	Researcher	Description
		Smulders published *Periodike Onthouding in het Huwelijk, Methode Ogino* with the Dutch Roman Catholic Medical Association. This highly controversial work promoted the official Calendar/Rhythm Method over the next few decades.
1938	Rudolf Vollman, Swiss gynaecologist	**Start of study to dispel the myth of the 28-day cycle** Vollman started collecting cycle information in response to Knaus' assertions that "the percentage of regularly menstruating women seems to be very high" and that "ovulation occurs spontaneously on the 15th day prior to the onset of menstruation." He believed that women with "a regular menstrual cycle" exist only in gynaecology textbooks. [601] He considered other indicators for gathering the required evidence including 24-hour urine collections, but settled on waking temperature. Vollman's data gathering continued for the next 39 years until he published his monograph in 1977. [601]
1939	Adolf Butenandt, German biochemist	**Nobel Prize for work on sex hormones** Butenandt was awarded a Nobel Prize for his discovery of estrone (weak estrogen), progesterone and androsterone (weak androgen).
1945	A.F. Clift English gynaecologist	**Spinnbarkeit effect** Clift studied the rheology (viscosity) of cervical secretions and the relationship with hormone levels. He observed the effect of estrogen on cervical secretions facilitating sperm penetration. He first described the "spinnbarkeit" (spinnability) effect – the capacity of thin, transparent cervical secretions to be drawn out into a long thread – an effect which is most marked at the time of ovulation.
1947	Jacques Ferin, French gynaecologist	**Waking temperature** Ferin suggested the use of waking temperature to time intercourse for avoidance of pregnancy, noting that "practically – the sterile period begins 48 hours after the temperature shift." [416]
1948	Edward Keefe, American gynaecologist	**Forget the temperature "dip" – look for the rise** Keefe designed an open-scale thermometer which demonstrated that: • the temperature rise to the higher level confirmed ovulation; and • the dip before the rise (as some authorities asserted) seemed to be an artefact.
1951	Arthur Campos da Paz, Brazilian gynaecologist	**Fern pattern of cervical secretions and sperm penetration** Da Paz first proposed studying the fern pattern of cervical secretions (drying effect of sodium chloride and mucin) to determine its receptivity to sperm penetration.

(*Continued*)

Table 1.1 (Continued)

Date	*Researcher*	*Description*
1957	Gerhard Döring, German gynaecologist	**Döring rule to identify the start of the fertile time** Döring confirmed Vollman's research on temperature as an effective marker of the *end* of the fertile time, but a more effective method was needed to identify the *start* of the fertile time. He advised the subtraction of six days from the earliest temperature rise (over the course of a year). He later added an extra day: *earliest temperature rise minus 7* to identify the first fertile day. [132]
1957	Erik Odeblad, Swedish gynaecologist, pioneer in NMR imaging	**Studies of the biophysical properties of cervical secretions** Odeblad used a nuclear magnetic resonance (NMR) spectrometer to study mucus membrane. He isolated cervical secretions from individual crypts, identifying several different types of secretion along the length of the cervical canal.
1958	Maxwell Roland, American gynaecologist	**Fern pattern in other bodily fluids including saliva** Roland reviewed the work of da Paz and others on the fern effect in cervical secretions. He noted the presence of ferning with estrogen activity approaching ovulation, but its absence by the mid-luteal phase. Other bodily fluids, including saliva, were found to show this fern pattern – a phenomenon which led to the development of a number of saliva-based home kits as predictors of ovulation. [509]
Late 1950s	JGH Holt, Dutch gynaecologist	**Temperature Method: practical use** Holt presented the Temperature Method to couples in an intelligible manner. He demonstrated that ovulation is confirmed, and the end of the fertile time is identified, by a clear rise of 0.2 deg.C or more for three consecutive days after six low temperatures – the *3 over 6 rule.* Holt devised a simple card with two windows to identify the relevant three high and six low readings. His only condition was that the woman measured her temperature once a day, preferably in the morning before getting up but always at a fixed time. [288] **Calculo-thermic Method: temperature and calendar calculation** Holt combined temperature with Ogino's calendar calculation, *Shortest cycle minus 18,* to identify the *start* of the fertile time – thus giving a clear set of rules for identifying the temperature rise and the limits of the fertile time.
1959	John Marshall, British neurologist	**Marshall introduces Temperature Method to CMAC** Marshall introduced Holt's approach to the Catholic Marriage Advisory Council (CMAC) in London, designing special charts and instructions. He began instructing couples by postal correspondence and wrote a textbook on NFP for doctors. [385]

Date	*Researcher*	*Description*
1962	Edward Keefe, American gynaecologist (Keefe 1962)	**Cervical self-examination methodology developed** Keefe described the cyclic changes in the cervix. He noted that the fertile cervix was higher in the pelvis, soft and open, whereas the infertile cervix was lower, firm and closed. He developed the methodology for self-examination of the cervix, first recommending use of a speculum, but later recognising that self-palpation was more accurate. [321]
1962	Carl Hartman, American zoologist and authority on mammalian reproduction	**Reviewing the evidence for different indicators of fertility** Hartman reviewed the evidence for (and correlation between) 11 different indicators of fertility. These included hormone assays, analysis of the corpus luteum, changes in vaginal smears, liquefaction of cervical secretions, endometrial biopsies, direct observation and recovery of oocytes (during laparoscopy and laparotomy), mittelschmerz pain and temperature rise. [268]
1964	John Billings, Australian neurologist	**Early days of *The Ovulation Method*: use of combined indicators** Billings published the first edition of *The Ovulation Method,* in which he recommended couples use a combination of indicators. To identify the start of the fertile time, he advised: • a calendar calculation (based on three- or five-day sperm survival); • changes in the cervical secretions; and • checking the glucose content of cervical secretions with test tape. Billings also advised charting waking temperature to identify the end of the fertile time. [52]
1967	WHO, Geneva	**WHO Scientific Report Group identifies research needs** A WHO Scientific Group evaluated the biological basis of fertility control by periodic abstinence. They suggested further studies including: • the determination of: "a formula that may give a better estimate of the time of ovulation than the current formulae"; and • "simple tests for the accurate prediction of ovulation". [613]
1968	Pope Paul VI encyclical *Humanae Vitae*: On the Regulation of Birth	***Humanae Vitae:* reaffirmation of orthodox teaching of Catholic Church** The Pope's encyclical *Humanae Vitae* reaffirmed Catholic orthodoxy on marriage and prohibition of contraception. It supported the use of NFP (with abstinence during the fertile time). Pope Paul VI called for "Doctors" and "Men of Science" to "succeed in providing a sufficiently secure basis for the regulation of birth founded on the observation of natural rhythms". [599]

(Continued)

Table 1.1 (Continued)

Date	*Researcher*	*Description*
1968	John Marshall, British neurologist	**Temperature Method: first effectiveness study** Marshall published the first prospective effectiveness study (field trial) of the Temperature Method in the *Lancet.* This demonstrated a high level of contraceptive effectiveness when couples restricted intercourse to the late (post-ovulatory) infertile time. [380]
1968	Erik Odeblad, Swedish gynaecologist, pioneer in NMR imaging	Odeblad's NMR studies demonstrated the mosaic of different secretions (which he defined as S, L and G-type) and their changing ratios throughout the menstrual cycle. Odeblad observed the potential for rapid sperm transport through highly estrogenised secretions and the blocking effect of progestogenic secretions synthesised in the lower part of the cervical canal. He made detailed analysis of the spinnbarkeit and ferning effects. [434]
1970	John Marshall, British neurologist	**Psychological experiences** Marshall published the psychological experiences of couples in the field trial. [384]
1972	Kamran Moghissi, US gynaecologist	**Correlation between hormonal changes, temperature and secretions** From the early 1970s, temperature changes were being linked directly to ovarian hormones and pelvic ultrasonography. Moghissi studied the inter-relationship between reproductive hormones, waking temperature, cervical secretions and endometrial biopsies (in 10 women). He observed that the properties of cervical secretions showed a remarkable relationship to the estrogen peak just before ovulation. He demonstrated that the temperature rise begins two days after the LH surge and coincides with the rise in plasma progesterone. [410]
1972	WHO	**WHO call for accurate home test to predict the limits of the fertile time** The WHO established a task force on methods for the prediction and detection of ovulation. A major objective was to develop an accurate, easy and cheap test that could be used in the home to predict the start and end of the fertile time. Research on numerous markers of fertility found that the most accurate determinant of the start of the fertile time was the increase of oestrone-3-glucoronide (E-3-G) in urine. The LH surge provides the most accurate marker of ovulation and prediction of the end of the fertile time.
1972	Drs John and Evelyn Billings, Australia	**The Billings reject other indicators and rely on cervical secretions** John and Evelyn Billings developed the understanding of cervical secretions into a practical method of family planning. They changed their thinking on the Ovulation Method, rejecting temperature and calendar calculations and believing that women could use cervical secretions as a single indicator.

Date	*Researcher*	*Description*
1972	The Billings in collaboration with James Brown and Henry Burger	***Ovulation Method* renamed *Billings Method*** John and Evelyn Billings compared women's observations of cervical secretions with urinary LH, estrogen and progesterone to gain scientific credibility for their method. Billings renamed the Ovulation Method (secretions only) the Billings Method then later renamed it again as the Billings Ovulation Method. Billings asserted that their observations provided a basis for a natural method based solely on the changes in cervical secretions. The guidelines to avoid pregnancy recommended avoiding intercourse from the *first* sign of secretions until the morning of the fourth day after peak day. Billings concluded that women need to be taught to recognise their cervical secretions. They suggested that widespread application of the method required confirmation of its reliability in practice and that the research needs identified by WHO (1967) could be met by simple clinical means. [51] [613]
1976	WHO Special Programme of Research in Human Reproduction	**WHO initiates research into the Ovulation Method** The Special Programme of Research in Human Reproduction initiated a multi-centre study of the Ovulation Method (cervical secretions as a single indicator) to determine: • the percentage of women of widely differing characteristics who could be successfully taught to recognise changes in cervical secretions; and • the effectiveness of the Ovulation Method to avoid pregnancy.
1976	Thomas Hilgers, American gynaecologist	**Hilgers Method/Creighton Model Fertility Care** Hilgers worked with Billings in Australia and then introduced the method into the US. He developed a more standardised approach to teaching – grading secretions according to sensation, colour and consistency. This was originally called the *Hilgers Method,* then renamed the *Creighton Model Fertility Care* system after Hilgers moved to Creighton University. [284]
1977	Rudolf Vollman	**Pattern of ovulatory and anovulatory cycles over reproductive life** Vollman's studies spanning almost 40 years showed the effectiveness of temperature as an indicator of fertility. He demonstrated the changing nature of temperature curves over the reproductive lifespan, noting the importance of gynaecological age (the duration of time from menarche) rather than chronological age. [601]
1979	International seminar on NFP, Dublin	**Divergent philosophies on crucial family planning definitions** Thomas Hilgers (who introduced his adaptation of the *Billings Method* into the US) presented his paper: "A critical evaluation of effectiveness studies in natural family planning". He criticised NFP studies for using the same measure of contraceptive effectiveness as other methods of contraception, suggesting that NFP is unique in that it is not singularly contraceptive, but can be used to plan a pregnancy. In the ensuing

(*Continued*)

Table 1.1 (Continued)

Date	*Researcher*	*Description*
		discussion, Jeff Spieler, a WHO scientist, challenged Hilgers on his definitions of: • method discontinuation; • planned and unplanned pregnancies; and • method and use effectiveness (correct and typical use). Many proponents of the Hilgers/Billings Method assert that if a couple's stated intention is to avoid pregnancy but they have intercourse at the fertile time (take a risk) then this was a planned pregnancy. Most authorities would categorise this as a typical use failure. [119]
1980	WHO	**Relationship between ovulation and hormonal markers** A WHO study of 177 women defined the changes in E2 luteinising hormone, follicle-stimulating hormone and progesterone in relation to the temperature rise and direct evidence of ovulation (at laparotomy). It concluded that the first significant rise in estradiol was the best marker for the start of the fertile time and LH was the best marker of *impending* ovulation. [614]
1981	WHO multi-centre study on the Ovulation Method (New Zealand, India, Ireland, the Philippines and El Salvador)	**Results of WHO multi-centre study on the Ovulation Method** • Ninety-three percent of women were able to record an interpretable ovulatory pattern of cervical secretions. Most women needed three cycles of observation before recognising the changes with confidence. • The typical use failure rate (Pearl Index) was 10–25%. The majority of unplanned pregnancies was related to conscious departure from the rules (took a chance). [616]
1983	Anna Flynn, British gynaecologist	**Subjective assessment of fertility compared with objective markers** Flynn studied the reliability of women's subjective assessment of the fertile time in relation to urinary hormones and pelvic ultrasonography. She demonstrated the importance of a calculation to identify the start of the fertile time, and the difficulty with identifying the first subtle changes in cervical secretions. [178]
1986	James Boyer Brown, endocrinologist, New Zealand	**First home urine test kit** Brown, who had done extensive laboratory work on ovarian activity, introduced the first home urine test kit to the public: the electrically powered Ovarian Monitor required the user to collect, measure and heat urine in test tubes. It had laboratory accuracy but was not easy to use and took 40 minutes per test. [66]
1988	Kathleen Dorairaj, gynaecologist, India	**Modified Mucus Method in India – a simplified method** While some authorities were making the observation of cervical secretions more complex, Dorairaj recognised the need for a simplified approach of relevance to specific communities.

Date	Researcher	Description
		Dorairaj introduced the Modified Mucus Method in India to reduce the number of abstinence days and so improve its acceptability among rural and illiterate women with low status within the family. Dorairaj used a cascade teaching system: women who had learnt the method became teachers and then supervisors. Acceptance among non-users of contraception was high. There was a high acceptance amongst Hindus but lower acceptance amongst Sikhs. Fertility education helped to empower women and enabled them to understand their potential to regulate their own fertility. [130]
1988	The Bellagio Conference on Lactational Infertility, Italy	**LAM** The Bellagio Conference published a consensus statement on LAM, defining the three criteria for its effective use: less than six months postpartum, fully breast-feeding and amenorrhoeic. [327]
1989	Elizabeth Clubb, general practitioner, Oxford	**FAMs are cost-effective in NHS Primary Care** Clubb demonstrated that FAMs are cost-effective to teach in NHS Primary Care in the UK. She used standardised teaching materials, including audio-visual aids. [94]
1994	International Conference on Population and Development, Cairo, Egypt	**The Cairo Conference on Population and Development** The conference focused on meeting the needs of individuals, rather than achieving demographic targets, by: • the empowerment of women through education and health services; • the provision of family planning as part of a broader package of reproductive health care, with high quality, client-centred services; and • access to informed choice – which includes *all* methods of family planning (including FAMs). [490]
1995	Allen Wilcox and the North Carolina team	**Fertile time: from five days before until the day of ovulation** Wilcox used hormonal assays to define the fertile time, showing that conception can occur only during a six-day window that ends on the day of ovulation. The day of ovulation and the day before ovulation have the highest probability of pregnancy. [631]
1996	John Marshall, Postal Correspondence Service, London	**Consequences of abstinence** Marshall published work on abstinence, focusing on its positive and negative effects on couples and their relationships. This was based on his correspondence with over 10,000 couples spanning 40 years. Marshall, a "Man of Science", was criticised by the Catholic community for his stance and breaking the silence on the difficulties of abstinence. [383]
1996	Unipath Diagnostics	**First computerised direct hormone-monitoring device** Persona, a hand-held computerised device which measures changes in estrone-3-glucoronide and LH by a simple urine dipstick, was launched to the public. [56]

(*Continued*)

Table 1.1 (Continued)

Date	*Researcher*	*Description*
1997	Joint International Conference, IRH, Georgetown University; US Agency for International Development; Society for the Advancement of Contraception	**NFP and Reproductive Health Awareness: Expanding options and improving health** The meeting focus was on the role of NFP as a component of reproductive health and expanding its availability through a variety of service delivery structures. The IRH stated its policy to improve the acceptability, availability and effectiveness of FAMs in developing countries. The US Agency for International Development (USAID) declared that family planning is a key reproductive health intervention and supported natural methods as part of informed choice. [153]
1998	Didi Braat, Dutch gynaecologist	**Home tests for salivary ferning must be discouraged** In response to increasing demand for cheap self-tests to predict the fertile time, Braat studied the reliability of small microscopes to detect estrogen-related fern patterns in saliva. The study included women with regular menstrual cycles, post-menopausal women and men. Eight out of ten post-menopausal women and all of the men tested positive for ovulation. These kits are unreliable and their use should be discouraged. [61]
1999	Richard Fehring, PhD Nursing, Marquette University	**Marquette Model** Fehring introduced the Marquette Model, which combines observation of cervical secretions with a fixed calculation and a fertility monitor measuring estrogen and LH to identify the fertile time. [167]
1999	IRH, Washington DC	**Standard Days Method (SDM)** The Institute for Reproductive Health introduced SDM (fixed fertile time days 8–19) as a simplified method suitable for women with cycle lengths of 26–32 days. This easy-to-teach method has applications for global use. [10]
2001	IRH, Georgetown University, Washington DC	**TwoDay Method (TDM)** The IRH introduced the TDM based on the presence or absence of secretions. This simplified form of observing cervical secretions (as with SDM) is appropriate for teaching in low-resource settings. [11]
2007	Petra Frank-Herrmann, University of Dusseldorf	**Combined-indicator method is more than 98% effective** Frank-Herrmann demonstrated that using a standardised teaching protocol and a combination of indicators, FAMs are more than 98% effective (over 17,500 cycles including the learning phase). [189]
2008	Software developers	**Apps for smartphones** Introduction of application software for smartphones, tablet computers and other mobile devices. These use a number of different methodologies, but there have been no effectiveness studies to date.

A woman's ability to identify her fertile time depends on an understanding of three key things: the time of ovulation, the length of time after ovulation during which the egg can be fertilised and the length of time after intercourse that sperm can survive in her body. FAMs are diverse. They can be categorised as observation-based methods, which rely on the woman's ability to recognise her subjective symptoms; calendar-based methods, which rely on the regularity of the menstrual cycle; or technology-based methods, including urine-testing kits and fertility monitors. Some methods use a single indicator, whereas others use a combination of indicators:

- Single-indicator methods such as temperature, cervical secretions and calendar calculations.
- Combined-indicator methods, which may combine temperature, cervical secretions, cervical changes, cycle length calculations and other "minor" indicators. Some women combine different technologies with their observations.
- Personal hormone monitoring such as the Clearblue natural contraception monitor (Persona), which uses a dipstick to analyse urinary hormone levels.
- Computerised thermometers, some of which allow input of other fertility indicators.
- Saliva testing kits, including low-power microscopes which analyse a characteristic fern-like pattern, caused by the crystallisation of sodium chloride.
- Simplified methods which include the SDM (calculation-based) and the TwoDay Method (TDM), which is cervical secretion-based. These methods may provide options for low-resource settings and our emerging multicultural society.
- LAM, a transitional postnatal method for the first six months while a woman is fully breastfeeding and her periods have not returned. LAM does not strictly fit the WHO definition of FAMs as it is not based on identifying the fertile time; however, it is viewed alongside FAMs.

There are three key aspects to identifying the fertile time:

1 Observation: has the woman been taught to observe her indicators correctly?
2 Recording: is she using a clear and reliable means of recording her indicators?
3 Interpretation: is she using evidence-based guidelines to interpret the information?

The indicators of fertility will be described in turn (chapters 4 through 8) as single-indicator methods and also as part of a combined indicator approach. The indicators are combined to provide the most effective guidelines for avoiding pregnancy for normal fertile women and in special fertility circumstances (after hormonal contraception, postpartum and approaching the menopause). Test kits and monitors are discussed in chapter 9 — Some are marketed as aids to conception and others for avoiding pregnancy, with varying levels of evidence to support their use.

PAPER-BASED AND ELECTRONIC CHARTING SYSTEMS

FAM users need a reliable system to record fertility indicators. The charting system needs to be accessible, it needs to be easy to enter daily information and it needs to have the capacity to store past cycle history. It should also allow a clear and accurate interpretation of the fertile time. Most systems involve paper-based charting (appendix A) but for ease-of-use, many women are now turning to online systems such as apps for mobile phones and tablets.

Undoubtedly, electronic charting is the way forward, but current technologies are varied: some allow the input of a single indicator (such as cycle length); others accommodate a combination of indicators. Many systems provide computerised interpretations of charts, which is appealing, but although there are some theoretical efficacy finding studies comparing the results of apps to a set of test cycles, to date there have been no effectiveness studies, so they cannot be recommended for couples avoiding pregnancy.

MODIFICATION OF SEXUAL BEHAVIOUR

FAMs have largely evolved outside mainstream medicine, with information passed down predominantly through two distinctly different groups: devout Catholics and women's health activists. This has implications for the way the method is viewed and how couples modify their sexual behaviour to accommodate the fertile time. Some couples abstain from intercourse, some use withdrawal and others use barrier methods. The effectiveness is dependent on the level and type of sexual activity, consistency of use and the reliability of the method used. A clear distinction between FAMs and NFP is important when considering effectiveness, as there may be a significant difference in efficacy rates for couples using barrier methods or withdrawal at the fertile time compared with couples who abstain during the fertile time.

Abstinence

NFP, often thought of as the "pure" form of FAMs, is defined by WHO as a method for planning or preventing pregnancies. NFP always implies abstaining from intercourse during the fertile time if pregnancy is to be avoided. NFP specifically excludes the use of barriers or withdrawal during the fertile time. NFP is therefore not a contraceptive method in the strictest sense of the word. The Oxford dictionary defines contraception as "the deliberate use of artificial methods or other techniques to prevent pregnancy as a consequence of sexual intercourse". The difference may be subtle, but for some groups it may be an important distinction; for example, NFP is the only method approved by the Catholic Church as each act of intercourse is "open to life".

Barrier methods

Many couples combine their FA knowledge with barriers during the fertile time (mixed-method users). This can work well, provided couples are properly instructed and use barriers consistently and carefully. Intelligent use of this combined approach allows for unprotected intercourse during the infertile time, protected intercourse at the times of *relative* infertility and complete avoidance of penetrative sex during the few highly fertile days. This level of commitment is highly effective.

Withdrawal method

Withdrawal (coitus interruptus) is widely practiced either on a regular basis or as an "emergency" measure during the fertile time. The debate about whether pre-ejaculatory fluid contains sperm lives on (page 248) but withdrawal during the fertile time is most unforgiving of imperfect use.

EFFECTIVENESS AND COST-EFFECTIVENESS OF FAMS

The range of effectiveness for FAMs is very wide due to the diverse nature of the methods and the conditions under which they are learnt and used. Randomised controlled trials are generally considered to be the gold standard, but these have been fraught with variability and limitations. A large European prospective study demonstrated that combined-indicator methods provide the most accurate information about the limits of the fertile time; and when couples are well-taught and follow the appropriate guidelines over 98% effectiveness is achievable (page 240). [189]

A cost-effectiveness study in general practice in Oxford showed a similar effectiveness. The study confirmed that audio-visual materials reduce teaching time and group-teaching is feasible for some couples. The time/cost compared favourably with other methods. Although the cost in the first few months was higher, due to the nurse's teaching time, once a couple understood the method they no longer needed to attend the clinic on a regular basis, and the ongoing cost of charts and thermometers was minimal. [94]

SELF-ASSESSMENT QUESTIONS

Answers are at the end of this section.

1 Define fertility awareness (FA).
2 How would you explain the difference between FAMs and NFP? Why might this be significant?
3 What is the outer limit of sperm survival in the female reproductive tract?
4 What is the outer limit for egg survival?
5 What is the most secure age (biologically) to have a child?
6 What are the two key variables which impact on the effectiveness of FAMs to avoid pregnancy?

HEALTH PROFESSIONALS' ATTITUDES TO FAMS

Health professionals are not generally well-informed about FAMs and understandably shy away from methods outside their expertise. The attitude of health professionals towards physiological methods is often negative – they are generally dismissed as unreliable.

In the late 1990s, physicians in the US were asked whether they included FAMs as an option when discussing family planning choices with their female patients. Of the 375 physicians who responded:

- thirty percent made no mention of FAMs;
- almost 50% mentioned FAMs as an option to some women; but
- only 11% mentioned FAMs as an option to most or all of the women.

There was a correlation between physicians' awareness of local FAM instructors and the likelihood of referral to these services. The responses imply that the better informed physicians are about these methods, and the closer their perception is to the actual effectiveness, the more they are prepared to inform women of their availability. Physicians who were aware of local FAM services were more likely to have information in the form of books or leaflets, but the majority felt more confident discussing medically related methods. [559] Likewise, a survey in 1997 found Italian doctors favoured a "medical" rather than a "behavioural" approach in their treatment preferences. [227]

The knowledge gap related to FAMs is not limited to doctors. In the US, 514 nurse/midwives completed a survey about their levels of knowledge and promotion of NFP and LAM. They ranked NFP as the ninth most used and the eighth most effective method in their practice, with an average perceived method-effectiveness of 88% and use-effectiveness of 70%. Although most nurse/midwives felt they had received training to provide NFP for couples avoiding pregnancy, only 22% would offer it as an option for child spacing. [165]

In the US, when women were provided with positive information about FAMs, 20% expressed an interest in using these methods to avoid pregnancy, however, only about 2% of women were currently using a FAM. The majority of users were white, with high-school education, above-average income, in long-term committed relationships and predominantly Catholic. This may be at least partly because doctors have a limited knowledge about FAMs and instruction is generally through faith-based groups. [444]

ANSWERS TO SELF-ASSESSMENT QUESTIONS

1 See definition on page 3
2 "FAM" is the broad term and includes NFP. NFP always implies abstinence from intercourse during the fertile time. This is the only method approved by the Catholic Church. It is important to understand whether a couple intend to use abstinence during the fertile time (NFP) or whether they will regularly or occasionally use barrier methods or withdrawal. Couples who use their FA knowledge in combination with another method need to understand how to use the method consistently and carefully, how the method could affect the observation of the fertility indicators and the effectiveness of the method if it fails during the fertile time.
3 Seven days
4 48 hours
5 20–35 years
6 The woman's ability to accurately identify her fertile time and the partners' ability to modify their sexual behaviour to accommodate the full width of the fertile time.

INTEGRATING FA INTO FAMILY PLANNING SERVICES

Health professionals are in a key position to provide objective information about fertility and reproductive health awareness as part of comprehensive family planning services.

It is well-recognized that there is no ideal method of family planning, but integrating FAMs as part of the full range of contraceptive choice helps to meet the needs of more couples. Many general practice and family planning clinics in the UK now successfully integrate FAMs into contraception and sexual health services. Couples who are satisfied with their method of family planning are more likely to use it carefully and consistently, and therefore achieve a high degree of effectiveness.

ACTIVITY

Consider how you might integrate various aspects of fertility knowledge into your existing practice. If you require further training or resources, contact FertilityUK, which provides access to a network of trained practitioners and Advanced Skills courses for health professionals (see www.fertilityuk.org).

The starting point for FA education is an understanding of reproductive anatomy and physiology. FAM users need only know the essentials which are of practical significance, but it is vital for health professionals to have a good understanding of reproductive function to be able to provide relevant client-focussed information and advice.

MALE FERTILITY

2

Most men are fertile from puberty, which starts around 12 years of age, and remain fertile throughout their adult lives. Sperm are produced in a continuous process, from puberty onwards with each individual spermatozoon taking around three months to reach maturity. Although there is no equivalent to female menopause, men do experience a gradual decrease in testosterone and normal age-related physiological changes.

It is important to distinguish between fertility and potency as the two do not necessarily correlate. A man may be sexually potent, with the capacity to perform sexually – to achieve an erection and ejaculate inside a woman's vagina – but be infertile. Alternatively, he may have perfectly healthy sperm but an inability to perform. Sexual potency can be affected by physical or psychological factors at any age; similarly, male fertility can be adversely affected by a number of factors. For the purposes of FA we need to assume that the man is always fertile and, if pregnancy is to be avoided, we assume he is producing viable sperm on a round-the-clock basis.

REPRODUCTIVE ORGANS

The male reproductive organs comprise the penis and the scrotum, which contains the two testicles. The testicles hang asymmetrically with the left testicle normally hanging slightly lower than the right (the reverse being indicative of dextrocardia). The right testicle is normally slightly larger than the left. From each testicle runs a narrow tube, the vas deferens, which opens into the urethra. The urethra runs from the bladder, through the prostate and then through the length of the penis to convey urine from the bladder to the outside. The male accessory glands (prostate and seminal vesicles) also open into the urethra, so forming a common pathway for urine and seminal fluid (figure 2.1).

The testicles

The terms "testicles" and "testes" (singular: testis) are often used synonymously, even though their definitions are slightly different. The testicle *contains* the testis (male gonad) along with its ducts including the epididymis and scrotal portion of the vas deferens with its coverings, muscle layer, blood, lymph and nerve supply. The boxed insert in figure 2.1 shows a longitudinal section of the testicle. There are around 500 fine seminiferous (sperm producing) tubules, divided by fibrous septa into about 200 lobules. The testis is enclosed by a tough covering (tunica albuginea) surrounded by an outer capsule (tunica vaginalis). Between these two coverings there is a small amount of serous fluid, which allows movement of the testis within the scrotum.

The highly convoluted seminiferous tubules straighten, converge and amalgamate to form the wider channels of the rete testis. About 15 efferent ducts convey sperm from the rete testis to the epididymis. The epididymis is divided into three parts: the head (caput), the long coiled tubule of the body (corpus) and the wider tail (cauda), where sperm are stored prior to

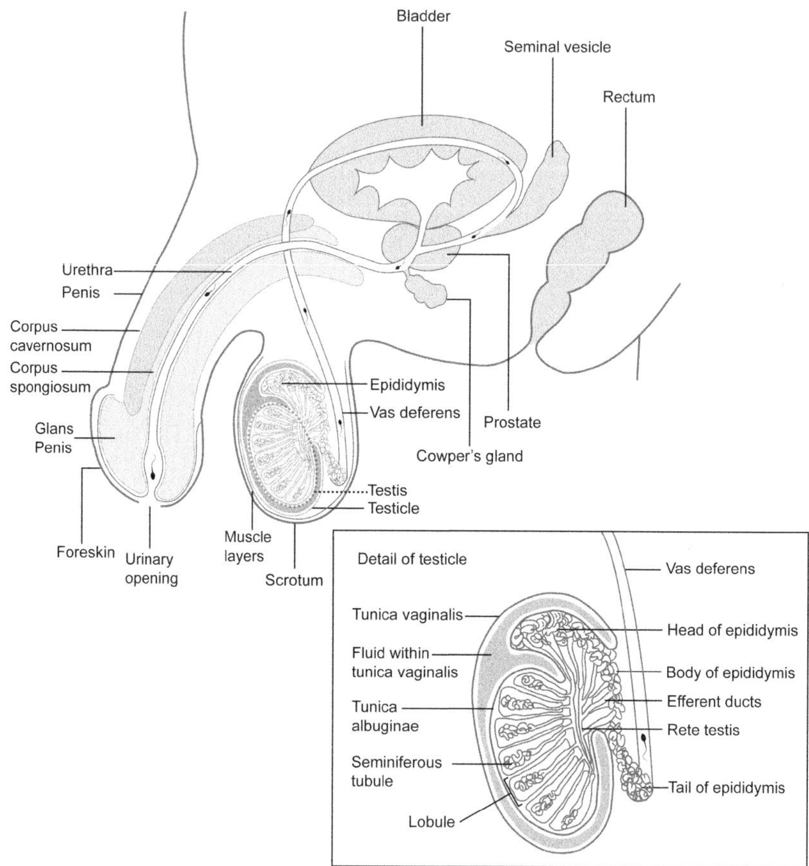

Figure 2.1 Male reproductive system including details of the testicle (adapted from Reiss 1998) [502]

ejaculation. The vas deferens conveys sperm from the epididymis to the male accessory glands at the base of the bladder.

The testes have two main functions:

- The seminiferous tubules produce the male gametes (spermatozoa or sperm) – the man's genetic contribution to his child.
- The Leydig cells in the interstitial tissue between the seminiferous tubules produce the male sex hormones (androgens), including testosterone. These in turn are responsible for the development and maintenance of the male secondary sex characteristics such as deepening of the voice plus growth of facial, pubic and body hair.

The penis

The external appearance of the penis shows the long body (shaft) and the bulbous glans with the urethral opening (meatus) at the tip. The glans is covered by the foreskin (prepuce), a separate hood of retractable skin which retracts during erection to expose the glans. The foreskin is sometimes removed by circumcision for cultural, religious or medical reasons. The skin around the penis has a great number of sensitive nerve endings, concentrated on the underside of the shaft and over the surface of the glans which, when stimulated, cause a build-up of sexual excitement and erection of the penis.

On the underside of the penis, a band of elastic tissue known as the frenulum runs backwards in a small cleft in the glans from just behind the urethral opening. It acts as a tether preventing the foreskin from being retracted too far. The rounded border which slightly projects round the circumference of the base of the glans is known as the corona. The corona and the frenulum are the two extremely sensitive areas that many men find particularly responsive to stimulation.

Internally the root of the penis originates in the perineum, so almost half of the penis is concealed but, despite its internal placement, this area (crus) is extremely vulnerable to injury. The body of the penis has three columns of spongy erectile tissue: two corpora cavernosa which lie on the upper-side, acting as blood storage chambers, and one corpus spongiosum which lies between them on the under-side and helps to regulate blood flow. The urethra extends from the bladder through the centre of the prostate, through the corpus spongiosum and to the external meatus. [235]

The average length of the visible penis is 3–4 inches (7.5–10 cm) when soft and relaxed (flaccid) and 6–8 inches (15–20 cm) or longer when hard and erect (tumescent). The larger the penis when non-aroused, the less it increases in length. Anxiety about penis size is common, particularly amongst adolescents, but although the size of a man's penis may be linked to his pride it is not related to his sexual performance or fertility potential.

Physiology of erection

An erection is a physiological phenomenon in which the penis becomes firmer, engorged and enlarged. It occurs as a result of a complex interaction of psychological, neural, vascular and endocrine factors. An erection requires a high pressure supply of arterial blood, relaxation of the smooth muscle and a functioning blood storage mechanism. These physiological changes occur as part of sexual arousal and are a necessary precursor to intercourse. A problem in any of these areas will ultimately result in erectile difficulties.

Although erections are usually associated with sexual arousal or sexual attraction, they can also occur spontaneously and are observable in new-borns. Erections also occur during rapid eye movement (REM) sleep and are particularly common in pre-pubescent boys due to their increasing testosterone levels. It is normal for a man to have a number of spontaneous erections during the day, between one and five erections at night, and to wake with an early morning erection (so called morning glory). The erection reflex can be adversely affected by physical, emotional or mental influences, drugs or alcohol.

Male sexual functioning and sexual intercourse

During sexual intercourse (coitus) the erect penis enters the woman's vagina where pelvic thrusts produce frictional stimulation between the penis and the vaginal walls; this normally leads to ejaculation in the upper part of the vagina. Successful sexual functioning requires more than just adequate reproductive physiology: it requires the right stimulation (physical and emotional) and the absence of stress symptoms, fatigue, distracting thoughts or feelings of hopelessness or depression. Past sexual experiences create a mental framework that can either enhance or sabotage successful sexual functioning.

The physiological process from erection to ejaculation is under the control of the autonomic (involuntary) nervous system, which works most successfully in a state of relaxation. Most men have occasional times when they cannot get an erection: for example, if they are tired or stressed, or have drunk too much alcohol. Erectile problems are increasingly common with advancing age. Persistent or recurring erectile difficulties may have a physical cause (such as testosterone deficiency or degenerative changes in nerve fibres in diabetic men) or be linked to psychosexual problems. Many men struggle if they are feeling pressured to conceive or being asked to have sex "at the right time". The issue of erectile difficulties frequently arises during FA consultations and requires discussion with appropriate investigation and referral.

Male sexual response

The nature of human sexual response was first described by Masters and Johnson in the early 1960s. The sexual response cycle has four stages which are almost identical in men and women: excitement, plateau, orgasm and resolution. [391] Most sexual encounters, however, go through five stages – the first stage, sexual attraction or desire was not included by Masters and Johnson. Sexual attraction is the most individualised stage of human sexual response, and the only two variables of attractiveness that appear to be universal and related to reproductive success are youth and health. [273]

During sexual excitement (arousal) blood flow increases to the genital area, the penile arteries open up, the smooth muscle relaxes, the penis fills with blood and stores it in the spongy erectile tissue, so becoming firm and erect. The scrotum darkens due to increased blood supply.

As excitement increases, the plateau phase is reached, the penis is firmer and longer, the testicles are drawn towards the perineum and a drop of clear lubricating pre-ejaculatory fluid (from the Cowper's glands) appears at the urethral opening. Fluids are expelled into the prostatic urethra and the man can feel he is about to ejaculate. In healthy men, once the plateau phase has been reached, ejaculation and orgasm are almost inevitable.

Ejaculation normally occurs at the height of orgasm and is typically experienced as an intense, pleasurable feeling of a sudden build-up and explosive release of sexual tension. Almost every man will ejaculate at orgasm, but the intensity of orgasm may vary. Men report greater pleasure with a greater volume of ejaculate. Men (and women) experience 3–12 contractions at orgasm. In men the contractions originate in the superficial muscles of the perineum and are felt in the penis prostate and pelvic region. The rhythmic contractions of orgasm initially occur at 0.8-second intervals, gradually slowing in speed and intensity.

During the resolution phase, the blood flow which had increased the congestion in the pelvic organs drains away and a man loses his erection, the testicles descend and the scrotum becomes softer and looser. As the intense pleasure of orgasm is past, there is usually a sense of total relaxation and calm attributed to the release of oxytocin, prolactin and endorphins. The time taken before a man is able to become sexually aroused again (known as the refractory period) will vary from a few minutes for a young man to hours and longer as a man gets older. Women do not have a refractory period in the same way as men and if stimulated appropriately may have another orgasm or series of orgasms.

SPERMATOGENESIS

Spermatogenesis is the highly complex process of multiple cell divisions resulting in sperm formation in the seminiferous tubules of the testes. This takes place under hormonal control in a continuous process from puberty throughout adult life.

Early in embryonic development, the primordial germ cells (spermatogonial stem cells) migrate to the area where the testes will be situated, settling in the seminiferous tubules in the developing testes. These ancestral cells containing 46 chromosomes (diploid) lie dormant until puberty. From puberty onwards, follicle-stimulating hormone (FSH) and luteinising hormone (LH) from the pituitary gland stimulate the testes to produce testosterone and initiate spermatogenesis. The Sertoli (nurse) cells lining the seminiferous tubules, which are activated by FSH, control sperm production and nourish the developing sperm cells.

Sperm production involves an orderly sequence of mitosis (producing two identical daughter cells) and meiosis (a specialised two-stage process of reductive division resulting in four daughter cells, each with half the number of chromosomes). The spermatogonial stem cells proliferate to become spermatogonia, replicating their DNA, then proceed through primary and secondary spermatocyte stages to form spermatids. The round spermatids, each containing 23 chromosomes (haploid) then start to differentiate (spermiogenesis), becoming elongated then forming the head, mid-piece and tail of the spermatozoa, the male gametes (figure 2.2).

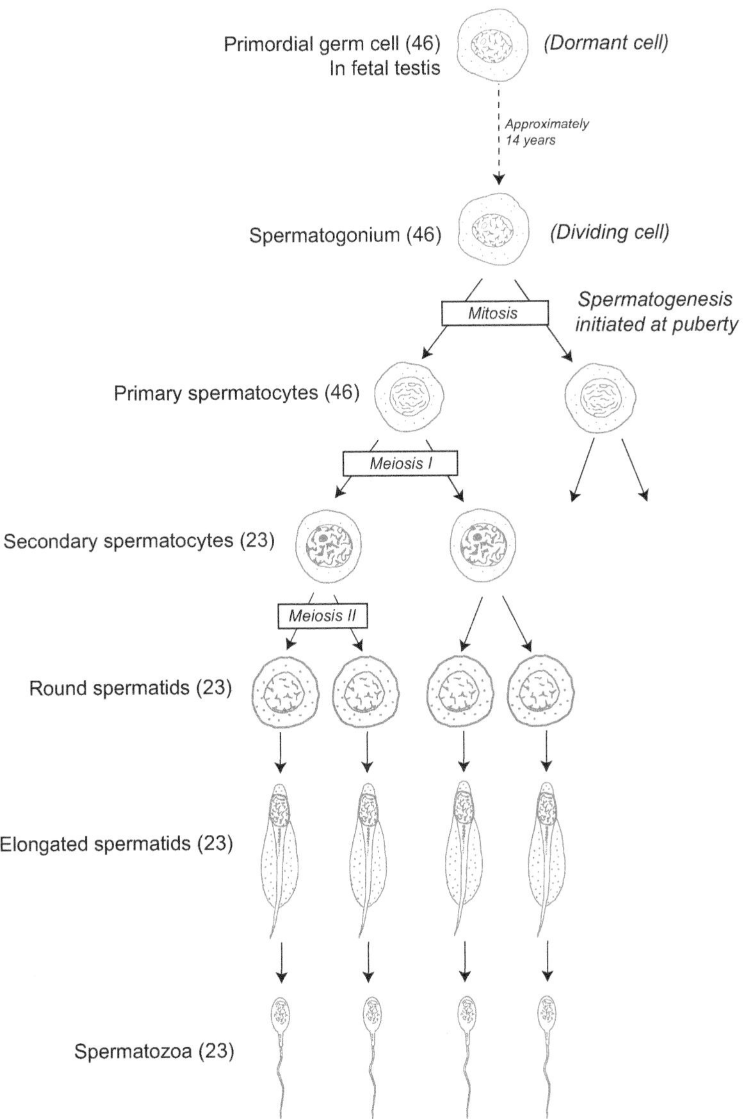

Figure 2.2 Stages of spermatogenesis – development of mature sperm (adapted from Reiss 1998) [502]

Fully formed sperm pass from the seminiferous tubules, via the rete testis and the efferent ducts, into the head of the epididymis, where they mature, acquiring their potential for motility and fertilising ability. The maturation process continues along the length of the epididymis to its tail where they are stored waiting to be ejaculated.

The testicles produce sperm in a continuous process with around 100 million sperm produced by each testicle every day and around 250 million sperm released at each ejaculation. The time from the beginning of the development of an individual spermatozoon to the time it is ready for ejaculation is around three months (64 days for sperm development and another

10–14 days to pass through the epididymis). Any changes to preconception health and lifestyle therefore take around three months for the benefits to be noticeable.

Scrotal temperature

Optimum sperm production requires the testicles to be maintained at a temperature of around 35 deg.C – that is about two degrees lower than normal body temperature. It is the function of the scrotum, the loose pouch of deeply pigmented skin, to control testicular temperature. If the temperature is too high, the scrotum gives off heat by sweating and by relaxing its muscle layer so that the surface area expands, allowing the testicles to move further away from the body and to cool down. In colder ambient temperatures the muscle layer contracts, making the surface area of the scrotum smaller and drawing the testicles in closer to the warmth of the body. The temperature-regulating mechanism of the scrotum can be affected by prolonged exposure to heat – a significant lifestyle factor for men during the preconception time.

SPERM STRUCTURE

Antonie van Leeuwenhoek, the Father of Microbiology, discovered the first living cells by using one of the first microscopes. In 1678 he studied his own semen and discovered spermatozoa which he described as "parasites invading semen; animals in the semen moving forward with a snake-like motion of the tail, as eels do when swimming in water." [416]

The spermatozoon (figure 2.3) is microscopic in size. It has a spheroid head measuring about 3.5 microns wide and 5 microns long, plus a neck and tail contributing to a total length of about 50 microns. It is the smallest cell in the human body.

A spermatozoon (figure 2.3) comprises:

- Head – a normal-shaped head is spheroid with a smooth contour. About half of the head region is covered by a cap-like structure – the acrosome, which is rich in enzymes, including hyaluronidase to penetrate the zona pellucida (outer covering) of the oocyte. The head contains the nucleus with the father's tightly packed genetic material – 22 chromosomes plus either an X or Y sex chromosome.
- Mid-piece – this contains the spirally arranged mitochondria (Jensen's spiral body) which provide some of the energy to power the tail
- Tail (flagellum) – this contains the axial filament (complex array of micro-tubules) to propel the sperm

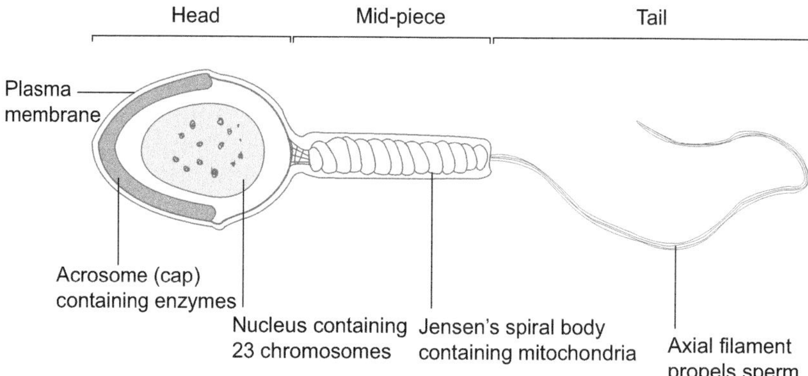

Figure 2.3 Structure of a spermatozoon (surface view)

Mature sperm do not reach their full motile capacity until they are mixed with seminal fluid from the male accessory glands, and they do not achieve their full fertilising capacity until after ejaculation when they go through a process known as "capacitation" in the female reproductive tract.

X and Y chromosome-bearing sperm

The sex of the child is determined at fertilisation and is dependent on whether the egg is fertilised by a spermatozoon bearing an X or Y chromosome. The two different types of sperm show subtle yet significant differences. There is some evidence, but not strong evidence, to suggest that X-bearing sperm are larger (with 3% more DNA), slower-moving and more resistant to acidic conditions. Y-bearing sperm are smaller, swim faster and are less tolerant of acidic conditions. These physical differences have led to much research on the association between the timing of conception and the sex ratio at birth, plus endless innovative ways to try to influence the child's sex, including dietary changes, sexual position and intercourse timing (page 336).

MALE ACCESSORY GLANDS AND PRODUCTION OF SEMINAL FLUID

Seminal fluid (semen) acts as a buffer and the medium for transporting sperm to the female reproductive tract. It is produced by the male accessory glands, principally comprising the prostate and seminal vesicles. The male accessory glands must be healthy for normal sperm function.

Prostate gland

The prostate gland is a solid chestnut-sized gland situated at the base of the male bladder with the urethra running through its middle. Secretions from the prostate contribute about one-third of the volume of seminal fluid and its main nutritive content. Prostatic secretions are slightly acidic and rich in zinc, which is required to maintain the sperm DNA integrity (prevent DNA damage). The prostate also produces an enzyme known as prostate specific antigen (PSA) which, following ejaculation, liquefies the coagulated seminal fluid to release the sperm. The prostate enlarges progressively throughout life (from around 40 onwards), causing compression of the urethra and reduced urinary flow. It is also susceptible to inflammation (prostatitis), a cause of male subfertility, and to prostate cancer, one of the most common cancers in men. The condition of the prostate gland can be assessed by estimating the serum PSA level.

Seminal vesicles

The seminal vesicles are a pair of glands situated above and behind the prostate gland with ducts opening into the upper part of the urethra. The secretions from the seminal vesicles are slightly alkaline and rich in fructose, the main source of energy for the sperm. These secretions contribute about two-thirds of the volume of seminal fluid.

Cowper's glands and pre-ejaculatory fluid

The Cowper's (bulbo-urethral) glands are a pair of pea-sized glands situated near the prostate. They are the male equivalent of the female Bartholin's glands. During sexual arousal the glands secrete a small amount of clear, sticky fluid into the urethra – the pre-ejaculate. This helps to prepare the urethra for the passage of sperm by both lubricating it and neutralising any traces of acidic urine. A man has no warning sign of this lubricative pre-ejaculatory fluid (pre-cum). Although the fluid itself does not contain sperm, research into the presence of sperm in pre-ejaculatory fluid is conflicting. One study showed that over 40% of men had motile sperm in the pre-ejaculate despite passing urine more than once since their previous ejaculation. The effectiveness of withdrawal method is therefore highly variable (page 248).

Composition of seminal fluid

Seminal fluid is a greyish-white, viscous, alkaline fluid (pH 7.2–8.0) with a distinct odour which acts as a transport medium for sperm. At ejaculation the male accessory glands expel between 2 and 5 ml of seminal fluid, pushing the sperm through the urethra. Seminal fluid comprises a minute amount of clear secretion from the Cowper's glands, a small amount of acidic secretions from the prostate (containing zinc and PSA), secretions from the epididymis and vas containing sperm, and alkaline secretions from the seminal vesicles contributing most of the semen volume (with fructose providing the energy source for sperm motility). The first part of the ejaculate contains the highest concentration of sperm with the highest sperm motility and lowest DNA fragmentation.

Many men worry about the amount of fluid they produce, but volume does not necessarily correlate with sperm count. Semen volume is affected by the time interval since the previous ejaculation with larger semen volumes following longer abstinence. The intensity and duration of stimulation leading to ejaculation can also affect volume and potentially sperm count (normal semen analysis: page 342).

EMISSION AND EJACULATION

Ejaculation is the release of seminal fluid (ejaculate or cum) from the penis during male orgasm. Ejaculation involves coordinated muscular and neurological events with two main phases: emission and expulsion. During emission, under adrenaline control, smooth muscles in the prostate, vas deferens and seminal vesicles contract sequentially to expel secretions from the male accessory glands and sperm from the epididymis into the posterior (prostatic) urethra. The bladder neck is occluded to prevent retrograde ejaculation. The rhythmic muscular contractions of the tubes from the epididymis, the muscular part of the prostate and the urethral muscles help to expel the seminal fluid through the urethral opening – ejaculation. Semen is ejaculated with some force (average 10 mph) in a series of 5–10 spurts, often with a pelvic thrust between each spurt. [389] As a man gets older and his testosterone level declines, the amount of seminal fluid as well as the force with which it is ejaculated decreases.

SPERM TRANSPORT IN THE FEMALE REPRODUCTIVE TRACT

During intercourse, approximately 250 million sperm are deposited in the anterior vagina, just a few thousand reach the Fallopian tubes, around 30 make it to the outside of the egg and one spermatozoon successfully penetrates the zona pellucida to achieve fertilisation. This sperm selection process helps to optimise the chance that the successful spermatozoon will have vigorous motility and normal morphology (shape). Suarez and Pacey's paper gives a comprehensive description of sperm transport in the female reproductive tract. [568]

Andrologist Allan Pacey's research formed the basis of the script for the highly acclaimed Channel 4 documentary *The Great Sperm Race,* which portrayed the tortuous journey of sperm in their quest to fertilise the egg. Sperm meet numerous obstacles along the way from the acidic vaginal environment, the complexities of the cervical canal and its secretions, the narrow utero-tubal junction, the white blood cells of the woman's immune system which view sperm as "foreign invaders" and through to the final barrier, the zona pellucida. There are a number of mechanisms which aid the process, including chemical and temperature signals, a sperm reservoir in the lining of the tubes and the ovulation process, which helps to activate the sperm.

Site of sperm deposition

Seminal fluid ejaculated into the upper vagina during intercourse creates a sperm pool near the cervical os in the form of a loosely coagulated gel. The viscous nature of semen helps to keep it in contact with the woman's cervix, and its alkalinity protects sperm from the harsh acidic environment of the vagina. Within minutes, semen starts to liquefy due to the action of PSA, freeing the sperm to swim towards the cervix. There is noticeable "flow-back" of seminal fluid almost immediately after intercourse which often causes concern for women who are trying to conceive. Zoologists Baker and Bellis examined the flowback of 11 women and found that this occurred in 94% of the acts of intercourse, with the average flowback time of 30 minutes. They estimated that about 65% of sperm were retained, but in 12% of intercourse acts almost 100% of the sperm were eliminated. [22] This supports the notion that only a minority of sperm enter the cervical mucus and ascend higher into the female reproductive tract.

Vaginal defences and mechanisms to protect sperm

Sperm have the ability to travel from the hostile vagina to the haven of the Fallopian tube very rapidly, however, sperm which remain lower down in the female reproductive tract are vulnerable. The vagina is open to the outside and therefore exposed to the risk of infection especially during sexual activity. It has good defence systems, including lactic-acid-producing bacteria and immunological responses (including leucocytes) to combat infectious micro-organisms, but these can also damage sperm. Both males and females have protective mechanisms against the vaginal defences:

- Sperm are deposited close to the external cervical os to allow rapid escape from the hostile vaginal conditions.
- The alkaline pH of seminal fluid helps to neutralise the acidic vaginal secretions.
- At the fertile time alkaline cervical secretions have an additional neutralising effect.
- Seminal plasma protects sperm from the vaginal immune response.
- The sheer numbers of sperm help to overcome the vaginal defence system.

Sperm transport through the cervix and cervical mucus

A woman's cervix acts as a gateway to the uterus. Scanning electron microscopy shows the potential passageways for sperm through the cervical canal. Large primary mucosal grooves extend from the external os, branching into smaller secondary grooves deep in the cervical canal. Although the primary grooves appear to form a preferential pathway for sperm, it is not known whether the secondary or even tertiary grooves could end blindly and entrap sperm.

The glandular epithelium lining the cervical canal produces cervical mucus, a gel structure with semi-solid and liquid phases. The characteristics of cervical mucus change under hormonal control to either encourage or impede sperm penetration. [152] Approaching ovulation, under the influence of estrogen, the cervical os is open and the cervical canal wider. As sperm swim toward the dilated os, they encounter the alkaline cervical mucus, which accepts, filters, prepares and then releases them. The concentration of sperm in the mucus column is maximal from 15 minutes to 2 hours after vaginal deposition. Rapid penetration into cervical mucus favours sperm survival because of its optimal pH. [180]

Transmission electron microscopy shows that cervical mucus has a heterogeneous mosaic-like micro-structure with interstices (small gaps) between the mucus macro-molecules. The gaps in this "mesh-like" structure are larger around the time of ovulation, but they are still smaller than the sperm head, so advancing sperm must thrust their way through the mucus micro-structure. [317] Estrogenised cervical mucus is highly hydrated and can exceed 96% water content; the higher the water content, the lower the viscosity, and the easier for sperm to penetrate. [318]

Chretien has confirmed Odeblad's earlier work [436] showing the close relationship between the three-dimensional arrangement of the mucus framework and the ability of sperm to move rapidly in a given direction. Sperm entering the cervical canal appear to be constrained to follow the oriented micellar lines of strain, akin to "swimming lanes for sperm". [90] Cervical mucus acts as a means of sperm selection, encouraging the progression of vigorously motile and morphologically normal sperm and filtering out sperm with reduced motility and abnormal morphology.

Sperm storage in the cervix

Little is known about how long sperm take to get through the cervix or whether they are stored there. Vigorously motile sperm have been recovered from the cervical canal up to five days after artificial insemination but it is not known whether sperm still present in the canal this long after deposition would reach the Fallopian tube and be capable of fertilisation. [237] Odeblad, a pioneer in nuclear magnetic resonance in Sweden, describes the anatomy of the cervix with folds and clefts terminating in "grape-like" structures, crypts and tunnel clusters. He prefers the term "secretory units" to "crypts" as this more appropriately describes the assembly of epithelial cells producing a certain type of mucus, however, "crypts" is commonly used. Odeblad has observed sperm moving directly to the uterus, but the majority "hibernating" for 20 hours on average (and up to several days) in the secretory units before migrating to the uterine cavity. [436]

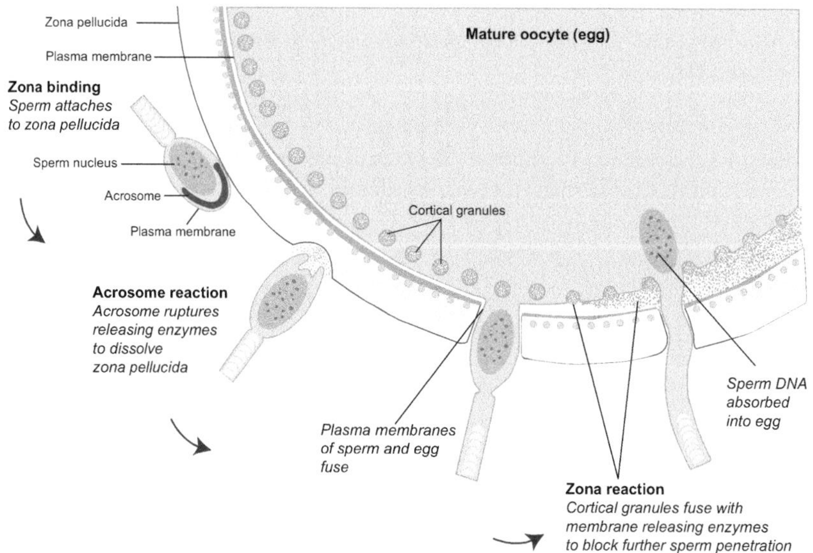

Figure 2.4 Stages of fertilisation

Sperm migration through the uterus and tubes

The sperm that survive the journey through the cervical canal are assisted by muscular contractions of the myometrium which enhance their passage through the uterine cavity. A few thousand sperm swim through the utero-tubal junctions to reach the Fallopian tubes, where they are possibly stored in a reservoir, or at least maintained in a fertile state, and around 30 will eventually reach the egg.

As the time of ovulation approaches, sperm go through capacitation acquiring their fertilising ability; they become hyperactive, swimming more erratically towards the widest part of the tube (ampulla). The contractions of the wall of the tube assist the passage of sperm and egg. The tube is also lined by cilia which contribute to the transport and protection of the gametes.

Sperm may be guided to the egg by changes in thermal and chemical gradients – they may "smell" the egg when they get close to it. It has been shown that bourgeonal, a component of the Lily of the Valley scent, attracts sperm by altering their calcium balance – "The Lily of the Valley phenomenon" [555] although some authorities are less convinced by this now. The midpiece of sperm contains some of the same olfactory receptors as those present in the nose. One very small study compared the olfactory sensitivity of 14 men with unexplained infertility to 23 controls. The men with unexplained infertility were less sensitive to the smell of bourgeonal. [548] A possible link between olfactory receptor disorder and sperm function is interesting, but much larger studies are needed to confirm these findings.

FERTILISATION

Fertilisation is the process during which the spermatozoon fuses with the egg, normally in the intermediate part of the Fallopian tube. The process takes about 24 hours, during which time the spermatozoon penetrates the external membrane of the egg (zona pellucida) and the genetic material of the two gametes is combined to form the zygote. Fertilisation should not be confused with *conception*, the process from fertilisation to implantation, which takes a number of days.

For fertilisation to take place, the spermatozoon has to be able to recognise the mature egg and bind to it (zona binding). When the spermatozoon attaches to the zona, it initiates the acrosome reaction during which the acrosome gradually ruptures, releasing its enzymes to dissolve a hole through the zona pellucida. The plasma membranes of the spermatozoon and egg then fuse and the egg initiates the zona reaction, a chemical reaction which prevents the entry of additional sperm: the egg depolarises its membrane and the cortical granules near the surface of the egg fuse with the membrane, releasing their enzymes and rendering the zona pellucida impenetrable to further sperm (figure 2.4).

Once inside this gelatinous outer membrane, the hyperactivated spermatozoon becomes immotile and separates from its tail; the DNA of the spermatozoon is then absorbed into the egg. The mature spermatozoon and egg cell each contain 23 chromosomes (gametes are haploid cells). Following normal fertilisation, two haploid pronuclei will be visible – one from the fertilising spermatozoon and the other from the egg (figure 3.5). The chromosomes then pair up (syngamy) to form 46 chromosomes (23 pairs), the full chromosomal complement.

If two sperm fertilise the egg, which is not uncommon, this results in triploidy, or higher numbers of sperm (tetraploidy or polypoidy). In IVF if more than two pronuclei are present, although the embryo may develop to blastocyst stage, it will not be transferred as it is incompatible with normal development and nearly always results in miscarriage. Polyspermy can also cause a molar pregnancy, a condition where there is usually no fetus, but an abnormality of the placenta which carries a risk of choriocarcinoma.

Sperm that are abnormally shaped or have a defective or missing acrosome will not be able to bind to the egg or dissolve the egg coat. Sperm morphology (shape) therefore forms an important component of a semen analysis.

SPERM SURVIVAL

Sperm survival depends on the presence of estrogen-primed cervical secretions. In the absence of alkaline secretions, the acidic vaginal environment rapidly destroys sperm. [180] [436] The evidence for sperm survival can be assessed in one of three ways: by measuring the time from a single act of intercourse to the estimated day of ovulation in a conception cycle, by retrieving sperm at time intervals from the female genital tract to observe sperm motility and fertilising capacity, or by observing the fertilising capacity of sperm in vitro.

Sperm survival is longer than previously thought. In the early days of the Calendar/Rhythm Method, sperm survival in the female genital tract was considered to be less than 48 hours. [332] Based on the Barrett and Marshall data on the risk of conception on different days of the menstrual cycle, [34] Royston estimated that the mean survival time of sperm was 1.47 days. [518]

A motile sperm does not mean it is capable of fertilisation because sperm lose their fertilising ability before they lose their motility. Sperm have been shown to retain their ability to undergo the acrosome reaction and penetrate the zona pellucida for up to 80 hours after insemination and vigorously motile sperm have been retrieved from the cervix up to five days after insemination. [237]

In a study using LH and cervical secretions as markers of ovulation, three pregnancies out of 91 conception cycles were attributed to a single act of intercourse six days before the LH surge. [184] Research using estrogen:progesterone ratios to estimate ovulation (221 conception cycles) concluded that sperm retain their fertilising capacity for up to five days in the female genital tract. [631] Women who produce good-quality cervical secretions for a longer interval of time are more likely to provide optimum conditions for lengthy sperm survival times.

A number of mathematical models have been developed to investigate the probability of conception on different days of the menstrual cycle. Ferreira-Poblete estimated sperm have a 5% probability of surviving more than 4.4 days and a 1% probability of surviving more than 6.8 days. [174] The most well-established figures for sperm survival suggest an average of 2–3 days, but with the possibility of surviving in optimum conditions for up to a week – a message which should be communicated consistently.

SELF-ASSESSMENT QUESTIONS

Answers are at the end of the chapter.

1 What are the two main functions of the testes?
2 What is the average sperm survival time and the extreme limit for sperm survival?
3 Name the male accessory glands and explain their function.
4 Explain the role of pre-ejaculatory fluid and the possibility of it containing sperm.
5 A woman who is trying to conceive is anxious about losing sperm after intercourse. How would you explain the nature of seminal fluid, liquefaction and flowback?

MALE SEX HORMONE SYSTEM

The male sex hormone system, which controls testicular function and sperm production, is fundamentally similar to the female sex hormone system. The hypothalamus (master endocrine gland) located at the base of the brain is closely linked anatomically to the pituitary gland. The hypothalamus secretes a number of releasing hormones including gonadotrophin-releasing hormone (GnRH) which is also known as luteinising hormone releasing-hormone (LHRH). From puberty onwards, GnRH controls the release of the gonadotrophins, FSH and LH, from the anterior pituitary. GnRH is produced in a pulsatile manner and its release is influenced by circulating hormone levels and factors including body weight and exercise intensity.

In men, FSH and LH act on the testes to promote the secretion of androgens (including testosterone) and to maintain spermatogenesis. The male hypothalamic-pituitary-gonadal axis is a finely controlled system: hormone production should remain relatively constant throughout a man's life, resulting in a continuous supply of sperm from puberty into old age. Figure 2.5 shows the hypothalamic-pituitary-gonadal axis with similar pathways in men and women.

Androgens are produced primarily by the Leydig cells located in the interstitial tissue of the testis, in response to pituitary LH. Androgens are also produced in small amounts in the

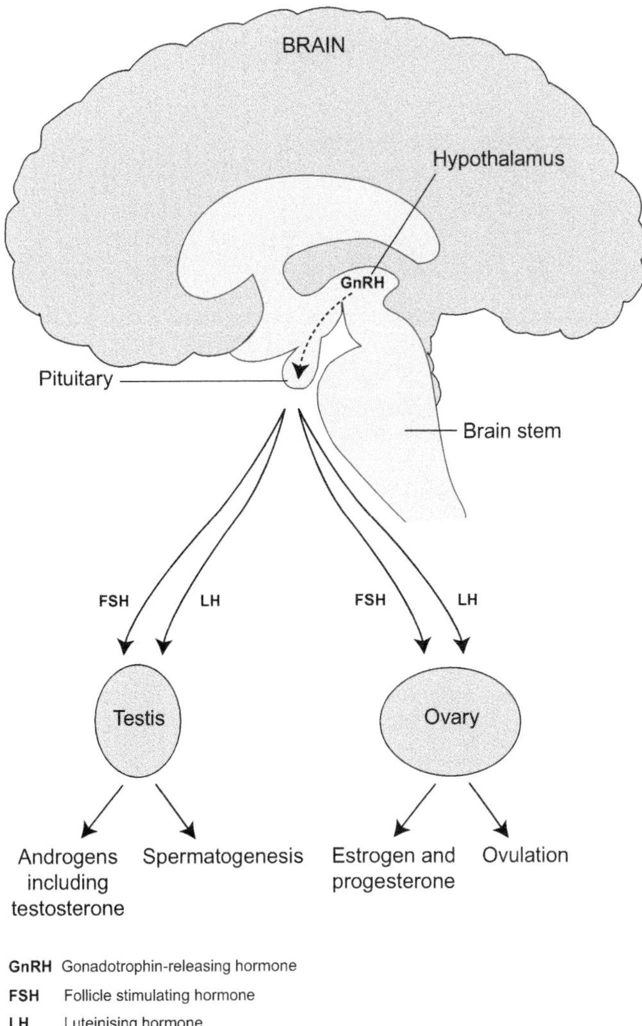

Figure 2.5 Hypothalamic-pituitary-gonadal axis (adapted from Reiss 1998) [502]

adrenal glands. High concentrations of testosterone are required in the testes to maintain sperm production.

Testosterone levels have a circadian rhythm with significant differences between morning and evening levels. Peak testosterone levels are reached between 07:00 and 10:00, whereas the lowest levels are at 19:00. [220] This peak in testosterone means that men are generally more ready for sex in the mornings. This is important information for couples who are trying to conceive because it is often the woman who dictates the sex schedule and this may work against her partner's natural hormonal fluctuations.

Testosterone levels vary with age, the peak being reached at around 18 years old followed by a gradual decrease due to ageing of the Leydig cells. Reduced testosterone levels are linked to declining sexual function and to diminished energy, muscle function and bone density. There is no evidence of a sudden drop or male menopause, but there is some evidence, in older men, of variability in testosterone levels dependent on the amount and quality of sleep. [458]

ANSWERS TO SELF-ASSESSMENT QUESTIONS

1. Functions of testes
   a. Production of male gametes (spermatozoa)
   b. Production of male hormones (androgens) including testosterone
2. Sperm survival
   a. Average 2–3 days
   b. Allow up to seven days for extreme life of sperm in optimum conditions
3. Male accessory glands
   a. Prostate gland produces acidic fluid providing nutrients including zinc, which is required to maintain the sperm DNA integrity (prevent DNA damage).
   b. Seminal vesicles produce alkaline fluid, which includes fructose, the energy supply for sperm. The combined fluids from the prostate and seminal vesicles make up the seminal fluid.
   c. The Cowper's (bulbo-urethral) glands secrete a small amount of clear lubricating fluid during sexual arousal.
4. Pre-ejaculatory fluid (from the Cowper's glands) lubricates the urethra and neutralises traces of acidic urine in preparation for ejaculation. The fluid itself does not contain sperm, but the research shows conflicting results regarding the presence of sperm in the pre-ejaculate. One study found that more than 40% men had motile sperm in the pre-ejaculate despite passing urine more than once since their previous ejaculation.
5. When seminal fluid is first ejaculated it is greyish-white and viscous, which helps it to stick to the cervix. Within a few minutes the semen becomes transparent and more liquid as it releases the sperm. It is very normal for a woman to lose some of the fluid after intercourse, but millions of healthy sperm will already be on their way through the cervix.

FEMALE FERTILITY

A woman has a finite number of eggs, which are present from birth and released on a cyclical basis during her fertile years. There are only a few days during each menstrual cycle which are potentially fertile, but the accurate identification of these days allows a couple to use FAMs to either plan or avoid pregnancy.

Health professionals need an in-depth knowledge of the menstrual cycle and female fertility to be able to explore a client's understanding of reproductive anatomy and physiology, and correct any myths or misunderstanding. FAMs, by their nature, also require a dialogue about sexual activity, the timing of intercourse and the potential impact of modifying sexual behaviour to accommodate the fertile time. Open communication is encouraged between health professionals and clients about normal sexual functioning and any related sexual difficulties.

REPRODUCTIVE SYSTEM

The female reproductive system comprises:

- the external genitalia (genitals); and
- the internal reproductive organs – ovaries, Fallopian tubes, uterus, cervix and vagina – protected by the bony pelvis.

External genitals

The external genitals, known collectively as the vulva, consist of the area enclosed by the mons pubis, labia majora and the perineum, and include the labia minora, clitoris, introitus (vestibule) and the vaginal opening (figure 3.1).

The mons pubis or pubic mound is a soft, fatty pad lying over and protecting the pubic bone. After puberty it is covered by the typically triangular-shaped female pubic hair. The mons continues backwards to form the labia majora (outer vaginal lips). These two soft fleshy hair-covered skin folds, which develop from the same embryological tissue as the male scrotum, extend backwards either side of the vaginal opening to the perineum (area between the vaginal opening and anus). If the outer vaginal lips are parted, the labia minora (inner vaginal lips) become visible extending from the clitoris above and joining at the fourchette (lower border of the vaginal opening). The inner lips are thinner and skin-covered on the outer aspect but with a silky-smooth epithelium on the inner aspect. They are homologous to the penile skin and male urethra. The labia minora have a rich blood supply and are highly sensitive.

The clitoris is formed of highly sensitive erectile tissue, the female counterpart of the male penis. It is a much larger organ than is often assumed as it has a visible portion (glans or head) and a hidden part (crus or root) which extends into the anterior vaginal wall. The clitoral glans, which is roughly the size and shape of a pea, is covered by a prepuce (hood) corresponding to

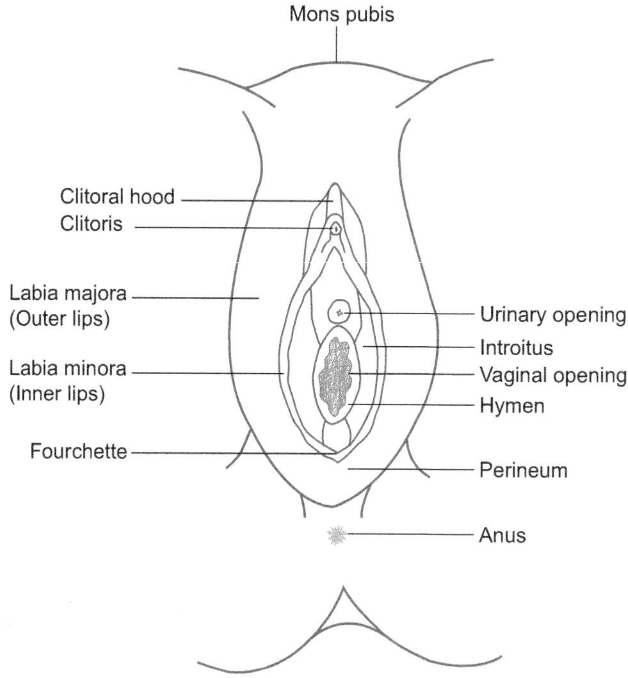

Figure 3.1 Female external genitals

the male foreskin. The clitoris is a woman's most sensitive erogenous zone and plays a major role in sexual pleasure but, unlike the male penis, it does not contain the urethra and so has no urinary function.

The introitus is the area between the labia minora. It is perforated by the urethral and vaginal openings, and the ducts of the Bartholin's and Skene's glands. The Bartholin's glands (greater vestibular or bulbo-urethral glands) are a pair of a pea-sized mucus-secreting glands, located one on each side of the vaginal opening in the lower part of the labia majora. They produce a colourless lubricative fluid in response to sexual stimulation to lubricate the entrance to the vagina thus allowing comfortable penetration. The Bartholin's glands are homologous to the male Cowper's glands. The Skene's glands (lesser vestibular or peri-urethral glands) are a pair of small glands located on the anterior wall of the vagina at the lower end of the urethra, forming part of the highly erogenous area known as the G-spot (Grafenberg spot). The Skene's glands (increasingly referred to as the "female prostate") drain into the urethra near the urethral opening and may be the source of female ejaculation (squirting). Skene's glands are homologous to the prostate gland and the ejaculatory fluid has a similar composition to male prostate fluid. [477]

The hymen is a thin membrane covered on both sides by mucosa that surrounds or partially covers the vaginal opening. It doesn't seem to have a specific function, but remains as a vestige of embryological vaginal development. In most girls the hymen is gradually stretched by physical exercise or the use of tampons. The majority of women are not aware of the hymen tearing at any stage and it is often relatively non-existent by the time of first intercourse, although the frilled edge remnants (carunculae myrtiformes) may still be visible. The hymen can vary in size, thickness and elasticity. A tough inelastic hymen can cause difficulties with intercourse and may not be discovered until starting fertility investigations. If the hymen is imperforate, then menstrual blood cannot escape, resulting in haematocolpos (distension of the vagina) which requires surgical incision. The physical state of the hymen is *not* an indicator of a woman's virginity.

The external genitals vary between women. The labia minora may be quite large, protruding from the labia majora and often of uneven size. The colour of the outer and inner lips will also vary, with the outer lips darker and the inner lips appearing pinker or red. The appearance of the genitals will change during pregnancy, after birth and following the menopause.

During vaginal birth the first area to be injured tends to be the fourchette at the lower part of the vaginal opening. If it is considered necessary to enlarge the vaginal opening to facilitate birth, then the perineum may be cut by a surgical incision (episiotomy) to avoid an extensive tear.

Female sexual function and the sexual response cycle

The physiology of sexual response was first described by Masters and Johnson, after direct observation of almost 700 men and women in around 10,000 sexual response cycles. The female sexual response cycle can be divided into four phases: the excitement (arousal) phase, plateau phase, orgasm and resolution. [390]

During sexual arousal, nerve endings are stimulated, causing increased blood flow to the genital area. The erectile tissue of the clitoris becomes engorged and the erect clitoris emerges from the clitoral hood; the vaginal lips become engorged and darker in colour; and the vaginal walls and Bartholin's glands produce a clear lubricating fluid. The uterus rises slightly, drawing up the cervix, the vagina increases in length and the upper part of the vagina distends.

As sexual stimulation and arousal increase, the woman reaches a plateau phase with the inner vaginal lips becoming softer and more engorged. The clitoris has now doubled in size but is less visible as it is covered by the swollen tissues of its hood. The vagina becomes wetter, the cervix is pulled up further and the top part of the vagina balloons (forming an area where seminal fluid collects during intercourse).

A woman may or may not reach orgasm, the intensely pleasurable climax of sexual activity. Orgasm is usually accompanied by a series of pleasurable contractions of the uterus, vagina and possibly the anus. The 3–12 rhythmic contractions initially occur at intervals of less than one second, gradually losing their intensity and becoming more widely spaced. Most women require stimulation of the clitoris in order to become sexually aroused and achieve orgasm; only about 50% of women experience orgasm from vaginal penetration alone. Masters and Johnson showed that the physiology of orgasmic response was identical whether stimulation was clitoral or vaginal, and proved that some women were capable of being multi-orgasmic.

A woman may have a short plateau phase followed by a single orgasm, a longer plateau and multiple orgasms, or a plateau phase with no orgasm and a much slower resolution phase. This pattern will vary from one woman to another and within the same woman from one sexual response to another, but all of these experiences can be deeply satisfying.

During the resolution phase, blood drains away from the congested pelvic area and the genital organs return to their non-aroused state. As the all-consuming intense pleasure of orgasm passes there is usually a sense of deep relaxation and calm due to the release of oxytocin (love/bonding hormone), prolactin (hormone of satiation) and endorphins (feel-good factor). Women do not have a refractory period in the same way as men and if stimulated appropriately may have another orgasm or series of orgasms.

Female ejaculation: Fact or fiction? Although female ejaculation does occur, the vast majority of women do not ejaculate at orgasm. Unlike a physiologically normal man who cannot urinate at orgasm, it is physically possible for a woman to leak urine during sexual stimulation and orgasm, which is partly why female ejaculation has been so controversial. [477]

An international online survey analysed data from 320 women (average age 34) who experienced female ejaculation. The average age of first ejaculation was 25 years and most women ejaculated a few times a week, ejaculating 2 oz. fluid (approx. 50 ml). The fluid was usually described as transparent and the majority of women felt ejaculation enriched their sex lives and that of their partners. [633]

A systematic review aimed to clarify the aetiology of fluids released during female orgasm to distinguish between normal arousal fluid, female ejaculation and urinary incontinence. Female ejaculation at orgasm manifests as either ejaculation of a small quantity of whitish secretions from the female prostate or squirting of a larger amount of diluted and changed urine with the possibility of both phenomena occurring simultaneously. There was only objective evidence of female ejaculation in tens of cases, but subjective reporting was much higher.

Urinary incontinence affects women more commonly than men. Stress incontinence can cause leakage during penetration (coital incontinence) due to pressure on the bladder and weak pelvic floor muscles. Urinary leakage may also occur at orgasm due to other urethral disorders. [455] Women who do release fluid during sexual activity may feel embarrassed by it, but should recognise that this may be quite normal; however, any suspected form of incontinence should always be investigated.

Vaginal "flowback" Baker and Bellis have studied the architecture of the female reproductive tract and the controversial phenomenon of human sperm competition. They studied 150 flowbacks from 11 women. The flowback (loss of fluid following intercourse) is a mixture of seminal fluid, sperm and other cells (originating from the male and the female). The flowback emerges from the vagina in a series of three to seven white globules and normally measures up to 3 ml. Flowback occurs either while the woman is still horizontal after intercourse, when she next starts to walk or possibly when she next urinates. The average time to flowback is 30 minutes (range 5–120 mins). All flowbacks contained sperm and 94% of intercourse acts were followed by flowback. [22]

Ancient Greeks may have been convinced by the benefit of sneezing and jumping backwards, and many women still believe vigorous exercise or urinating might help to expel unwanted fluids, but these measures are unlikely to reduce the risk of pregnancy. Women who are trying to conceive often prefer to lie flat for 10–15 minutes to feel as if they have given the sperm a chance, but they can be assured that there is no "best position" to conceive or any need to perform gymnastic feats to retain sperm.

Libido and the menstrual cycle

The hormones testosterone and estrogen are generally linked to increased libido whereas progesterone is linked to decreased libido, so from an endocrinological perspective one might anticipate a heightened libido around ovulation and a diminished libido during the luteal phase. Indeed, an often-cited disadvantage of FAMs is that couples need to abstain from intercourse at the time when a woman's libido is at its highest.

The research on libido is conflicting. Psychologist Anne Walker discusses a review of 32 studies where eight reported increased sexual activity around ovulation, 17 reported increased activity premenstrually, 18 postmenstrually and four during menstruation. Thirteen studies reported peaks pre- and postmenstrually, which may partly be explained by increased levels of abstinence during a period. Women generally reported increased libido in the latter part of the follicular phase and again just before a period. [604]

Some of the controversy surrounding female sexual arousal across the menstrual cycle may be due to the variety of ways that self-reports are elicited and whether participants are aware of the purpose of the research. Women have been shown to respond with cultural expectations of the cycle if they are "aware" but show a pattern which fits a hormonal basis if they are "unaware" of the study purpose. [156]

There is no clear correlation between ovarian hormone levels and libido, although estrogen may have a role in vaginal lubrication, particularly after the menopause. Some women report a loss of libido related to increased progestogen in the early days of combined hormonal contraception. The relationship between testosterone and libido is unclear, but some women with testosterone deficiency experience improved libido and well-being with testosterone replacement. [114]

A study measuring FSH, LH, estrogen, progesterone and testosterone in more than 250 women found an increase in sexual activity and specifically female-initiated sexual activity around the time of ovulation which is consistent with some earlier studies. [471] Women who complain that their libido is at its highest around ovulation and feel little desire in the luteal phase may not be suited to FAMs to avoid pregnancy, however, in practice this is rarely an issue. There is undoubtedly a physiological component to libido, but the psychological aspects cannot be ignored. Relationships are complex, and conscious (or subconscious) motives around pregnancy and risk-taking may need to be explored.

Internal reproductive organs

The internal organs of the female reproductive system, which lie in the pelvic cavity, consist of two ovaries from each of which runs a Fallopian tube which opens into the uterine cavity. The cervix at the lower end of the uterus opens into the vagina. The cervix and its secretions are of particular significance for FA.

Figure 3.2 shows a front view of the female reproductive organs (for a side view, see figure 3.6). The organs are enveloped in the broad ligament – the wide folds of peritoneum which extend from the sides of the uterus to the pelvic walls enclosing the blood vessels, lymphatics

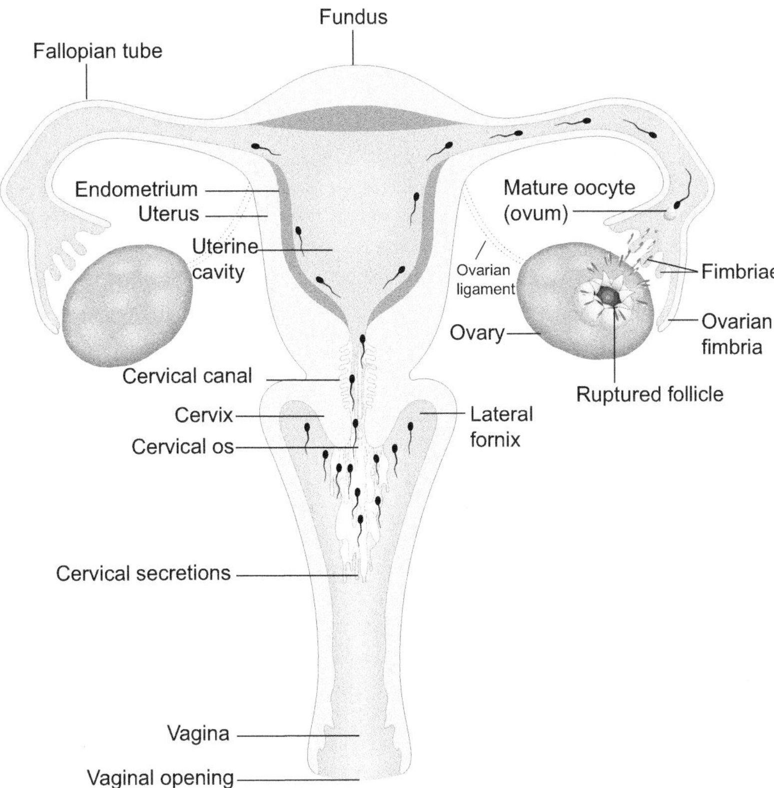

Figure 3.2 Female reproductive organs, front view (© Pyper & Knight, FertilityUK 2016)

and nerves that supply the uterus. The Fallopian tubes are enclosed in the upper border of the broad ligament (not shown in figure 3.2).

Ovaries

The ovary is the female gonad (equivalent of the male testis). In an adult woman the two ovaries are flattened oval structures measuring about 3.5 cm long, 2 cm wide and 1.25 cm thick (about the size and shape of an almond). They are situated one on each side of the uterus, supported by ligaments. A fibrous ligament (ovarian ligament) connects it to the lateral surface of the uterus just below where the Fallopian tube joins the uterus (dotted lines in figure 3.2) and a fold of peritoneum (suspensory ligament) extends in the opposite direction to the pelvic wall (not shown).

The ovaries have two distinct, but inter-related, functions:

- the production of female gametes or oocytes (ova, singular: ovum) and
- the synthesis of the female sex hormones estrogen and progesterone.

Oogenesis The ovarian follicles first form in the female fetus from the fourth month of gestation, when developing primordial germ cells migrate to the fetal ovary. These oogonial stem cells multiply by mitosis to form several million precursor cells, the oogonia. The oogonia enter the first phase of meiosis (reductive division) but soon this arrests resulting in primary oocytes, which become surrounded by a small group of flattened ovarian cells forming primordial follicles. About 7 million primordial follicles are formed initially. By the time of birth their number has declined to around 2 million (1 million per ovary), and by menarche, there are about 400,000 viable follicles left, some of which will eventually be recruited during a menstrual cycle. Primary oocytes contain 46 chromosomes (full genetic complement) and can remain in this state for many years.

The final maturation of a primary oocyte takes place within a pre-ovulatory follicle in response to the LH surge. The oocyte completes its first meiotic division to form the secondary oocyte or ovum (with 23 chromosomes), which will be released at ovulation. The second meiotic division only occurs in response to fertilisation (figure 3.3).

As the oocyte matures, it extrudes two polar bodies – small structures consisting of nuclear material with a tiny amount of cytoplasm. The first polar body, released at the end of the first meiotic division, contains half the recombined genetic material of the egg. The second polar body, which is released in response to fertilisation, contains a haploid chromosome complement. The extrusion of the polar bodies allows the oocyte to retain virtually all of its cytoplasm whilst reducing its chromosome content from 46 to 23. Polar bodies perform no known further function in the body, but they can be used to test for chromosomal abnormalities in a form of pre-implantation genetic screening. Array CGH (comparative genomic hybridisation) has the potential to analyse the full chromosomal content without damaging the egg or embryo.

Follicular atresia After puberty, a constant small proportion of follicles start growing each day. From about 12 years of age when a girl reaches her menarche (first menstrual period) up until about 52 when, as a mature woman, she reaches her menopause (final menstrual period) she will release approximately one egg (ovum) per menstrual cycle at the time of ovulation; this totals the loss of less than 500 eggs over the course of her reproductive life (roughly one egg per cycle for 40 years). The vast majority of eggs will therefore never be released; the follicles will not fully develop and mature, and they degenerate without rupturing – a process known as "atresia". The menopause occurs when the ovarian reserve has been depleted to less than about 1,000 eggs. The rate at which the ovarian follicles degenerate (rate of attrition) is the key factor which determines a woman's age at menopause. A poor complement of follicles at birth and/or a rapid rate of attrition could result in premature ovarian insufficiency (leading to premature menopause).

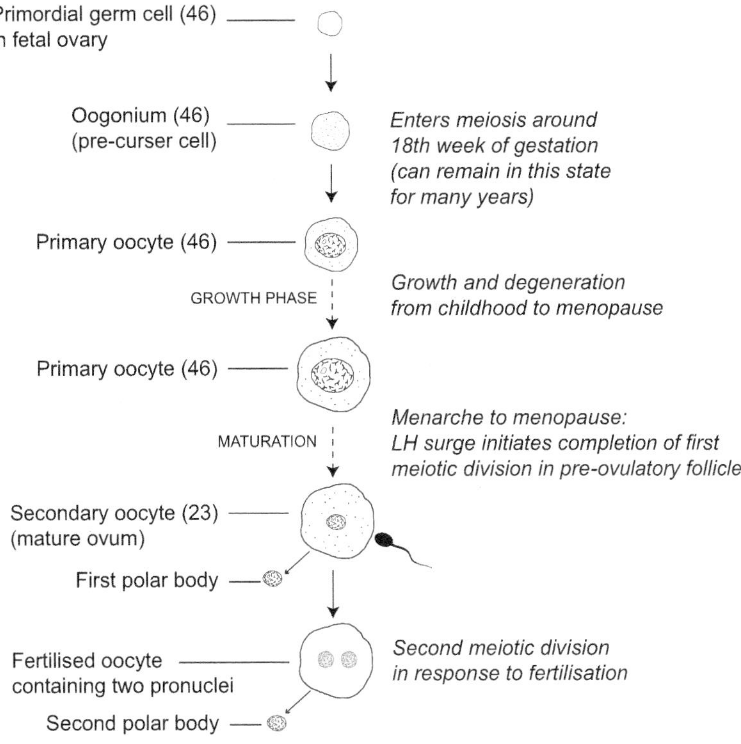

Figure 3.3 Stages of oogenesis – development of the mature oocyte (ovum) (adapted from Reiss 1998) [502]

Follicular development The ovarian follicles are at different stages of development. The earliest stage of follicular selection starts about 150 days before the cycle in which the egg will be released. There is a constant progression in the development of follicles, from early stage development to antral follicles (resting stage), which are potentially ovulatory and available at the start of a menstrual cycle. Little is known about what initiates the resumption of follicular development after many years in the resting stage or why one primordial follicle resumes development and proceeds to ovulation, yet a neighbouring follicle might remain in the resting state for decades. Initially follicular growth is independent of pituitary control but in larger follicles, growth and development is regulated by FSH and LH. The larger follicles are both gonadotrophin-sensitive and gonadotrophin-dependent. [194]

Growing follicles go through various stages: from primordial (oocyte with a single layer of granulosa cells around it) through primary, secondary and pre-antral (with increasing layers of granulosa cells), to antral stage (containing a fluid-filled cavity or antrum), to a fully fledged pre-ovulatory or Graafian follicle (with an enlarged fluid-filled antrum and the oocyte at the side of the follicle, surrounded by the nourishing and protective cumulus and corona cells which prevent premature maturation). As the follicles grow they become surrounded by a collar of theca cells which produce androgens that are then converted to estrogens by the granulosa cells.

A cohort of up to 20 gonadotrophin-sensitive antral follicles (resting follicles 2–8 mm in diameter) are recruited in the late luteal phase of the cycle and begin to develop further. These growing follicles produce increasing amounts of estrogen. The recruitment phase lasts from the end of the luteal phase of the previous cycle until about day 5–7 of the current cycle. A single follicle is then selected from this cohort to become the dominant follicle (selection) – this is the follicle which is most sensitive to FSH. The dominant follicle produces the most estrogen; it also develops LH receptors in the late follicular phase in preparation for the LH surge and impending ovulation. As it enlarges, the area between the follicle and the surface of the ovary becomes thinner and weaker, creating the stigma through which the egg will be released. The dominant Graafian follicle reaches 18–20 mm in diameter before it ruptures (figure 3.9). Occasionally follicles do not rupture, but persist and enlarge to form ovarian cysts. If a follicle is greater than 20 mm, it is known as an ovarian cyst.

Ovulation Ovulation is the process during which a Graafian follicle ruptures to release the egg along with follicular fluid. Ovulation follows a brief surge in LH which matures the egg and prepares the follicle for rupture. Ovulation usually occurs around 36 hours after the initiation of the LH surge. Before 2008, ovulation was considered to be a sudden, explosive event, but laparoscopic images by Donnez show that the protrusion of the mature follicle and release of the egg into the peritoneal cavity takes around 15 minutes. [361] Ovulation usually occurs 10–16 days before the start of the next period and may be accompanied by temporary abdominal discomfort or pain (mittelschmerz) (page 161). [409]

Side of ovulation There has been considerable controversy as to whether ovulation occurs on alternate sides, as a random event or more frequently on the right side. The first study to use ultrasound to determine the side of ovulation concluded for the first time that ovulation occurs on random sides, but this study was conducted on women with fertility problems. [80] A European multi-centre collaborative study of normal fertile women used hormonal assays and pelvic ultrasound to observe 205 cycles from 81 women during at least two consecutive ovulatory cycles and reached the same conclusion: in normal fertile women, the side of ovulation is a random event independent of the side of the previous cycle. [148]

Second ovulation If two or more follicles mature almost simultaneously, then more than one egg may be released and there is the possibility of conceiving dizygotic (fraternal) twins. As soon as one egg has been released, the rapidly increasing progesterone (from the corpus luteum) prevents estrogen from stimulating another LH surge. The positive feedback to the hypothalamus reduces GnRH pulses stopping further ovulation – so when a second ovulation occurs, it always occurs within a 24-hour window. Ultrasound studies clearly show that there is no evidence of a second follicle developing to the size of one that will rupture and release an egg later in the same cycle. When there is more than one ovulation this always occurs within the same ovulatory phase – that is, within the same episode of cervical secretions. [507]

Multiple follicles and dizygotic twins At the start of each menstrual cycle, FSH stimulates a new wave of follicle growth among the antral follicles, then as the growing follicles produce increasing amounts of estrogen this signals back to the pituitary causing FSH levels to fall. Usually, when FSH levels reach a certain concentration early in the cycle, one follicle becomes dominant, but when the level of FSH is higher or exceeds the critical threshold at the time of follicle selection, multiple follicle growth results which increases the chance of dizygotic twins. It is thought that the increased incidence of naturally conceived twins in older women is due to the higher concentrations of FSH driving the selection of more follicles. [287]

Mature oocyte The ovum is the mature oocyte. It is the largest cell in the human body, measuring about 0.1 mm in diameter (i.e. about 120 microns). The ovum is ready to burst into action after contact with the sperm. The mature egg is similar in structure to those of other species, including the hen's egg. In the centre of the egg is the nucleus containing 23 chromosomes, the mother's genetic contribution to her child. Surrounding the nucleus is jelly-like cytoplasm which contains the energy source and nourishment to support the embryo during its early stages of development before it becomes attached to the placenta. The outer part of the egg has an internal and external membrane. The transparent external membrane or zona pellucida (equivalent to the shell of a hen's egg) contains glycoproteins that bind the sperm to the surface of the egg. The internal plasma membrane which surrounds the cytoplasm has a layer of cortical granules beneath its surface. These small membranous particles contain enzymes (equivalent of the acrosome in sperm) which, immediately after fertilisation, fuse with the membrane rendering the zona pellucida impenetrable to further sperm. The egg

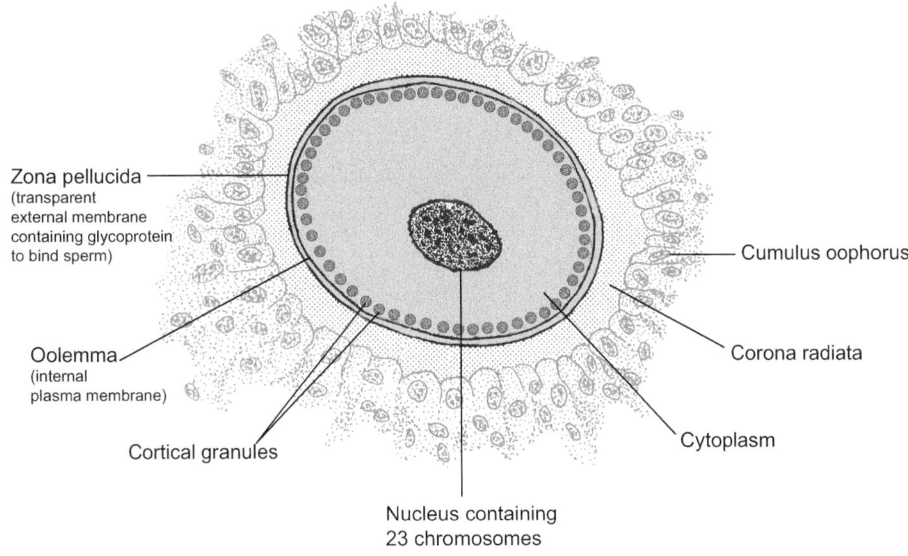

Figure 3.4 The mature oocyte (ovum)

is surrounded by a luminous halo of nutrient cells (corona radiata and cumulus oophorus) (figure 3.4).

Lifespan of the egg The average fertilisable lifespan of the egg is 17 hours. [518] This is generally rounded up to 24 hours, plus another 24 hours to allow for the possibility of a second ovulation. Thus the potential fertilisable lifespan of the egg is 48 hours after ovulation.

Corpus luteum After the follicle has ruptured, the stigma heals and the residual granulosa and theca cells are transformed (through luteinisation) into the corpus luteum – a yellowish structure with a rich blood supply and accumulation of fats. The corpus luteum (yellow body) is a temporary endocrine structure which produces significant amounts of progesterone and also some estrogen which suppresses further ovulation. The fully formed corpus luteum is approximately 2 cm in diameter with a normal lifespan of 10–16 days. If there is no conception, the cells degenerate, the production of progesterone ceases and menstruation follows. Eventually all that remains of the corpus luteum is a small white scarred area on the ovary known as the "corpus albicans". If conception occurs, the corpus luteum remains active for three to four months of pregnancy.

Under normal conditions the ruptured follicle is transformed into the corpus luteum, but occasionally a corpus luteum forms from a ripe follicle which failed to rupture – a luteinised unruptured follicle may be a cause of "unexplained" infertility (page 349).

Can sex trigger ovulation? Ovulation is technically referred to as "spontaneous ovulation", meaning that ovulation occurs as a result of the changing dynamics of the menstrual cycle and *not* as the result of sexual excitement or other events. It is unfortunate that colloquial use of the term "spontaneous" can imply the opposite, which may explain why women often fear that sex can induce a *spontaneous* ovulation. [507]

Although intercourse in mammals can accelerate ovulation, this trigger-effect has not been observed in humans. [628]

Some women say that their cycles are more regular when they are having sex, but sexual activity or inactivity may involve complex relationship issues or social factors. Regular sex may help to reduce stress. Research on llamas and bulls has found that a component in seminal fluid elicits an ovulatory response. [482] Similarly, work on fruit flies has shown that proteins in seminal fluid affect sexual receptivity and fecundity (reproductive rate). [226] It is not known whether there may be any similar mechanisms associated with human sperm.

There is some suggestion that women who are (or have been) sexually active have improved reproductive function, compared with women who have never been sexually active (controlling for factors including age). A study of 259 regularly menstruating women (18–44 years) observed higher levels of estrogen, mid-cycle LH and mid-luteal progesterone amongst the women who were sexually active. The sexually inactive women had a higher incidence of sporadic anovulatory cycles. There was, however, no evidence of sex triggering ovulation. [471]

Evidence of ovulation Women frequently talk convincingly about whether or not they are ovulating and the timing of ovulation, however, it is useful to consider the levels of evidence confirming ovulation as this is particularly relevant for women who are trying to conceive. Moghissi defines the levels of evidence as follows.

- Definite proof of ovulation:
  - establishment of pregnancy
  - surgical retrieval of an egg from the Fallopian tube
- Strong evidence:
  - direct observation of the corpus luteum by laparoscopy or laparotomy with the presence of a stigma
- Presumptive evidence:
  - serial ultrasound scans monitoring follicular growth, rupture and development of the corpus luteum
  - direct hormone monitoring (LH, estrogens or progesterone) in blood or urine
  - peripheral changes in the reproductive tract which include changes in temperature and cervical secretions [408] [409]

In practice, most evidence of ovulation is presumptive. Women being investigated for fertility delays may be offered mid-luteal phase progesterone assays and possibly cycle monitoring using ultrasound and direct hormone monitoring; however, the only evidence of ovulation available to most women is either urine test kits or observation of fertility indicators, the latter being more subjective.

Direct hormone monitoring: objective markers Direct hormone assessment (blood or urine) provides an objective marker of ovulation and circulating reproductive hormone levels. A raised mid-luteal phase progesterone level is used to confirm ovulation during fertility assessment for women with delays in conceiving. Although there have been attempts to produce home kits to test progesterone metabolites, including some new developments using urinary pregnanediol-3a-glucuronide (PDG), [149] there are currently no home kits which *confirm* ovulation.

The rise in estrogen to a peak level followed by a sharp drop provides circumstantial evidence, although not proof, that a ripe follicle is ready to burst. Usually a surge of LH from the pituitary follows the estrogen peak causing the follicle to rupture, but ovulation may still fail to occur despite the LH surge. [614] [618] [98] OPKs and fertility monitors which measure LH (and estrogen) may have a role for women using FAMs, either alone or in conjunction with subjective indicators, but they do not prove the occurrence of ovulation.

Indicators of fertility: subjective assessment The more indirect indicators of fertility provide secondary markers reflecting the changing ovarian hormone levels. [178] [618] A raised temperature level is a retrospective sign indicative of the thermogenic action of progesterone from the corpus luteum. Symptoms such as the build-up of a characteristic pattern of cervical secretions reflect the rising estrogen levels which occur with increasing follicular size approaching ovulation, but this does not always result in ovulation. So, **despite signs and symptoms normally associated with ovulation, there are no guarantees of ovulation.**

Use of terms pre- and post-ovulation Vollman, a pioneer of the Temperature Method, advised avoiding the use of "pre- and post-ovulation" as this supposes a knowledge about ovulation, preferring the terms "postmenstrual" and "premenstrual", defining the premenstrual phase as starting at the first high temperature. As most women associate "premenstrual" with the few days just before a period, this terminology would seem confusing. The terms "early" and "late" infertile times are used here to define the "pre-" and "post-ovulation" infertile times of the cycle. If the terms "pre- or post-ovulation" are used loosely, this implies *presumed* ovulation based on subjective indicators. Similarly, reference may be made to "anovulatory" cycles implying *presumed* absence of ovulation, based on monophasic cycles where the temperature remains on the low level throughout the cycle.

Follicular waves There is some evidence that follicular activity occurs in waves. Fifty women with normal menstrual cycles had daily ultrasound scans to observe follicular development for an interval between one ovulation and the next (i.e. starting in the luteal phase). All the women had more than one wave of follicular development: 68% had two waves and 32% had three waves of activity. Although waves of follicular development were observed in the luteal phase, these never resulted in ovulation and there is no possibility of an LH surge to trigger ovulation in the luteal phase due to its suppression by progesterone. Most of the waves involved small antral follicles of less than 8 mm diameter. Whether there were two or three waves, there was still only one ovulatory event and it was always the final wave which culminated in ovulation (this occurred at the anticipated time at the end of the follicular phase).

Reports of this research created a media storm in 2003 as the waves were erroneously equated with ovulation and assertions that women can ovulate more than once and at any time of the menstrual cycle. This was not helped by one of the authors who was reported to have commented that up to 40% of women may not be able to use FAMs because there is no "safe" time. These serial ultrasound scans spanning one inter-ovulatory interval showed **no evidence of more than one ovulation.** [17] Increasing evidence of the wave theory was published in a review of more than 200 studies on follicular development. [18]

Fallopian tubes

The Fallopian tubes (named after the 16th century Italian anatomist Gabriele Fallopio) are also known as the "uterine tubes", "oviducts" or "salpinges" (singular: salpinx, Greek for trumpet). The two long, thin, mobile, hollow tubes run outwards from the upper angle of the uterus *toward* the ovaries (they are not "fixed" to the ovaries). Each tube is about 10 cm long and consists of the interstitial part which runs through the uterine musculature, the narrow isthmus, wider ampulla and the funnel-shaped infundibulum with about 10–15 slender finger-like projections or fimbriae projecting from its rim.

The infundibulum opens into the peritoneal cavity, with the fimbriae lying close to, but not touching, the ovaries. The ovarian fimbria of each tube is elongated and can reach the ovary. The tubal mucosa is arranged into longitudinal folds which become increasingly convoluted towards the outer end of the tube. The mucosal folds have ciliated cells mostly on the apex of the folds.

The inside diameter of the tube decreases along its length with the widest part at the fimbriated end and the narrowest part (about 1 mm diameter) in the interstitial portion. The tube communicates with the lower genital tract via the uterine cavity and with the peritoneal cavity via the abdominal opening. This allows a direct pathway for ascending infection.

The Fallopian tubes perform the following functions:

- Sperm transport to achieve fertilisation
- Egg pick-up and transport – minute oscillations of the fimbriae guide the egg into the tube
- Fertilisation in the ampulla (Latin: flask)
- Nutrition, protection and transport of the zygote – the zygote is delivered to the uterine cavity at blastocyst stage at precisely the right time for implantation.

Just before ovulation the fimbriae position themselves over the area where the egg will be released (stigma), the beating cilia providing a gentle suction drawing the egg into the tube, contracting rhythmically to create a peristaltic wave (towards the uterus) which draws the egg further into the tube. Tubal transport is complex and requires an interaction between muscular peristaltic contractions, ciliary activity and the flow of tubal secretions. The microscopic cilia are easily damaged by external factors including infection, endometriosis and smoking, which can result in tubal problems and infertility. [370]

Fertilisation Fertilisation describes the process whereby the spermatozoon fuses with the egg. This must take place during those few hours after ovulation if pregnancy is to occur. Fertilisation normally occurs in the intermediate part of the tube and takes around 24 hours (page 41).

The Fallopian tube on the side of ovulation is normally the one to collect the egg, but a healthy tube is highly mobile and can often reach almost across to the other ovary so, in situations where a woman has lost a tube on one side and an ovary on the opposite side, it is known that the egg can cross over to the opposite tube and achieve conception. The mobility of tubes can be severely impaired following infections such as chlamydia, which causes the formation of adhesions and either prevents the tube from capturing the egg or blocks it completely.

Sex of the child The sex chromosome from the spermatozoon determines the child's sex. The egg contains 22 chromosomes plus an X sex chromosome and the spermatozoon contains 22 chromosomes plus either an X or Y sex chromosome.

X egg + X spermatozoon = XX zygote = female
X egg + Y spermatozoon = XY zygote = male

When the two haploid gametes are combined, the fertilised egg contains the normal diploid chromosome complement of 23 pairs. Despite the fact that there are equal numbers of X- and Y-chromosome-bearing sperm in each ejaculate, giving a 50:50 chance in terms of the child's sex, this does not slow the ongoing debate about whether you can influence the sex of the child (page 336). To date **there is no reliable scientific evidence to support any natural means of sex selection.**

Monozygotic and dizygotic twins In the first few days after fertilisation the embryo can split into two or more genetically identical parts, forming monozygotic (identical) twins who will be of the same sex with identical characteristics. However, if two or more eggs are released and fertilised, the result is dizygotic (non-identical or fraternal) twins, who may be of like or different sex. If the woman had intercourse with two different men during her fertile time the twins could have different fathers. Bi-paternal twins may be more common than is known.

Conception – from fertilisation to implantation Conception describes the process which starts with fusion of the spermatozoon and egg (fertilisation) and continues through the early development of the embryo to the implantation of the blastocyst (figure 3.5).

Embryo development The fertilised egg (single-celled zygote) normally has two haploid pronuclei (one from the spermatozoon and one from the egg) forming the full chromosome complement. This is the first stage in embryo development. The embryo then starts to progress by cleavage (dividing by mitosis) to form two, four, eight cells to reach the solid cluster of about 16 undifferentiated cells, the morulla (mulberry) stage.

The blastocyst stage has about 100 cells which have differentiated into the inner cell mass and the outer single cell layer, the trophoblast. The blastocyst contains a fluid-filled cavity (blastocoele) which creates a micro-environment for embryonic development. The inner cell mass will develop into the fetus and the trophoblast forms the trophectoderm cells which will eventually form the placenta and the fetal membranes.

The quality of the embryo is equally dependent on the genetic material from spermatozoon and egg. **A healthy-looking embryo (observed in-vitro), which appears to be dividing normally and may reach blastocyst stage, is not guaranteed to be chromosomally normal (euploid).** Embryos which have an abnormal chromosome complement are more likely to miscarry or

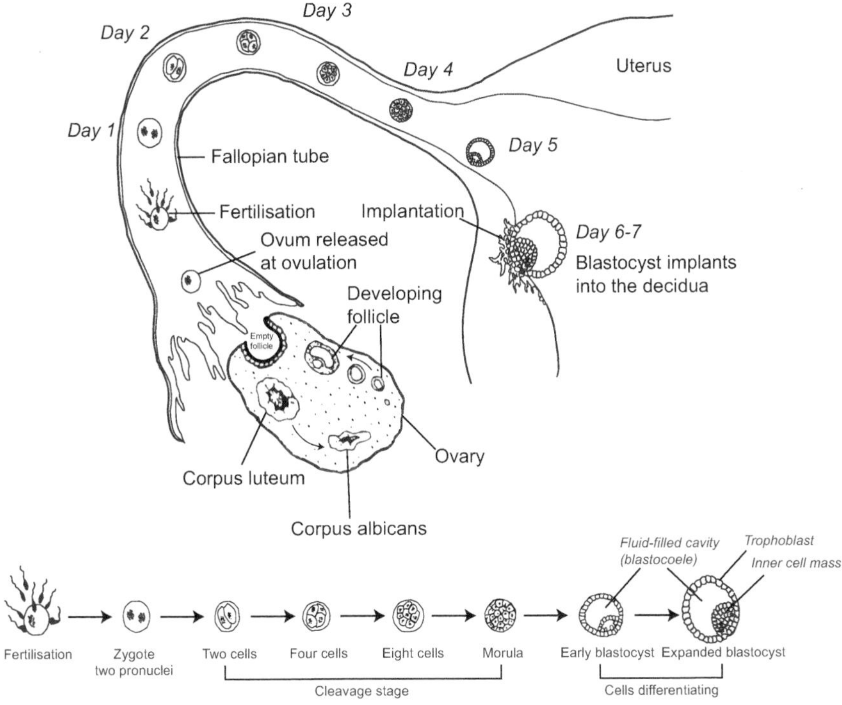

Figure 3.5 The process of conception: from fertilisation to implantation showing the stages of embryo development

result in a child with a chromosomal abnormality such as Down's syndrome. Couples who are going through assisted conception, such as IVF, are often acutely aware of the stages of normal embryo development. Some couples may require pre-implantation genetic (aneuploidy) screening to try and select chromosomally normal embryos.

The early embryo is normally transported from the tube to the uterus in around 80 hours, whence it can start to implant. The term "embryo" describes the developmental time-span from fertilisation until about eight weeks after fertilisation (10 weeks after the last menstrual period) when most of the organs are formed, after which time it becomes the *fetus* until the time of birth.

Uterus

The uterus (womb) is a thick-walled potentially hollow organ situated in the pelvic cavity between the bladder and the rectum. It is shaped like an inverted pear and measures about 8 cm long, 6 cm wide (side to side) and 4 cm deep (front to back) in a non-pregnant woman. The uterus is divided into three areas: the corpus (body), the isthmus (narrower section) and the cervix.

At the top of the uterus (opposite the cervical opening) is the fundus. During pregnancy the fundus is palpated to establish fetal lie and presentation. Uterine size and fetal growth is assessed by measuring the fundal height in centimetres from the pubic bone to the fundus which, from 20 weeks onwards, is roughly equivalent to the number of weeks gestation.

At the lower end of the uterus, the cervix projects into the upper part of the vagina. The space around the cervix is divided into four fornices: anterior fornix (between the cervix and bladder), posterior fornix (between the cervix and rectum) and two lateral fornices (right and left adnexae) – the space where the ovaries and Fallopian tubes lie. The triangle-shaped uterine cavity connects with the Fallopian tubes at the cornua (upper outer angles) and at the lower end with the vagina via the cervical canal.

Anteversion, retroversion and its relevance for cervical palpation About 80% of women are born with an anteverted anteflexed uterus – the "normal" position. The uterus is approximately at right angles to the vagina with its long axis tilted forwards towards the pubic bone and anteflexed (curved forwards on itself) from a pivot point at the level of the internal cervical os. A healthy uterus is mobile. The anteverted uterus lies on the urinary bladder and moves backwards as the bladder fills.

About 20% of women are born with a retroverted uterus with its long axis tilting backwards towards the spine. The retroverted uterus may also be retroflexed (curved backwards on itself). Provided the uterus is mobile (on internal palpation), its position is of little significance to fertility. Figure 3.6 shows a side view of the female reproductive organs to demonstrate the angle of the vagina and relative position of the uterine body and cervix. The main image shows an anteverted uterus within the pelvic cavity with the dotted lines showing the uterus in a retroverted position with the relative position of its cervix.

The uterus can sometimes be abnormally "fixed" in a retroverted position as a result of endometriosis, a cyst, fibroid or tumour pushing it backwards, or due to adhesions from pelvic inflammatory disease or pelvic surgery. A naturally positioned retroverted uterus is asymptomatic, but if it is abnormally "fixed" in a retroverted (and possibly retroflexed) position, it may cause back-ache, chronic pelvic pain or deep pain on penetration. These symptoms are a result of the condition, not the uterine position.

The cervix is in direct line for the sperm in a normally positioned anteverted uterus, but in a deeply retroverted or retroflexed uterus the cervix may be pointing upwards slightly and out of direct line. It is controversial whether this has any impact on sperm penetration.

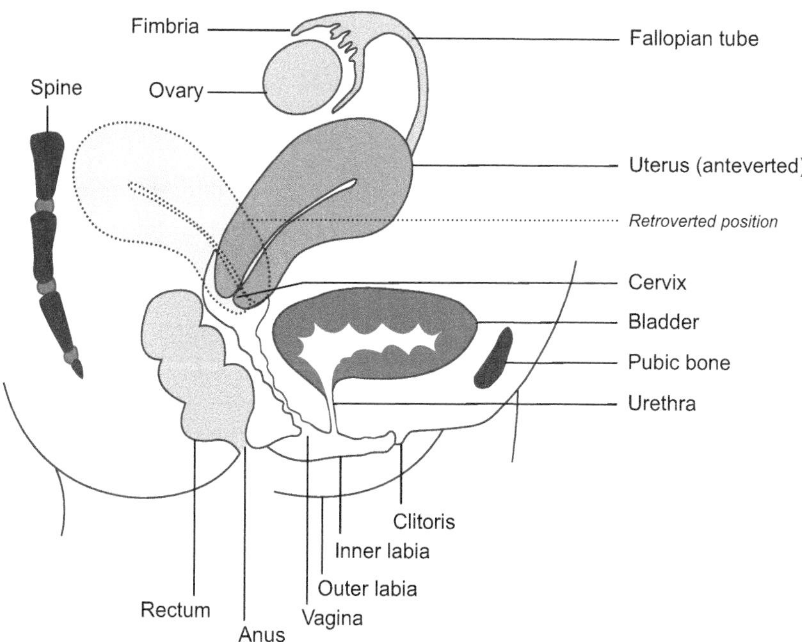

Figure 3.6 Female reproductive organs: side view showing a normally positioned anteverted uterus (dotted lines show relative position in retroversion)

Uterine position and location of the cervix is most significant when teaching cervical self-palpation. With an anteverted uterus, the cervix points slightly forward (anteriorly) and the os is easily felt by the examining finger (figure 3.6). If the uterus is very anteverted and anteflexed the cervix may point backwards towards the posterior vaginal wall and the os will be harder to reach. With a retroverted and retroflexed uterus the cervix points slightly upwards into the anterior vaginal wall, the os may lie against the vaginal wall and be difficult to reach behind the pubic bone (page 149).

Layers of the uterus The uterus has three layers – the outer perimetrium (serous membrane), the myometrium and the endometrium. The bulk of the uterus is composed of the myometrium – bundles of smooth muscle fibres which, during pregnancy, are capable of enormous expansion in size and number to accommodate the growing fetus. The myometrial layer is the strongest muscle by weight in the female body. During labour these muscle fibres contract and shorten leading to effacement and dilatation of the cervix and subsequent delivery. The criss-cross arrangement of the muscles compresses the blood vessels after placental separation to reduce blood loss.

The uterine cavity has a highly specialised lining called the endometrium, which is composed of two layers: basal and functional. The functional layer is highly responsive to ovarian hormones. It has a complex system of spiral arteries, veins, capillaries and branching vessels. When fully developed it is thick, spongy, nutritious and capable of sustaining pregnancy, then it is completely shed and regenerated each menstrual cycle. The basal layer, a thin layer next to the myometrium, is essential for the growth and regeneration of the functional layer. The basal layer has its own blood supply of small straight arteries and is less responsive to hormonal changes so is always preserved.

Endometrial changes during the menstrual cycle The functional layer of the endometrium goes through three distinct phases during the cycle: menstrual, proliferative and secretory.

Menstrual phase During the menstrual phase the functional layer of the endometrium is shed – menstruation (menses, menstrual period). About 14 days after ovulation if there is no conception the corpus luteum stops functioning, and the decreasing progesterone (and estrogen) levels cause the endometrium to degenerate. The spiral arteries become increasingly coiled, restricting blood flow to the functional layer and forcing blood through the complex branching network of vessels, which subsequently rupture. The haemorrhage and uterine contractions caused by increased prostaglandins help the uterus to expel the necrotic endometrial tissue consisting of blood, mucus, endometrial glands, cellular debris and the unfertilised egg.

Menstrual bleeding is usually heaviest on the second and third days of the cycle with 90% of loss occurring within the first three days. The amount of loss can vary from woman to woman and from one menstrual period to the next in the same woman. Estimates of blood loss are highly subjective. Studies of menstrual loss estimate an average loss of 35 ml during each period. Menstrual loss is only considered excessive and requiring treatment if it exceeds 80 ml (page 77).

Biologically, menstruation occurs at the end of a cycle in which the egg has not been fertilised; however, because the first day of a period is an easily recognised landmark, for practical purposes it is taken as day 1 of the cycle (with the menstrual cycle lasting from day 1 of the period up to the day before the next period starts). The first menstrual period a girl experiences is known as the "menarche" and the final menstrual period is the "menopause".

Ovulatory and anovulatory bleeds Bleeding will occur both in ovulatory and anovulatory cycles. If ovulation occurs but there is no conception, the next period will follow around 14 days later due to the decrease in progesterone (and estrogen). This progesterone withdrawal bleed is normal – it is a "true period".

If there is no ovulation, the ovaries still produce enough estrogen to stimulate endometrial growth. Bleeding occurs when the estrogen levels fall and can no longer maintain the endometrium. Bleeding in anovulatory cycles is varied: it may be irregular, painless, heavy and sometimes prolonged, or infrequent and light. Some women will have amenorrhoea. An anovulatory bleed is technically an estrogen withdrawal bleed (not a true period) – this is not normal. This detail is relevant for women using FAMs whether to plan or avoid pregnancy.

Proliferative phase During the pre-ovulatory phase of the cycle the increasing level of estrogen from the developing ovarian follicles stimulates endometrial growth and regeneration. The epithelial cells on the surface of the endometrium multiply (proliferate) profusely and the mucus-secreting endometrial glands proliferate and elongate. The small muscular spiral arteries grow inward from the basal layer between the elongating glands. This phase of endometrial thickening continues until ovulation and will be of *variable* length.

Secretory phase Immediately after ovulation, progesterone starts to exert its effect on the estrogen-primed endometrium. Blood flow and glandular growth is greatly increased. The glands now start secreting watery mucus, rich in glycogen and lipids, which assist in sperm transport through the uterus. The secretory phase has a *fixed length*.

If fertilisation occurs, the endometrium develops further into the decidua, which is even thicker and more vascular with more prominent glands and greater secretory activity to sustain the blastocyst during implantation and early development. The implanting blastocyst in turn produces human chorionic gonadotrophin (hCG) which stimulates the corpus luteum to continue its production of progesterone, thereby preventing menstruation.

If there is no fertilisation, falling estrogen and progesterone levels from the failing corpus luteum result in the degeneration of the endometrium leading to menstruation and the cycle starts again.

Implantation Implantation is a highly complex (and only partially understood) process involving a number of stages during which the blastocyst embeds itself into the decidua. The blastocyst needs to be in close contact with the endometrium (apposition) to initiate a complex interaction between its trophoblast and the decidua. The blastocyst and decidua secrete adhesive molecules (including phospholipids) using a glue-like mechanism for initial attachment. Complex growth factors are also involved to encourage rapid growth and development.

The trophectoderm starts to penetrate through the layers of the decidua to establish contact with the maternal circulation. Successful implantation requires the blastocyst to escape from the zona pellucida (hatching), and the specialised villi of the trophectoderm to secrete hCG, sending signals to the mother and beginning two-way communication between the embryo and the mother's circulation – **this is the start of pregnancy**. There is a specific window of implantation: in most successful pregnancies, the blastocyst implants eight to 10 days after ovulation. [627]

Implantation starts around four to five days after ovulation, but it requires at least 10 days to complete the early stages of the process. Around 40% of blastocysts fail to implant and the unimplanted blastocyst will be washed away with the next period unless it secretes enough hCG to maintain the life of the corpus luteum and prevent menstruation.

Ultrasound imaging of early pregnancy A trans-vaginal scan of a normal pregnancy will identify the gestational sac from about four to five weeks. The first anatomical structure seen within the gestational sac is the yolk sac (which provides nutrients). The first visible evidence of the embryo is the fetal pole, which is seen as a clearly defined thickening on the edge of the yolk sac. The very early heartbeat is seen as a subtle flicker. This increases to 120–180 beats per minute from about six weeks. Abnormalities in this process may indicate miscarriage.

Cervix

The cervix is the lower part of the uterus which projects into the upper vagina. The cervical canal runs through the cervix from its opening into the uterus at the internal os to its opening into the vagina at the external os. The canal, which is lined by mucus-secreting columnar epithelium, is about 3 cm long. In a nulliparous woman the external os is shaped like a circular dimple; after childbirth it is a transverse slit which may be sufficiently open to admit the finger-tip.

The upper part of the cervix is composed largely of muscle fibres which play a major role in retaining a pregnancy. The lower part is mainly collagen (connective tissue). In the first stage of labour (and in miscarriage) uterine contractions cause the cervix to shorten and dilate. The cervix is capable of stretching during birth to around 10 cm in diameter to accommodate the circumference of the baby's head.

The vaginal aspect of the cervix (ectocervix) is covered by thick stratified squamous epithelium and the portion facing into the cervical canal (endocervix) is lined by mucus-secreting columnar epithelium. The cervical epithelium is sensitive to infections including chlamydia, herpes and human papilloma virus (HPV). The immature cervix is particularly vulnerable, so women who have sex at an early age and women who have many sexual partners are at high risk for cervicitis, which may lead to ascending infection, pelvic inflammatory disease (PID) and subsequent infertility.

The transition between the squamous and columnar (glandular) epithelium is known as the squamo-columnar junction. The position of this zone changes over reproductive life and in response to exogenous hormones such as hormonal contraception. Columnar cells, which naturally migrate downwards onto the vaginal aspect of the cervix, may result in a reddened area of columnar epithelium around the cervical os – this is a cervical ectropion (page 215). Columnar cells which become exposed to the acidic vaginal secretions are replaced by the more acid-resistant squamous cells. This is the transformation zone. This whole area is a common site for cellular changes which, if left untreated, can lead to cervical intra-epithelial neoplasia (CIN) – hence this is the area targeted by cervical screening (page 218).

Effect of estrogen and progesterone on the cervix The cervix goes through distinct changes in its level (height), position, consistency and opening throughout the menstrual cycle. For a woman with an anteverted uterus the infertile cervix is low, firm, closed and tilted; the fertile cervix is high, soft, open and straight. About one week before ovulation, in response to increasing levels of estrogen, the cervix starts to change very subtly from its infertile to fertile state. After ovulation, due to the action of progesterone, the fertile cervix reverts back quite rapidly to its infertile state (within about 24 hours).

Cervical mucus

Cervical mucus is a complex gel structure with semi-solid and liquid phases. Its main constituents are mucin molecules, water, chemical and biochemical compounds (sodium chloride, amino acids, simple sugars and enzymes) which nourish sperm and influence sperm penetration. The fluid content and composition of cervical mucus varies throughout the menstrual cycle under hormonal control. [89] [317] [318]

The principal functions of cervical mucus are:

- to admit sperm from the hostile vaginal environment, protecting them against the acidic conditions and the antimicrobial activity of leucocytes;
- to be receptive to sperm penetration at or near ovulation and prevent sperm entry at other times;
- to act as a means of sperm selection, encouraging the progression of morphologically normal sperm and filtering out sperm with abnormal morphology (shape) which characteristically have reduced motility;
- to nurture sperm biochemically and initiate capacitation (sperm's fertilising ability);
- to entrap and store sperm for later release closer to ovulation; and
- to protect the uterine cavity against infection. [151] [406]

During pregnancy, cervical mucus has unique physical and immunological properties distinct from the properties in a non-pregnant state. [38] Although the viscous mucus plug inhibits the ascent of most bacteria during pregnancy, it does not block the passage of ureaplasma which is commonly found in the vagina of healthy women. If ureaplasma ascends to the amniotic cavity it may cause premature rupture of the membranes and preterm labour, thus having implications for antenatal care. [263] This protective mucus plug is normally lost as "the show" during cervical effacement shortly before or during labour.

Effect of estrogen on cervical secretions The ovarian hormones estrogen and progesterone influence the quantity and quality of cervical secretions. The different types of secretion either encourage or impede sperm penetration and this determine the state of fertility (page 39). [52] [88]

When estrogen levels are low (during menstruation and the early pre-ovulatory phase), there are minimal thick, sticky, white secretions at the cervix which impede sperm penetration. At this stage, the woman feels dry and is not aware of any secretions at the vulva.

About five to six days before ovulation, the ovarian follicles start to grow, estrogen levels rise and the fluid content of the cervical mucus increases. Secretions start to flow into the vagina and the woman experiences a sensation of moistness at the vulva followed by the appearance of sticky white secretions. At this stage, sperm may start to penetrate through the cervical canal.

As estrogen levels increase further, the cervical secretions become highly hydrated and the water content can exceed 96% – the higher the water content, the lower the viscosity and the easier for sperm to penetrate. [73] [318] Cervical mucus has a mesh-like micro-structure with small gaps between the mucus molecules. As ovulation approaches the gaps become larger, facilitating sperm penetration. The secretions, now easily recognised by a slippery or lubricative sensation at the vulva, are more profuse, wetter, slippery, transparent (or translucent/cloudy) and stretchy (the spinnbarkeit effect, see figures 3.7 and 3.8). If these secretions are dried, allowed to crystallise, and then viewed under a microscope, a pattern resembling fern leaves is seen (the ferning effect, see figure 3.8).

Spinnbarkeit effect The spinnbarkeit effect describes the capacity of thin, transparent (or translucent) cervical secretions to be drawn out into a long thread. [93] Spinnbarkeit of 10–20 cm has been shown to provide optimal conditions for sperm survival. [95] Although the spinnbarkeit thread may show crystal-clear secretion along its length, it may also show an uneven thread with different types of secretion. Detailed study has shown that thin parts of the thread contain stringy "S-type" secretion with thicker parts showing "L-type" (loaf) secretions. There may also be occasional white or milky parts containing "G-type" secretions (figure 3.8). [435] [436]

Ferning effect Cervical secretions that are allowed to dry in air and observed under a low-powered microscope, show clearly discernible patterns of crystallisation due to the effect of sodium chloride on the mucin molecules. The fern pattern has been suggested as an indirect test for ovulation and for estrogen activity. [509] This ferning effect is also observable in other bodily fluids, including saliva – hence the plethora of home tests which purport to identify ovulation using cheap plastic microscopes (page 171). Insler demonstrated that the first positive ferning in cervical secretions appeared five to seven days before ovulation. He also showed that scant amounts of cervical secretion, with a trace of spinnbarkeit and ferning, may still be found in post-menopausal women and in amenorrhoeic women with very low estrogen levels (but in those circumstances the external os was almost invariably closed). [298]

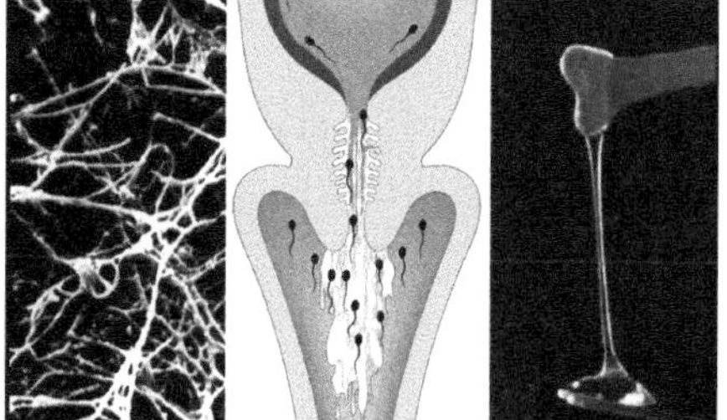

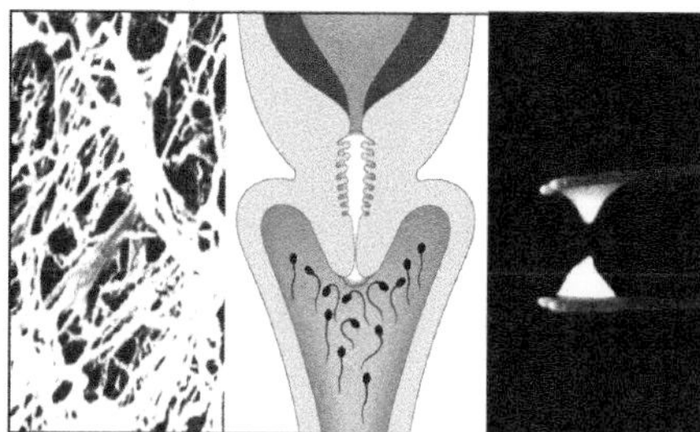

Figure 3.7 Effect of estrogen and progesterone on cervical secretions (© Pyper & Knight, FertilityUK 2016)

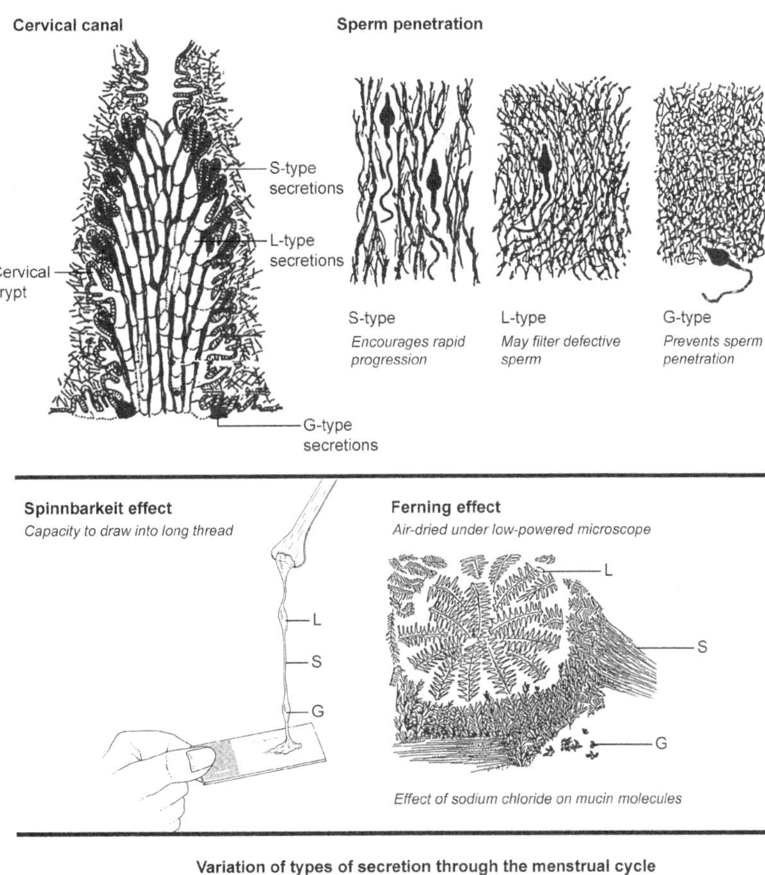

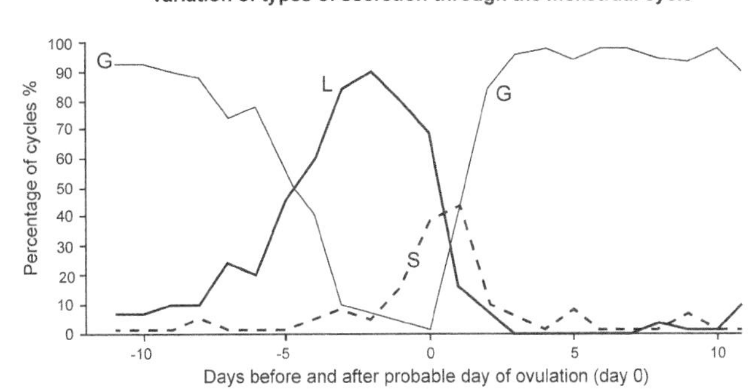

Figure 3.8 Structure of the cervical canal and cervical mucus demonstrating sperm penetration and the changing ratios of different mucus types through the menstrual cycle. Note the spinnbarkeit and ferning effect of estrogenised secretions. [435] [436] Reproduced with kind permission from Erik Odeblad

Detailed study of the fern pattern has shown different types of secretion contributing to the fern pattern: L-type mucus showing large palm-like crystals, S-type mucus showing thin parallel needles and G-type mucus showing irregular-shaped crystals or no crystals (figure 3.8). [435] [436]

Effect of progesterone on cervical secretions Immediately after ovulation, under the influence of progesterone, the cervical secretions decrease in quantity, become thicker, white and sticky forming a dense plug in the cervical canal which prevents sperm penetration (figure 3.7).

Function of different types of cervical mucus Odeblad used nuclear magnetic resonance imaging to describe four morphologically different types of cervical mucus isolated from single crypts in different zones in the cervix over the course of a menstrual cycle. He initially named them G (produced in response to progesterone) and E (crypts responding to estrogen stimulation), but after further study he divided the E-type into L-type (referring to the oval loaf-shaped rods) and S-type (referring to long narrow string-shaped rods or sperm-conveying mucus). Odeblad's microscopy studies also identified another pattern of crystallisation in mucus which he labelled "P-type" (peak) as it showed maximum volume on the days of peak fertility. The four different types of mucus are described as follows:

- G-type mucus contains varying numbers of cells, with increased density after ovulation. Its high viscosity and glue-like characteristics create a mechanical plug blocking the cervical canal, acting as a natural barrier to sperm. G-type mucus has small irregular crystals or no crystals when allowed to dry and observed under a microscope. G-type mucus contains leucocytes, lymphocytes and gammaglobulins, suggesting it provides a protective barrier against infection. G-type mucus is predominantly produced in the lower part of the cervical canal and is present throughout the cycle apart from during menstruation and the fertile time.
- L-type mucus has an intermediate viscosity and is produced throughout the fertile time. It forms a flexible mechanical support structure for the string-like S-type mucus. It may filter out defective sperm which deviate from the S-type mucus during sperm ascent. The L-type mucus is responsible for the palm-leaf-like "ferning" when allowed to dry and crystallise. L-type and S-type secretory units are found along the entire length of the cervical canal and both types are necessary for maximum fertility.
- S-type mucus appears one to three days after the L-type. It shows tiny crystals, with long, thin needle-like structures, aligned as parallel bundles with large spaces between them containing a watery fluid – the natural medium for swimming sperm. Some sperm enter S-type mucus at the cervical os moving directly to the uterine cavity, others travel to an S-type crypt where they seem to "hibernate" for around 20 hours before progressing through the reproductive tract. When sperm enter the crypts, the S-type mucus secretion appears to diminish. Some women who are trying to conceive report this temporary reduction in the clear, slippery secretion the day after intercourse.
- P-type mucus is very similar to S-type but shows a specific branching. Its role may be to liquefy any mucus that is blocking sperm from entering the S-type crypts. P-type mucus is confined to the upper part of the cervical canal. P-type mucus may also have an immunological function at the cervix. [435] [436]

Cyclic variation Following menstruation, G-type mucus predominates. As estrogen stimulation of the cervix increases, L-type mucus increases; with maximum estrogen stimulation S-type mucus is synthesised. The S-mucus flows continuously as long strings of watery fluid between the loafs of L-mucus "as water in a brook streams between pebbles". [436] This streaming effect causes the parallel orientation of the mucin molecules forming micelles (bundles). Following ovulation, the G-type mucus is secreted by the lowest crypts in the cervical canal, which blocks the cervical os, helping to retain the sperm and block further sperm penetration.

Figure 3.8 shows the cervical canal with complex secretory units (crypts) producing different types of mucus, sperm penetration through the different types and the changing proportions of the mucus types throughout the menstrual cycle. The spinnbarkeit and ferning effect are also shown.

Other studies have confirmed a mosaic of the four distinct mucus types in various proportions during the cycle, with the mucus types corresponding well to Odeblad's original work: Type I (G-type mucus), type II (L-type mucus) type III (S-type mucus) and type IV (P-type mucus). The results confirmed the changes in the diameter of gaps between the glycoprotein mesh and the parallel nature of the "swimming lanes" under estrogen influence. Cervical mucus differs from the follicular to the luteal phase of the cycle, whilst around ovulation several types of mucus co-exist, with secretions from different secretory units mixed in different proportions in the cervical canal. [400] This mosaic of mucus types constitutes what a woman sees as the changing pattern of her cervical secretions.

Cervical secretions: Practical aspects

Start of the fertile time The first day that a woman observes *any* sign of cervical secretions indicates the start of the fertile time – this is the earliest opportunity that sperm could survive in the female genital tract. She then observes the progressive build-up of secretions to *peak day* (the last day of wet, slippery, transparent, stretchy secretions) which correlates closely with ovulation. [51] [281] [118] Peak day can be recognised only retrospectively on the day following peak when the secretions have reverted to sticky or dry again.

End of the fertile time The fertile time ends three full days after peak day. The woman will be aware of dryness or only scant sticky secretions until the start of the next period. Some women may observe one or more days of wetter, transparent, stretchy secretions just before the period starts. This is related to the falling progesterone levels (and slight increase in estrogen) premenstrually (page 117).

Vagina

The vagina is a muscular elastic canal which leads from the external genitals (vulva) into the pelvis in an upwards and backwards direction (roughly towards the small of the back). The vaginal entrance lies between the urethral opening and the anus. The anterior and posterior walls of the vagina normally lie in contact, making the vagina a potential cavity. It is normally closed by the apposition of the labia and in some women it may be partially occluded by the hymen.

The widest diameter of the vagina changes along the length of its canal. From the vaginal entrance, the lower third of the canal is wider from front to back (antero-posterior) but above this the transverse diameter is wider. This is important knowledge for introducing a speculum. It may also be especially important information when working with couples with sexual difficulties. An understanding of the vaginal anatomy allows a woman and her partner to learn to explore the vagina more sensitively if she is having difficulties with penetration – if two fingers are introduced into the vagina, they should first be inserted vertically ("handshake" position) and then the wrist is twisted through 90 degrees (palm up) so that the fingers are horizontal. This follows the natural shape of the vagina which is an "H"-shape in cross-section.

The vaginal canal is approximately 9 cm long. The anterior vaginal wall is around 7 cm long, with the cervix projecting at its upper end; whereas the posterior wall extends the full 9 cm. At the upper end the vagina ends blindly in the vaginal vault which is divided into four areas in relation to the cervix – the shallow anterior fornix, the capacious posterior fornix (the most common site of semen pooling following intercourse) and the two shallow lateral fornices.

The vaginal canal has an outer muscular layer and an inner epithelial lining which forms a number of rugae (folds) giving it a characteristic ridged texture. These rugae allow expansion during sexual stimulation to accommodate the erect penis. During labour the hormonal changes of pregnancy allow enormous expansion as the vagina forms the lower part of the birth canal.

Some women may fear that their vagina is not big enough to accommodate a tampon or penis but, apart from those who have congenital abnormalities or have had vaginal surgery, this is rarely true. About 1% of women suffer from involuntary muscular spasms of the muscles around the vaginal entrance (vaginismus) when penetration is attempted. This psychosomatic condition results from severe anxiety and fear of penetration. It may be related to sexual abuse or other childhood trauma and is a common cause of sexual dysfunction or non-consummation of a relationship. Vaginismus may only be diagnosed during cervical screening or as part of fertility investigations. Most cases of dyspareunia (painful intercourse) are psychosomatic, but always require physical examination. The anatomical size of the vagina may vary slightly but functional size is largely determined by muscle tone and the contraction of surrounding muscles.

Pelvic floor muscles The lower end of the vagina is surrounded by a sling of voluntarily controlled muscles which support the pelvic organs. They form a figure-of-eight shape around the vagina and anus. A woman can learn to identify these muscles either by squeezing the muscles as if to stop a flow of urine, or by inserting one or two fingers into the vagina then squeezing the vaginal muscles. Muscular tightening is felt about half way up inside the vagina. The vaginal muscles can be tightened intentionally to increase sexual arousal or partner stimulation. At orgasm these muscles can be felt contracting at intervals of less than one second.

The muscular perineal body (which lies under the perineum) is essential for the control of the pelvic floor, particularly in women. Damage during vaginal delivery can lead to weakness in the pelvic floor. Pelvic floor exercises, first described by American gynaecologist Arnold Kegel, [323] are especially important following childbirth and around the menopause to strengthen the pelvic floor, improve bladder control, and prevent stress incontinence and prolapse. These exercises also help to increase awareness of the sensation at the vulva to distinguish the presence or absence of secretions (page 121).

Vaginal secretions and vaginal acidity During the reproductive years, the vagina is kept moist by cervical and vaginal secretions. The vagina is lined by squamous epithelium (continuous with that of the vaginal aspect of the cervix). Vaginal epithelium is under cyclic hormonal control and produces transudate which seeps out between the cells to moisten the vagina. Superficial epithelial cells are constantly exfoliated, releasing glycogen. Doderlein's bacilli (lactobacilli which are normal vaginal inhabitants) feed on the glycogen in the shed vaginal cells producing lactic acid. The vaginal acidity ($pH < 5$) inhibits the growth of other bacteria and protects the vagina from infection.

The vagina has a self-cleansing mechanism. Women should be discouraged from vigorous cleaning or the use of vaginal sprays or douches as this alters the pH and reduces the vagina's natural resistance to infection. The acidic vaginal environment kills sperm in a matter of hours; however, during the fertile time, in estrogenised cervical secretions, sperm can survive for up to seven days. A healthy vagina depends on sufficient estrogen. If estrogen levels are too low, vaginal dryness may result – this is common during the peri-menopause and for some women who are breastfeeding.

Sexual activity and vaginal lubrication During sexual stimulation the Bartholin's glands produce a colourless fluid which is secreted around the vaginal opening to act as a lubricant. The increased blood flow to the vaginal tissues during sexual excitement causes increased secretion of tissue fluid through the membranous vaginal walls (transudate). These secretions help to lubricate the vagina in preparation for intercourse. At the culmination of intercourse, the ejaculate is deposited as a seminal pool in the upper part of the vagina. The cervix dips into this pool during female orgasm establishing an interface between the seminal fluid and cervical secretions, thus encouraging sperm penetration through the female genital tract.

Awareness of different secretions Vaginal moistness or wetness originates from a number of sources: cervical mucus, vaginal transudate, arousal fluid, female ejaculatory fluid (not to be confused with stress incontinence) and seminal fluid (following intercourse). A woman who uses FAMs learns to distinguish between these different secretions. Women are normally aware when they are sexually aroused or have intercourse and arousal fluid can be distinguished from fertile secretions as it has no stretch. Women should be encouraged to report any unusual vaginal discharge that is discoloured, has an offensive odour or causes irritation. It is important to exclude pathology and treat promptly.

SEX HORMONE SYSTEM

The female reproductive system is under the control of hormones. The hypothalamus (master gland) is in overall control of the cascade of hormones which result in changes in the target organs – the endometrium, cervix (and its secretions) breasts and vaginal tissue.

Hypothalamic-pituitary-ovarian axis

The hypothalamus, a region in the brain roughly behind the eyes, produces releasing and inhibiting hormones in response to bodily signals. These hormones act on the pituitary, the pea-sized gland which hangs from the hypothalamus on a stalk. The pituitary and hypothalamus effectively function as one unit: the hypothalamic-pituitary axis.

The menstrual cycle and ovarian function are controlled via the hypothalamic-pituitary-ovarian axis (HPO-axis), which works in a very similar way to the male sex hormone system (page 42). The hypothalamus is involved in the control of autonomic (involuntary) bodily functions including temperature, sleep, thirst, appetite and fluid balance. Disturbances to these processes can affect hypothalamic function and cause menstrual disturbance.

The hypothalamus secretes GnRH which, from puberty onwards, controls the release of the gonadotrophins, FSH and LH, from the anterior pituitary. The pulsatile release of GnRH is influenced by circulating sex hormone levels, plus factors such as body weight and exercise. Women who exercise intensively or have extremely low body fat levels such as with anorexia nervosa are likely to have reduced GnRH production causing ovulation disorders, menstrual disturbance and weight-related amenorrhoea (page 331).

Follicle-stimulating hormone (FSH)

Follicle-stimulating hormone stimulates the recruitment of antral follicles. It initiates the growth and differentiation of the granulosa cells, promoting the action of the enzyme aromatase which converts androgens to estrogens. FSH also acts on the dominant follicle to help trigger ovulation. FSH levels reach a peak around day 3 of the cycle and decline in the late follicular phase, with a temporary rise at the time of the LH surge. FSH then remains low until the end of the luteal phase when the levels start to rise as the corpus luteum function declines, stimulating the recruitment of the next batch of antral follicles. FSH levels rise to extremely high levels as ovarian function declines approaching the menopause.

Luteinising hormone (LH)

The main function of LH is to mature the egg and trigger ovulation. LH also has a role in ovarian hormone production: stimulating the production of androgens (which are then converted into estrogens). The level of LH is consistently low throughout the cycle except for the significant rise (to about 10–20 times the baseline level) immediately before ovulation. The surge in LH is initiated by positive feedback as estrogen levels reach a critical level in the late follicular phase. The LH surge matures the follicle and the egg, and triggers ovulation. The surge lasts 36–48 hours, with ovulation typically occurring within 24 to 36 hours of the start of the urinary surge (LH is detectable in serum about 12 hours before its detection in urine). [97] [40] After ovulation, LH initiates the transformation of the collapsed follicle into the corpus luteum and helps to maintain luteal function.

Once the LH surge is underway it becomes increasingly difficult for sperm to penetrate the cervical mucus as the estradiol levels fall and progesterone levels starts to rise. [317] It is therefore important for women who are trying to conceive to understand the importance of intercourse *in advance of* the LH surge – delaying intercourse until a positive urine LH test may be counterproductive.

High levels of LH may indicate endocrine disturbance such as polycystic ovary syndrome (PCOS), and very low levels of LH (and FSH) may be found in women with amenorrhoea due to disturbances of the HPO-axis. Ovulation does not occur in the absence of an LH surge. [388]

Estrogens

Estrogens (the WHO preferred spelling of "oestrogens") are a group of sex steroid hormones including estrone, estradiol and estriol. Estrogens are produced in various tissues in both men and women from the conversion of androgens (male hormones). There are essentially three forms of estrogen:

- Estrone (E1) – produced mostly by the adrenal glands and in body fat (hence the importance of body fat percentage in fertility). Estrone is a weak estrogen, but can still stimulate proliferation of the endometrium. It is the major source of estrogen in post-menopausal women.
- Estradiol (E2) – the most important estrogen and main form of estrogen of relevance for fertility (often referred to generically as "estrogen"). Under the influence of FSH, granulosa cells in the developing follicles convert androgens into estradiol in large quantities. Increasing amounts of estradiol are produced at puberty, leading to the development and maintenance of female secondary sex characteristics. Estradiol promotes proliferation of the endometrium and, along with progesterone, produces secretory endometrium. Increasing estradiol in the pre-ovulatory phase is responsible for the softening of the cervix, dilatation of the os and the liquefaction of cervical secretions. The concentration of estradiol gradually increases from the start of the cycle and reaches its peak around 24 hours prior to ovulation. [97] The critical threshold of estradiol triggers the LH surge, which in turn triggers ovulation. Estradiol is the most commonly measured type of hormone for non-pregnant women – the level varies through the menstrual cycle and after menopause it drops to a very low but constant level. Estradiol has other widespread functions, including deposition of bone and relaxation of smooth muscles in the coronary arteries, which is why post-menopausal women are at increased risk of osteoporosis and coronary heart disease.
- Estriol (E3) – an estrogen produced in large amounts by the placenta (the precursor comes from the fetal adrenals and liver). Estriol may have a role in keeping the uterus inactive during pregnancy. Estriol can be detected from around the ninth week of pregnancy with the levels increasing throughout pregnancy. Estriol can be used to monitor the well-being of a pregnancy.

Progesterone

Progesterone is the hormone of pregnancy (literally: for pregnancy). It is produced by the corpus luteum following ovulation, at which time the rapidly increasing progesterone levels prevent further ovulation. Progesterone transforms the endometrium from its estrogen-primed proliferative state to its secretory state to encourage implantation. If pregnancy occurs, the trophectoderm of the implanting blastocyst produces hCG, which maintains the corpus luteum and the production of progesterone. At around 12 weeks the placenta begins to take over the production of progesterone – this is the luteal-placental shift. If ovulation occurs but there is no pregnancy, the corpus luteum disintegrates, the progesterone levels fall and a "true period" follows. If there is no ovulation, there will be no corpus luteum; progesterone levels remain low and the ensuing bleed will be anovulatory (page 59).

Progesterone has a significant effect on the indicators of fertility. It causes the cervix to be firm and closed, and it thickens the secretions to block sperm penetration. Progesterone also has an effect on blood vessel walls, causing peripheral vessels to contract. Diminishing blood flow through constricted capillaries reduces heat loss, resulting in a rise in waking temperature of around 0.2 deg.C. [194]

Table 3.1 Effect of ovarian hormones on target organs and indicators of fertility

Target organ	*Estrogen effect*	*Progesterone effect*
Endometrium	Promotes repair, growth and thickening (proliferation)	Promotes increased blood flow, glandular growth and secretory activity to support implantation
Cervix	High, soft, open and straight	Low, firm, closed and tilted
Cervical secretions	Liquefies mucus producing wetter, slippery, stretchy secretions assisting sperm penetration	Increases viscosity creating thick sticky plug impenetrable to sperm
Waking temperature	Maintains at lower level	Increase of about 0.2 deg.C
Breasts	Tenderness or tingling sensation particularly around the nipples	Increase in size, fullness and heaviness due to increased blood flow and fluid retention
Mood	Possible positive effects, but varied	Possible negative effects, but varied
Libido	May increase sexual desire, but varied	May reduce sexual desire, but varied

Inhibin

Inhibin is a protein hormone which exists in a number of forms. It is produced by the granulosa cells in ovarian follicles. Inhibin B plays a role in follicular development and the regulation of FSH. It is secreted by developing pre-antral and antral follicles and in larger quantities by the dominant follicle, where its action (along with estrogen) suppresses FSH and initiates the atresia of the other developing follicles.

Anti-mullerian hormone

Anti-mullerian hormone (AMH) is secreted by granulosa cells in both late pre-antral and small antral follicles (i.e. in follicles that have been recruited from the primordial follicle pool but not yet selected for dominance). Ultrasound studies of healthy women with regular menstrual cycles show that AMH is produced substantially only by follicles up to 8 mm diameter, which correlates with rapidly increasing estrogen levels and selection of the dominant follicle. AMH levels are relatively stable throughout the menstrual cycle. Their significance in fertility is as a measure of ovarian reserve, with levels becoming undetectable approximately five years before the menopause (page 345).

MENSTRUAL CYCLE

The menstrual cycle describes the rhythmic sequence of physiological changes in the ovaries, uterus and cervix under the influence of the female sex hormones. It is essential for the release of mature eggs and to renew the endometrium in preparation for implantation. **The days of the menstrual cycle are numbered from the first day of the period (first day of fresh red bleeding) until the day before the next period starts.** Physiologically, menstruation (breakdown of endometrium) indicates the *end* of the menstrual cycle, but as menstruation is such an obvious event it is always considered the *start* of the cycle.

1 **Hormonal control** The menstrual cycle is controlled by the pituitary hormones FSH and LH. FSH stimulates the growth and development of ovarian follicles and production of estrogen; the LH surge matures the egg, and it triggers ovulation and the production of progesterone by the corpus luteum (collapsed follicle). Estrogen and progesterone influence changes in the endometrium (womb lining), cervix, cervical secretions and waking temperature.

2 **Ovarian activity** Growing follicles produce increasing amounts of estrogen. As estrogen rises, it stimulates a surge in LH which matures the egg and causes the follicle to rupture at ovulation. This phase takes a variable number of days. The egg lives for around 24 hours. After ovulation the collapsed follicle forms the corpus luteum (yellow body), which produces progesterone. It has a fixed lifespan of 10–16 days.

3 **Endometrium** The endometrium (womb lining) is shed during the period. Then, as the follicles grow, the estrogen regenerates the endometrium in preparation for pregnancy. Estrogen also produces wetter secretions to nourish sperm and encourage them to penetrate the cervix. After ovulation, progesterone thickens the cervical secretions to prevent further sperm penetration. Progesterone creates a soft, thick, nourishing endometrium to encourage implantation of a fertilised egg.

4 **Cervix** The cervix changes under the influence of estrogen from low, firm, closed and tilted to high, soft, open and straight when a woman is fertile. After ovulation, under the influence of progesterone, the cervix reverts to its infertile state of low, firm, closed and tilted. The change from infertile to its most fertile state takes about a week, whereas the change back to the infertile state takes place within 24 hours.

5 **Cervical secretions** At first the secretions feel moist and appear white or cloudy. As estrogen levels rise, they become thinner, wetter, more transparent and stretchy – this is the most fertile time. After ovulation the secretions change back to sticky and then dry again. Any secretions indicate fertility.

6 **Fertile time** Sperm can fertilise a woman's egg up to seven days after intercourse when cervical secretions are present. Allowing for the lifespan of the egg, the fertile time lasts around nine days.

7 **Infertility and relative infertility** The days before the fertile time starts are only *relatively* infertile as ovulation may occur earlier, or sperm may survive longer than anticipated. The days after the fertile time ends are considered *infertile* and the most effective in avoiding pregnancy.

8 ***Recording the indicators of fertility*** The days of the menstrual cycle are numbered from the first day of one period to the day before the next period starts. Days of the period are marked by shading in the appropriate box, followed by dry days, then days of moist, white, sticky secretions and then the wetter, transparent, slippery stretchy secretions. The last day of wetness is peak day (vertical shading to correlate secretions with temperature) – this is the closest time to the presumed ovulation. The secretions then change back abruptly to sticky white, or dryness until the next period starts. Progesterone causes the waking temperature to rise by about 0.2 deg.C after ovulation and then stay at the higher level until the next period. The fertile time (shown by the white block and the arrow) starts at the first sign of secretions and ends after the third high temperature past peak day. Additional calculations can be used to increase the effectiveness of FAMs for avoiding pregnancy.

Figure 3.9 The menstrual cycle and indicators of fertility (© Pyper & Knight, FertilityUK 2016)

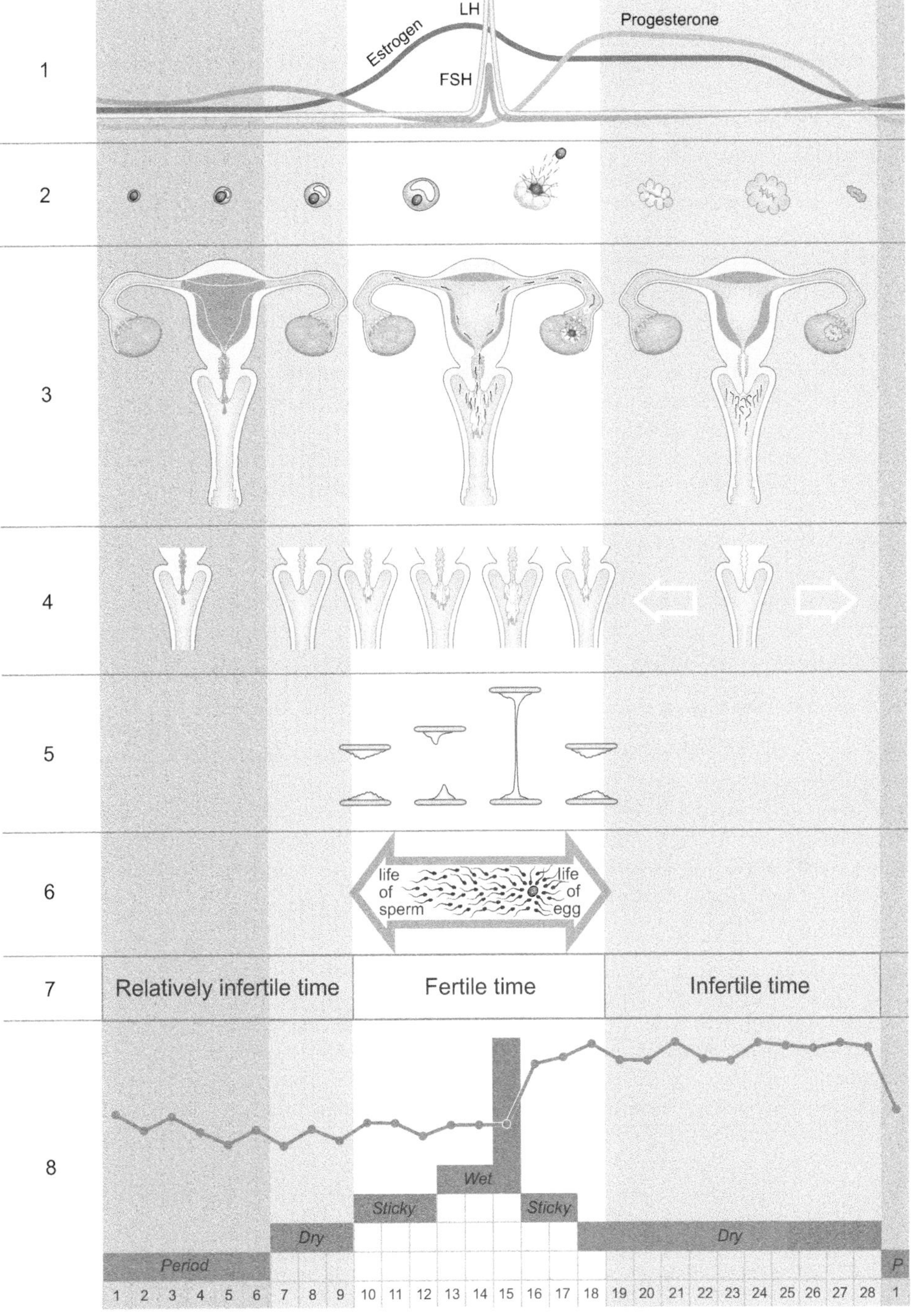

Figure 3.9 (Continued)

Key events in the menstrual cycle

The cycle of ovarian changes starts in the late luteal phase about three days before the start of menstruation. A small rise in FSH initiates the recruitment of a cohort of up to 20 antral follicles, one of which is destined to ovulate during the next menstrual cycle.

In the follicular phase, FSH stimulates increased growth and development of the follicles which in turn produce estradiol. The dominant follicle is selected around day 7 and its granulosa cells produce increasing amounts of estradiol (and inhibin B), which suppresses FSH production and causes the other follicles to degenerate. When estradiol levels reach a critical level for sufficient time, it initiates a surge in LH which matures the egg and triggers ovulation. A smaller FSH peak accompanies the LH surge. Following ovulation, the corpus luteum produces progesterone, which is maximal about seven days after the LH surge. Progesterone (and inhibin) levels fall in the last few days of the cycle, leading to feedback to the brain to initiate the next ovulatory cycle and the degeneration of the endometrium (the start of menstruation). [73]

Figure 3.9 shows the hormonal control of the cycle, the changes in the endometrium, cervix and cervical secretions, and the identification of the fertile time based on the observed indicators. These images were developed by Dr Cecilia Pyper, Jane Knight and FertilityUK in collaboration with IRH. They have been extensively consumer-tested and work well for teaching purposes.

Length and variation of the menstrual cycle

The concept of the 28-day menstrual cycle is still prevalent in both scientific and popular literature, yet it is well-documented that cycle length varies between women and throughout reproductive life. A wide variation in cycle length is normal.

Variability in the follicular and luteal phases

The main variability in the menstrual cycle is related to the follicular phase (pre-ovulation), which averages 13–15 days but shows wide variation due to the variable time for follicular selection and growth. **The luteal phase (post-ovulation) is constant at 10–16 days** due to the fixed lifespan of the corpus luteum. [96] Baird looked at the variability in the menstrual cycle using estrogen and progesterone metabolites on daily urine samples from more than 200 healthy women (mostly aged 25–35). The follicular phases ranged from 9 to 55 days; the luteal phases ranged from 6 to 18 days with more than 70% lasting 12–15 days. [20] [626]

Luteal phase and its adequacy

The luteal phase represents an undisturbed and competent follicular maturation process and is vital for successful implantation. The endometrium is most receptive 8–10 days after ovulation, [627] so the luteal phase needs to be at least 10 days long for the blastocyst to successfully implant. **If the luteal phase is less than 10 days, there is insufficient time for implantation and the cycle will be infertile.** The length of the luteal phase (and hence the fertility potential of the cycle) can only be determined retrospectively based on the timing of the next period. Cycles with short or inadequate luteal phases are more likely at the extremes of reproductive life (see figure 4.14 in chapter 4) and at times of stress (page 346).

Lenton used the LH surge as a marker of ovulation in 327 apparently ovulatory menstrual cycles. The majority showed a normal luteal phase of 14 days, but 5% had abnormally short luteal phases. Lenton estimated that all cycles with a luteal phase of less than or equal to 9 days were abnormal. Some cycles with luteal phases of 10, 11 and 12 days were also considered abnormal. [352] This confirmed the findings of Döring, who used temperature as a marker for ovulation and noted that cycles with fewer than 10 raised temperatures were generally infertile. [133]

Many women who are trying to conceive express concerns about short luteal phases and/or premenstrual spotting. These issues are controversial but could indicate prematurely declining progesterone levels or endometriosis (pages 207 and 346).

Studies on menstrual cycle length

Studies on menstrual cycle length show similar results with *average* (mean) cycle lengths around 27.7 days ± 3 days. [96] The word *average* in statistics is a loose term as studies report in different ways. The average generally refers to the mean value. The *mean* is the number found by adding up all the values, then dividing it by the sum of the total number of values; the *median* is the middle value of a list of numbers and the *mode* is the value that occurs most often.

The need to understand the variability in cycle length was heightened by the development of the Calendar/Rhythm Method in the 1930s. Ogino suggested that the method should not be used by women with a cycle variation of more than *10* days. Tietze later suggested that this should be reduced to *eight* days. [579] A number of large studies were initiated in the 1930s and 1940s (the heyday of the Calendar/Rhythm Method) to ascertain the range of normal variability in cycle length. Some studies such as the Tremin Trust, set up by Treloar at the University of Minnesota, have spanned decades and are ongoing. A recent analysis of a subset of Treloar's data concluded that variable menstrual cycle histories are most common. Gorrindo and colleagues (amongst others) suggested the need for a redefinition of normal and abnormal cycles. [236] Some of the studies on cycle length are summarised in table 3.2.

The records collected by Latz from 2,000 women using the Calendar/Rhythm Method in the mid-1930s clearly demonstrate cycle length variability. All women showed variation. The most common variation was four days, shown by 25% of women, with 1% of women showing a variation of 10 days or more (figure 3.10). [347]

Table 3.2 Variation in cycle length: results of large studies spanning decades

Study	*Key findings on cycle length variation*
Latz (Chicago) 2,000 women, 24,908 cycles Calendar/Rhythm Method [347]	– All women showed variation in cycle length. – One in four showed a four-day variation (the most common). – One in five showed a five-day variation.
Matsumoto (Japan) 701 women (ages 13–52), 18,213 cycles [392]	– The most common length was 28 days, but this occurred in 12% of cycles. – The majority of cycles were longer than 28 days (median of 29 days and mean of 30 days). *Note:* Vollman commented on the imbalance in the age groups.
Treloar (University of Minnesota) 2,702 women, 275,947 cycles 30-year study [583] This research is ongoing through the Tremin Research Programme, Pennsylvania State University.	– Mean cycle length was 28.6 days. – The first few years after menarche and last few years before menopause show the most cycle variation (long and short cycles). – Median cycle length gradually shortened from 29 to 27 days in women aged 20–40 years.
Chiazze (US and Canada) 2,316 women (age 15–44) 30,655 cycles [84]	– The most common cycle length was 27 days (12% of cycles). – Adolescent cycles are highly variable. – Variability decreases steadily until the minimum at 35–39 years.
Vollman (Switzerland) 691 women, 31,645 cycles Cycle length and temperature Used "gynaecological" age 40-year study [601]	– The most common cycle length was 28 days, but only about 12% cycles were 28 days. – The first few years after menarche and last few years before menopause are the most variable. – Cycle length changes with age through reproductive life, forming a U-shaped curve (conforming closely with Treloar).

(Continued)

Table 3.2 (Continued)

Study	*Key findings on cycle length variation*
WHO (multi-centre) 725 women, 7514 cycles [616]	– The mean cycle length was 28.6 days. – Ninety-six percent of cycles were in the range of 23–35 days. *Note:* the SDM was based on this dataset. (Fertile time = days 8–19, provided cycles are 26–32 days.)
Colombo and Marshall (London) 2,355 sets of temperature charts (at least 13 consecutive cycles) [99]	– Twenty-three percent of women had cycle variation of more than 10 days. – Forty-two percent of women had a variation of more than seven days. – Only one in four women had six consecutive menstrual cycles within a six-day range.
Meunster (Denmark) 3,743 women epidemiological (postal survey) [420]	– Two out of three women showed more than a five-day variation in cycle length over the course of a year.
Gorrindo (Washington, DC) 628 women (15–45 years) Analysis of sub-set of Treloar data [236]	– Five categories (types) of menstrual history were defined: 1 Very stable 2 Stable but great variability in cycle length 3 Oscillating. Erratic cycle lengths. Downward trend. 4 Oscillating. Erratic cycles. No downward trend. 5 Highly erratic and variable histories – Only 28% women had stable histories (types 1 and 2). – Seventy-two percent of women had erratic histories (types 3–5).

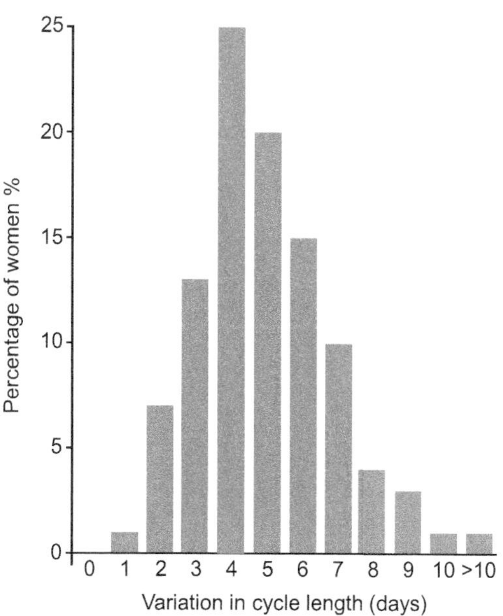

Figure 3.10 Variability in menstrual cycle length (2,000 women, 24,908 cycles), Latz Foundation (adapted from Murphy 1959 [418]; first published in *JAMA*, 1935, Vol. 105 [236])

Table 3.3 Suggested normal limits for menstrual parameters in the mid-reproductive years (adapted from Munro 2012 [417]; FIGO system for abnormal uterine bleeding, *Am. J. Obstet. Gynecol.* 2012)

Dimensions of menstruation and menstrual cycle	*Descriptive term*	*Normal limits (5th–95th percentiles)*
Frequency of menstruation	Frequent	< 24 days
	Normal	24–38 days
	Infrequent	> 38 days
Regularity of menstruation	Absent	No bleeding
(Cycle-to-cycle variation over 1 year)	Regular	Variation 2–20 days
	Irregular	Variation > 20 days
Duration of menstrual flow	Prolonged	> 8 days
	Normal	4.5–8 days
	Shortened	< 4.5 days
Volume of menstrual flow	Heavy	> 80 ml
	Normal	5–80 ml
	Light	< 5 ml

Matsumoto tried to establish normal cycle length in Japanese women. He assumed 25–38 days was the "normal range" and declared cycles shorter than 25 days as polymenorrhoea (frequent menstruation) and cycles longer than 38 days as oligomenorrhoea (infrequent menstruation). [392] This definition almost fits with the recommendations by the International Federation of Gynecology and Obstetrics (FIGO) for normal limits for menstrual parameters (normal menstrual frequency: 24–38 days; see table 3.3).

Treloar reported on the cycle lengths of more than 2,700 women (mostly university students) from the mid-1930s to 1960s. He noted that women used the terms "regular" or "28 days" to indicate their belief that their cycles were normal, but variation was the rule. He showed how each woman had her own central trend in cycle length, which varied with age: the first few years after menarche, similarly the last few years before menopause, showed a pattern of mixed long and short cycles, but variations in cycle length were still common during the relatively stable mid-reproductive years. [583] Figure 3.11 shows the gradual shortening of cycles at the time when women have their most stable cycles (20–40 years). Fifty percent of women have cycle lengths with minimal variation over reproductive life (grey shaded area). Some women show much greater variation with cycle length forming a U-shaped curve. The contours show all recorded menstrual cycles, including abnormal cycles with medical conditions and interventions.

Vollman collected information on cycle length and temperature for nearly 40 years. [601] In this vast dataset the 28-day cycle was the commonest length, but **only about 12% of cycles were 28 days.** He found that **cycles of 25–32 days were more likely to show a biphasic temperature** (presumed ovulatory) whereas very short or very long cycles were more likely to be monophasic possibly indicating anovulation. Vollman used the concept of "gynaecological age" based on the time from menarche (rather than chronological age), which meant that his data was physiologically comparable.

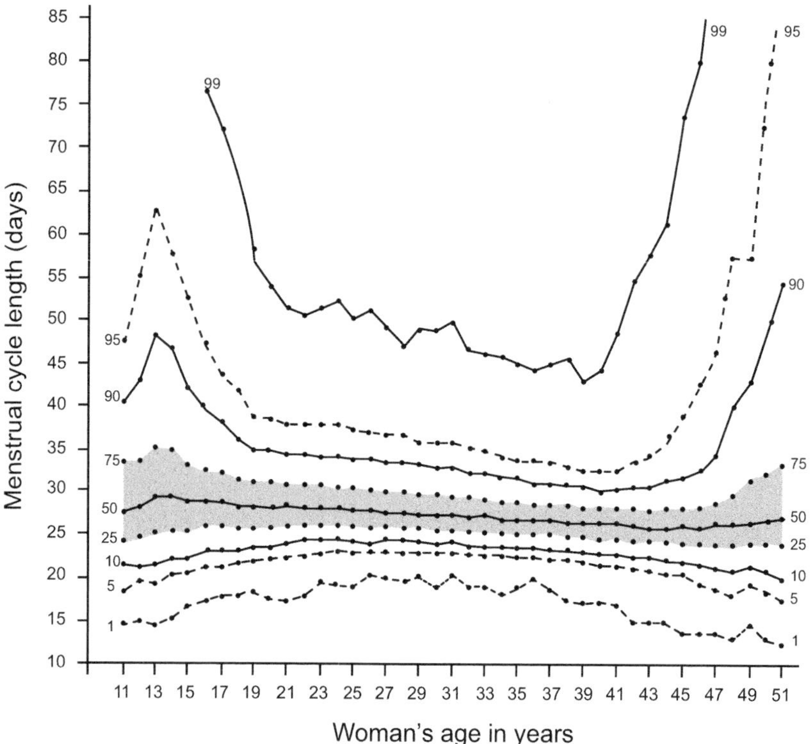

Figure 3.11 Variability in menstrual cycle length by age (2,702 women, 275,947 cycles) (adapted from Treloar 1967 [583])

Gynaecological age and its impact on cycle length Vollman's findings demonstrated that:

- Fifty-five percent of girls had their first period at 13–14 years (range 9–21 years).
- There were similarities in menarche between mothers and daughters, and between sisters.
- Cycle length was most variable in the first few years after menarche and in the years preceding the menopause.
- Cycle length changes with age forming a U-shaped curve from menarche to menopause (similar to the Treloar data).
- Mean cycle length decreases steeply from 35 days to 30 days between gynaecological ages 0–4 years. It then descends slowly reaching a minimum of 27.2 days at gynaecological age 29 (around age 43) then increases to 44 days at gynaecological age 40 years (around age 53).
- The average length of the follicular phase declines with age as cycles shorten, while the luteal phase remains relatively constant.
- The average length of the luteal phase is around nine days for the first five years after the menarche. It then begins to lengthen, averaging 12 days through reproductive maturity.

Marshall's database of charts included cycle length and temperature (with some women recording cervical secretions). The charts, collected through Marshall's correspondence service in London, were analysed by Colombo in Padua. **Only 25% of women had six consecutive cycles within a six-day range.** [99]

Classification of menstrual terms

There has been major international discussion about a new classification system for menstrual terms. In 2010, FIGO formally accepted the new classification. Bleeding that can be considered a "period" is described according to the following parameters: frequency of onset (in days, over an interval of a year), regularity of onset (in days), duration of menstrual flow (in days) and heaviness of flow (volume in ml). Table 3.3 shows the suggested normal limits for the different menstrual parameters for women in their mid-reproductive years. **The normal limits for frequency of menstruation (cycle length) are 24–38 days.**

FIGO suggests that terms with Greek or Latin roots, such as "menorrhagia" (heavy bleeding), "polymenorrhoea" (frequent bleeding), and "oligomenorrhoea" (infrequent bleeding) should be abandoned and replaced with simple descriptive terms that are easily understood by women and can be used in clinical practice or for collaboration on international research. The recommendation is that the four parameters of the menstrual assessment require explicit exploration in a structured clinical history and that simple key words should be used to describe the most important features (for example, "heavy, irregular menstrual bleeding"). Any additional abnormality should be specified (for example, change in the menstrual pattern, inter-menstrual bleeding, premenstrual spotting). [191] *Note:* The current FIGO definition of irregular bleeding (> 20 days) is taken from population studies which include women of varying ages with no known disease or hormonal therapy. This undoubtedly includes women with ovulatory disorders but with no formal diagnosis of PCOS. This definition is being re-evaluated.

Implications of cycle length variations

Variations in cycle length have significant implications for women using FAMs to avoid pregnancy. It is vital that any calculations made on past cycle length are not based on a woman's *perception* of her cycle length, but on clearly documented records of her last 12 cycles. Couples who use combined-indicator methods to avoid pregnancy can use different calculations to identify the start of the fertile time (page 77).

FERTILITY CYCLE

The menstrual cycle focuses around menstruation as the key event during the cycle; but for the purposes of FA it is more appropriate to place the emphasis on *fertility,* so the term "fertility cycle" is preferred, with the focus on identifying the limits of the fertile time. It is more practical to divide the cycle into three phases rather than the customary pre-and post-ovulation phases, hence:

- the **early *relatively* infertile time;**
- the **fertile time** (when intercourse can result in pregnancy); and
- the **late infertile time.**

Figure 3.12 shows a fertility cycle of about 28 days. The early *relatively* infertile time (pre-ovulatory) includes the period and a few days after the period. **The fertile time starts at the earliest opportunity that sperm could survive in the female genital tract.** After ovulation, time is allowed for the fertilisable lifespan of the egg and the possibility of a second ovulation (within 24 hours). **The fertile time ends when the egg is no longer fertilisable.** After the fertile time ends the rest of the cycle will be completely infertile – the late infertile time (post-ovulatory).

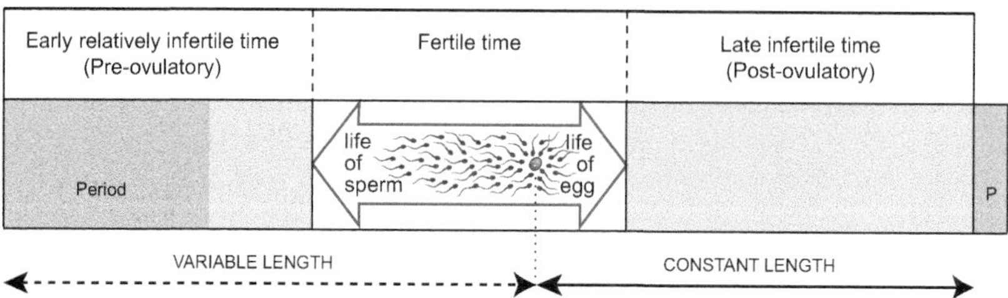

Figure 3.12 The fertility cycle (the arrow demonstrates the life of sperm and egg) (© Pyper & Knight, FertilityUK 2016)

Early *relatively* infertile time

The early infertile time varies most. It is only ever *relatively* infertile due to the possibility of early ovulation/longer sperm survival. Couples who use FAMs to avoid pregnancy need to understand the distinction between *relatively* infertile (pre-ovulation) days and *infertile* (post-ovulation) days and consider whether they are willing to accept the risk associated with unprotected intercourse in the early part of the cycle.

The most accurate prediction of the start of the fertile time is made by using a combination of the changes in cervical secretions and a calendar calculation (with optional cervical changes). OPKs identify only the short-lived LH surge and are of no value in identifying the *start* of the fertile time. A fertility monitor which combines urinary estrogen and LH gives more advance warning of the fertile time, but is not as effective as combined indicators. Figure 7.1 (in chapter 7) describes the correlation of indicators to identify the first fertile day and increase the effectiveness of the early infertile time.

Fertile time

Intercourse can result in pregnancy only on a limited number of days in each cycle.

- The **fertile time starts** as soon as there is a possibility of sperm survival, which is shown by the first sign of cervical secretions, the first change in cervix or the first fertile day by calculation – whichever comes *first*.
- The **fertile time ends** when the egg is no longer fertilisable, which is confirmed by the progestogenic nature of cervical secretions and a significant and sustained rise in waking temperature.

Physiologically, the fertile time only lasts six days – the day of ovulation and the preceding five days [631] (page 81) – but precise limits of the fertile time are not easy to define without the use of direct hormone markers. The fertile time perceived by the woman depends on the method used to identify its limits, but is around 10 days.

Length of the fertile time

The length of the fertile time has implications for couples planning and avoiding pregnancy. Keulers studied the fertile time in 410 subfertile couples, using ultrasound to determine ovulation and post-coital tests to detect the first normal sperm-mucus interaction day. The length of the fertile time varied considerably in this group, from less than one day to more than five days. **The longer the fertile time, the higher the probability of conception and ongoing pregnancy.** [328]

When women use subjective indicators, the *potential* fertile time is longer than the *actual* physiological fertile time. This is due to the less precise nature of the observed indicators and allows for user error. The fertile time starts at the first change from dryness (first sign of any secretions) and lasts until there are observable progesterone-related changes in cervical secretions which correlate with a rise in temperature. An additional calendar calculation may be used to identify the start of the fertile time. In a large European prospective study of new FAM users, the **average length of the fertile time was 13 days.** This was less after the first year as more personalised cycle information became available. [189]

Variations in the fertile time in relation to cycle length

The relative position of the fertile time varies dependent on the length of the cycle and specifically the timing of ovulation. The time from ovulation to the *next* period (post-ovulatory) is constant. The time from the period to ovulation (pre-ovulatory) constitutes the most variable length of the cycle. The fertile time starts earlier in a short cycle and later in a longer cycle.

Figure 3.13 shows a short cycle (22 days), an average cycle (29 days) and a long cycle (36 days). In all cycles the interval from ovulation to the next period remains constant at around 14 days, but the time before ovulation is varied. The fertile time arrow covers 10 days – seven days before ovulation for sperm survival and three days after ovulation to ensure the egg is no longer fertilisable.

- Short cycle: ovulation occurs around day 8, fertile secretions could be present during the period and bleeding would mask their appearance. There are no early *relatively* infertile days and intercourse during a period could result in pregnancy.
- Average length cycle: ovulation occurs around day 15 and there would be a few early *relatively* infertile days.
- Long cycle: ovulation does not occur until around day 22, so there are potentially many early *relatively* infertile days.

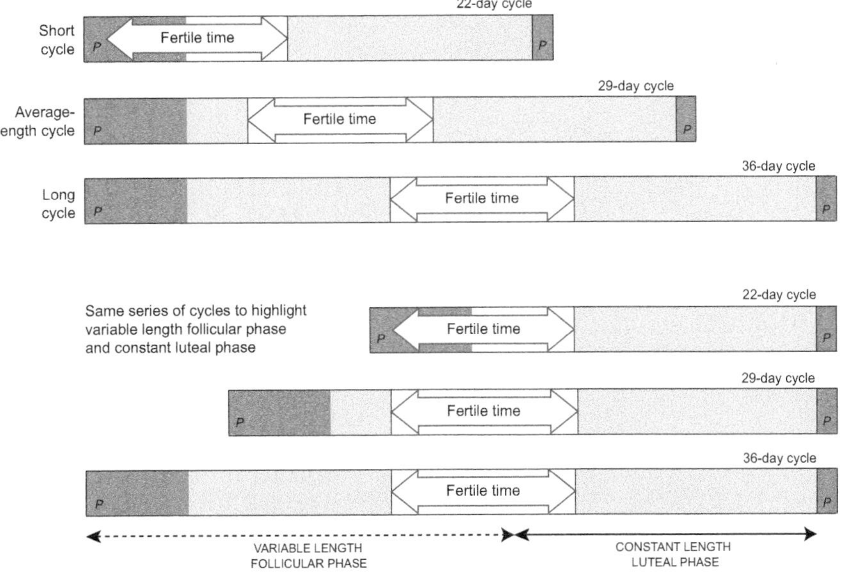

Figure 3.13 Variations in the fertile time in relation to cycle length (© Pyper and Knight, FertilityUK 2016)

The days during and just after a period are notorious for unintended pregnancies because women mistakenly believe they are "safe". **All women need accurate information about cycle length variability and the risk of pregnancy from intercourse during a period.**

Figure 3.13 shows why the term "day 21 progesterone test" should be abandoned. A progesterone assay to confirm ovulation needs to be taken approximately one week after ovulation when progesterone has reached its plateau. For example, a correctly timed *mid-luteal phase* progesterone would be taken about day 29 in the 36-day cycle. A prospective indicator such as cervical secretions helps to optimise the timing of these tests (page 344). In the second series of images in figure 3.13, the same three cycles are positioned so that the start of the next period correlates. This clearly shows the difference between the constant-length luteal phases and the variable-length follicular phases.

Late infertile time (post-ovulatory)

The late infertile time has a constant number of days due to the relatively fixed lifespan of the corpus luteum. The end of the fertile time is confirmed by a combination of indicators (temperature and secretions with optional cervical changes). Couples who are avoiding pregnancy generally have about **10 days in the late infertile time when they can have unrestricted intercourse with a high level of effectiveness.** [189]

PROBABILITY OF CONCEPTION

The day-specific probability of conception is defined as the probability that intercourse on a particular day relative to ovulation will result in pregnancy. This describes the *fecundability* of a couple. A number of factors affect fecundability: the timing of intercourse relative to ovulation, viability of the egg(s) and survival of sperm (which depends on the presence and quality of secretions). Age and lifestyle also play a part.

The earliest marker of pregnancy is hCG, which is produced by the implanting blastocyst about 6–12 days post-fertilisation. [627] It is not possible to identify the time of fertilisation precisely, but it occurs within hours of ovulation, so ovulation is used as a surrogate measure for the timing of conception. Fecundability studies have used a number of different markers for ovulation, some more precise than others.

Barrett and Marshall Study

The first study on the probability of conception was by Barrett and Marshall in the UK in the 1960s: 241 couples of proven fertility were recruited when seeking advice about NFP. The women (aged 20–50 years with 90% aged 20–39) kept daily temperature records. The *3 over 6 rule* confirmed the temperature rise and the day before the rise was assigned the day of ovulation. [34] The usable data consisted of 2,192 cycles with 103 pregnancies. All conceptions occurred during the fertile time extending from five days before to one day after the temperature rise (figure 3.14). The risk of conception approximated to zero, six days before and two days after the rise. However, a report on an additional 14 conception cycles suggested that conception can result from intercourse as early as the ninth day before ovulation and up to the fourth day after (by temperature rise). This seminal study confirmed the need to wait for three high temperatures to avoid pregnancy. It demonstrated that **the late infertile time is the most effective for avoiding pregnancy, but the time before ovulation is unpredictable and is only *relatively* infertile.** In this study daily intercourse resulted in a 68% probability of conception, which was reduced to 14% with weekly intercourse. This is important information for couples planning pregnancy (page 311).

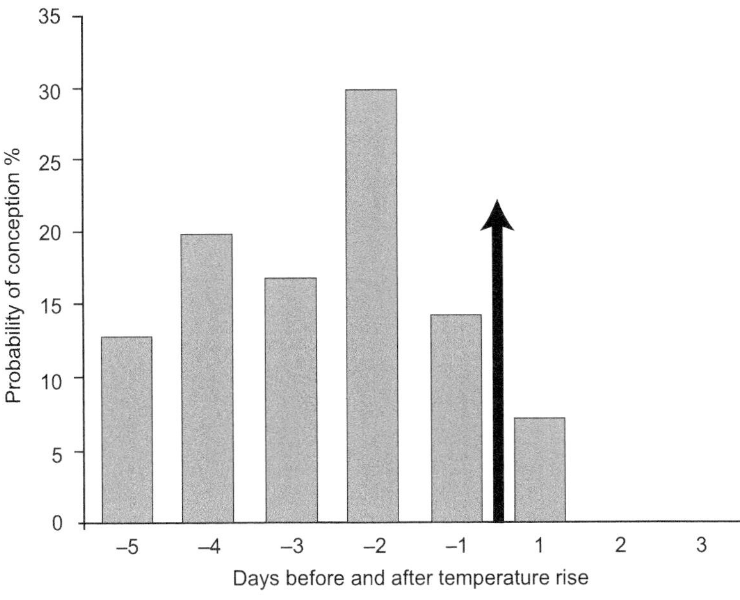

Figure 3.14 The risk of conception relative to temperature rise (adapted from Barrett and Marshall 1969 [34])

North Carolina Early Pregnancy Study

The North Carolina Early Pregnancy Study [631] recruited 221 healthy women at the time they discontinued contraception with the intention of planning pregnancy. The women were aged 21–42 years with 80% aged 26–35. The day of ovulation was estimated by measuring estrogen and progesterone metabolites in urine, the ratio of which decreases abruptly with luteinisation of the follicle. This changing ratio correlates closely with the LH peak and ovulation. [20]

Wilcox identified a **six-day fertile window starting five days before ovulation and ending on the day of ovulation.** Figure 3.15 shows the daily probabilities of conception. The solid line shows probabilities based on all 625 cycles and the bars represent probabilities calculated from data on 129 cycles in which intercourse was reported to have occurred on only a single day during the six-day interval. The probability of conception drops rapidly after ovulation due to the short lifespan of the egg, with the longer time approaching ovulation showing the ability of sperm to retain their fertilising capacity. Note that **the highest probability of conception is from intercourse one to two days preceding ovulation,** not on the actual day of ovulation – sperm need time for capacitation in the female genital tract and to arrive in the tubes in advance of ovulation.

The chances of a healthy ongoing pregnancy were higher in the days immediately preceding ovulation. The clinical pregnancy rate increased from around 4% five days before ovulation to 29% two days before and 27% one day before ovulation, dropping to 8% from intercourse on the day of ovulation. [632]

Dunson compared the North Carolina data with the Barrett and Marshall data using a statistical model to correct for errors in estimating the day of ovulation. He suggested that estimates based on basal body temperature (BBT) are not perfect but have a high probability of being ± one day of the true ovulation day. After controlling for errors, he estimated the same six-day fertile window in both studies. He also estimated that the highest probability of conception resulting in clinical pregnancy occurs on the day before ovulation. [140]

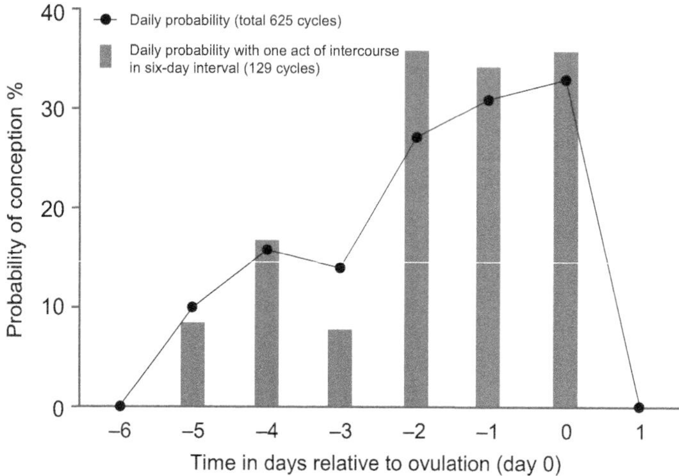

Figure 3.15 Probability of conception in relation to ovulation using hormonal assays (adapted from Wilcox 1995 [631])

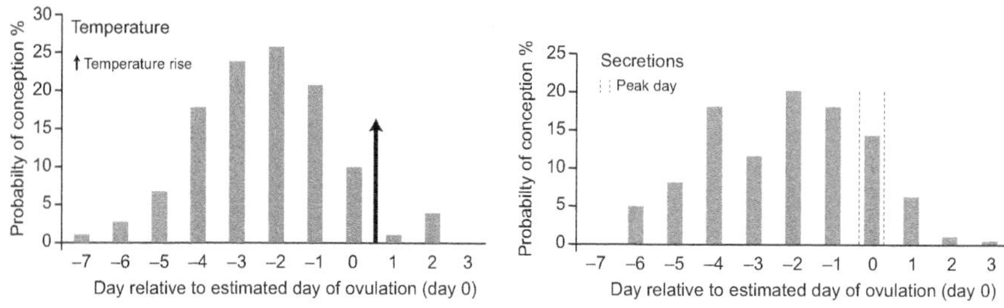

Figure 3.16 Probability of conception in relation to ovulation using temperature and cervical secretions (adapted from: Colombo 2000 [101])

European multi-centre (fecundability) study

A large multi-centre study recruited 782 couples from seven European centres providing FAMs: Milan, Verona, Lugano, Dusseldorf, Paris, London and Brussels. [101] Women were aged 18–40 years, healthy (with no known fertility problems) and in committed relationships. Women kept daily records of temperature, secretions, bleeding, disturbed sleep and intercourse. The study incorporated two surrogate markers for ovulation: temperature (last day before the rise) and peak day (last day showing the most fertile secretions). The study protocol was in line with the Barrett and Marshall study and used the *3 over 6 rule* to establish the temperature rise. Data from 99 women from a prospective study in Auckland [185] of couples trying to pre-select the sex of their child were subsequently added to increase the sample size.

A total of 7,017 cycles were available for analysis (881 women). Eighty percent of the women recorded both temperature and secretions. The day-specific probabilities of conception presented in figure 3.16 show daily estimates of conception probabilities in cycles with one or more acts of intercourse. These results (analysed using the Schwartz model) [532] show similar results to others. Further analysis of this data using a different statistical model demonstrated that **the quality of cervical secretions was a stronger predictor of conception than the day relative to ovulation** (page 139). [49] The main weakness of the study was its reliance on subjective indicators as surrogate markers for ovulation, but although there will be variation between observed indicators and more objective markers, the data has significant practical importance for the application of FAMs.

Practical application

The European multi-centre study was able to provide clear guidance which is applicable in everyday practice:

- Couples planning pregnancy should maximise intercourse frequency in the four days preceding peak day (and temperature rise).
- The highest chance of conception is two days before peak (20% chance) and two days before the temperature rise (26%).
- Couples who use FAMs to avoid pregnancy need to recognise that the fertile time could extend up to 11–12 days.
- There is still a risk of conception up to six days before peak and up to eight days preceding the temperature rise.

This clearly demonstrates the need for additional markers to identify the start of the fertile time – hence the use of calculations based on personal cycle length and other cycle characteristics (discussed on page 155).

Current state of knowledge on probability of pregnancy

A review of day-specific probabilities of pregnancy [368] described the application of different statistical models and the implications for epidemiological research (table 3.4). The findings show conceptions occurring from seven days before to four days after ovulation – the wide variation being related to the subjective nature of the indicators.

Table 3.4 Summary of studies on the probability of conception using different markers for ovulation [368]

Potential days when intercourse can result in conception	*Ovulation marker*	*Study*
From: 5 days before ovulation To: the day of ovulation	Direct hormone assessment: estrogen/progesterone ratio with or without LH	Wilcox 1995 [631] Dunson 2001a [142]
From: 4–7 days before ovulation To: 1–4 days after ovulation	Waking temperature	Barrett 1969 [34] Schwartz 1980 [532] Royston 1982 [518] Colombo 2000 [101]
From: 5–7 days before ovulation To: 3–4 days after ovulation	Peak day (cervical secretions)	Colombo 2000 [101] Stanford 2002 [563] Stanford 2003 [561]

FERTILITY THROUGH REPRODUCTIVE LIFE

A woman is at risk of pregnancy throughout her fertile life (menarche to menopause). During this time period (around 40 years) she is likely to experience 400–500 menstrual cycles, some of which will be normal fertile cycles while others will be infertile as a result of anovulation or luteal phase deficiency (LPD). An understanding of these normal physiological changes helps to reassure a woman that her symptoms are normal or alert her to warning signs indicating the need for medical advice.

From puberty to reproductive maturity

A basic understanding of puberty, normal physiological changes and the time-frame to reproductive maturity is important for health and educational professionals working with young people, whether for specific health advice or for general health education in group settings such as schools (page 359).

Adolescent changes

The vague term *puberty* describes the "growing up" time of adolescence when the reproductive organs mature and secondary sex characteristics appear. The adolescent growth spurt is the first sign of puberty, which begins in girls from about nine years old. Over the next few years, the breasts enlarge, pubic and axillary hair appear, the pelvis broadens, the uterus and vagina undergo further development, and the girl has her first menstruation (menarche) about three years after the start of her growth spurt. Although there is some estrogen activity from body fat and adrenals before the ovaries become active, ovulation frequently does not start until about two years after menarche. It must be assumed that **a girl could be fertile as soon as she starts menstruating, which means she could be potentially fertile about two weeks *prior to* menarche.**

Menarche

Menarche is a highly significant event for girls, but reproductive maturity is not reached until regular ovulatory cycles are established. During the first few cycles, the HPO-axis is immature; this means that estrogen is produced from developing follicles, but the positive feedback required to trigger ovulation starts later. Irregular cycles with variable menstrual flow are common in the first few years after menarche because the endometrium is primed by variable amounts of estrogen but is unopposed by progesterone (gynaecological age: page 76). [556]

Menarche and the body fat connection

In the late 1960s, while researching adolescent growth spurts, Frisch [205] [206] discovered that menarche is closely related to a critical body weight and sexual maturity is more closely linked to body weight than to chronological age. Rapid growth in girls is accompanied by a large increase in stored and easily mobilised energy: **"sex fat"** which is **essential to cope with the energy demands of reproduction**. If a girl diets or exercises intensively during her growth spurt, her menarche and sexual maturity will be delayed. Frisch reported that the average weight at menarche was 47 kg, which was consistent whether girls matured early or late age-wise. Frisch's research on fatness as a trigger for menarche is widely accepted, but has been criticised by Trussell for statistical flaws. [584]

Normal menstrual cycles in young women

The American Academy of Pediatrics guidelines [438] for normal menstrual parameters in young women state the following:

- Median age of menarche: 12.43 years
- Mean cycle length: 32.2 days (in the first gynaecological year)
- Menstrual cycle lengths: typically 21–45 days
- Menstrual flow: less than eight days
- Menstrual product use: three to six pads or tampons per day

Health professionals need to be able to reassure young women (and their parents) about what to expect leading up to reproductive maturity.

Brown's concept of the continuum

Brown and colleagues in Melbourne have studied ovarian activity in women at all stages of reproductive life. They looked at the relationship between ovarian hormone levels and biological responses, including the frequency and degree of vaginal bleeding. Ovarian activity was measured by urinary estrogen and pregnanediol using 24-hour urine specimens. The research included five-year studies of adolescent girls, postnatal and peri-menopausal women. During these reproductive phases, five types of ovarian activity were encountered. Brown suggested that as these cycle types are part of a normal physiological process, they cannot be considered abnormal.

Cycle types: steps of the continuum

Brown described the process of ovarian activity in response to pituitary stimulation as the "continuum", which can be conceptualised as steps or cycles, with each one merging into the next, progressing from 1 to 5 or in reverse sequence:

1 No ovarian activity
2 Anovulatory follicular activity, but raised estrogen (constant or fluctuating levels)
3 Luteinised unruptured follicle (LUF) syndrome
4 Ovulation followed by a deficient or short luteal phase
5 Full ovulatory cycle

The cycle types are numbered purely for ease of reference. Only the full ovulatory cycle (cycle type 5) would be a potentially fertile cycle (with ovulation and a normal length luteal phase) capable of producing a pregnancy. Cycles can move unpredictably from fertile to infertile types and back at any time during reproductive life, stress being a major disruptive factor.

The effect of pituitary hormones on the ovaries can be observed in a fertility clinic setting during ovarian stimulation with gonadotrophins. A sub-optimal dose will not produce a full ovulatory cycle, but may result in other cycle types, confirming that it is the level of gonadotrophin stimulation on the ovary which determines the cycle type.

Start of reproductive life

At the start of reproductive life, Brown found that the time taken to progress from childhood to reproductive maturity was very variable. For one girl in the study, estrogen activity became more significant at age 12 with observable secretions; her first bleed occurred at 13 and her first ovulation at 16. The researchers commented that this pattern is also observable in chimpanzees, which start copulating with oestrus caused by estrogen peaks before menarche, but may not conceive until four years after menarche.

End of reproductive life

Brown's study demonstrated how, at the end of reproductive life, the ovulatory mechanism fails first before follicular activity ceases – the reverse of the sequence at the start of reproductive life. Follicular activity and ovulation can reoccur erratically before it ceases entirely. A woman will often continue to notice signs of estrogen activity in the form of cervical secretions and vaginal bleeds long after ovulation ceases (page 286). [67]

SELF-ASSESSMENT QUESTIONS

Answers are at the end of the chapter.

1 What are the two main functions of the ovaries?
2 Can a woman ovulate twice?
3 What is the fertilisable lifespan of the egg?
4 According to research based on the estrogen:progesterone ratio [631] how many days in a cycle could intercourse result in pregnancy?
5 What is the normal range for cycle length for women in their mid-reproductive years? [416]
6 What is the length of a normal luteal phase?
7 What is conception?

AGE AND DECLINING FERTILITY

The issue of age and fertility is complex. It is included here as it is relevant for both planning and avoiding pregnancy. Knowledge about the impact of age on fertility is patchy and public health messages can be confusing (page 11). This can affect the way some couples view contraception (often taking risks) and the unrealistic expectations of others about their chances of achieving a healthy pregnancy.

Fertility decline in different populations

Female fertility declines with age, although there may be slight variation between different populations. Figure 3.17 shows declining fertility in three populations: Hutterites (very fertile), Swedes (moderately fertile) and Chinese (least fertile). The Hutterites, a North American Protestant sect similar to the Amish, have been studied repeatedly in view of their high levels of natural fertility, [277] but they show a similar age-related decline in fertility. The dotted line on the graph shows the decline in fertility based on 10 studies in different populations not using contraception. [428]

Factors contributing to reduced fertility

A number of factors contribute to reduced fertility in older women:

- Less frequent intercourse
- Irregular cycles, less frequent ovulation, anovulatory cycles and short luteal phases

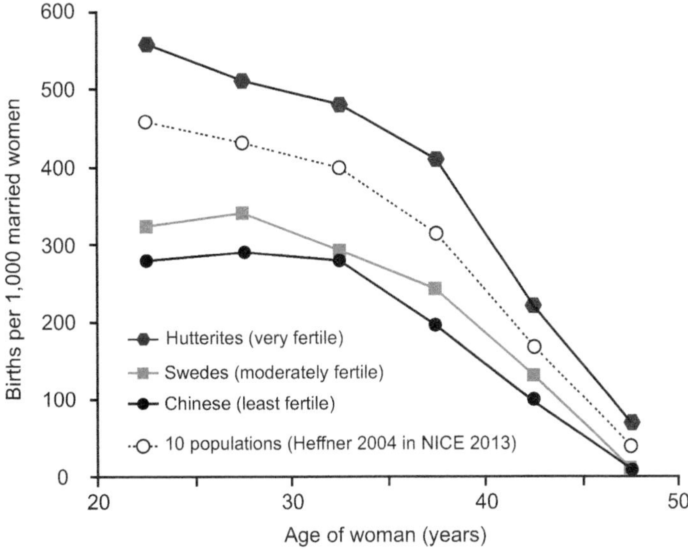

Figure 3.17 Declining fertility in different populations (adapted from Lockwood, G. in McPherson, A 1998)

- Reduced quantity and quality of secretions
- Increased vaginal dryness and use of lubricants which may reduce sperm motility
- Higher incidence of gynaecological problems such as fibroids or endometriosis
- The male partner tends to be older so more likely to have reduced semen quality
- Increased risk of miscarriage due to chromosomal abnormalities with the egg

The "time of uncertainty"

A woman may be permanently infertile for up to 10 years before she reaches her menopause (figure 3.18). The years when a woman continues to bleed, but ovulates only infrequently, cause confusion and uncertainty because women generally assume that having a period means that they must be ovulating (pages 87 and 206). During this ten-year interval, referred to here as "the uncertain years" (shaded area in figure 3.18), some women notice changes in cycle length but others have regular cycles which are anovulatory. Ovulation may occur sporadically but the luteal phase may be deficient. The release of a chromosomally normal egg (or two) will result in a normal pregnancy, but there is a high chance that an egg will be chromosomally abnormal, resulting in miscarriage or congenital abnormalities. Women who do not wish to conceive must use family planning until medically advised otherwise – usually one year post-menopause if over 50 and two years if under 50.

Impact of age on the probability of conception

Colombo's European dataset [101] was analysed to assess the impact of age on the probability of conception, using temperature and secretions as the markers for ovulation.

Woman's age The probability of pregnancy was twice as high for young women (19–26) compared with 35–39-year-olds (figure 3.19). The researchers concluded that a woman's fertility begins to decline in her late 20s, with a substantial decrease by her late 30s. Fertility for men

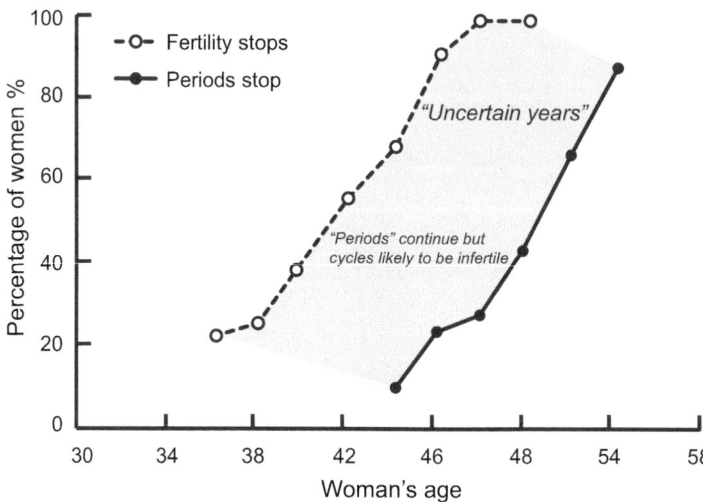

Figure 3.18 Biological infertility starts on average 10 years before menopause in British women (adapted from Lockwood in Mcpherson 1998 [358])

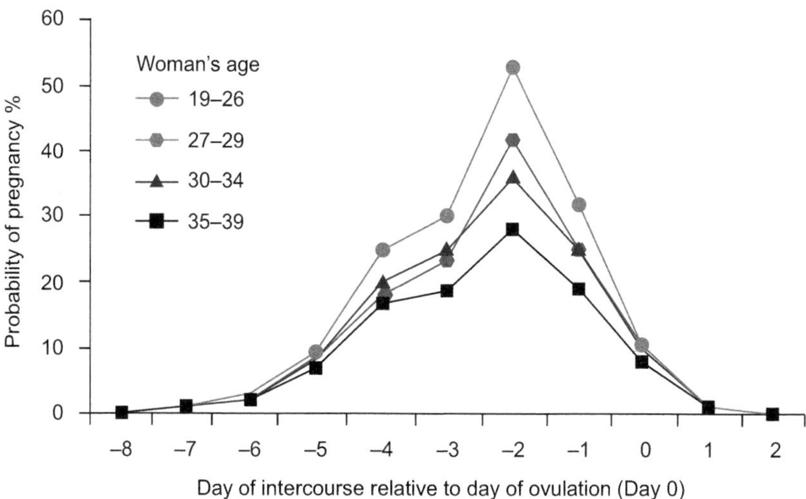

Figure 3.19 Probability of clinical pregnancy following intercourse on a given day relative to ovulation: impact of the woman's age (5,860 menstrual cycles recorded by 782 women aged 18–40 years, with 433 pregnancies; adapted from Dunson 2002) [145]

was less affected by age but showed a significant decline by the late 30s. They found no evidence for a shorter fertile time in older women. [145]

Man's age Figure 3.20 shows the analysis for male age, which was made on the assumption that intercourse occurred at the peak time for conception (two days prior to ovulation). Women aged 19–26 had around a 50% chance of pregnancy per cycle if their partner was the same age. This fell to around 40% for women aged 27–34 and less than 30% for women aged

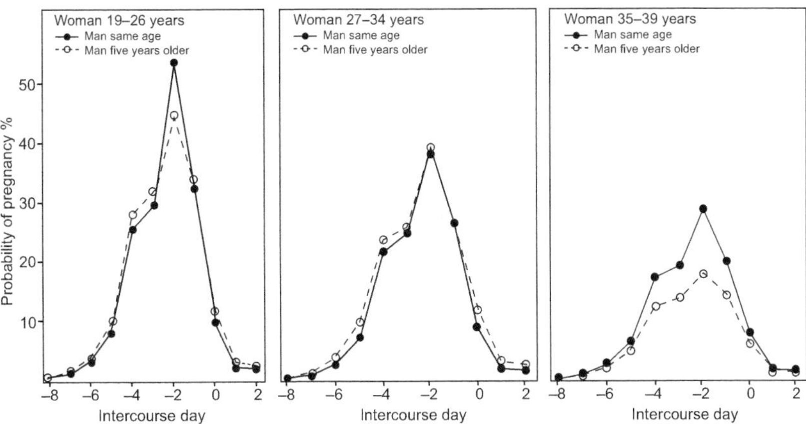

Figure 3.20 Probability of clinical pregnancy following intercourse on a given day relative to ovulation: impact of the man's age (adapted from Dunson 2002) [145]

35–39. There was an additional fall in the older age group to around 20% if the man was five years older. Thus after adjusting for the woman's age, fertility was significantly reduced for men over 35. [145]

Age and time to pregnancy

As fecundability is reduced in older women it follows that the time to pregnancy is increased. A French study on reproductive ageing was able to control for both male and female age, and the level of sexual activity. More than 2,000 nulliparous women with azoospermic partners who were undergoing artificial insemination with frozen donor sperm were divided into age categories: younger than 25 years, 26–30, 31–35 and older than 35. Figure 3.21 shows the cumulative success rate over 12 cycles, demonstrating a slight but significant decrease in fecundability after 30 and marked decrease after 35. [533]

Dunson used Colombo's European dataset [101] to estimate the effects of ageing on time to pregnancy:

- One percent of couples were estimated to be infertile (unable to conceive without assisted reproduction) – this percentage did not change with age.
- The rate of subfertility (inability to conceive within a year of unprotected intercourse) was estimated at 8% for women aged 19–26, 14% for women aged 27–34 and 18% for women aged 35–39 years.
- Male age was an important factor from the late 30s onwards, with the percentage of couples failing to conceive within 12 cycles increasing from an estimated 18% to 28% between 35 and 40 years.
- The estimated percentage of subfertile couples that would conceive after an additional 12 cycles varied from 43% to 63% depending on age.

This study confirmed that the increased rates of subfertility in older couples are attributable primarily to declines in fertility rates rather than to absolute infertility and that many subfertile couples will conceive if they try for an additional year. [143] Note that in the scientific paper Dunson used the terms "sterile" for couples who were unable to conceive without assisted

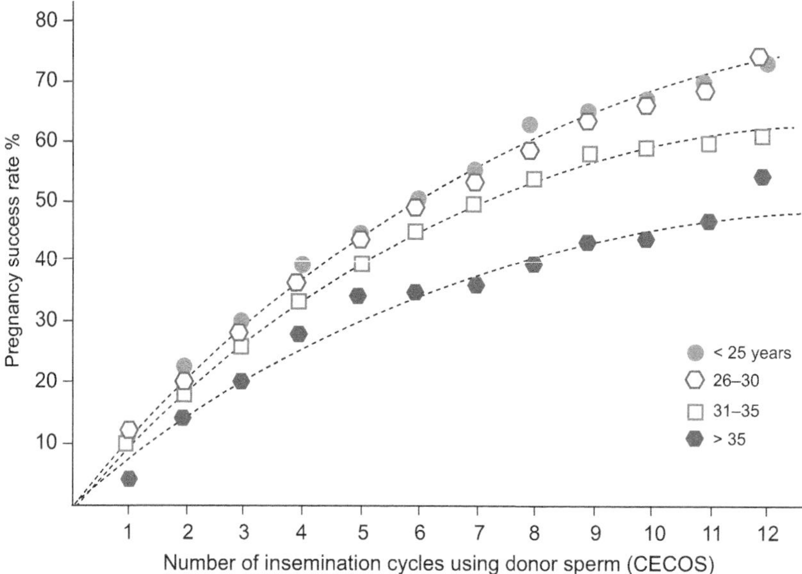

Figure 3.21 Cumulative success rates for 2,193 nulliparous women of different ages (donor insemination) [533]

reproduction and "infertile" for those unable to conceive within a year of unprotected intercourse – the respective terms "infertile" and "subfertile" are preferred.

Realities of reproductive ageing

There are currently no reliable ways to predict a woman's age at menopause or to accurately predict her chances of conceiving. The message is clear: although assisted reproductive techniques are improving, they cannot compensate for delayed conception. [353] [375] [637] Some women may manage to delay childbearing by freezing their eggs, but they need to understand that IVF is required to use frozen-thawed eggs and there are no guarantees of success. Some older women may consider IVF using donated eggs, but others will remain childless by circumstance, not by choice. RCOG urges health professionals to remind young people of the biological realities of reproductive ageing and suggests that sex education in schools should include fertility alongside contraception and STIs (page 359). [493]

INDICATORS OF FERTILITY

There are three different approaches to identifying the fertile time:

- observing the physiological indicators (observed indicators), which includes recording waking temperature and/or monitoring changes in secretions with optional cervical changes;
- using cycle length calculations based on either a fixed formula or derived from personal records of cycle length; and
- using a fertility monitor.

The different indicators of fertility can also be categorised as:

- prospective markers (reflect follicular growth), which identify the start of the fertile time;
- immediate markers (appear when ovulation is imminent), which identify maximum fertility; and
- retrospective markers (evident after follicular rupture), which confirm ovulation and the end of the fertile time. [388]

The following chapters discuss the methodology, use and effectiveness of indicators alone and in combination. This information can be used to plan or avoid pregnancy.

ANSWERS TO SELF-ASSESSMENT QUESTIONS

1 Function of the ovaries:
   a The production of oocytes (female gametes)
   b The synthesis of female sex hormones estrogen and progesterone
2 Yes, a woman can ovulate twice (dizygotic twins). The second ovulation always occurs within 24 hours because the increasing progesterone suppresses a second LH surge.
3 The egg is fertilisable only for about 17 hours. For FAM purposes, allow 24 hours plus another 24 hours for a possible second ovulation: total 48 hours for egg survival.
4 Wilcox identified a six-day fertile window starting five days before ovulation and ending on the day of ovulation.
5 Normal range for cycle length (frequency of menstruation) is 24–38 days. [417]
6 A normal luteal phase lasts 10–16 days.
7 Conception is the process which starts with fertilisation (fusion of egg and spermatozoon) and continues through the early development of the embryo to the implantation of the blastocyst whereby direct communication is established with the mother.

4 TEMPERATURE

First indicator

The first indicator of fertility is the temperature – the temperature taken first thing upon waking, before getting out of bed or doing anything. In the follicular phase, estrogen has a suppressant effect maintaining body temperature at its lower level. After ovulation, the thermogenic action of progesterone (from the corpus luteum) causes an increase in temperature of around 0.2 deg.C, producing a biphasic curve.

If there is no conception, the corpus luteum disintegrates, the progesterone level falls and the temperature drops back to the lower level around the start of the next period.

If conception occurs, the corpus luteum continues to produce progesterone, the endometrium is maintained and the temperature may reach an even higher level (figure 4.1).

Temperature cannot *predict* ovulation or give any indication of the start of the fertile time. The **temperature rise confirms ovulation and determines the *end* of the fertile time**. Temperature forms a key part of combined-indicator methods.

PHYSIOLOGY OF TEMPERATURE

The most commonly accepted average core (internal) temperature is around 37 deg.C (slightly lower for an oral temperature). Temperature is varied throughout the day with the lowest (basal) point around 04:30 am. For practical reasons, most women record their temperature on waking, which is likely to be several hours after the basal level. Daily temperature charting is therefore more correctly referred to as *waking* temperature. An oral waking temperature is usually around 36.5 deg.C rising to around 36.7 deg.C after ovulation (a rise of around 0.2 deg.C).

The rise in temperature is caused by increased progesterone following ovulation. Within six hours of the start of the LH surge, the granulosa cells luteinise and start secreting progesterone, initially into the follicular fluid and later into the ovarian vein. This initial rise in progesterone slightly precedes ovulation, making it first an indicator of imminent ovulation and then a marker of the end of the fertile time. [388] Changes in the progesterone level define the occurrence of ovulation and the adequacy of the corpus luteum. A significant rise in temperature (0.2 deg.C) occurs when the circulating progesterone level reaches 12.75 nmol/l. [410] This can be compared with a normal pre-ovulatory progesterone level lower than 3 nmol/l, a mid-luteal phase level between 16 and 30 nmol/l, which is suggestive of ovulation, and a level higher than 30 nmol/l, which confirms ovulation.

The first high temperature normally occurs one to two days *after* ovulation. Using LH and progesterone, Moghissi determined this interval to be about 1.75 days. [410] A study using ultrasound with LH found the temperature rise occurred on the day of ovulation or up to two days after ovulation in over 80% of cycles (see figure 10.1 in chapter 10). [230]

The exact mechanism for the action of progesterone is unknown. It was thought to be caused by its action on the temperature-regulating mechanism of the hypothalamus, but is now considered to be due to vasoconstriction of peripheral vessels. Reduced capillary blood flow leads to diminished heat loss, hence the rise in core temperature. [194]

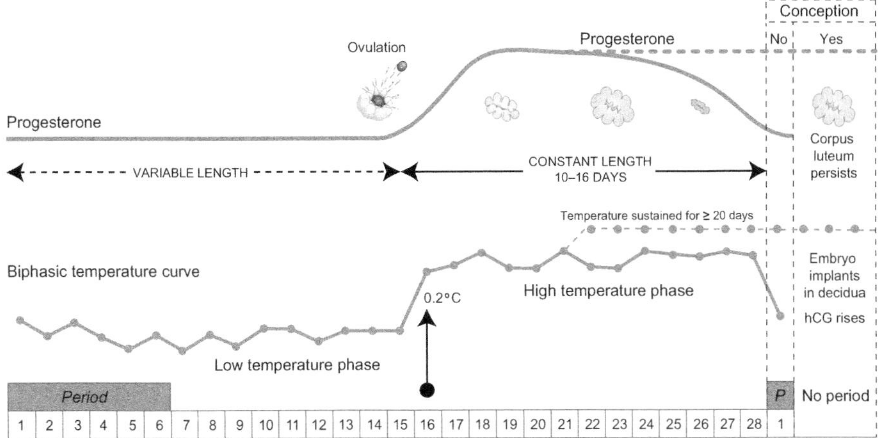

Figure 4.1 Effect of progesterone on waking temperature in conception and non-conception cycles

EQUIPMENT: THERMOMETERS AND CHARTS

The only equipment needed to record an accurate waking temperature is a reliable thermometer, a simple chart, a black and red pen, and a ruler. These are all readily available and inexpensive.

Thermometers

There are two main types of thermometer suitable for fertility purposes: liquid-in-glass and digital. Digital thermometers are generally recommended due to concerns about breakage with glass. Thermometers can be prescribed for FAM purposes.

Liquid-in-glass thermometer

A traditional thermometer is a calibrated sealed glass tube containing a glass capillary with a column of liquid that expands and contracts with temperature change. As the temperature rises the expanding liquid is forced through a constriction in the neck, close to the bulb, and along the capillary tube. When maximum temperature is reached the level of the liquid can be read. As the temperature drops, the liquid column breaks at the constriction so remaining static in the tube. The thermometer can be read and recorded at leisure, provided that it is kept out of direct sunlight and away from direct heat. The liquid must be shaken back down into the bulb prior to its next use.

Basal body thermometers, designed specifically for fertility purposes, have an expanded narrow scale usually ranging from 35.5 to 38.5 deg.C. The narrow range makes it easier to read and detect the subtle changes. Classic clinical thermometers (which range from about 35 to 42 deg.C) are designed to detect extremes of temperature change and are not suitable.

Mercury thermometers were the reference standard and performed well for fertility purposes but mercury was banned for medical use in 2009 due to its toxicity. There may still be some mercury thermometers in circulation but these can no longer be recommended.

Some manufacturers use alcohol with added red or blue dye. Another alternative is Galinstan (a liquid alloy of gallium, indium and tin). The accuracy of Galinstan thermometers for fertility purposes is not known but in a study using axillary temperatures in children, Galinstan compared well to mercury and performed better than digital. [531]

Digital thermometer

Most women use battery-operated digital thermometers because, although they may be more expensive, they are safer than glass and virtually unbreakable. A digital thermometer consists of an electronic probe and a digital display. There are a number of brands available and no research to compare reliability, but Omron, Becton Dickinson, and Boots thermometers appear to give consistent results. The manufacturer's instructions should be followed.

Features:

- On/off button – most also switch off automatically after a few minutes
- Easy-to-read display
- Fast recording time (less than one minute)
- Audible bleep when the temperature has stabilised
- Last memory recall (so that temperature can be recorded when convenient)
- Low-battery warning light

Computerised thermometers

Some devices combine an electronic thermometer with a hand-held computer which uses temperature data in combination with a calculation based on cycle length. This provides information about the start and end of the fertile time, but prospective effectiveness studies are lacking (page 170).

Tympanic membrane thermometers

Many women ask about the use of ear thermometers. Infrared tympanic membrane thermometers have the advantage of ease of use, safety and speed, however, there are concerns about their accuracy. They may work well for identifying fever and are particularly useful for children, but studies show differences of up to 2 deg.C and variations in the measurements in both ears. Ear thermometers have not been tested for fertility purposes but, even with training, they are not considered to be sufficiently reliable. Similarly, liquid crystal (forehead) thermometers are not suitable for fertility purposes as they perform less well than tympanic thermometers. [120] [464] [442]

Fertility awareness chart

Various charts are available for recording waking temperature. Each small box on the chart should be a square, rather than a rectangle, because a "flattened" graph is difficult to read and causes errors. It is common to see women confused by temperature readings simply due to poorly designed charts, but when temperatures are transposed onto a well-designed chart (appendix A) the pattern is apparent.

The FA chart includes space for recording the name, age, chart number (new or experienced user), dates and days of the week, current and past cycle length, target temperature time, temperature route and days of intercourse. Waking temperature is recorded on the centigrade grid. Changes in secretions, cervix (optional) and readings from a fertility monitor (optional) are recorded in the appropriate boxes. Days of intercourse are shown by circling the appropriate day of the cycle. A comments box allows free text to note factors disturbing the readings. The user is encouraged to mark the chart clearly in black ink (figure 4.2).

A blank chart (with instructions for use) is included in appendices A and B. Electronic versions can be downloaded (free) from the FertilityUK website (www.fertilityuk.org). These specially designed combined indicator charts have been tested over many years; they are easy-to-use and highly readable.

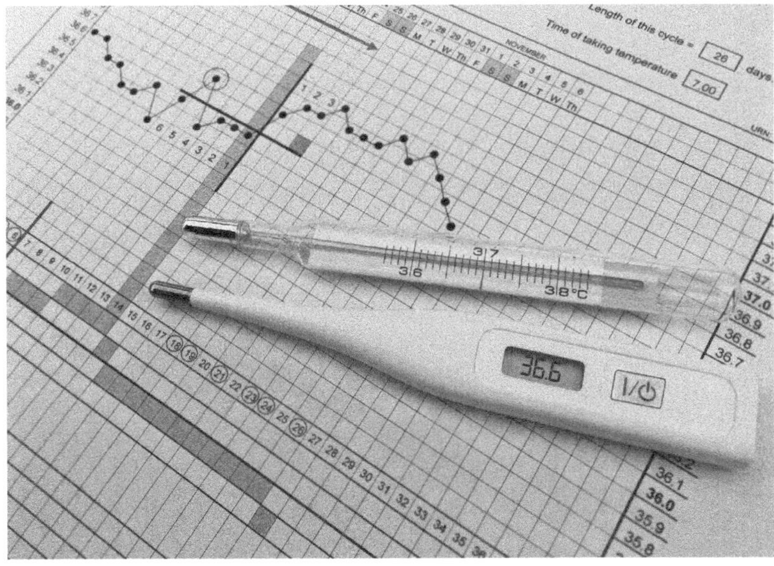

Figure 4.2 Fertility awareness chart with a liquid-in-glass thermometer and a digital thermometer

RECORDING PERIOD AND CYCLE LENGTH

The days of the cycle and menstrual bleeding are recorded as follows:

- Days of the cycle are numbered starting with the first day of the period (day 1).
  - If red bleeding starts at any time during the day before the woman goes to bed, that is considered day 1.
  - If bleeding starts overnight and is first noticed the next morning, then that morning is counted as day 1.
- The days of the period are indicated by shading in the appropriate box.
- The length of the cycle is measured from the first day of one period to the day *before* the next period starts. The cycle length is then recorded in the box at the top of the chart.
- A record of past cycle length is kept to enable an ongoing calculation based on the last 12 cycle lengths.

Common errors in recording cycle length

Two errors are commonly made when calculating cycle length: The first is to count the number of days from the *end* of one period to the *beginning* of the next, so effectively counting only the days when there is no bleeding (hence reporting a short cycle). The second error is to include the first day of the *next* period in the calculation, so adding an extra day. It is important to clarify terms to ensure the accuracy of recordings. The menstrual *period* is the number of days of bleeding. The menstrual *cycle* is the number of days from the first day of one period (fresh red bleed) to the day *before* the next period starts. Any days of spotting should be included in the previous cycle.

RECORDING AND CHARTING WAKING TEMPERATURE

Women require clear instruction in recording and charting an accurate waking temperature under standard conditions. Errors in recording technique, reading the thermometer or charting the readings may result in errors of interpretation and potential user failure.

Temperature route

The temperature can be taken orally, vaginally or rectally. Oral temperatures are the most common and are usually accurate provided they are taken as instructed. Some women prefer to take their temperature vaginally believing it is more discreet (particularly with small children around). Rectal temperatures are now rarely used. An axillary reading is not sufficiently reliable.

Oral Advise the woman to place the temperature probe under her tongue to the right or left of its root, ensuring that it remains in contact with the floor of the mouth. She should keep her lips closed and breathe normally through her nose. [104]

Vaginal Advise the woman to insert the thermometer gently into her vagina for about 4.5 cm. Recommend that she slides a finger alongside the thermometer to ensure its correct positioning. There has been a report of a glass thermometer being inadvertently inserted into the urethra, necessitating surgical removal from the bladder. The surgeon reminded professionals that it is unreasonable to expect lay people to have a detailed knowledge of anatomy and that if internal temperatures are suggested, clear unequivocal instructions must be given. [459] Incorrect positioning should not be possible with a wider digital thermometer.

Rectal Advise the woman to smear the probe with a little lubricant and gently insert it into her rectum for about 2.5 cm. while lying on her side with knees drawn up. Although rectal temperatures were advised in the early days of the Temperature Method, oral and vaginal routes provide equally satisfactory sites for FAM purposes, hence there is rarely a reason to use rectal temperatures. [519]

Changing temperature route

Oral and core (internal) temperatures parallel each other quite closely, the core temperature being slightly higher. [268] In some situations, if an oral route does not give a consistent reading it may be advisable to suggest switching to an internal route, provided this is acceptable. Advise the woman to test the impact of the temperature route by using two thermometers simultaneously for about two weeks. Record on the chart with two different colours. An internal temperature may give a more stable pattern which is easier to interpret. Any change in temperature-taking route should be made at the start of a cycle as there may be slight discrepancies in the readings.

Temperature-taking time: influence of circadian clock

Body temperature, along with many other physiological processes, is influenced by the circadian rhythm, so women using temperature as an indicator of fertility need to make allowances for this. Body temperature is at its highest at about 19:00 and drops to its lowest (basal point or nadir) between 03:00 and 06:00 (average 04:30). Waking temperature is commonly taken around 07:00 hence at a time when it is still steadily rising from its basal point.

A woman should take her temperature at about the same time every morning, immediately on waking, before she gets out of bed or any other physical activity. Ideally this should be after an uninterrupted night's sleep, but if she has to get up during the night then she should aim to have three undisturbed hours back in bed before taking her temperature – one hour may be sufficient but this should be noted (regarding shift work, see page 198).

Adjusting temperature readings to allow for waking time The dates and days of the week should be clearly marked on the chart, with the weekends highlighted to help discern changes from routine. Similarly holidays or any known disturbances should be clearly marked. The most appropriate time to take the temperature is usually the time the alarm is set on weekdays – the target time. If the temperature is taken within an hour of target time (30 minutes either side) then this is still within target: e.g. if the alarm is normally set for 07.00, from 06:30 until 07:30 is within target time. If the temperature is taken more than 30 minutes either side of the target time, the temperature may be affected by the circadian rhythm and an adjustment needs to be made.

It is recommended to use an adjustment factor of 0.1 deg.C per hour for each hour that the waking time differs from the target time (equivalent to one square on the chart). [520] To make the adjustments, do the following:

- **If the temperature is taken later than usual:** count *down* one square for each hour later that the temperature has been taken (e.g. if the alarm is normally set for 07:00 on weekdays, but the woman sleeps until 09:00 at weekends, the temperature is adjusted *downwards* by two squares).
- **If the temperature is taken earlier than usual:** make the adjustment by counting *up* one square for each hour earlier (e.g. if the same woman has an early start at 06:00, she will need to adjust the reading *upwards* by one square).

It is not known whether this adjustment factor works for temperatures taken before 05:30 or after 11:00.

Women should be encouraged to make a note on the chart if the temperature is taken outside the target time. It is helpful to highlight disturbed readings (e.g. with a red pen). New users should note disturbances, but not attempt to make adjustments. With time and experience, these adjustments can be made with confidence.

Missed temperatures

A new user should be encouraged to take her temperature every morning and to try to avoid missed readings. She should, however, understand that it is normal to forget to take her temperature, especially during the learning phase – and never feel pressured to make up false readings. If the temperature is missed, she should leave a gap and join only consecutive dots. Drawing a line between non-consecutive dots confuses the interpretation as the level of the missing temperature(s) is unknown. If a "crucial" reading is missed (around the temperature rise) then there may be insufficient information to interpret the chart – the chart should be clearly marked "Uninterpretable: insufficient information". Experienced users may be able to reduce the number of temperature readings to about 10 days of the cycle (see page 164 and figure 8.1 in chapter 8).

Instructions on taking and recording temperature

Advise the woman on appropriate thermometers and charts (page 93) and how to take and record her waking temperature accurately. Instructions are provided in appendix B.

Taking waking temperature

The woman needs to understand the standard conditions required for temperature taking:

- Use a centigrade thermometer and follow the manufacturer's instructions.
- Keep the thermometer by the bed within arm's reach.

- Take the temperature immediately on waking, before getting out of bed or any other activity.
- Place the bulb of the thermometer under the tongue in contact with the floor of the mouth, close the lips and wait for the required time. A digital thermometer takes less than one minute to register, but a glass thermometer takes about five minutes by mouth and around three minutes for internal temperatures.
- Glass thermometer: if the liquid stops between two readings, record the *lower* reading to minimise the chance of creating a false rise (e.g. if the liquid stops between 36.7 and 36.8 deg.C record it as 36.7 deg.C).
- Digital thermometer: if the thermometer gives readings to two decimal places, ignore the second decimal place (to ensure that the temperature is always averaged down).
- Remove the thermometer. Read it carefully and record the reading on the chart immediately.
- Rinse the thermometer with cold water and return it to its storage place.
- Any change in temperature route should be made at the start of the cycle.
- Any change in thermometer (loss or breakage) should be noted on the chart.
- Keep a spare battery for a digital thermometer.
- Glass thermometers:
  - Shake down below 35 deg.C (ready for use next morning) by grasping the top of the thermometer and shaking down the column of liquid using a sharp flick of the wrist away from the body and any hard surfaces.
  - Do not use if a fever is suspected (leave a gap on the chart).
  - Store out of direct sunlight and away from radiators or direct heat.
  - Do not put in hot water.
  - Keep glass thermometers away from children.

Recording temperature on the chart

The woman should be instructed in how to record her temperature clearly on the chart. She should:

1. Mark the temperature reading with a dot in the *centre* of the relevant square. Do not place dots on the lines.
2. Join the dots to form a continuous graph.
3. If a reading is missed, leave a gap on the chart. Do *not* join non-consecutive dots.
4. Make a note if the recording time varies by more than 30 minutes either side of target time.
5. Start a new chart on the first day of the period (fresh red bleed). If the period starts during the day, that day's temperature reading is transferred to the new chart.
6. Note anything unusual on the chart, such as a late night, alcohol or stress.

ACTIVITY CHART-BUILDING EXERCISE, COMBINING INDICATORS

This activity consolidates learning related to recording and interpreting indicators. Add the following information to a blank chart (available in appendix A or downloadable from www.fertilityuk.org).

Step 1 Recording the period and temperature readings

1. Jo is 26 years old. She wants to avoid pregnancy for the next two years. Her partner John dislikes condoms so they abstain from penetrative sex during the fertile time. This is Jo's sixth chart and she is starting to feel more confident.
2. Notice the days of the cycle numbered consecutively across the bottom.

3 Add the dates (with days of the week) at the top starting on Wednesday 8 March (day 1). Clearly indicate the weekends.
4 Shade in the relevant boxes to denote the days of the period. The first day of her cycle (start of period) is on Wednesday 8 March and she has a five-day period. Her next period starts on Thursday 6 April.
5 Starting with day 1 and moving consecutively through to day 30, add the following daily temperature readings (dots) in the centre of the appropriate squares: 36.7, 36.6, 36.5, 36.8, 36.8, 36.6, 36.4, 36.5, 36.5, 36.6, 36.6, 36.5, 36.5, 36.7, 36.5, 36.5, 36.8, 36.9, 36.9, 36,9, 36.9, 37.0, 37.0, 36.9, 36.9, 36.9, 36.9, 36.8, 36.7, 36.6 deg.C
6 Jo had a lie-in until 09:00 on Saturday 11 and Sunday 12 March, otherwise she was consistent with her temperature-taking time.
7 Join the dots to form a continuous graph.
8 Set the activity aside for now.

This exercise is continued on page 128 and at specific intervals until completion by the end of part I.

INTERPRETING TEMPERATURE READINGS

A cycle in which ovulation is presumed to have occurred is characterised by a biphasic temperature curve. The temperature remains on the lower level until the time of ovulation when a rise (shift) occurs of about 0.2 deg.C. It remains at the higher level until the start of the next period. The rise in temperature may take place abruptly (from one day to the next), slowly or in a series of steps.

3 over 6 rule

Holt first demonstrated that the *end* of the fertile time can be identified by a clear rise of 0.2 deg.C or more for three consecutive days after six low readings – the *3 over 6 rule*. [288] This allows 48 hours for the outer limit of ovum survival (24 hours for one egg and the possibility of a second ovulation within 24 hours). The original rule allowed the temperature rise to be 0.1 deg.C provided that at least *one* of the three high temperatures was a minimum of 0.2 deg.C, but it is now recognised that the *third* high temperature is most significant to ensure that the rise is sustained.

Importance of third high temperature The third high temperature must be at least 0.2 deg.C above the six low readings. [189] In practice this means that the third reading must have a gap of at least one square (see hatched box in figure 4.3). If the third high temperature is not at least 0.2 deg.C above the six low readings, wait for a fourth high reading to ensure that the temperature is staying at the higher level. The fourth high temperature need only be above the coverline (figure 4.4).

Identifying the temperature rise

To identify the relevant temperatures when applying the *3 over 6 rule*, a horizontal coverline is drawn on the line immediately above the highest of the low-phase temperatures. A vertical line is then drawn, forming a cross on the chart between the two days when the temperature shift from the lower to the higher phase occurred.

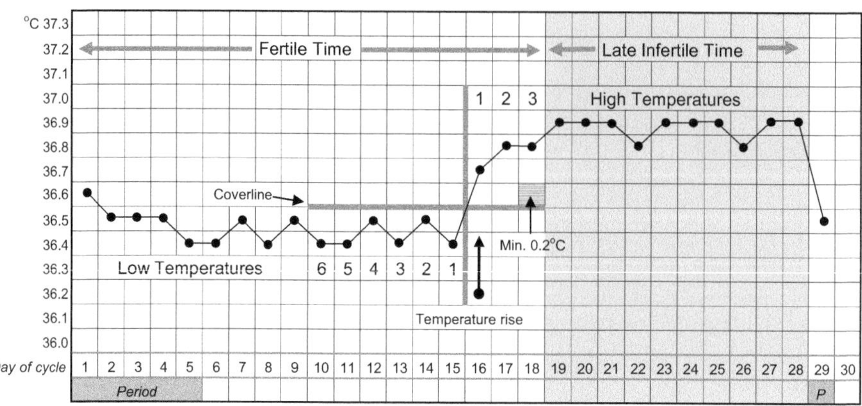

Figure 4.3 Biphasic chart showing fertile time, late infertile time and *3 over 6 rule*

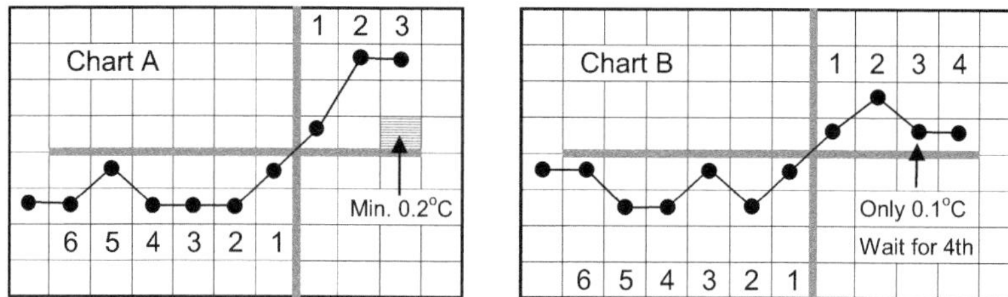

Figure 4.4 Importance of the third high temperature: in chart A, the fertile time ends after the third high temperature (it is at least 0.2 deg.C). In chart B, the third high reading is only 0.1 deg.C, so wait for the fourth high temperature (which is above the coverline).

In figure 4.3 the coverline is drawn between 36.5 and 36.6 deg.C showing that the temperatures for days 16, 17 and 18 are all above the coverline, hence above the low-phase temperatures. The six low temperatures are therefore in the lower left quadrant and the three high temperatures in the upper right. The first high temperature (day of the rise) is on day 16. Using temperature as a single indicator, the fertile time starts on day 1 and lasts until the third high temperature has been recorded (day 18). The remainder of the cycle is then infertile – the late infertile time.

Use of teaching aids The *3 over 6 rule* is efficient and simple to teach, with most new users grasping the concept quickly. One of a number of different techniques can be used to help the learner identify the relevant temperatures:

- Slide a ruler upwards from the bottom of the chart, keeping the top edge parallel with the horizontal lines on the chart, until the high temperatures appear above the ruler (a coloured semi-transparent ruler works best).
- Use a sheet of paper instead of a ruler, moving it in the same direction.
- Move a sheet of paper across from left to right to reveal the high readings (the way a cycle would naturally unfold).
- Use a simple card with two windows removed to identify the relevant high and low readings (the original "Holt window").
- Lay a "plastic cross" (black cross on clear plastic) over the temperatures to determine the appropriate readings.

The woman should be instructed in how to draw the cross on her chart and to number the high-and low-phase temperatures. She should:

1 Draw the coverline on the line immediately above the highest of the low temperatures to extend across the width of the six low and three high temperatures.
2 Draw the vertical line to separate the low- and high-phase temperatures.
3 Hatch some lines in the box above the coverline on the day of the third high temperature, to ensure that the third high reading is at least 0.2 deg.C (there should not be a temperature reading in the hatched box).
4 If the third high temperature is *not* 0.2 deg.C then wait for a fourth high temperature which just has to be above the coverline (figure 4.4).
5 Number the high temperatures 1–3 *above* the readings in the upper right quadrant.
6 Number the low temperatures 1–6 (from right to left) *below* the readings in the lower left quadrant. Writing the numbers in this way emphasises the high and low readings and allows for later adjustments to accommodate the other indicators.

Level of coverline Keefe found that in most women who recorded an oral temperature at 7.30 am (after 8 hours sleep), the temperature before ovulation was below 36.5 deg.C rising to about 36.7 deg.C after ovulation. He suggested that this was so consistent that charting may not be needed. [320] Undoubtedly, with experience, users become accustomed to the expected level of their low and high-phase temperatures, but the temperatures should still be charted to observe for any disturbance and to allow correlation with other indicators. Although the normal coverline will usually be between 36.5 and 36.6 deg.C, this will vary between women and from one cycle to another in the same woman depending on temperature time and route. The temperature gives a more objective marker which is visible for a partner or health professional. An abnormally low or high coverline could indicate thyroid disease (page 213).

Extended coverline (coverline technique)

The *3 over 6 rule* provides the most effective way to identify the *end* of the fertile time for women of normal fertility. In circumstances where there may be doubt about the accuracy of the six low temperatures, for example after stopping hormonal contraception or during breast-feeding, then the **coverline technique** is used. This extends the horizontal coverline over all the low-phase temperatures, excluding the first four days of the cycle (figure 15.2). The extended coverline is unnecessary in most situations.

Different methods to interpret temperature

A number of different methods have been used to interpret temperature readings. McCarthy's computer analysis of more than 8,000 charts compared several methods used to identify the rise: the *3 over 6 rule*, the average of the temperatures around the rise, and a smoothed curve which used the average of all the readings. The smoothed curve produced the highest proportion of biphasic charts, but was limited by its requirement for the readings for the entire cycle. The *3 over 6 rule* identified a biphasic curve in 76% of charts. [394]

Computerised thermometers and Web-based programmes use different analyses to interpret temperatures. Although theoretically these should be accurate, there is little reliable evidence of their effectiveness (page 170). Women who understand their fertility learn to understand their own personal pattern and how to handle disturbances such as alcohol or disrupted sleep, but computerised systems are unable to effectively manage disturbances. Ongoing research into computerised management of severe and multiple disturbances could change this. [200]

Keep it simple

The concept of *3 over 6* is simple, yet effective. It does not require a high level of education – in fact the more sophisticated user is at risk of over-complicating it. The case study of the keen physicist reminds of the need to follow instructions and stick to simple rules.

CASE STUDY THE KEEN PHYSICIST

Penny and David had relied on their own version of the Calendar/Rhythm Method since their marriage six months earlier. Penny wanted to pursue further studies so thought they should learn to use a more "reliable" natural method. They were open to a pregnancy but ideally wanted to wait three years. They were both instructed in the *3 over 6 rule* as part of a combined indicator approach. Penny started observing her secretions; meanwhile David, a physicist, was keen to take charge of temperature recording. They failed to attend their first follow-up appointment. By the third cycle, Penny was pregnant. On discussion David had entered the temperature readings into his computer and applied a number of mathematical models to predict when they were safe to have intercourse – with unexpected results.

Variations in type of rise

The temperature rises from the lower to the higher level in one of three ways: an abrupt rise (most common), a slow rise or a step rise (figure 4.5).

- **Abrupt rise** The temperature rises sharply between one day and the next.
- **Slow rise** The temperature rises slowly over several days.
- **Step rise** The temperature rises by 0.1 or 0.2 deg.C then stays at that level for 48 hours before advancing another step.

The frequency of the different types of temperature rise was observed in over 1,000 cycles from 155 healthy fertile women: 83% of cycles showed an abrupt (acute) rise, 14% a slow rise and 3% a step rise. [377] A saw-tooth rise (series of peaks and troughs) has previously been described – but, because this is rarely seen and is often associated with stress, it is not advisable to attempt to interpret such a rise. If the *3 over 6 rule* does not fit, the chart cannot be interpreted.

Significance of type of rise

The type of temperature rise and the way this is measured is of most relevance for research purposes to ensure consistency of data. Bailey (and Marshall) showed that when a slow or step rise is measured from the *start* of the rise, the post-ovulatory (hyperthermic) phase was significantly

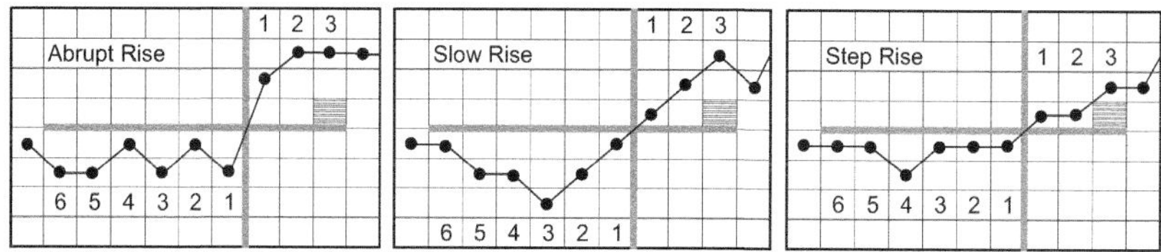

Figure 4.5 Types of temperature rise showing the *3 over 6 rule* (note the hatched box which ensures that third high temperature is at least 0.2 deg.C)

longer than that measured from the first high temperature following an abrupt rise. [19] They suggested that ovulation may not always have occurred before the start of the slow rise, hence Marshall's advice for couples to avoid intercourse until there were *five* consecutive temperatures from the foot of a slow or step rise, instead of the usual three after an abrupt rise. [379] This is of academic interest only because when temperature readings are observed above a coverline and correlated with peak day (last day of most fertile secretions) this overrides the need for counting extra days to accommodate the type of rise.

Value of combining indicators There will always be slight variability in the observed indicators when compared with more objective markers of ovulation (page 183). In most cycles, the temperature rise occurs *after* ovulation, but it can occur before. Correlating the temperature rise with peak day (last day of most fertile secretions) provides the most accurate confirmation of the *end* of the fertile time. **The fertile time ends when there are three high temperatures *after peak day*.**

The "dip" before the rise

The concept of the "dip" before the temperature rise causes considerable confusion. There is some evidence of pre-ovulatory temperatures dropping to their lowest point a day or two before ovulation. This low point (nadir), which may coincide with the peak in estrogen levels, was first observed in the early 20th century and promoted as a way to help gynaecologists *predict* ovulation. It has been widely publicised as a way for women to pinpoint ovulation, with numerous illustrations showing a temperature chart with an arrow labelled "ovulation" pointing to a strategic dip.

In the 1940s Keefe designed the first expanded narrow-scale mercury thermometer (Ovulindex) specifically for fertility purposes. Its easy-to-read scale and accuracy (to 0.1 deg.C) helped to overcome the problems with ordinary fever thermometers. Keefe commented that the temperature dip seemed to be an artefact. [320]

The temperature dip is rarely seen in practice. Numerous dips are observable in fertile and subfertile women due to the nature of day to day changes or more significant disturbances. A dip was observed in only 18% of charts kept by 130 subfertile women (50 out of 271 charts) (Halbrecht 1945 in Marshall 1963) and 10% of charts kept by 155 fertile women (112 out of 1,134 cycles). [385] It is better to ignore the dip completely. [414] [601]

In the 1990s Martinez reassessed the reliability of temperature in fertility management, concluding that **waking temperature can provide a relatively accurate *retrospective* marker of the time around ovulation.** Martinez found that the temperature nadir was within one day of the LH surge in 75% of cases and within two days in 90% of cases. [387] **The best prospective marker for optimising conception is the cervical secretions** (pages 128 and 139) with the rise in temperature *confirming* ovulation retrospectively.

Temperature spike

A temperature spike is a single recording which is 0.2 deg.C or more above its immediate neighbours on each side (figure 4.6). A spike may result from a disturbance caused by alcohol the night before, a late night, oversleeping, minor illness or stress. At times there may be no obvious cause for a spike. It is helpful to circle the spike using a red pen so that the disturbance is easily recognised. It can also help to cover the outlying temperature with a thumb so that it does not distract from the overall pattern of readings. Toni Weschler, women's health educator, and author of *Taking Charge of Your Fertility* terms this the "rule of thumb". [610]

One temperature spike can safely be ignored when determining the six low temperatures, but where possible there should be an explanation for the disturbance. **If there is more than**

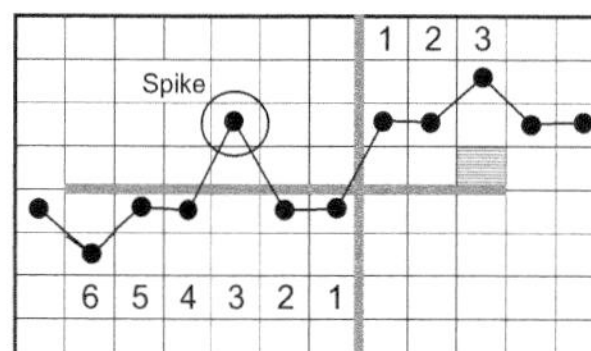

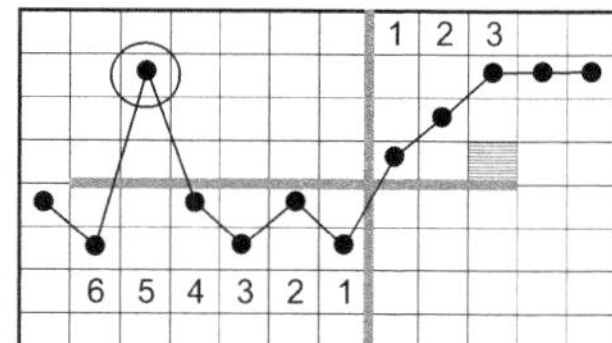

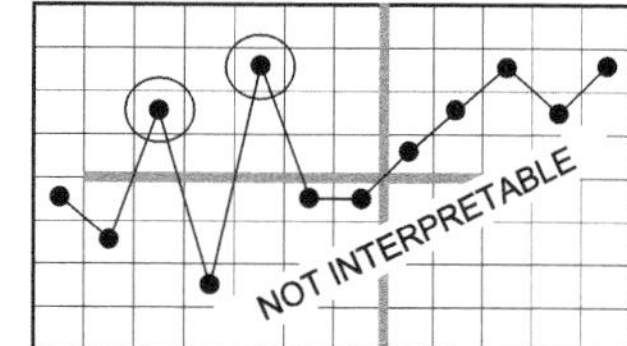

Figure 4.6 Temperature spike: one spike in the six low temperatures can safely be ignored (charts A and B) but more than one spike in the six low readings (chart C) renders the chart uninterpretable

one spike in the six low temperatures, the *3 over 6 rule* **cannot be applied.** A woman should consider her other fertility indicators and wait until the position becomes clear – the chart may be uninterpretable (figure 4.6). If there is a disturbed reading in one of the three high temperatures, it is advisable to wait for a fourth high temperature to ensure that the fertile time has ended.

Note on terminology: Confusion exists between the terms *spike* (meaning a sharp increase or rise) and *peak* (meaning the maximum point of something – the point of maximum fertility). A peak is sometimes thought of as the pointed top of something (like a mountain), hence potential confusion between spikes and peaks. As these two terms relate to different indicators, there should be a clear distinction in the terminology: a *temperature spike* and *peak secretion day* (last day of most fertile secretions).

DISTURBANCES AFFECTING TEMPERATURE

Erratic temperatures are common. They may be a feature of disruptions to routine, illness, stress or poor temperature-taking and recording technique.

Faulty technique

During the learning phase it is common to see erratic temperatures due to faulty technique. This is characterised by subnormal readings as well as abnormally high readings and may be due to either user error or equipment failure (figure 4.7). Consider the following:

- faulty thermometer;
- poor-quality equipment, e.g. calibrations on card (glass thermometers) can become detached and move around;
- battery failure (digital thermometer);
- failure to keep thermometer in the same position in the mouth with lips closed;
- failure to leave the thermometer in place for the required time;
- alterations in recording time (with no explanatory note);
- failure to shake the liquid down properly (glass thermometer);
- change of thermometer mid-cycle;
- changes in temperature taking–route mid-cycle; and
- temperatures may not be recorded accurately with dots in the centre of the square and lines joining consecutive readings.

If the thermometer is in question, consider changing it. A woman can then use both thermometers (one after the other) for a few days to observe the difference, then continue with the more

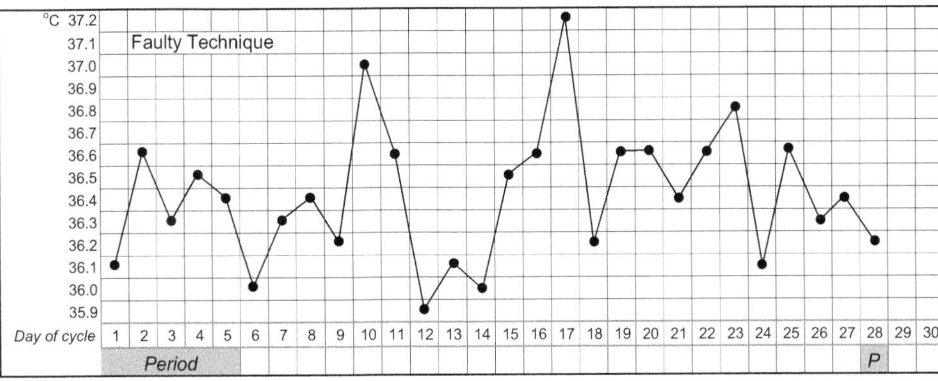

Figure 4.7 Erratic temperature readings with large swings due to faulty technique

reliable thermometer. If careful enquiry reveals that the equipment is not faulty and the temperature is being taken accurately, suggest changing the route (page 96).

Common disturbances affecting temperature

If it has been established that the temperature-taking and recording technique is correct, then consider other reasons for disturbed readings. A single disturbed reading is likely to produce a temperature *spike* but consecutively disturbed temperatures may cause disruption for more than one day. Common disturbances include:

- Changes in temperature-taking time (for example, oversleeping) can affect the temperature reading.
- A late night can affect the following morning's temperature.
- Alcohol can affect the following morning's temperature
- Weekends – a combination of factors including alcohol, late evening meal, later to bed and/or a lie-in may result in consecutively higher readings on Saturday and Sunday morning ("weekend syndrome").
- Disturbed nights (for example, getting up for children) can affect the following morning's temperature.
- Changes in the sleeping environment (for example, going away on holiday) can affect the following morning's temperature.
- Shift work – night shifts, "late" and "early" shifts present challenges (page 198).
- Changing the clocks can disrupt temperatures for several days (page 197).
- Illness such as a cold or sore throat may cause a temperature spike or mildly raised temperatures for a few days.
- Illness causing a fever (pyrexia) may produce temperatures outside the normal range – these are unlikely to be confused with the ovulation rise (page 220).
- Analgesics such as aspirin or paracetamol are anti-pyretic so may cause a lower temperature than normal if taken within four hours prior to the temperature reading.

Any disturbances should be noted on the chart alongside the affected reading or in the comments box. A coloured (red) pen can help to highlight possible disturbances. If the disturbance affects crucial readings in the fertile time the chart will not be interpretable and should be clearly marked as such, for example: "Uninterpretable: Too much disturbance". Factors affecting the chart are discussed in chapter 12 with a checklist on page 224.

Male partner as a control

One way of getting around common disturbances, such as ambient room temperature or sleep disturbance, is for the woman's partner to take his temperature too, thus acting as a control. A small study which used LH kits to estimate the day of ovulation highlighted the difference between the man's monophasic temperature and the increased temperature difference in the luteal phase of a biphasic cycle ("Gap" technique). [137] [138] Increased male involvement could be viewed as positively contributing to the couple's commitment to the method, but much larger studies are required to confirm these findings. This degree of male involvement is impractical for most couples.

NORMAL AND ABNORMAL TEMPERATURE PATTERNS

Temperature charts show a number of variations, some of which are typical of normal fertile cycles; others, whilst less common, may indicate fertility problems including anovulation or a deficient luteal phase. The temperature rise confirms ovulation and determines the *end* of the fertile time for avoiding pregnancy. It also has a role as a diagnostic aid for subfertile couples (page 309).

Normal fertile cycles

A cycle with a biphasic temperature curve is indicative of ovulation. A normal length luteal phase of 10–16 days allows adequate time for implantation, so indicates a potentially fertile cycle – the only cycle type which can result in conception (figure 4.3).

Variations in day of rise

Overall cycle length is variable, with the follicular phase showing the most variation, particularly at the extremes of reproductive life (page 72). The temperature rise occurs about 14 days before the start of the next period, hence it will occur earlier in shorter cycles and later in longer cycles.

If the first day of the temperature rise is on or before day 8, the *3 over 6 rule* cannot be applied. [385] This proviso ensures that the rise is occurring at a biologically feasible time and prevents a co-incidental finding of three high and six low readings which are not related to ovulation.

Figure 4.8 shows short, average and long cycles, with the vertical arrow indicating the temperature rise (first high temperature). The pre-ovulatory phase is varied in length while the post-ovulatory phase is relatively constant. The grey shaded area indicates the late infertile time following the third high temperature – the safest time for intercourse for couples avoiding pregnancy.

Women should be instructed that they must **always assume that there will be a temperature rise** (however late in the cycle) and **wait for the rise** (and the following three days) to ensure that the fertile time has ended. Unintended pregnancies occur when couples fail to wait for the rise and resume intercourse believing that they have never had such a late temperature rise before so assume that either they missed the rise or they must be pregnant.

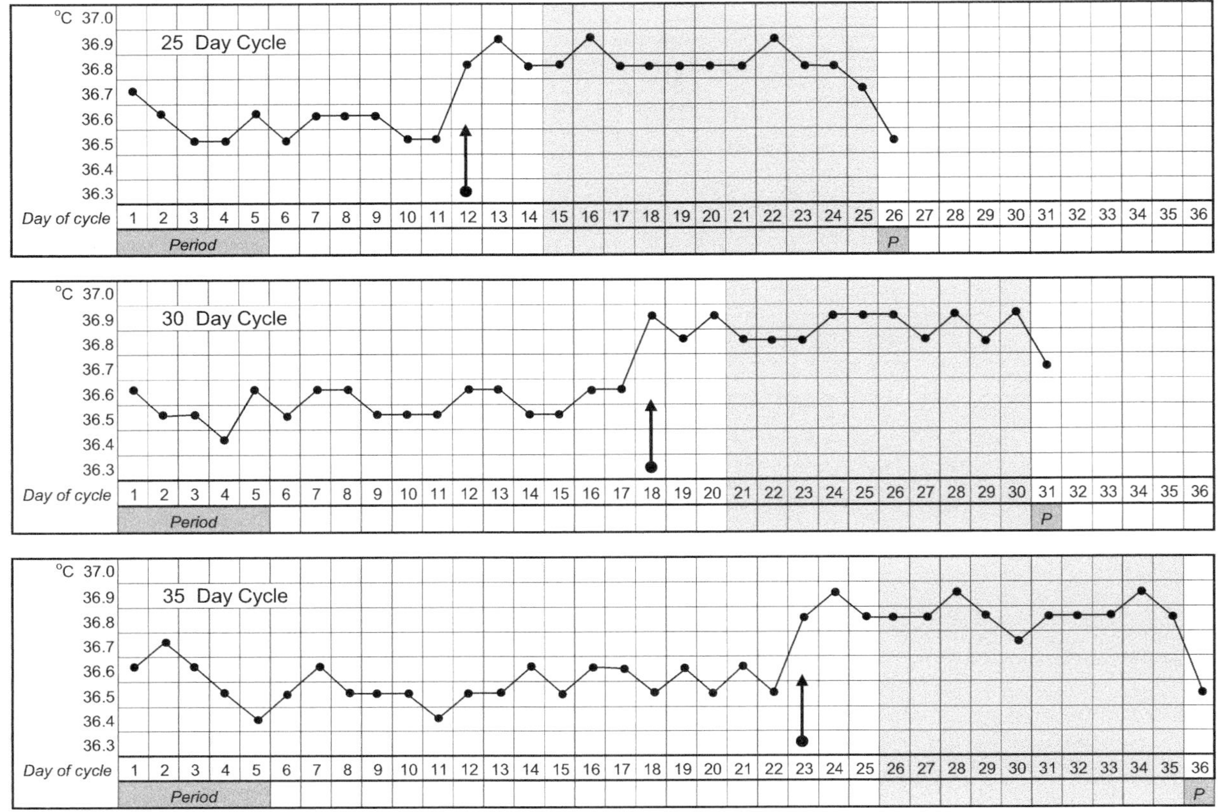

Figure 4.8 Variations in the day of the temperature rise in cycles of 25, 30 and 35 days. Note the variable number of low-phase temperatures with the more constant number of high-phase temperatures.

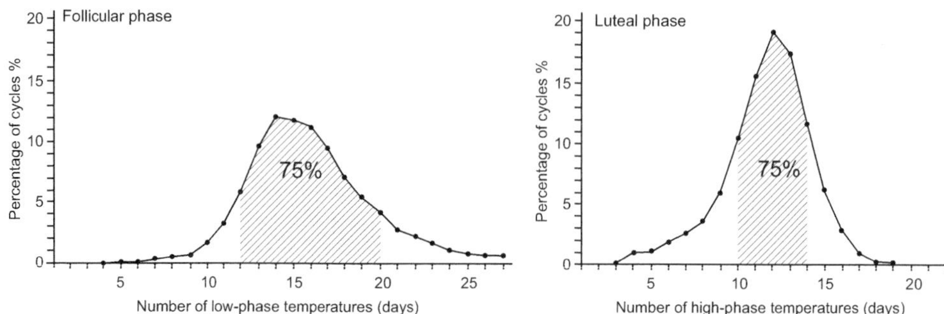

Figure 4.9 Variability in the length of the follicular and luteal phases by temperature (656 women: 20,672 cycles). Note the wide variability in the follicular phase compared with the luteal phase. The hatched areas represent 75% of cycles (adapted from Vollman 1977). [601]

Length of follicular and luteal phases

Vollman studied the temperature curves in more than 20,000 cycles. In 75% of cycles the luteal phase varied by four days only (10–14 high temperatures), whereas the follicular phase varied by 8 days (12–20 low temperatures) – see figure 4.9.

Colombo found similar results in his analysis of Marshall's data (2,913 cycles). In 74% of cycles there were 11–16 raised temperatures (most commonly 12), while 4% of cycles had a luteal phase greater than 16 days. [99] Colombo's analysis of the European multi-centre study (5,426 cycles) found that the mean length of the follicular phase was 16.6 days and the mean length of the luteal phase was 12.4 days. [101] The luteal phase length by temperature shows a close correlation with the North Carolina study using the estrogen:progesterone ratio, in which the luteal phase lasted 12–15 days in more than 70% of cycles. [20]

Conception cycles

In a cycle in which conception occurs, the corpus luteum continues to produce progesterone and the temperature is sustained at the higher level. Some women notice a second rise in temperature about 7–10 days after the ovulation rise (triphasic pattern). This occurs around the start of implantation and may occasionally be accompanied by light spotting.

Vollman showed that the normal luteal phase lasted 10–16 days with an absolute outer limit of 19 days. He noted that all women whose charts showed a raised temperature for 20 days or longer turned out to be pregnant. [601] Colombo confirmed these findings: **a luteal phase of 20 days or more indicates with a high degree of probability that conception has occurred.** [99] In some circumstances, the temperature stays at the higher level, there is no period, but a pregnancy test is negative. This can occur either in the case of a luteinised unruptured follicle or a persistent corpus luteum cyst.

Figure 4.10 shows the chart for a woman who was planning pregnancy. The usual coverline is between 36.6 and 36.7 deg.C The temperature rises to the higher level (day 13) and remains at the higher level for about a week. It then shows a further rise to around 37 deg.C (day 21). The first sign of pregnancy is usually a missed period but some women continue to have intermittent bleeds through pregnancy – these always need investigating, but may not be pathological. A sustained high temperature may be the first indication of pregnancy as in the following case study.

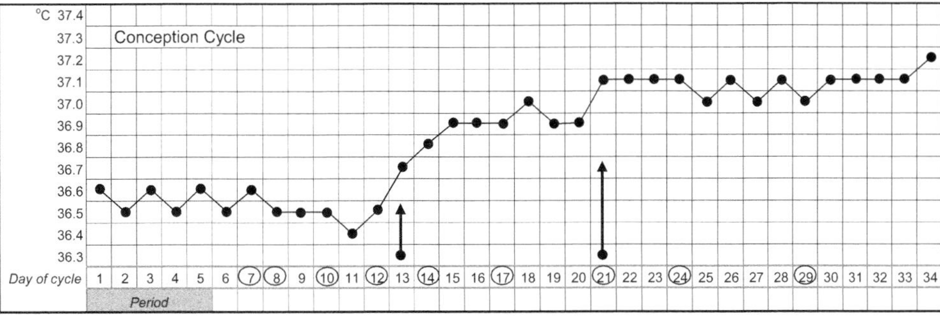

Figure 4.10 Conception cycle: note the ovulatory rise on day 13 followed by a further rise about a week later indicative of implantation. A sustained rise for 20 days or more indicates pregnancy.

CASE STUDY SUSTAINED TEMPERATURE IN PREGNANCY

Ali had recently stopped combined oral contraceptives (COCs) due to worsening migraines. She and her partner of two years were about to go travelling but were keen to learn FAMs in conjunction with condoms. At her follow-up, Ali's charts showed that she had two "periods" while she was away, however, her temperatures were consistently raised at around 37 deg.C. On further questioning, she had experienced nausea and felt tired but assumed this was travel-related. A pregnancy test confirmed the suspicion about the elevated temperatures and a scan dated the pregnancy at 11+ weeks. Ali remembered one night when they had concerns about a split condom. Although the timing was not ideal, she decided to continue with the pregnancy. Ali felt confident about her body's natural signs and went on to be a confident FAM user.

Short luteal phase

Cycles in which the luteal phase is less than 10 days have insufficient time for implantation. This can be recognised only in retrospect at the start of the next period. Döring observed that **cycles with fewer than 10 raised temperatures were generally infertile.** [133] Figure 4.11 shows a short cycle with a short luteal phase. There are less than 10 high temperatures, so the cycle is likely to be infertile.

A short luteal phase can occur in a cycle of any length, so the overall cycle length will not necessarily be short. For example, if the temperature rise occurred on day 27, but the next period started on day 36, the overall cycle length is long, but the cycle may still be infertile as there are less than 10 raised temperatures.

Cycles with short luteal phases are more common at the extremes of reproductive life (figure 4.14), postnatally, and at times of stress. Women who are using FAMs to avoid pregnancy may report frustrations with short luteal phases as this reduces the number of days available for intercourse in the late infertile time. Short luteal phases are of particular significance for women who are trying to conceive (page 346).

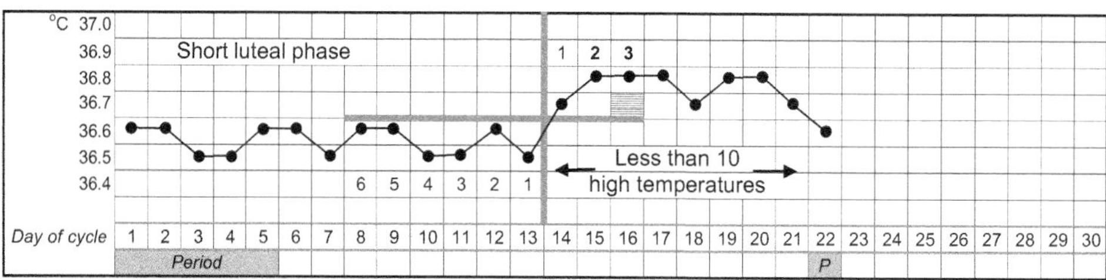

Figure 4.11 Short luteal phase in a 21-day cycle. Note the temperature rise on day 14. As there are only eight high temperatures this is likely to be an infertile cycle.

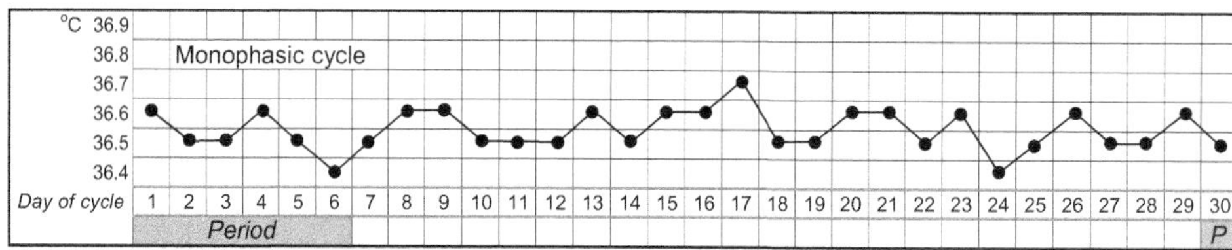

Figure 4.12 Monophasic cycle: absence of temperature rise may indicate anovulation

Monophasic chart (anovulatory cycles)

If there is no ovulation there will be no temperature rise: the temperature remains on the same level throughout in a monophasic cycle. A monophasic temperature chart does not conclusively show the absence of ovulation, but is a good indication. Anovulatory cycles are more common at the extremes of reproductive life – during adolescence and approaching the menopause. They may also occur after childbirth, after miscarriage and after hormonal contraception. Anovulatory cycles also commonly occur during times of stress, whilst extreme stress may result in amenorrhoea.

Figure 4.12 shows a 29-day cycle with a monophasic temperature. The bleeding, which starts on day 30, could be masking secretions and the "period" (technically an estrogen withdrawal bleed) could be associated with ovulation (page 206). The monophasic temperature in figure 4.12 shows relatively small day-to-day variation, but sometimes there will be greater variation – this is typically seen in the basic infertile pattern (BIP) experienced by breastfeeding women who are not yet ovulating (figure 16.4).

The entire monophasic cycle is likely to be infertile, but this cannot be known until the end of the cycle because there is always the possibility of a delayed temperature rise. Some would argue that ovulation occurs in *every* menstrual cycle, but in some cycles there is an intermittent bleed before the delayed ovulatory rise.

Frequency of monophasic cycles in relation to cycle length

Vollman observed the characteristics of nearly 15,000 cycles in relation to gynaecological age. He found that throughout reproductive life **an average of around 7% of cycles were monophasic.** The likelihood of the cycle being monophasic varied with cycle length, with **very short or very long cycles** being significantly **more likely to be anovulatory.** Vollman's dataset showed that:

- In very short cycles (7 to 17 days), 57% were monophasic.
- The percentage of monophasic cycles decreased as cycle length increased.

- In 24-day cycles, nearly 6% were monophasic.
- In 25–32 day cycles, the rate of monophasic cycles was at its minimum (3%).
- In cycles of more than 33 days, the percentage of monophasic cycles increased.
- In cycles of 60 days or more, more than 41% of cycles were monophasic.

The *average (median)* cycle length of the monophasic cycle was 28.0 days compared with 27.5 days for all cycles studied, hence a **28-day cycle cannot be assumed to be ovulatory.** [601]

Frequency of monophasic cycles by gynaecological age

The percentage of monophasic cycles varies with age. Figure 4.13 shows the distribution of monophasic cycles by gynaecological age. In the year of the menarche 56% cycles were monophasic, decreasing sharply during the adolescent years to 6.6 % at a gynaecological age of eight years. The minimum rate of monophasic cycles was at gynaecological age 29. The percentage of monophasic cycles then rises in the pre-menopausal years to 34% at gynaecological age 40–45 years.

Cycle characteristics throughout reproductive life

The characteristics of menstrual cycles vary throughout reproductive life (page 76). Döring used waking temperature to estimate the frequency of monophasic cycles (presumed anovulatory), short luteal phases and normal biphasic cycles (presumed ovulatory) in women aged 12–50 years (> 3,000 cycles). The highest rate of anovulatory cycles was in 12–14 year olds, with an almost continuous decrease until the minimum number in the 26–30-year age group. The percentage of anovulatory cycles increased again in women over 40 (figure 4.14).

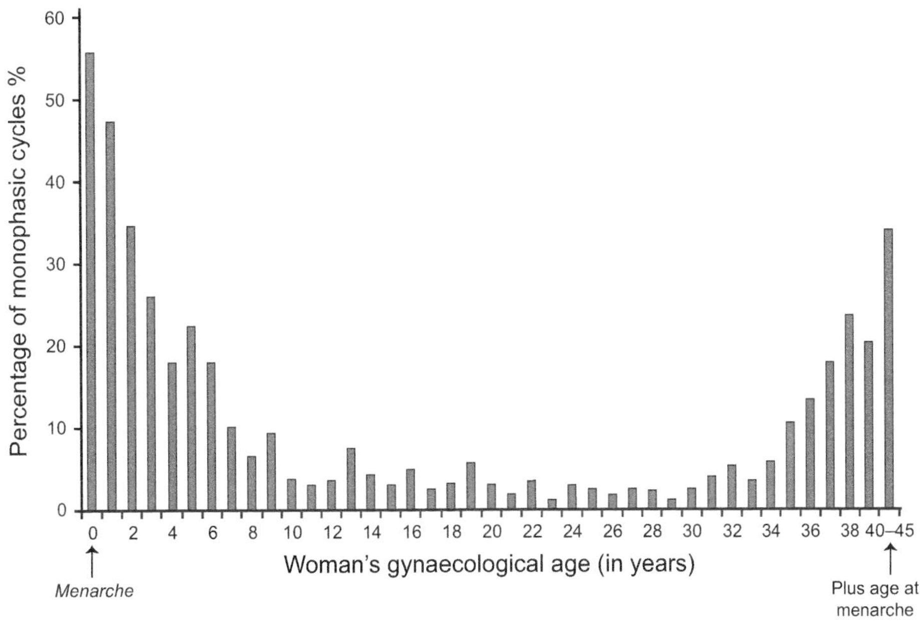

Figure 4.13 Monophasic temperature curves by gynaecological age (total 14,848 cycles) (adapted from Vollman, 1977) [601]

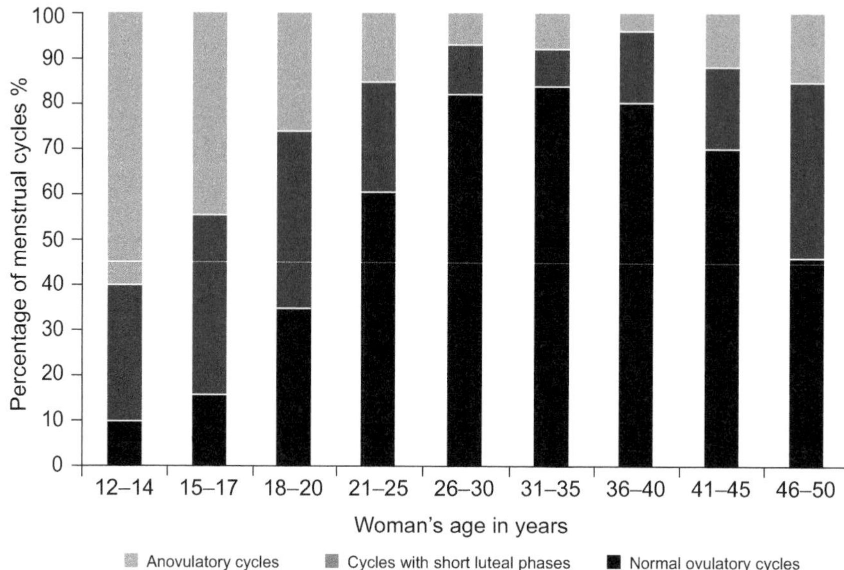

Figure 4.14 Distribution of normal ovulatory cycles, short luteal phases and anovulatory cycles in 3,264 cycles from 481 women (adapted from Döring 1969) [133]

Döring reported on the different stages of reproductive life:

- **Post-menarche:** Döring most striking finding was the high percentage of inadequate cycles (monophasic or short luteal phases) in the early years after the menarche, which explains the comparative subfertility of young girls (page 359).
- **Subfertile women:** Döring commented that in subfertile couples, cycles with short luteal phases were possibly of greater importance than anovulatory cycles as these were more prevalent in the 25-40–year age group. In more than 1,200 women undergoing fertility investigations, cycles with short luteal phases were 2.5 times as common as anovulatory cycles (page 346).
- **Postpartum women:** A high percentage of postpartum cycles were inadequate. Ninety-five women recorded temperatures from the first until the fourth period after childbirth (285 cycles). Twenty-two percent of cycles were presumed anovulatory, and 32% had short luteal phases. The first cycle was biphasic in only a few cases, but, with cycles 2–4, 46% showed normal biphasic curves with adequate luteal phases, and 54% were still considered inadequate for conception by the fourth cycle postpartum (page 269). [133]
- **Peri-menopausal women:** In the oldest age group (46–50 years), many women still showed apparently normal ovulatory cycles and therefore remained at risk of unintended pregnancy (page 291).

TEMPERATURE IN FERTILITY PRACTICE

FA helps to identify monophasic cycles, LPD, irregular bleeding and reduced quantity or quality of cervical secretions. There is some evidence that putting women in control of their fertility may improve adherence with medical treatment. [190] Daily temperature recording is well-accepted by the majority of women, possibly due to the active involvement in investigation and treatment and increased awareness of physiological changes. [387] However, temperature charting is not recommended by NICE fertility guidelines (pages 303, 307 and 350). [428]

TEMPERATURE CHARTING TO AVOID PREGNANCY

The main use of temperature charting is by couples using FAMs to avoid pregnancy. The temperature chart alone cannot identify the start of the fertile time, so there is no early relatively infertile time, but it has a key role in identifying the end of the fertile time.

Reliability of temperature to confirm ovulation

In Marshall's collection of 36,641 charts from 1,798 women (each with at least one sequence of six charts), a temperature rise could be determined and the *3 over 6 rule* applied in 81% of charts. The remainder had an undetermined temperature rise, were monophasic, had critical temperatures missing, or were illegible. One percent of charts were affected by illness. [407] These statistics serve as a reminder that not all charts are interpretable. **It may not be possible to apply the *3 over 6 rule* in up to 20% of cycles.** The biggest mistake users (and new practitioners) make is to try and make the rules fit the desired outcome.

SELF-ASSESSMENT QUESTION

Answers are at the end of the chapter.

Figure 4.15 represents six cycles (labelled A–F). Each shows a five-day period at the start of the cycle and then the first day of the next period to denote cycle length. The grey line represents the temperature curve with the 0.2 deg.C rise followed by the drop in temperature a number of days later. For each cycle, comment on the total cycle length, the day of temperature rise and the length of the luteal phase. Add any other comments to explain the characteristics of the cycle.

GUIDELINES: TEMPERATURE AS A SINGLE INDICATOR

The following guidelines apply for women who are using temperature as a single indicator.

- The fertile time starts on day 1 of the cycle (first day of period).
- The fertile time ends after the third high temperature has been recorded, provided it is at least 0.2 deg.C above the highest of the preceding six low readings (the other temperatures need only be 0.1 deg.C). Intercourse can be resumed on the evening of the third high temperature.
- If the third high temperature is not at least 0.2 deg.C above the six low readings, wait for a fourth high temperature – which has only to be above the coverline. Intercourse can then be resumed from the *fourth* evening.
- The late infertile time lasts until the start of the next period.

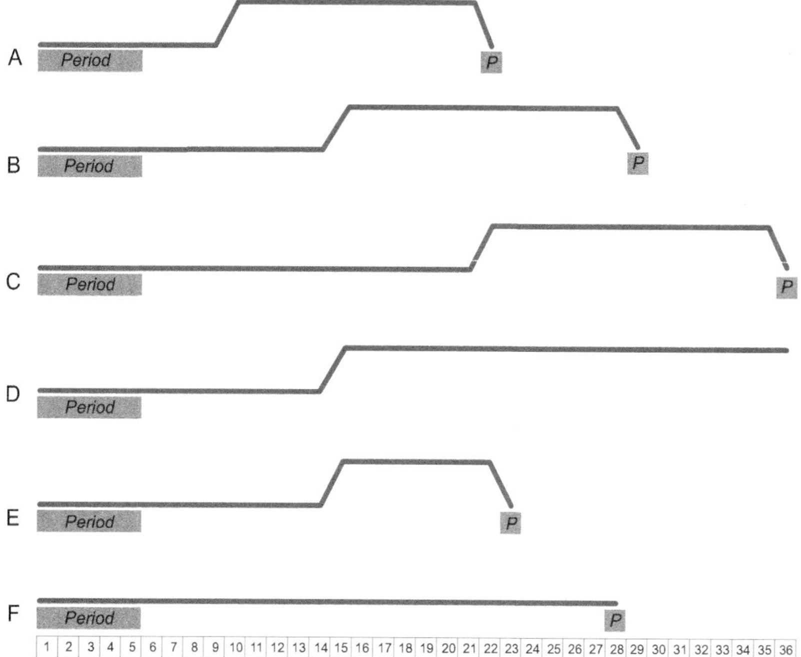

Figure 4.15 Series of six temperature curves for comments

Temperature is not normally used as a single-indicator method, because it requires lengthy and unnecessary abstinence. When used in combination with changes in cervical secretions, **the fertile time ends on the evening of the third high temperature after peak day** (guidelines: pages 114 and 227).

RISK OF CONCEPTION IN RELATION TO TEMPERATURE RISE

Barrett and Marshall demonstrated the risk of conception in relation to the temperature rise and the effectiveness of the late infertile time. All conceptions occurred from five days before to one day after the temperature rise with the risk of conception approximating to zero six days before and two days after the rise (page 80). [34] The European multi-centre study used a similar protocol. The daily estimates of the probability of conception were largely similar to the Barrett and Marshall study, but the European data showed a risk of conception for up to eight days preceding the temperature rise and two days after (page 82). [101] When discussing the probability of pregnancy with couples, it depends on whether the information is being used to plan or avoid pregnancy as to whether pregnancy is considered a "chance" or a "risk". The majority of couples in the Barrett and Marshall study were using the information to avoid pregnancy, hence the focus was on the "risk" of conception.

EFFECTIVENESS OF TEMPERATURE

Using temperature as a single indicator requires an average of 16 days of abstinence because couples have to abstain from the start of the cycle until after the third high temperature. It is therefore effective only if used by highly motivated couples who can tolerate prolonged abstinence. Ideally temperature should always be combined with other indicators.

Marshall showed a distinct difference between the effectiveness of the pre- and post- ovulation phases (total: 8,294 cycles). Thirty-two couples used temperature as a single indicator and a further 255 used temperature plus a calculation (shortest cycle minus 19) to identify the first fertile day (allowing pre-ovulatory intercourse). This highlighted the increased effectiveness of the post-ovulatory phase (6.6 vs. 19.3 per 100 women years). [380]

Marshall studied a further 108 couples (2,109 cycles) who were using cervical secretions in combination with temperature and calculation. The first fertile day was identified by the shortest cycle minus 18 or first appearance of secretions, whichever was *earlier*. The last fertile day was identified by the third high temperature (0.1 deg.C rise). There was an overall failure rate of 3.9% (Pearl Index). All unintended pregnancies occurred in couples having intercourse in both the pre- and post-ovulatory phases. There were no pregnancies amongst the 36 couples who restricted intercourse to the post-ovulatory phase. Of the seven unintended pregnancies, three were user failures (couples knowingly broke rules) and four were method failures (couples followed the guidelines but still conceived). [382] Guidelines for both pre- and post-ovulatory intercourse are now more conservative, hence show increased effectiveness, but **couples who require the highest level of effectiveness may wish to restrict intercourse to the late infertile time (post-ovulatory)** (page 234).

SUMMARY: ROLE OF TEMPERATURE

A temperature chart:

- provides good presumptive evidence of ovulation;
- identifies the late infertile time as the most effective for avoiding pregnancy;
- identifies irregular cycles and the length of the pre- and post-ovulatory phases;
- identifies cycles with a short luteal phase (fewer than 10 raised temperatures);
- identifies monophasic cycles (absent temperature rise);
- identifies early pregnancy (raised temperature for 20 days or longer);
- helps to time investigations such as mid-luteal phase progesterone;
- highlights times of illness, stress or the impact of drugs;
- indicates the frequency and timing of intercourse; and
- can be used to monitor the effect of drugs used for ovulation induction.

There are both advantages and disadvantages to temperature charting – first the advantages:

- It is a simple, inexpensive, non-invasive and reliable method for confirming ovulation.
- It is easy to learn – readings are generally reliable even in the first cycle of charting.
- It is the least subjective of all the observed fertility indicators.
- It provides a visual sign for the woman, her partner and the health professional.
- It provides a reliable indicator at all stages of reproductive life.
- It is well-accepted by most women despite the commitment required.
- Experienced users can limit recordings to about 10 days of the cycle (figure 8.1).

The disadvantages of temperature are that:

- It requires an accurate thermometer and proper instruction.
- It requires a time commitment (both in teaching and for daily recording).
- It requires standardised conditions and a stable lifestyle.
- Factors such as disturbed sleep, illness or drugs may affect the readings.
- There is a risk of becoming too introspective (particularly for subfertile couples).
- There is a possibility of user error in recording or charting.
- There is a lack of standardised protocols for interpretation, hence inter-observer variation.

ANSWERS TO SELF-ASSESSMENT QUESTION

Cycle A Short cycle (21 days). Temperature rise on day 15. Adequate luteal phase (10+ raised temperatures). The first high temperature is on day 10 so the *3 over 6 rule* can be applied (rise occurs after day 8). This is a normal fertile cycle (likely to confirm ovulation).

Cycle B Average length cycle (28 days). Temperature rise on day 15. Adequate luteal phase. Normal fertile cycle.

Cycle C Long cycle (35 days). Temperature rise on day 22. Adequate luteal phase. Normal fertile cycle. This cycle demonstrates why a progesterone test to confirm ovulation would be inaccurate if taken as a routine "day 21 progesterone" as this occurs before the temperature rise, hence is likely to be pre-ovulation.

Cycle D Conception cycle. The temperature rise occurs on day 15. Temperature stays at a sustained high level for 20 days or longer. There is no following period. This is highly likely to indicate pregnancy.

Cycle E Short cycle (22 days). Temperature rise on day 15. Short luteal phase. There are fewer than 10 raised temperatures, so this is likely to indicate an infertile cycle as there is insufficient time for implantation.

Cycle F Average length cycle (27 days). There is no temperature rise in this monophasic cycle. If the temperature has been taken accurately and consistently, this could indicate anovulation.

CERVICAL SECRETIONS

5

Second indicator

All women have a right to understand their menstrual cycle. Women need to be able to distinguish between normal physiological secretions and abnormal vaginal discharge which may require prompt medical attention. The changes in cervical secretions provide the best prospective marker of the fertile time for women planning pregnancy. This knowledge may be of particular value for those with irregular cycles and for subfertile couples. Women who are using FAMs to avoid pregnancy observe changes in secretions as part of a combined-indicator method. Cervical secretions can be used as a single indicator, but couples must understand and accept the reduced effectiveness (page 134).

Note on terminology: The cervical/vaginal secretions a woman observes at the vulva comprise mucus from the columnar epithelium lining the cervical canal, endometrial secretions, and cellular sloughing of superficial squamous cells from the vaginal walls. The term "mucus" has negative connotations, being linked to nasal discharge, and translating in many languages as "phlegm" or "slime". Some use the term "cervical fluid" (female equivalent of seminal fluid with properties of sperm transport), but because the gel structure in question has semi-solid phases this term may be less appropriate at times. This mixture of substances which a woman observes will be referred to as "cervical secretions".

CHANGES IN CERVICAL SECRETIONS DURING THE CYCLE

Cervical secretions are produced continuously by the columnar epithelium lining the cervical canal, but the quantity and quality varies throughout the menstrual cycle under the influence of the ovarian hormones. Different types of secretion either encourage or impede sperm penetration and determine the state of fertility (see physiology section on page 61). This chapter focuses on cervical secretions as an indicator of fertility.

Figure 5.1 shows the effect of estrogen and progesterone on cervical secretions. It demonstrates the limited number of days when the secretions allow sperm penetration, with the mesh-type secretion preventing sperm penetration, and the parallel "swimming lanes" encouraging sperm penetration. The day of the cycle is not important: focusing on cycle days only adds confusion. If hospitable secretions are present, sperm can penetrate the cervical canal and survive in the female genital tract for up to seven days prior to ovulation. These days will be earlier in shorter cycles and later in longer cycles and will vary between women and from one cycle to the next.

A woman can conceive only on days when cervical secretions allow sperm penetration (the fertile time). There are a variable number of days prior to the start of the fertile time (early relatively infertile time) and a more constant number of days after the fertile time has ended (late infertile time).

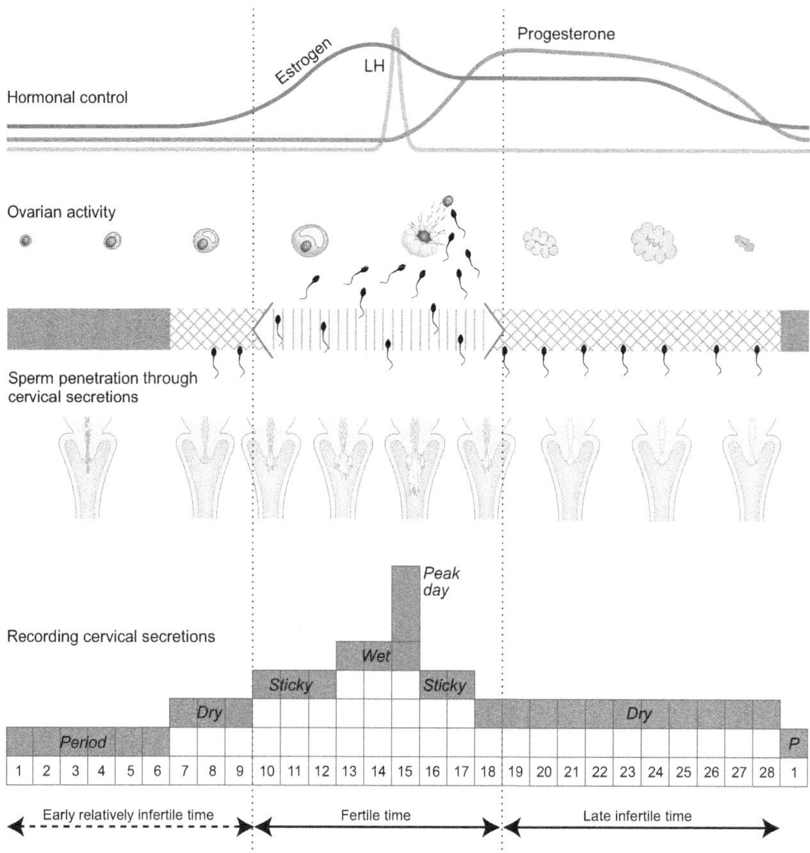

Figure 5.1 Changes in cervical secretions under hormonal control, demonstrating the fertile time when secretions allow sperm penetration (© Pyper & Knight, FertilityUK 2016)

Early relatively infertile time (pre-ovulation)

Following menstruation, there may be several dry days. These days may be absent from short cycles and numerous in long cycles. The woman is aware of a feeling of dryness or a positive sensation of nothingness at the vulva with no visible secretions. At this time estrogen levels are low and secretions at the cervix are sufficiently thick to prevent sperm penetration hence sperm are destroyed by the acidic vaginal environment.

Fertile time

As estrogen levels rise (reflecting increased follicular growth), the fluid content of the secretions increases and this is recognised at the vulva by a sensation of moistness or stickiness. There may be scant amounts of white or creamy-coloured sticky secretion which holds its shape due to its high cellular content (figure 5.2). This early secretion marks the start of the fertile time.

As the estrogen levels continue to rise, cervical secretions increase in amount, becoming wetter and cloudier in appearance, and slightly stretchy. As estrogen levels increase yet further, in the days approaching ovulation, the cervical secretions may be quite profuse with up to a

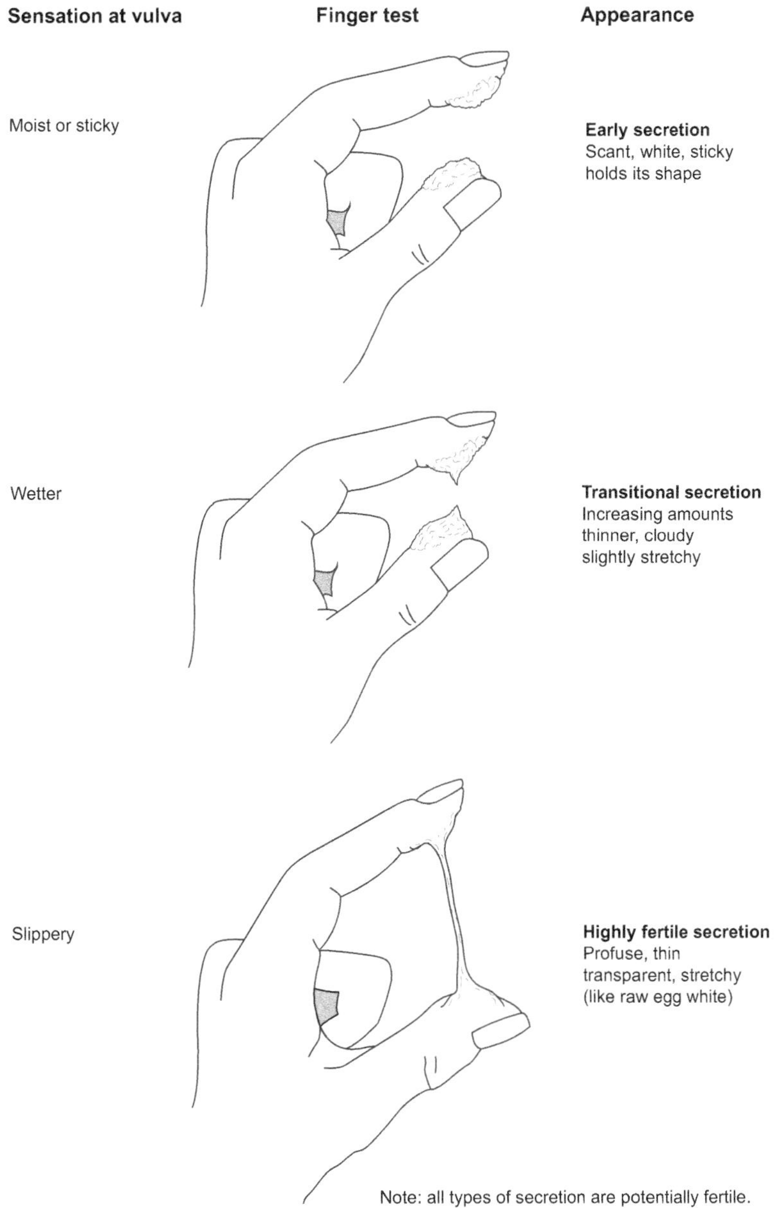

Figure 5.2 Characteristics of cervical secretions (reproduced with permission from Fertility, Clubb & Knight, D&C 1996)

ten-fold increase in volume. There will be a sensation of lubrication or slipperiness at the vulva. The appearance is similar to that of raw egg white: thin, watery and transparent. If stretched between the thumb and forefinger, it may stretch for several centimetres to form a thread before it breaks (the spinnbarkeit effect). Sperm move rapidly through these secretions, which provide the best prospective indicator for women trying to conceive. Not all women will be aware of the spinnbarkeit effect, observing only the increased wetness – this is quite normal.

Peak day is the last day of the wet, transparent, stretchy secretions. It can be recognized only retrospectively on the day following peak when the secretions have become sticky or dry again. Peak day correlates closely with ovulation and is so-called because it indicates maximum (peak) fertility during the menstrual cycle.

The fertile time starts at the first sign of secretions and ends three days after peak.

Late infertile time (post-ovulation)

Immediately after ovulation the increased progesterone causes the secretions to thicken again, forming a dense plug blocking the cervical canal and preventing sperm penetration. On the day after peak the slippery (lubricative) sensation is lost and there is a relatively abrupt return to stickiness or dryness again. Secretions at the vulva appear white and sticky and no longer stretchy.

COMPARING CERVICAL SECRETIONS WITH OBJECTIVE MARKERS

The changes in cervical secretions have been compared with objective markers of ovulation. Billings and Hilgers found that peak day correlated closely with LH, estradiol and progesterone. [51] [281] Fehring studied the relationship between peak day and urinary LH in 108 cycles with lengths ranging from 22 to 75 days (mean cycle length 29.4 days). Ninety-three of the cycles had both an identified peak day and an LH surge with 98% of the peak days occurring within ± four days of the LH surge. Fehring concluded that peak day very accurately identifies maximum fertility and fairly accurately identifies the day of ovulation and the end of the fertile time. [166]

In a study using serum LH and ultrasound, Depares found that the day of the *most abundant* (profuse) wetter transparent secretions correlated closely with the LH surge. Peak day occurred on or after ovulation (by ultrasound) in all of the cycles. [118] In Gnoth's study correlating the subjective indicators with urinary LH and ultrasound (total 87 cycles), peak day occurred within one day of objective ovulation in 82% of cycles and after ovulation in 21% (page 183). [230] [234]

Hormonal or ultrasonographic monitoring is cost-prohibitive in large population-based studies but, with simple written instructions, peak day can be used as an inexpensive method for estimating the day of ovulation/conception. A woman's subjective estimation of her peak day was compared with blinded daily hormone monitoring of estrone-3–glucuronide (E3G) and LH. The likely day of ovulation (± three days) was identified in 92% of cycles. It has been suggested that education about peak day may be appropriate as a marker for conception in studies of environmental exposure in very early pregnancy. [469]

WHO MULTI-CENTRE STUDY

A WHO multi-centre study of the Ovulation Method (cervical secretions as a single indicator) analysed 7,514 cycles from 725 women. WHO defined the fertile time as comprising any days on which cervical secretions were observed before peak day until three days after peak. The WHO study showed that:

- The average cycle length was 28.5 (± 3.18 days).
- The average length of the fertile time was 9.6 days (± 2.6 days).
- Peak day occurred on average on day 15 (± 2.6 days).

- The probability of pregnancy was maximal on peak day and declined on the days before and after peak. [617]
- Ninety-three percent of women were able to record an interpretable ovulatory pattern of cervical secretions in their first learning cycle. [615] [616]

MONITORING CHANGES IN CERVICAL SECRETIONS

There are three key stages to monitoring cervical secretions: **observing** the day-to-day changes, **recording** the characteristics on the chart and **interpreting** the pattern. The information gained can be used to plan or avoid pregnancy either as a single-indicator method or in combination with other indicators.

Observing cervical secretions

A woman is taught to recognise her cervical secretions by sensation (feeling at the vulva), appearance (colour) and by testing with the finger (consistency) (see figure 5.2):

Sensation Throughout the day, the presence or absence of secretions can be recognised by the feeling at the vulva in the same way that the beginning of a period is recognised. The sensation may be a distinct feeling of dryness, moistness (dampness), stickiness, wetness or slipperiness (lubrication). Sensation is important, but often the most difficult to learn; Kegel exercises can help (page 66). The woman is encouraged to alternately contract and relax her pelvic floor muscles periodically during the day. If there are no secretions present, the labia feel dry, giving a positive sensation of "nothingness"; sticky secretions give a sensation of moistness or stickiness; and wetter, slippery secretions give a sensation of lubrication as the labia slide apart smoothly.

Appearance The appearance of the secretions can be noted (mentally) each time the woman goes to the toilet. After urinating, soft white toilet tissue is used to wipe the vulva (from front to back). There may be a patch of dampness only on the tissue resulting from urine or normal vaginal moisture – this soaks into the tissue. Any cervical secretions will appear as a raised blob and the colour can be noted: white, creamy-coloured, translucent (opaque, cloudy) or transparent. Cervical secretions may be observed on underwear, where it will have dried causing some alteration in its characteristics, notably colour.

Finger-testing A finger-tip can be lightly applied to the secretion on the tissue and pulled away gently to test its capacity to stretch. The secretion may feel sticky and break easily, or it may feel smoother and slippery like raw egg white, stretching between the thumb and forefinger from a little up to about 20 cm – the spinnbarkeit effect.

The woman needs a consistent approach to monitoring the changes in her cervical secretions:

- The cervical secretions are observed at intervals throughout the day (at least three times a day – morning, noon and night) and recorded on the chart in the evening. This allows time for changes to become apparent during the day.
- If a woman is finding difficulty recognising secretions externally, advise her that they are often more noticeable after exercise, after a bowel movement, by using Kegel exercises or a slight bearing-down action.
- The amount and quality of secretions will vary from woman to woman and from one cycle to the next. A woman who is using cervical secretions as an indicator to avoid pregnancy needs to be alert to changes in sensation and to relatively small amounts of secretion.
- Most women can observe secretions externally, but if this is proving difficult, and the woman is comfortable with the idea, she can check by touching inside her vagina.
- Some women will be aware of a sensation of moistness, stickiness, wetness or slipperiness at the vulva but not necessarily observe any secretions. Sensation alone still indicates the presence of secretions.

- Women who monitor the changes in their cervix may find it easier to draw some secretions directly from the cervix, using the forefinger and middle finger.
- Every woman will find what works best for her, but the key thing is a consistent routine of checking.

Recording cervical secretions on the chart

A blank chart for recording secretions as a single indicator is included in appendix C. It includes an example chart, instructions for use and space to record four menstrual cycles. This is ideal for women who are planning pregnancy, whereas women using FAMs to avoid pregnancy should ideally record a combination of indicators on the combined chart (appendix A).

The characteristics of the secretions are recorded on the chart using shading in the appropriate box (figure 5.3). Box 1 for period, 2 for dry, 3 for moist white sticky and 4 for wet slippery and stretchy. Note the heavier line between box 2 (dry) and box 3 (moist) – this denotes the change from the early relatively infertile time to the start of the fertile time. As soon as there is any shading above the heavier line (i.e. the woman no longer feels dry) the fertile time has started. The woman is instructed as follows:

- The first day of the period (fresh red bleed) is day 1 of the cycle. Shade the box labelled "**Period**" (box 1).
- Each day of bleeding is marked by shading in the appropriate box. Heavier bleeding can be shown by solid shading whilst lighter bleeding or spotting can be shown by dots in the appropriate box.
- Each day when there is a dry sensation at the vulva (no secretions seen or felt) is marked in the box labelled "**Dry**" (box 2).
- Each day when there is a moist sensation with white or cloudy sticky secretions is marked in the box labelled "**Moist, white, cloudy, sticky**" (box 3).
- Each day when there is a wet or slippery sensation with transparent, stretchy secretions is marked in the top box labelled "**Wet, slippery, transparent, stretchy**" (box 4).
- **Peak day** is the *last* day when wet, slippery, transparent stretchy secretions are present (last day in box 4). It is not necessarily the day of the most profuse secretions, which frequently occurs one to two days before peak. Peak day is known only in retrospect when on the day following peak there is a change back to thick, white, sticky secretions again, or to complete dryness (change from box 4 to box 3 or 2). Peak is the *last* day when *any* characteristic would fit into box 4 (whether by sensation, appearance or finger-test). When peak day has been identified, the shading is extended upwards to highlight peak and to correlate with the temperature readings when using combined indicators.
- Each act of **intercourse** is marked by circling the appropriate day. Some couples may prefer not to record all intercourse. For couples avoiding pregnancy, the most significant intercourse acts to mark are the last intercourse before and the first after the fertile time – this helps to ensure that the guidelines are clearly understood. Couples planning pregnancy should mark all intercourse acts, particularly during the fertile time to ensure appropriate timing.
- **The day after intercourse** is marked as a "wet" day by putting a "X" in box 3. This is a non-intercourse day as seminal fluid could be masking secretions (figure 5.4).

In practice, the changes in secretions may not be well-defined. There may be a combination of more than one type of secretion: for example, cloudy secretions with some transparent stretchy secretions. The secretion possessing the more fertile characteristics (transparent stretchy) should be recorded, so effectively always shade the box with the higher number.

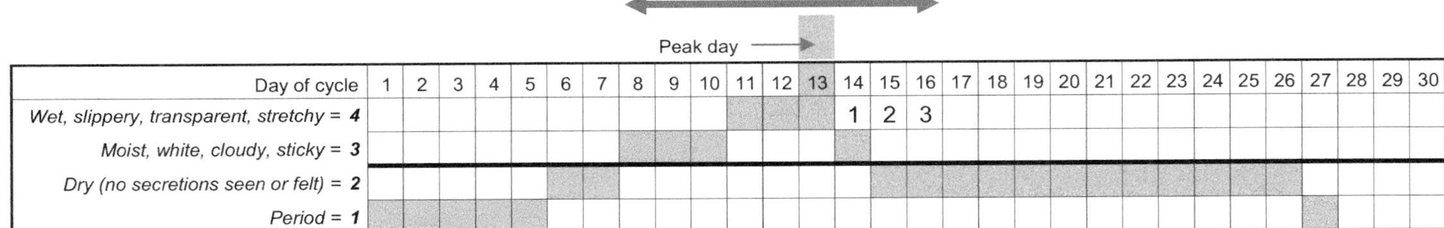

Figure 5.3 Typical pattern of cervical secretions throughout the menstrual cycle: period, early dry days, secretions with increasingly fertile characteristics approaching peak day, abrupt change back to less fertile characteristics, count of three after peak and dry days approaching the next period.

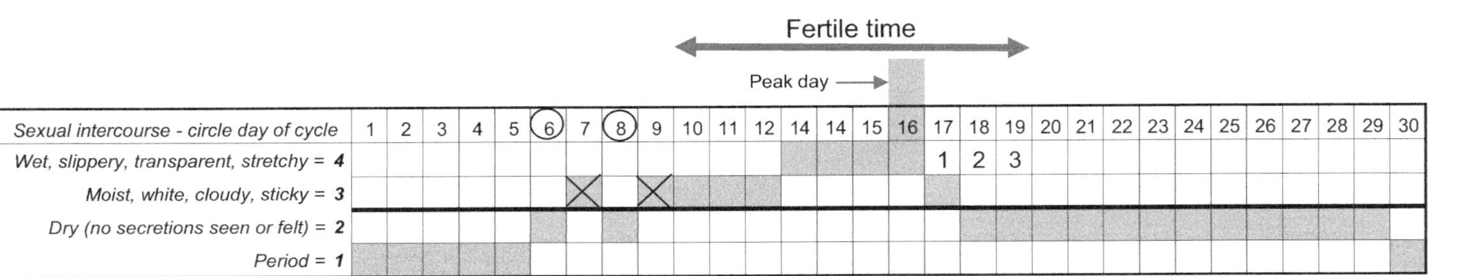

Figure 5.4 Recording a “wet” day the day after intercourse (note “X” in box 3)

Typical pattern of secretions throughout the menstrual cycle

The typical pattern of secretions comprises the period, early dry days, start of secretions with build-up to highly fertile secretions, peak day, the distinct change after peak and the dry days leading up to the next period.

Early dry days, start of secretions and build-up to peak day Figure 5.3 shows a typical pattern of cervical secretions throughout the cycle. This comprises a five-day period (box 1). Days 6 and 7 are dry (box 2). Day 8 is marked as moist, white, cloudy secretions (box 3) – this is the first sign of fertility (above the heavier black line). Days 9 and 10 still have sticky white secretions. By day 11, the secretions show more highly fertile characteristics: wetter, slippery and stretchy, so are marked in the top box (box 4). Days 12 and 13 are also marked in box 4. On day 14 there is a change back to sticky white secretions again (box 3) hence day 13 is peak day (the last day showing the most fertile characteristics). The shading on peak day is extended vertically upwards (chimney effect) and correlated with the temperature rise in a combined-indicator method.

Change after peak, *count of three* and days leading to next period The days after peak are numbered 1, 2, 3 (the *count of three)*. If the numbers are written in white space in box 4, this ensures that any other post-peak secretions are in box 3 or below. The fertile time ends three full days after peak day. Note the upward trend in the secretion pattern approaching peak day and the downward trend following peak. In this chart, the fertile time starts on day 8 (the first sign of *any* secretions), and the fertile time ends three days after peak day on day 16. This is shown by the fertile time arrow extending from day 8 until day 16 inclusive. The next period starts on day 27, hence this is a 26-day cycle.

Recording a "wet" day the day after intercourse in early dry days

Intercourse is marked on the chart by circling the appropriate day. In the early dry days, intercourse is restricted to the evenings to allow time for the woman to observe for any changes throughout the day. New users who are learning FAMs to avoid pregnancy should mark the day after intercourse as "wet" because of the difficulty with distinguishing cervical secretions from seminal fluid. This is necessary only during the early dry days when the first change from dryness is anticipated. The day after intercourse is marked with an "X" in box 3 as the origin of the moistness is unknown. A day marked with an "X" is a non-intercourse day. Couples should avoid intercourse on consecutive evenings until the woman feels confident she can observe the earliest change from dryness. A calculation to double-check the start of the fertile time is always advisable (page 155).

In the chart shown in figure 5.4, intercourse occurs on the evening of day 6. Day 7 is therefore marked as "wet" (a non-intercourse day). On day 8, after observing all day, the woman still feels dry so has intercourse again in the evening (a non-consecutive/alternate day), hence marks day 9 as "wet". By day 10 she is aware of a sensation of moistness during the day, but as there was no intercourse the evening before, this is the first sign of secretions – the fertile time has started. Peak day occurs on day 16 (note the change back to less fertile characteristics on day 17). In the *count of three* days post peak there are no further secretions marked in box 4 so the fertile time ends on day 19. The couple can then have unrestricted intercourse from day 20 until the start of the next period on day 30. Women who combine FAMs with barrier methods need to be able to distinguish between cervical secretions and spermicide (page 233).

Variations in pattern of cervical secretions

There are a number of normal variations on the typical pattern of secretions. These vary from woman to woman and from one cycle to the next.

Secretions immediately after period: no early dry days In some cycles, the secretions start immediately after the period, and may even be noticed during the period: this is more common in short cycles. There will be no dry early dry days, hence no relatively infertile days. Figure 5.5

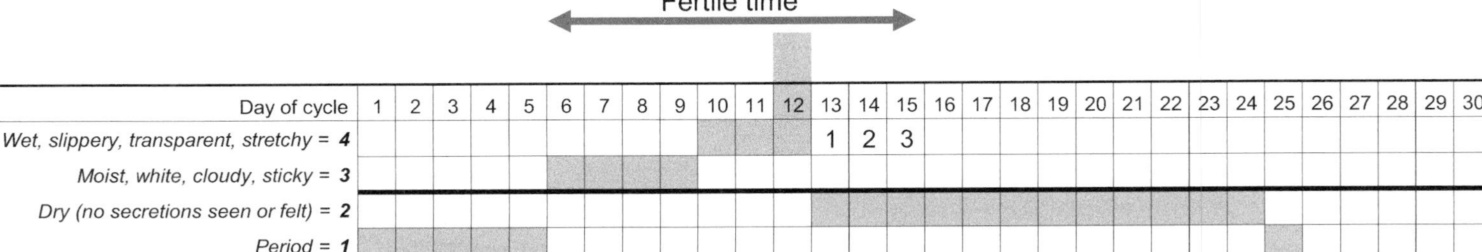

Figure 5.5 Start of secretions immediately after the period with no early dry days: 24 day cycle. Fertile time: days 6–15 inclusive.

shows a short cycle of 24 days with sticky white secretions starting on day 6 immediately after the period. The secretions are recorded in box 3 so the fertile time has started. Note peak day on day 12. The day after peak, there is an abrupt return to dryness. The count of three after peak is clearly written (in box 4). The fertile time arrow extends from day 6 until day 15 inclusive.

Couples who are trying to conceive often miss days of fertility if they have short cycles or the secretions start during or immediately after a period. Women tend to ignore those days, believing it to be "too early". It is important to get across the message about sperm survival: the secretions do not mean that the woman is ovulating on day 5 or 6, but if there are any cervical secretions, sperm can survive for up to a week.

Premenstrual secretions In the luteal phase of the cycle, due to the effect of progesterone, there may be continued dryness until the start of the next period (figure 5.5), but it is very common for women to observe several days of secretions (sometimes showing highly fertile characteristics) in the days approaching the next period. This is related to the falling progesterone levels, which result in a slight rise in estrogen. Any premenstrual secretions can be disregarded: they are not related to fertility and are of no practical significance. Couples who are avoiding pregnancy will feel more confident if it is apparent that the secretions are occurring towards the end of the high temperature phase (figure 5.6).

Interrupted pattern and multiple peaks Stress can have a disruptive effect on the menstrual cycle, delaying or suppressing ovulation. This can result in an interrupted pattern of secretions and more than one peak day. If there is more than one peak, ovulation does not occur until after the final peak. Waiting for the rise in temperature confirms the likely occurrence of ovulation and the end of the fertile time. There may be several attempts at ovulation, shown by the interrupted pattern of secretions reflecting fluctuating estrogen levels. Follicles may be developing, with estrogen levels increasing but not reaching the required threshold to trigger the LH surge and ovulation. This commonly occurs in women with PCOS, women who are breastfeeding (but reducing feeds), and in some women with long cycles (page 205).

Variations in peak day

Peak day may vary in the following ways:

- The change after peak may vary. There may be a distinct change to dryness (boxes 4 to 2) or a change to less fertile characteristics (boxes 4 to 3) with continued secretions. Provided there has been a distinct change, the peak day has passed and the count of three starts. During the three days after peak, if there is a return to *any* characteristics which would indicate higher quality secretions again, then peak day has not passed and the woman must continue to observe until she has had a distinctive peak. The fertile time is not over until she has had three full days after peak.
- Peak day normally occurs one to two days before the temperature rise, although this can vary. If peak day occurs on the day of the temperature rise or after the rise, to avoid pregnancy the user needs to wait until there are three high temperatures after peak day (guidelines: page 227).
- If there is no clearer, wetter, stretchy secretion then peak day will be the last day when the highest quality secretion is observed: for example, the secretions may change from sticky white to dry and the change from box 3 to box 2 would signal peak day. This may become normal for some women (for example, older women who have less of the highly fertile secretions) but exercise caution as this could be a disrupted pattern (for example, due to stress).

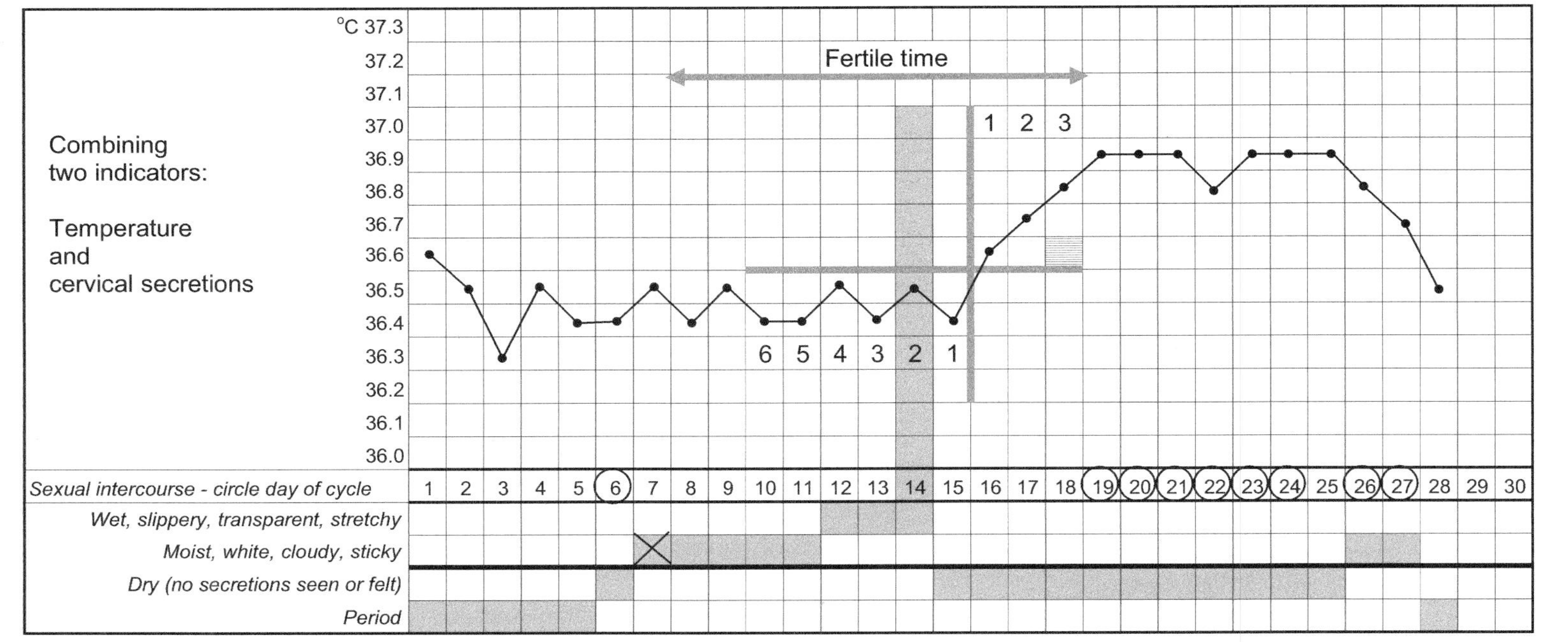

Figure 5.6 Correlating temperature and secretions on the combined chart. This shows a 27-day cycle with peak on day 14 and temperature rise following peak on day 16. The fertile time lasts from day 8 to 18.

ACTIVITY CHART-BUILDING EXERCISE (CONTINUED FROM PAGE 98)

Step 2 Recording the cervical secretions

1 The box labelled "Period" should by now have shading in days 1–5 and day 30 denoting the days of bleeding.
2 Shade in the appropriate boxes to show the changes in Jo's cervical secretions.
   a Days 6, 7, 8 and 9 are experienced as "Dry" (no secretions seen or felt).
   b Days 10, 11 and 12 are moist with white, cloudy, sticky secretions.
   c Days 13, 14 and 15 are wetter with clear, slippery, stretchy secretions.
   d Days 16, 17 and 18 have sticky white secretions.
   e Days 19–29 are dry.
   f Jo's period starts on day 30.

Set this exercise aside for now. To be continued on page 148.

GUIDELINES FOR ACHIEVING AND AVOIDING PREGNANCY

Cervical secretions provide the best prospective indicator of the fertile time for achieving pregnancy. Secretions can be used alone as a single-indicator method for avoiding pregnancy, but evidence clearly shows increased effectiveness when used in combination with a calculation to identify the start of the fertile time and temperature to identify the end of the fertile time.

Achieving pregnancy: optimising chances of conception

A woman who wishes to optimise her chances of pregnancy should understand that:

- Intercourse on any day when wet, transparent, slippery, stretchy secretions are present carries a high chance of pregnancy.
- The day with the most profuse secretions correlates closely with ovulation – this frequently precedes peak by one or two days.
- Peak day and the two days preceding peak are the days of maximum fertility.

Note: Secretions that show highly fertile characteristics are not always associated with ovulation; they are purely a reflection of estrogen levels. For example: women with PCOS who are not ovulating will still observe wetter secretions, often observing persistent and fluctuating transparent, stretchy secretions, but with reduced stretch (page 210).

Avoiding pregnancy using cervical secretions as a single indicator

A couple who are avoiding pregnancy using cervical secretions only should understand that:

- Intercourse must be avoided during a period (or any bleeding/spotting).
- Intercourse should be restricted to the evenings on non-consecutive early dry days.
- The day after intercourse is marked with an "X" to denote a "wet" day.
- The fertile time starts at the first sign of any secretions.
- The fertile time ends three full days after peak day.
- Intercourse is unrestricted from the fourth day after peak until the start of the next period.

It is always advisable to use a combination of indicators to increase the effectiveness of the method for avoiding pregnancy (page 124).

Combining temperature and secretions

Changes in secretions can be correlated with temperature readings on the combined chart. Each indicator is interpreted independently and then the two are combined. When combining temperature and cervical secretions:

- Intercourse must be avoided during a period (or any bleeding/spotting).
- Intercourse is restricted to the evenings on non-consecutive early dry days.
- The fertile time starts at the first sign of any secretions.
- The fertile time ends after the third high temperature past peak day (ensuring the third high reading is at least 0.2 deg.C above the highest of the six low readings).

Figure 5.6 (page 127) shows a chart from a couple who are avoiding pregnancy. The five-day period is followed by a dry day on day 6. Intercourse on the evening of day 6 (allowing all day to observe for any change from dryness) means that day 7 is marked as a non-intercourse "wet" day. On day 8 the woman experiences a moist feeling and observes scant amounts of white secretions, so the fertile time has started. The secretions build up to peak day. The distinct change to dryness on day 15 confirms day 14 as peak. Note the vertical shading extending upwards so that peak day can be correlated with the temperature.

The first high temperature is on day 16. The third high temperature on day 18 is at least 0.2 deg.C above the highest of the low-phase temperatures (demonstrated by the hatched area above the coverline). All three high temperatures occur after peak day, so the fertile time ends on day 18. Combining cervical secretions and temperature, the fertile time starts on day 8 and ends on day 18 (the fertile time arrow extends from day 8 to 18 inclusive).

The couple are now free to have unrestricted intercourse in the late infertile time – from day 19 until the start of the next period on day 28. Note the presence of premenstrual secretions on days 26 and 27. These are likely to be related to hormonal fluctuations and are not related to fertility. As the woman has recorded a distinct peak day which correlates with her temperature rise, the end of the fertile time was confirmed by at least two indicators and the rest of the cycle is infertile. The secretions on days 26 and 27 can be disregarded. Women should be reassured that after the fertile time has ended any secretions can be ignored – and to avoid confusion are often best unrecorded.

NEW USERS

At the first FA session, a woman is instructed in how to *observe* and *record* the changes in her secretions (usually in combination with temperature). A couple who are using FAMs to avoid pregnancy should not attempt to interpret indicators at this stage. A follow-up appointment is needed to *interpret* the chart and to start the process of putting the user in control of making her own interpretations: this can take 3–6 cycles.

Couples who are using FAMs to avoid pregnancy should avoid intercourse completely during the first cycle to allow the woman to observe her secretions without confusion from seminal fluid. If she can recognise a normal pattern of secretions in the first cycle, then intercourse can be resumed in the second cycle following the guidelines for avoiding pregnancy. It can take several cycles for a woman to be aware of the first change from dryness (first sensation of moistness) and to distinguish between different types of secretions, particularly to feel confident with identifying peak day and the change after peak.

Women's ability to detect changes in secretions

The majority of women can detect the characteristic changes in secretions. Roetzer's study of 180 women (3,542 cycles) showed that 90% could determine their fertile time by observing cervical secretions, but he advised that couples wishing to avoid pregnancy should combine secretions with temperature to increase the effectiveness. [505] The WHO multi-centre study of the Ovulation Method (cervical secretions alone) reported that out of 869 women 93% could detect secretion changes. Most women needed to observe their secretions for about three cycles before recognizing the changes with confidence. [615]

DIFFICULTIES WITH MONITORING CERVICAL SECRETIONS

Despite one-to-one teaching some women have difficulty using cervical secretions as an indicator of fertility. The woman may have:

- a normal pattern of secretions but difficulty observing, recording or interpreting the changes;
- changes in the quality, quantity or timing of cervical secretions;
- difficulties caused by confusion from other substances (e.g. seminal fluid, spermicide or lubricants);
- a confusing pattern of secretions caused by minor allergies (e.g. to bath products);
- an interrupted pattern or double peak (commonly due to stress);
- an abnormal vaginal discharge (e.g. candida) masking a normal pattern of secretions;
- menstrual disturbance and disrupted ovulation due to illness;
- an abnormal pattern of secretions due to a gynaecological condition (e.g. cervical ectropion); or
- a disturbed pattern of secretions due to medication (e.g. drying effect of antihistamines).

Table 5.1 provides a checklist for managing the client who is having difficulty distinguishing changes in secretions. The first thing to establish is the woman's monitoring technique.

Table 5.1 Managing difficulties with distinguishing changes in cervical secretions

Management of the woman with difficulties distinguishing changes in cervical secretions	
Observing secretions	**Monitoring technique for cervical secretions** – Is the woman's checking routine consistent? – Is she checking at least three times during the course of the day? – Is she considering sensation, appearance and finger-test? – Consider the use of Kegel exercises to increase awareness of sensation. – Is she checking on white toilet tissue/fingers/underwear? Is this consistent? – Is she varying her observations between internal and external monitoring? – Discuss her options and advise her to maintain a consistent routine. – Is she able to identify the first change from dryness? – Is she able to identify peak day (last day with the most fertile characteristics)?
Recording secretions	– Is she recording her secretions in the evening after observing all day? – Are the recordings on the chart legible in black pen? – Is she recording her observations clearly by shading in the appropriate box? – Is she shading in more than one box? – Remind her to record the secretions showing the most fertile characteristics only. – Is she identifying the first day of secretions (first day above the heavier black line)? – Is she using vertical shading for peak day? – Is she adding the *count of three* after peak day?

Interpreting secretions	– Is she is using an appropriate calendar-based calculation as a back-up to identify the start of the fertile time (change from dryness) if avoiding pregnancy? – Is she able to identify peak day? – Is she aware of earlier days with more abundant secretions? – Avoiding pregnancy: is she combining her observations with temperature to identify the end of the fertile time? – Is this an uninterpretable chart? If so, mark it clearly: *uninterpretable chart.* Women must accept that they will not always be able to identify the fertile and infertile times of the cycle. If the observations or recordings are unclear or the rules do not fit – the chart cannot be interpreted.
Amount and type of secretions will vary	**Quantity and quality of secretions** – Ask the woman to use her own words to describe her secretions. – Consider how her description fits with the boxes on the chart. – Some cycles will have more secretions than others due to hormonal fluctuations. – Older women will tend to have less cervical secretions. – Some subfertile women may have reduced quantity or quality secretions.
Persistent secretions	– A continuous and sometimes profuse pattern of secretions with no dry days may be due to a cervical ectropion (mucus-secreting columnar epithelium extending out through the cervical os).
Vaginal secretions	**Confusion with other fluids: the glass of water test** The vagina is naturally moist with secretions. It may be difficult to discern the difference between cervical secretions, other vaginal secretions and fluids such as semen, spermicide and artificial lubricants. One significant characteristic of cervical secretions is that they are insoluble in water. – Advise the woman to test the solubility of the secretion by inserting two fingers containing it into a glass of water: Mucilaginous secretions from the cervix will form a blob, dropping to the bottom of the glass whereas vaginal secretions will disperse. Some women may notice a string of secretions in the toilet bowl or in bath water.
Seminal fluid	Seminal fluid is viscous (gluey) and slightly rubbery. It breaks easily and dries more quickly than egg-white-type cervical secretions. – Advise the woman to do Kegel exercises after intercourse in the early dry days. This will expel seminal fluid making it easier to discern changes in cervical secretions. A woman who gains sufficient confidence in detecting subtle changes may not need to restrict intercourse to alternate dry evenings. A calendar calculation is always advisable as a back-up to identify the start of the fertile time.
Arousal fluid	Most women are aware of when they are sexually aroused, but arousal fluid might affect her observations, so explain that: – Arousal fluid is transparent and quite slippery but, unlike estrogenised cervical secretions, it has no stretch and will disperse in water. It is not possible to detect changes in secretions at times of sexual arousal.
Spermicide	Women who are combining FA with barrier methods may be confused by the effects of spermicidal gels. – Discuss the appearance and characteristics of the gel to ascertain any effect.

(*Continued*)

Table 5.1 (Continued)

Management of the woman with difficulties distinguishing changes in cervical secretions	
Vaginal lubricants	Vaginal lubricants, by definition, give a lubricative sensation. They are normally transparent and can be confused with cervical secretions. – Ask the woman about the use and timing of lubricants. – Women who are trying to conceive should be cautious about lubricants as some can be spermicidal.
Underwear and tight clothing	**Susceptibility to infection, skin sensitivity and allergic reactions** Warm, moist conditions provide a breeding ground for fungal and bacterial infections. – Advise breathable all-cotton pants as they are cooler and more absorbent. – Avoid nylon underwear, tights and restrictive clothing. – Avoid thongs because they provide a direct route for infections (such as E. coli) to pass from the rectum to the vagina and urethra, thereby increasing the risk of recurrent candidiasis (thrush) and cystitis.
Sanitary products	Excessive use of tampons results in vaginal dryness and increases the risk of thrush. If the flow is very light the tampon absorbs the natural vaginal moisture and the normal flora. This can cause a reactive discharge from the vaginal walls. – Is the woman using the appropriate absorbency for her menstrual flow? – Does she put in a tampon "just in case" if she is expecting a period? – Is she using pads excessively between periods? Sanitary towels and pads (even mini-pads) absorb secretions and may be chafing, causing a reactive discharge. Advise cotton pants and, if necessary, changing pants in the middle of the day.
Bath products	Scented and coloured soaps may cause sensitivity or allergic reactions of the delicate vulval skin. – Advise baby soap or simple, non-allergic soaps, shower gels and bath products. – Avoid talcum powders, vaginal deodorants and douches as they may affect the pH balance of the vagina and destroy the normal lactic acid-producing bacteria.
Washing powders	Washing powders (particularly biological) can cause sensitivity or allergic reactions. – Has she changed her washing powder recently? Advise non-biological powders and laundry products.
Interrupted pattern of secretions	**Effects of stress** Stress can delay or suppress ovulation and consequently cause disruptions to the normal pattern of cervical secretions. Temperature helps to clarify the situation. Consider whether the woman's chart shows: – a longer cycle; – an interrupted build-up to peak day (with return to dryness or secretions with less fertile characteristics; – a shorter time from peak day to the next period;
Double peak	– more than one peak day; or – a continuous pattern of dryness. Stress can lead to a suppressed immune system which affects both vaginal and general health. It may also increase the risk of candida (thrush).
Signs of infection	**Abnormal vaginal discharge** A woman who is aware of her normal pattern of secretions should be alert to any change which may indicate an abnormal (pathological) vaginal discharge. Warning signs of infection include: – a change in the colour or consistency of the secretions; – an excessive amount of secretions; – an offensive odour;

- vulval itching, redness or soreness; or
- unusual vaginal bleeding.

Abnormal discharges

Consider the possibility of sexually or non-sexually transmissible infections if the woman complains of:

- a watery or white cheesy discharge with intense itching and soreness and possibly a slightly yeasty smell – suspect candida (common after antibiotics or when the immune system is suppressed);
- a white or grey fishy-smelling discharge (particularly after intercourse) with no itching or irritation – suspect bacterial vaginosis (BV) – an imbalance of the normal vaginal bacteria (often as a reaction to scented bath products); or
- a green, yellow or frothy discharge with fishy smell, soreness, swelling and itching at the vulva with painful urination – suspect trichomonas (sexually transmissible).

Discourage self-diagnosis

Any sign of change from a normal pattern of secretions should be investigated and treated. Women should be discouraged from self-medicating, for example, with over-the-counter antifungal treatments because self-diagnosis may not be accurate.

Sexually and non-STIs

Symptoms of sexually and non-sexually transmissible infections are diverse. Some infections are accompanied by vaginal discharge, but with others the symptoms may be absent, short-lived or subtle. For example: chlamydia, a common STI (and significant cause of tubal infertility), can mimic cystitis or cause menstrual disturbance without any associated vaginal discharge.

Susceptibility to candida

A number of factors make women more susceptible to candida including pregnancy, diabetes, antibiotic use, clothing, hygiene practices and stress. Consider:

- Is the woman in good general health?
- Does she have a healthy work/life balance?
- Is she eating a balanced diet?

Some women with recurrent thrush benefit from a diet low in sugar and refined carbohydrates. Probiotic yogurts may be beneficial.

General illness

Illness

General illness can delay or suppress ovulation and disrupt the pattern of secretions.

- Ask the woman to indicate the duration of illness on the chart.
- Anticipate that there could be a variety of menstrual disturbances and changes in cervical secretions depending on the illness (and associated medication). The secretions may appear at unexpected times with changes in quality or quantity.

Gynaecological conditions

Cervical ectropion

- A persistent, and often profuse, pattern of secretions with few or no dry days may indicate a cervical ectropion.

PCOS

- Long cycles, an interrupted pattern of secretions, reduced spinnbarkeit and multiple peak days may indicate polycystic ovaries.

Medication

Over-the-counter and prescribed drugs

- Ask about the use (and timing) of medication including over-the-counter drugs.
- Is there a drying effect (e.g. over-the-counter antihistamines for hay fever)?
- Is there an increased amount of secretions (e.g. expectorant cough mixtures)?
- Is there a disrupted pattern?
- Consider the possibility of thrush related to antibiotic use.
- Consider the possible teratogenic effect if the woman is at risk of pregnancy

She may have a problem with observing, recording or interpreting the changes. If she is having difficulty observing secretions externally, she may be more successful if she monitors secretions directly from her cervix, with or without additional cervical palpation (page 148).

In chapter 12 the effects of stress, drugs, abnormal vaginal discharge and cervical ectropion plus other women's health issues are discussed alongside other factors which affect the menstrual cycle. For a list of drugs which affect the menstrual cycle see appendix G.

Women may be particularly susceptible to unintended pregnancies at times of stress and at any time that there is disruption to the menstrual cycle. If the pattern of secretions is significantly disturbed the chart may not be interpretable. This should be clearly stated and marked on the chart, e.g. *Uninterpretable: disrupted pattern of secretions.*

CERVICAL SECRETIONS AS A SINGLE-INDICATOR METHOD

The following discussion on single-indicator methods is included for completeness. Couples using FAMs will come across different methodologies or may be using one of these methods and feel dissatisfied. It is not uncommon in clinical practice to see women who have had an unintended pregnancy after being taught cervical secretions as a single-indicator method. Although women generally accept the pregnancy, this can put pressures on the relationship and economic pressures on the family. On checking their fertility knowledge and analysing their charts, it is often easy to see why conception may have occurred and for couples to see that with the additional checks offered by a combined indicator approach, pregnancy may have been avoided.

NFP teaching and Catholic philosophy

NFP has a long association with Catholicism and has been viewed by many as a "Catholic method". The Catholic Church's opposition to contraception dates back to the first century and is based on the teaching that all sexual acts must be open to life. In 1968 Pope Paul VI's encyclical *Humanae Vitae* reaffirmed the orthodox teaching of the Catholic Church and the continued prohibition on contraception. Many Catholic doctors responded to the Pope's call for more research in natural methods. Throughout the late 1960s and early 1970s most researchers were establishing the scientific credibility of combined indicator approaches, but others concentrated on single-indicator methods, using their own names to distinguish their particular method.

The knowledge base of physiological methods was greatly increased, but unfortunately alongside scientific progress NFP has remained largely connected to the Catholic Church with many organisations actively discrediting contraception. Instruction, particularly in methods which rely on cervical secretions alone, is often accompanied by the Church's teaching and aimed at Catholic married couples with insistence on abstinence during the fertile time. The religious orientation may or may not be appreciated.

Billings Ovulation Method

John and Evelyn Billings developed the methodology for using cervical secretions as a method of family planning in the early 1970s (timeline: table 1.1). They reported their findings in the *Lancet* in 1972 defining the main features of the pattern of secretions:

- Menstrual bleeding is followed by a variable number of days on which no vaginal loss is present (dry days).
- The onset of the mucus symptom is characterised by the appearance of increasing quantities of cloudy or sticky secretion; the duration of this phase is variable.

- This is followed by the occurrence of clear, slippery, lubricative mucus having the physical characteristics of raw white of egg (spinnbarkeit): this has been termed the "peak symptom". It characteristically lasts for one to two days and the last day of its occurrence is referred to as the day of the peak symptom (peak day).
- The peak symptom is followed by the presence of thick, tacky, opaque mucus, the duration of which is variable.

Guidelines To avoid pregnancy, women were instructed to abstain from intercourse from the *onset* of the mucus symptoms. Sexual activity could be resumed on the fourth day after the peak symptom. Couples trying to conceive were advised to concentrate their efforts on the days of the peak symptom.

Comparison of cervical secretions with objective markers The Billings compared women's observations of secretions with plasma LH, urinary estrogen and pregnanediol. They studied 22 Catholic women of proven fertility (between one and seven children) with cycles of 22–35 days. Peak day occurred in five women on the day of ovulation, in nine women one day before ovulation and in four women two days before ovulation. The temperature rise occurred one to two days after ovulation. Ovulation occurred an average of 0.9 days after peak day. The mean interval from the first sign of cervical secretions was 6.2 days before the estimated time of ovulation (range 3 to 10 days). The Billings concluded that the widespread application of the method required effectiveness studies in which women were taught to recognise their cervical secretions. [51]

Billings coloured stamp system The Billings introduced a system of coloured stamps for recording secretions: red for bleeding, white (with a picture of a baby) for wet secretions (fertile days) and green for dryness (infertile days). The original guidelines recommended that *any* secretions were potentially fertile. In 1973 they introduced a yellow stamp to indicate an "infertile pattern" of secretions. This was recommended for use by women with an unchanging pattern of secretions such as with very long cycles or during breastfeeding. [50] Within a short time early sticky white or cloudy secretions were being referred to generally as "infertile-type" secretions in the same category as dryness. This has caused considerable confusion. Many practitioners still teach in this way, hence putting women at risk of pregnancy.

> *Note:* **For women of normal fertility *any* pre-ovulatory secretions are potentially fertile** whatever their characteristics – only true dryness can be regarded as *relatively* infertile. The situation is different during breastfeeding, when a woman's ovaries may be relatively inactive for several months. A breastfeeding woman can be taught to recognise a BIP of secretions (an unchanging day-to-day pattern for at least two weeks) (page 276).

International teaching The Billings have taught their method to married couples with large-scale international teaching programmes and the method is still in widespread use. The Billings Ovulation Method (BOM) has a Catholic affiliation and accepts the use of NFP with abstinence only. The Billings philosophy differs from that of other methods when categorising pregnancy intention. Claims for the effectiveness of BOM have caused considerable controversy amongst the scientific community. For further information on BOM visit the Billings Life site: http://billings.life/en/.

Creighton model fertility care and NaProTechnology

In the mid-1970s Hilgers, an American gynaecologist, worked with the Billings' team in Australia before introducing the method into the US. Hilgers' independent investigation of the Billings system led him to develop a more standardised approach to teaching, grading different types of secretion according to sensation, colour and consistency. This rigorous checking and more detailed recording system, originally called the *Hilgers Method*, was renamed the *Creighton Model Fertility Care system* (CrM) in1977 after Hilgers moved to Creighton University. [284] In 1985, Hilgers established the Pope Paul VI Institute for the Study of Human Reproduction as a memorial to the late pope. CrM is seen as the family planning component of *NaProTechnology* (Natural Procreative Technology), a system that Hilgers terms a "new women's health science". NaProTechnology aims to monitor and maintain a woman's reproductive and gynaecological health, providing medical and surgical treatments that work with a woman's reproductive system and are endorsed by the Catholic Church. [280] As with BOM the use of other contraceptive methods is prohibited. Instruction is therefore generally limited to married Catholic couples who wish to use NFP with abstinence in accordance with the Church's teaching. For further information visit the Pope Paul VI Institute website: www.popepaulvi.com.

Note: many authorities would agree that this level of detail about the characteristics of secretions serves little practical purpose for most users and is unnecessary for women who combine indicators.

Marquette Model

The *Marquette Model* (MM), developed at Marquette University in the late 1990s, combines the observation of secretions with electronic hormone monitoring (Clearblue fertility monitor), which measures urinary estrogen and LH. The monitor is restricted to use by women with cycles of 22–42 days and provides the user with information about low, high and peak fertility. The monitor is designed for women planning pregnancy so does not give sufficient warning of the start of the fertile time for couples wishing to avoid pregnancy. MM therefore uses additional rules to increase effectiveness: for example, the fertile time starts on day 6 for new users, but after six months, monitor information is used to calculate the start of the fertile time. Women are encouraged to record cervical secretions as "L," low fertility (dryness or scant, thick white secretions); "H," high fertility (wetter, thinner, cloudy, slight stretch); or "P," peak fertility (clear, slippery stretchy) with Peak Day recorded as the last day of peak fertility.

Note: The MM has a Catholic philosophy recommending ways, including spiritual ways, that couples who have a serious need to avoid pregnancy can manage the time of abstinence. For further information, visit the Marquette University website: http://nfp.marquette.edu. [167]

Modified Mucus Method

While some authorities were making the original Billings Method more complex and technical, others recognised the need for a more simplified approach of relevance to specific communities. In the late 1980s, Dorairaj published the results of her work in India on the *Modified Mucus Method* (MMM) or *Fertility Awakening*, which she designed to reduce the number of days of abstinence and so improve acceptability among rural and illiterate women with low status within the family. She used a cascade teaching system: women who had learnt the method became teachers and then supervisors. The acceptance rate amongst non-users of contraception was high. This secular project had a high acceptance amongst Hindus but lower acceptance amongst Sikhs. FA education helped to empower women, gave them more information about their bodies and helped them to understand their potential to regulate their own fertility. [131]

Note: The MMM has largely been replaced by another similar simplified method: the TwoDay Method (TDM).

TwoDay Method

The TDM was developed by IRH at Georgetown University in the late 1990s. It is based on the presence or absence of secretions and provides a simplified family planning method which is easy to teach and learn. It may suit couples who are spacing their family and be particularly appropriate in low-resource settings and for populations with unmet family planning needs (full description: page 191).

EFFECTIVENESS OF CERVICAL SECRETIONS TO AVOID PREGNANCY

A number of studies using cervical secretions are summarised in date sequence in table 5.2. These cannot be directly compared due to the varied nature of the study populations and the different methodologies. The main section on the effectiveness of FAMs can be found on page 234.

Table 5.2 Effectiveness studies: cervical secretions as a single-indicator method

Study author	*Date*	*Description of study*	*No.*	*Cycles*	*Correct use*	*Typical use*
Weissman	1972	Ovulation Method (Tonga) [607]	282	2,593	1.4%	25%
Ball	1976	Ovulation Method (Sydney) [24]	124	1,635	2.9%	15.5%
WHO	1981	Ovulation Method Multi-centre trial (Auckland, Dublin, Bangalore, Manila and San Miguel) [616]	725	7,514	2.8%	19.6%
Dorairaj	1984	Modified Mucus Method (urban slums, Delhi) [129]		5,752	2%	2.6%
Hilgers	1998	Creighton Model Meta-analysis of five US studies (Omaha, St Louis, Wichita, Houston and Milwaukee) [284]	1,876	17,130	0.5%	3.2%
Arevalo	2004	TDM with abstinence or back-up method during the fertile time (Five culturally diverse centres in Guatemala, Peru and the Philippines) [11]				
		– *Abstinence*			3.5%	13.7%
		– *Condoms or withdrawal method*				6.3%
Fehring	2007	Creighton Model with Clearblue fertility monitor (five US sites in Atlanta, Madison, Milwaukee and St Louis) [169]	195	1,795	2.1%	14%
Fehring	2013	Internet-supported methods Comparing Clearblue fertility monitor with cervical secretions [170]	667			
		– *Monitor group*				7%
		– *Cervical secretion group*				18.5%

FAMs, unlike other contraceptive methods, can be used to achieve as well as avoid pregnancy, therefore a clear classification of desired outcomes is vital before a study starts. Participants should state their intention at the beginning of each cycle (to achieve or avoid pregnancy), but this does not always happen and many rely on recall to classify pregnancies. Some proponents argue that if intercourse occurs on a fertile day (even if the couple admitted that they took a risk) then the pregnancy was intentional, hence some of the difficulties with comparing studies.

First field trial of Ovulation Method The first prospective field trial of the Ovulation Method carried out by the Billings' team described the use of the method on the Pacific island of Tonga. The widely reported 1.4% pregnancy rate was based on three pregnancies which occurred with correct use, but there were also 50 pregnancies when couples stated that they had "taken a chance" by having intercourse on a day when they observed secretions, giving a typical use pregnancy rate of 25%. [607]

Study affected by concept of "infertile" secretions A prospective field trial conducted in Australia by Ball in the mid-1970s found a typical-use pregnancy rate of 15.5% [24] The study used the Billings' original guidelines (restricting pre-ovulatory intercourse to non-consecutive dry evenings), but while the study was ongoing the Billings introduced the "yellow stamp" and some teachers/study investigators started to teach that pre-ovulatory days, when sticky white or cloudy secretions were present, could be used for intercourse (yellow stamp days). These participants were reported on separately. Only four pregnancies occurred in couples who followed the study guidelines correctly, giving a correct use rate of 2.9%. Nine pregnancies resulted from couples taking a conscious risk, and eight pregnancies resulted from intercourse on yellow stamp days. This confirms the warning that *any* pre-ovulatory secretions are potentially fertile.

WHO multi-centre trial of Ovulation Method In the WHO cross-cultural five-centre study (New Zealand, India, Ireland, the Philippines and El Salvador) [616] 725 participants of proven fertility completed the three-cycle learning phase and entered the effectiveness phase. The study showed that if couples were well-taught and followed the instructions correctly, then cervical secretions used alone had a failure rate of approximately 3%, but such a low rate occurs only with correct use. The typical-use pregnancy rate was nearly 20%. The majority of unplanned pregnancies were related to conscious departure from the rules (took a chance on birthdays, holidays, etc.). There was a 36% discontinuation rate after 13 cycles. *All* secretions in the pre-ovulatory phase were regarded as days of potential fertility. [617]

Note: Trussell critically appraised the overall design of the WHO study, commenting that if used perfectly the Ovulation Method is very effective (3.2% life table analysis); however, it is extremely unforgiving of imperfect use. [587]

Cervical secretions and fertility monitor Fehring conducted a 12-month prospective efficacy trial involving 195 women. Women were taught to observe secretions in combination with the Clearblue fertility monitor (designed for planning pregnancy). The fertile time started on the first high reading or the first secretions, whichever came first, and ended on the last peak reading on the monitor or peak secretion day (whichever came last), plus three days. The typical use pregnancy rate was 14%, which is comparable with other methods based on secretions alone. [169]

Fertility monitor more effective than cervical secretions Fehring compared the efficacy and acceptability of two Internet-supported FAMs. In this study, 667 women were randomised into either the electronic monitor group or a cervical secretion group. The monitor group had a typical use pregnancy rate of 7% compared with 18.5% for the secretion group, demonstrating the increased efficacy of the monitor. This study was affected by a high drop-out rate. [170]

SELF-ASSESSMENT QUESTIONS

Answers are at the end of the chapter.

1 What is peak day?
2 Define the start of the fertile time if using cervical secretions as a single indicator.

3 Define the end of the fertile time if using cervical secretions as a single indicator.
4 How would you advise a couple who are planning pregnancy to optimise intercourse timing?
5 How would you advise a couple who are avoiding pregnancy about intercourse in the early dry days of the cycle?

USE OF CERVICAL SECRETIONS IN FERTILITY PRACTICE

The potential of cervical secretions to encourage or impede sperm penetration has been documented by gynaecologists since the 19th century. Sims conducted the first post-coital test in the 1860s, observing that the test was positive when the secretions were clear or translucent with the consistency of raw egg white. Cohen's studies of the spinnbarkeit effect concluded that profuse, thin transparent secretions with maximal spinnbarkeit (10–20 cm) provided optimal conditions for sperm survival. [95]

Cervical scoring

For many years, a cervical scoring system devised by Insler was used routinely in fertility practice. This was based on the quantity, spinnbarkeit and ferning capacity of cervical secretions plus speculum examination of the external cervical os. [298] This has largely been replaced by more precise – but costly – hormone monitoring and ultrasonography. A strong correlation has been shown between ovulation determined by cervical score assessment and by serial ultrasonography. Cervical scoring provides a simple, inexpensive and reasonably accurate method of ovulation prediction and detection, and may be highly appropriate for fertility management in low-resource settings. [2] [261]

Cervical secretions and chance of conception

Highest chance of conception from intercourse on peak day In a study of 524 pregnancies where peak day was used as a marker of the probable day of ovulation, 76% of the pregnancies were conceived from intercourse on one of three days: peak day, the day before peak and two days prior to peak. The study found that

- the highest chance of conception (39%) was from intercourse on peak day (estimated day of ovulation);
- 26% of conceptions occurred from intercourse on the day before peak (day of the most profuse secretions for most women); and
- 11% of conceptions occurred from intercourse two days prior to peak (figure 5.7).

The researchers recommended FA as a low-cost method for achieving pregnancy. [242]

Presence of secretions associated with twofold increase in probability of conception Bigelow used a subset of data from the European multi-centre study [101] to study the probability of conception in relation to the presence and quality of cervical secretions. The study sample contained 1,473 cycles with 353 confirmed pregnancies. The characteristics of secretions (sensation, appearance and finger-test) were scored from 1 to 4: dry sensation with nothing seen = 1; moist sensation but nothing seen = 2; moist sensation with thick, creamy, white or yellowish sticky secretions = 3; and wet, slippery sensation with watery or stretchy secretions like raw egg white = 4. (Note that many authorities, including FertilityUK, do not differentiate between days with moist sensation only and moist sensation with white secretions, that is, no distinction between types 2 and 3.) The last day of low-phase temperatures was used as the marker for

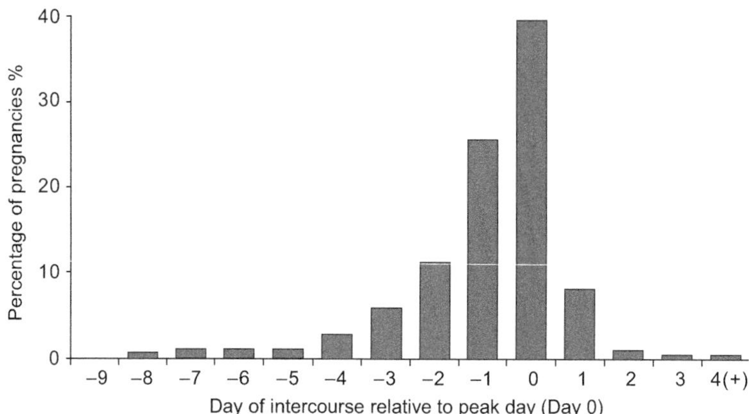

Figure 5.7 Timing of intercourse relative to peak day in 524 planned pregnancies (adapted from Gray 1995) [242]

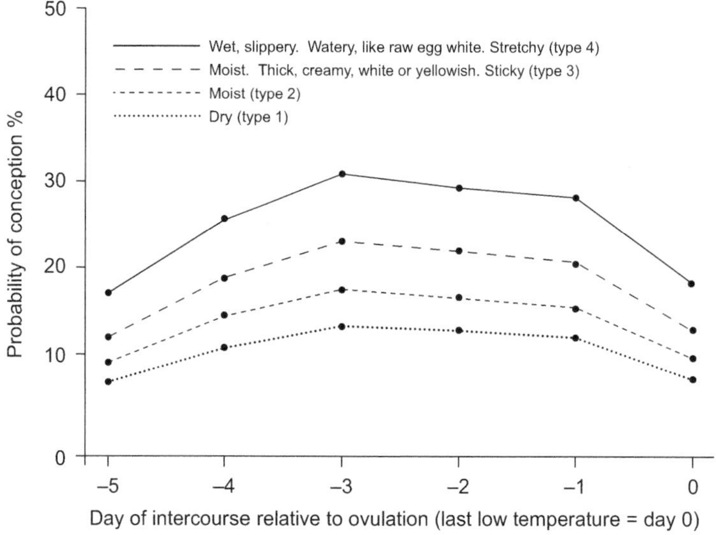

Figure 5.8 Estimated probability of pregnancy with a single act of intercourse in the fertile time, conditional on cervical secretions (adapted from Bigelow 2004) [49]

ovulation. Figure 5.8 shows the increase in pregnancy probability with higher quality cervical secretions. The day of lowest fertility was five days before ovulation, and the day of highest fertility was three days before ovulation.

Intercourse on *any* day in the six-day fertile time where the cervical secretions were described as type 4 (highly estrogenised) had a pregnancy probability of more than 17%. This can be compared with intercourse on the same day in relation to ovulation, which did not exceed 13% when no secretions were observed. Within the six-day fertile window (from five days before to the day of ovulation), the type of secretion observed on the day of intercourse was more predictive than the timing relative to ovulation.

If intercourse occurs on any given day relative to ovulation, the presence of cervical secretions was associated with a twofold increase in the probability of conception. Monitoring cervical secretions, therefore, provides a useful clinical marker of days with high conception probability. [49]

Studies on probabilities of conception require assessment of secretions Stanford analysed 81 conception cycles from 309 fertile couples (total 1,681 cycles) and 30 conception cycles from 117 subfertile couples (total 373 cycles). This showed that the cervical secretion score in the days preceding ovulation positively correlated with the cycle-specific probability of conception among couples of normal fertility. The highest probability of pregnancy was on peak day, with a 38% chance for normal fertile couples and 14% for subfertile couples. Stanford recommended that studies which aim to identify day-specific or cycle-specific probabilities of pregnancy may be incomplete without an assessment of the quality of cervical secretions. [561]

ANSWERS TO SELF-ASSESSMENT QUESTIONS

1. Peak day is the *last* day of the wet, transparent, slippery, stretchy secretions. It can be recognised only retrospectively on the day after peak when the secretions have reverted to sticky or dry.
2. The fertile time starts at the first sign of *any* secretions (the first change from dryness).
3. The fertile time ends three full days after peak day (the late infertile time starts on the fourth day after peak).
4. Aim to have intercourse on any day when the wetter, transparent, stretchy secretions are present. The day with the most profuse secretions has a high chance of pregnancy, as does the peak day. Any day with secretions of any kind is potentially fertile.
5. Guidelines for avoiding pregnancy in the early dry days:
   - No intercourse during a period, as bleeding can mask the start of cervical secretions.
   - Intercourse is restricted to non-consecutive dry days in the early relatively infertile time.
   - Intercourse is restricted to the evenings to allow observation of the first change from dryness.
   - The day after intercourse is marked with an "X" in box 3 to denote a non-intercourse "wet" day.

6 CERVIX

Third indicator

During the menstrual cycle the cervix goes through a series of changes in its level, position, consistency and dilatation. Many women who check secretions are aware of their cervix and its changes. These changes may be of particular value to women in circumstances where ovulation is delayed: for example, women with very long cycles, postpartum and during the perimenopausal years. Women who are planning pregnancy do not need to check their cervix, but those who are avoiding pregnancy can use cervical changes in conjunction with other fertility indicators to provide an effective method of family planning. Cervical changes are optional and some women will not wish to check their cervix for a variety of reasons – personal, religious or cultural.

PHYSIOLOGICAL CHANGES IN CERVIX

The ovarian hormones cause subtle changes in the muscle and connective tissue of the cervix (page 60). Women can learn to recognize these changes by gently palpating the cervix at approximately the same time each day, but uterine position will affect the relative height and position of the cervix.

At the infertile time of the cycle, with an anteverted uterus, the cervix is low in the vagina and easily within reach of the finger-tip. It appears long and may be off-centre, tilted to lie against the vaginal wall. It will feel firm (like the tip of the nose). The cervical opening (os) will be closed, giving the sensation of a dimple to touch. The cervix will feel dry. As the estrogen levels rise, the cervix rises higher in the vagina. It becomes shorter, straighter and more centrally positioned, and may be difficult to reach. It will feel softer (like the texture of the lip). It relaxes slightly, allowing the os to open enough to admit the finger-tip. The cervix feels wet and flowing with secretions. The changes in the level, position, consistency and dilatation of the cervix are gradual in the days approaching ovulation, but more dramatic following ovulation. The cervix starts to show fertile characteristics about six days before ovulation. After ovulation, with rapidly increasing progesterone, it returns to its infertile state within one to two days.

The main physiological difference between the cervix of an anteverted and retroverted uterus is that the cervix of a retroverted uterus will be high in the pelvis at the infertile time and low at the fertile time with the os pointing slightly upwards. Apart from this, signs of softness, openness and tilt are the same (page 148).

Nulliparous vs. parous cervix

The nulliparous cervix has a small round os (like the mouth of a small fish), which feels very tightly closed at times of infertility, relaxing enough to form more of a dimple at times of fertility. The os will dilate from about 1 mm in its closed position to up to 3 mm or more at the height of fertility. By comparison, the cervix of a woman who has given birth vaginally is slit-like and the os remains slightly dilated at all times. The parous woman will still be able to detect a definite change in the width of the os during the menstrual cycle and may detect dilatation exceeding 3 mm – sufficient to admit the finger-tip. Parenteau-Carreau found no difference between nulliparous and parous women in the time taken for the cervix to change during the cycle. [451]

DEVELOPMENT OF A PRACTICAL INDICATOR

Knowledge about cervical changes has been handed down through generations in some African and Asian cultures, with cervical self-examination being a strictly guarded secret amongst women that is passed down from mother to daughter at the time of marriage. [507] In the early 1960s Keefe taught 70 multiparous women both cervical palpation and self-examination using a speculum and took a series of photographs of the cervices of 10 of the women. His observations (> 1,300 cycles) showed that for three to four days preceding ovulation, the cervix softened progressively, the os dilated and the secretions became profuse, liquid and clear. Within three days, synchronous with a temperature rise, the cervix became firm, with a closed, dry os. Keefe concluded that cervical palpation was more reliable than observation with a speculum. [321] Some women noted significant changes in the level (height) of the cervix, describing its gradual ascent as the fertile time approached and its abrupt descent following. Keefe noted that the cervix shifted by 2–3 cm from its lowest to its highest level. [322] Parenteau-Carreau showed that in 85% of cycles there was a correlation of ± 1 day between peak day and the last day of the most fertile cervix. In 84% of cycles, the first high temperature occurred from two days before to one day after the last day of the most fertile cervix. It took an average of 2.6 days for the cervix to revert from its most fertile state to its infertile state (one to three days in 80% of the cycles). [451] Gnoth similarly found a close correlation between cervical changes and ovulation detected by LH and ultrasound (figure 10.1). [230] [234]

TEACHING SELF-EXAMINATION OF CERVIX

The subtle day-to-day changes in the cervix can be detected by self-palpation using a delicate finger-tip touch. Most women quickly recognise the more dramatic change which occurs around peak day (the last day when wet, slippery, transparent stretchy secretions are present) at which time the cervix changes quite abruptly from its high, soft, open, straight position to its low, firm, closed, tilted position. It takes longer for many women to recognise the more subtle changes in the early part of the cycle.

Cervical changes can be quite confusing at first, so it is not normally advisable to discuss self-examination with a user until she has charted her temperature and secretions for two to three cycles. Some women may be ready to check their cervix from the first session: for example, IUD users or those using a diaphragm or cervical cap.

Cervical changes indicating fertility and infertility

Figure 6.1 shows the difference in the cervix at the fertile and infertile times of the cycle. After the period, the cervix is low, firm and closed. It feels quite long and may be tilted to one side. It is generally quite easy to reach at this stage. As the estrogen levels rise, the cervix rises higher, becomes softer (spongier) and shorter in length. It is now harder to reach with the finger-tip and may feel straighter (more central) in position. The cervical os feels slightly open. Notice the dotted line on the image which indicates the relative height of the cervix. It takes almost a week for the cervix to change from its lowest position to its maximum height (and openness). After ovulation, under the influence of progesterone, the cervix changes back within one to two

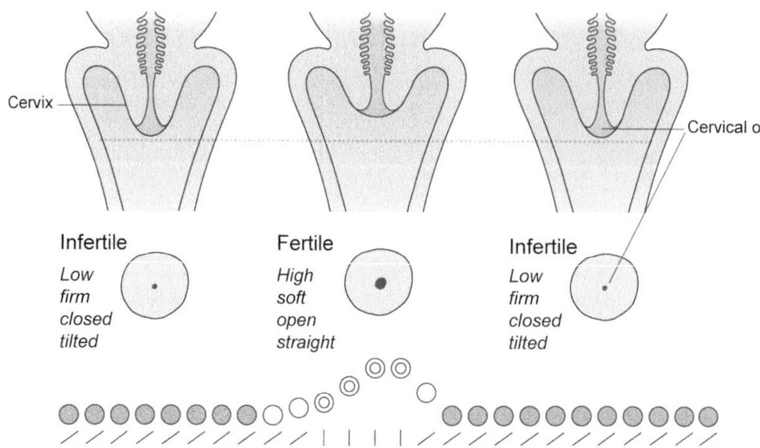

Figure 6.1 Changes in the cervix during the menstrual cycle (© Pyper & Knight, FertilityUK 2016)

days to its low, firm, closed, tilted position. The cervical changes are recorded on the chart using symbols. At the beginning of the cycle the cervix is low, firm and closed (solid black dot) and it feels tilted (angled line). The cervix then starts to soften (shown by the open circle). It rises higher in the vagina, becomes straighter in position (vertical line) and the cervical os feels open (circle within a circle). It then changes back within two days to low, firm, closed and tilted and remains so until the end of the cycle.

Examining the cervix

Advise the woman to follow these instructions:

- Examine her cervix at roughly the same time of day.
- Empty her bladder first (a full bladder makes the cervix more difficult to reach and alters the position of the uterus).
- Ensure her hands are washed and dried (and her fingernails are short).
- Use the same position for the entire cycle, whichever is more comfortable and easier:
  - squatting (as when sitting on the toilet);
  - lying on her back with knees bent and legs apart; or
  - standing with one leg resting on a chair or the side of the bath. (Right-handed people normally find it easier with the left leg raised and vice versa).
- Gently insert her index finger (or the index and middle finger) into her vagina until she can reach the top. The cervix will feel like a smooth indented ball (tip of the nose) compared with the vaginal walls, which feel soft, moist and ridged by comparison.
- Assess the height, consistency, dilatation and position of the cervix:
  - Height (level): use a straightened finger to assess the distance from the nearest part of the cervix to the lower border of the symphysis pubis, observing how far the perineum has to be indented to reach (height may vary by 2–3 cm). If the cervix is difficult to reach, use the other hand to press down just above the pubic bone through the abdominal wall onto the body of the uterus to bring the cervix within reach.
  - Consistency: with a delicate finger-tip touch, test the firmness or softness. (Does it feel like the tip of the nose or more like the texture of the bottom lip?)

- Dilatation (width) of the os: the cervix will feel more relaxed (less tightly closed) at the fertile time. The os dilates to more than 3 mm in a nulliparous woman and 6–8 mm in a parous woman.
- Position: determine whether the cervix is tilted or straight and whether it is lying against a vaginal wall. The length of the cervix can also be determined: the cervix shortens (becoming stubbier) as it rises higher in the pelvis.

■ Start checking the cervix on day 6 of the cycle, even if there is still slight spotting (Women who have very short cycles may need to start earlier to identify the earliest changes.)

■ Any secretions which naturally come away on the examining fingers should be recorded on the chart.

Difficulties with cervical palpation

Some women find it easier to palpate the cervix with one finger, but most women find using the index and middle finger helps to more easily identify the height, length and position of the cervix. A woman will rarely be able to determine all the characteristics. The height (upward shift) is often the easiest to detect (especially for nulliparous women), but other women will find the height the least conspicuous sign. The cervix is generally lower at night, hence the importance of a consistent time of day. Tilt is a sign that women either understand immediately or may never be able to detect. Women with a steeply anteverted or retroverted uterus may observe the most distinctive changes in tilt. Most women have some perception of consistency (firmness or softness) and dilatation. Teaching all the possible changes allows a woman to identify which is more noticeable for her. Cervical changes are highly subjective and individual, but most women will find two or three subtle changes which can be used as a practical guide.

If a woman is struggling to identify changes in her cervix, she may be more successful using her opposite (non-dominant) hand. This sometimes helps particularly if the cervical os is lying in close apposition to a vaginal wall. Her partner may sometimes be more in tune with her cervical changes and can be more actively involved by checking the cervix and sharing the responsibility of charting.

It is important that the observations are made by the same person over a complete cycle, in the same way, and at roughly the same time of day to ensure that the changes are genuine physiological changes and not due to the individual's perception. The examination should take only a few seconds each day, but it can take at least two to three cycles for the woman to feel confident in her observations. The easiest time to start checking is when there are highly fertile secretions approaching peak day – she may then observe the abrupt change from the fertile to infertile state. This often makes it easier to distinguish the more subtle changes in the early part of the next cycle.

Note: About one in five women have a retroverted uterus, which may cause difficulties or unexpected findings with cervical palpation (page 148).

Recording cervical changes on the chart

Changes in the cervix are recorded on the combined chart:

■ A solid black dot drawn on the baseline represents a low, firm and closed cervix. A slanted line below shows the tilt.

■ An open circle shows the softness.

■ An inner white circle shows the opening of the cervical os. A straight line below shows the cervix to be straight in position.

■ The symbols are placed in the box at a level to represent the relative height of the cervix.

Note: Most women do not need to check their cervix during their period. This is necessary only for a woman with very short cycles to ensure that she does not miss the earliest sign of change.

Guidelines for interpreting cervical changes

Cervical signs should *not* be relied on as a single-indicator method for avoiding pregnancy, but can be used in combination with other indicators for improved effectiveness. The guidelines for interpreting the changes in the cervix are as follows:

- A low, firm, closed, tilted cervix indicates infertility.
- A high, soft, open, straight cervix indicates fertility.
- The fertile time starts at the *first* sign of fertility – i.e. when the cervix shows the first sign of moving higher or becoming softer, more open or straighter.
- The fertile time ends when the cervix has returned to low, firm, closed and tilted, and remained so for three days.
- If the other indicators (temperature and secretions) correlate and determine that the fertile time has ended, there is no reason to wait for the cervix to remain closed for three days before resuming intercourse.

Cervical changes provide a useful double-check with secretions for women who are avoiding pregnancy, especially at times when the temperature may not be reliable (such as during illness). In such a situation it would be necessary to wait to have sex until the fourth day after peak and to ensure that the cervix had remained low, firm and closed for three full days. Couples who are avoiding pregnancy should always have a double-check for the start and end of the fertile time.

CORRELATING CERVICAL CHANGES WITH OTHER INDICATORS

Figure 6.2 shows the correlation between the temperature, secretions and cervix in a 27-day cycle. The first sign of fertility is on day 9 when the cervix becomes softer (open circle). Note that intercourse has been marked on days 5 and 7 (non-consecutive evenings) during the early dry days of the cycle. The day after intercourse is marked as a non-intercourse day. On day 9 the woman observes that her cervix has started to soften, so, although she still feels dry all day, the cervix has started to change giving the earliest warning of fertility. (The cervix often gives an earlier warning than the secretions, hence its value for avoiding pregnancy.)

The cervix starts to rise higher on day 12. On days 13, 14 and 15 the cervix is at its highest and the os is open. The last day of the high, soft, open cervix is day 15 (which correlates with peak day on this chart). On day 16 the cervix closes again and drops lower, but remains soft, and by the following day it has returned to its low, firm, closed, tilted position. Note the gradual build-up of cervical changes, over about a week, with the more abrupt return to the infertile state. The fertile time starts on day 9 (first change in cervix) and ends after the third high temperature past peak day (on day 19). The third high temperature is at least 0.2 deg.C above the highest of the low readings so the fertile time has ended.

Note the pattern of intercourse: non-consecutive evenings in the early dry days, with unrestricted intercourse from day 20 onwards. Observe too the temperature spikes (disturbances) on days 5 and 13. There is only one spike amongst the six low readings, so the *3 over 6 rule* can safely be applied.

In this example, the end of the fertile time by temperature and secretions coincides with the third day of a low, firm, closed cervix – but if this was not the case, provided the temperature and secretions correlate (double check), there is no reason to wait for the cervix to remain in its closed state for three days.

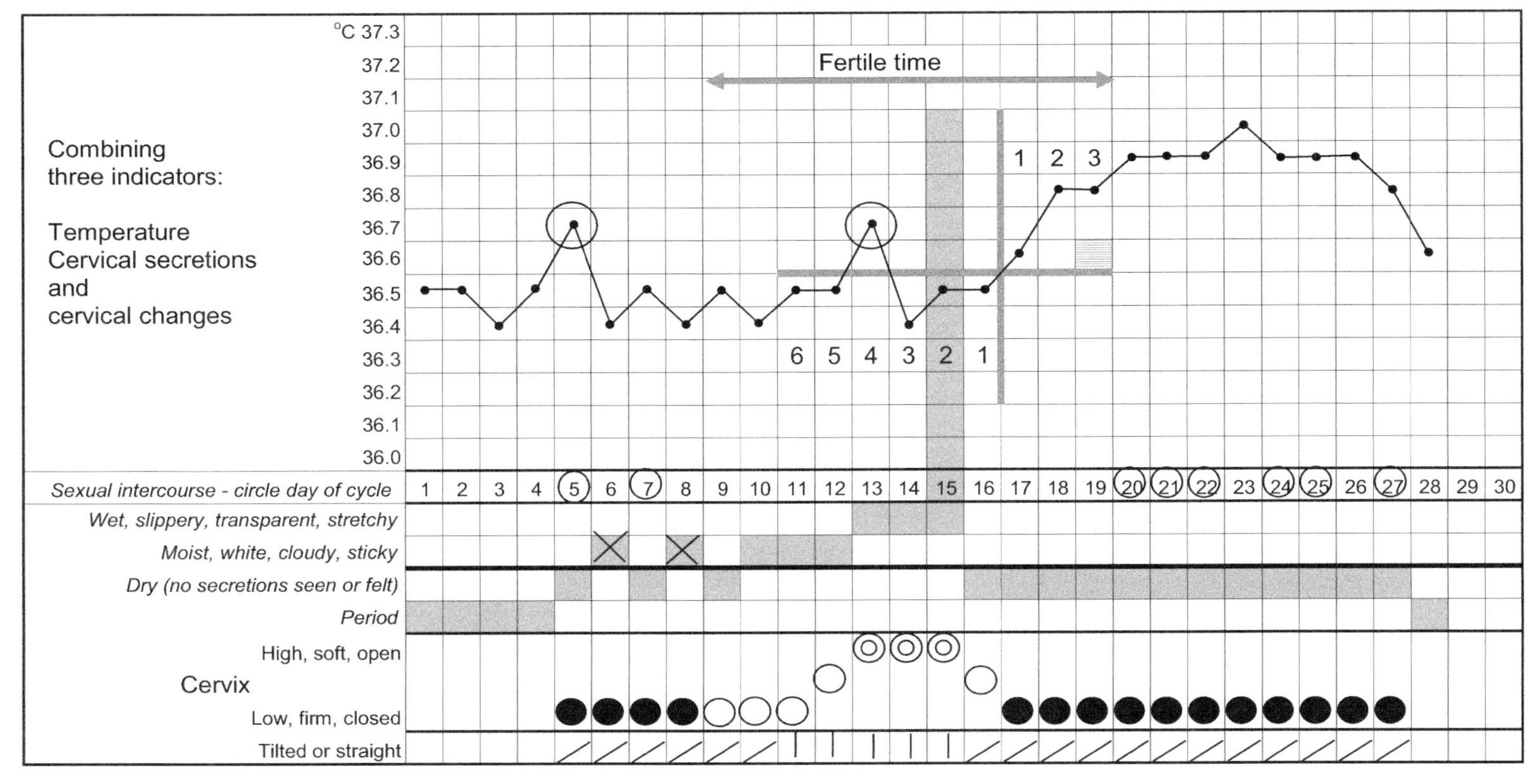

Figure 6.2 Correlation between temperature, secretions and cervical changes

ACTIVITY CHART-BUILDING EXERCISE (CONTINUED FROM PAGE 128)

Step 3 Recording the changes in the cervix

Jo likes the security of using cervical changes as an extra indicator and starts checking her cervix after her period has finished.

1 On days 6, 7 and 8 Jo records her cervix as low, firm, closed and tilted.
2 On day 9, it starts to feel softer and continues soft but still low on days 10 and 11. It still feels tilted.
3 On day 12 it still feels soft, but is a little higher and is starting to straighten.
4 On day 13 it feels very soft and now feels open. It feels much higher and straighter. It feels the same on days 14 and 15.
5 On day 16, it has dropped a little and is more closed and tilted.
6 On day 17, her cervix is low firm, closed and tilted again. It feels the same on days 18, 19 and 20 then she stops recording it.
7 Set exercise aside. To be continued on page 160.

Monitoring secretions at the cervix

Women who have a short build-up of secretions or difficulty distinguishing changes externally may find it easier to take secretions directly from the cervix. This gives an immediate picture of the conditions at the cervix and avoids the transit time while secretions pass along, and get caught up in, the ridged vaginal walls. For example: a woman may observe dryness at the vulva, but on palpating her cervix, there may be some sticky white secretions; or she may be aware of sticky white secretions externally, but on checking her cervix, there may be transparent stretchy secretions. It can take one to two days for thick, sticky secretions noted at the cervix to be visible externally, whilst the wetter highly fertile secretions normally appear at the vulva within hours. The most fertile characteristics must always be recorded at the end of the day.

If a woman wishes to take secretions directly from her cervix, advise her to position her index and middle fingers on opposite sides of the length of the cervix and firmly (but gently) squeeze the fingers together to express any secretions from the cervical canal. The characteristics of these secretions can then be recorded on the chart. This examination can be done morning and evening (and shortly before intercourse) – but not too frequently, or too vigorously. Internal monitoring should be avoided if there are any signs of infection.

Uterine position and its effect on self-examination

Anteverted uterus

The cervix in a woman with an anteverted uterus will feel low in the pelvis at the infertile time and high at the most fertile time. In a normally-positioned anteverted uterus, the cervix points slightly forward (anteriorly) and the external os is easily felt by the examining finger. In a steeply anteverted and anteflexed uterus, the cervix may point backwards towards the posterior vaginal wall and the os will be more difficult to reach.

Symbols The symbols representing cervical changes normally start off (at the infertile time) low on the baseline of the chart and rise higher with increasing fertility, dropping back to the baseline again after ovulation.

Retroverted uterus

The cervix of a woman with a retroverted uterus will feel high in the pelvis at the infertile time and low at the most fertile time (reverse of the anteverted uterus). In a retroverted and retroflexed uterus, the cervix may point slightly upwards into the anterior vaginal wall. If the cervix is lying against the vaginal wall behind the pubic bone, the os may be difficult to reach (page 58 and figure 3.6).

Symbols The symbols representing the cervix of a retroverted uterus may form a U-shaped curve. They start off (at the infertile time) high in the box showing the cervix as high, firm and closed; descend to low, soft and open (at the fertile time); then rise higher again, showing the cervix high, firm and closed (during the late infertile time).

Visualisation of cervix

Current guidelines for self-examination of the cervix recommend palpation alone. However, one pilot study looked at the feasibility of a woman using a mirror and lighted speculum to assess the dilatation of the os as a way to identify the days of maximum fertility. Although the cervix starts to show changes in height and consistency around a week before ovulation, the cervical os is open for a relatively short time only in the few days prior to ovulation. This has been described as the "pupil sign" (pupil as in the eye). In figure 6.2 days 13, 14 and 15 show the dilated os represented by a circle within a circle.

Twenty experienced FAM users (nulliparous and parous) compared their cervical rating with changes in secretions. The temperature rise was used as the estimated day of ovulation. The cervical os was scored as: 1 (estimated opening of 1 mm or less), 2 (1–3 mm) and 3 (> 3 mm). The pupil sign was determined as the number of days with a single or uninterrupted score of 3 preceded and followed by a lower score. The duration of the open os averaged 3.1 days (but with variation of 1–11 days). The open os (either a single day or the last day) coincided with ovulation (determined by waking temperature) in 71% of cycles. The researchers noted the need for supervised training plus difficulties with secretions, uterine retroversion and cervical lacerations which may have confused observation in some volunteers. Whether or not this sign is of any advantage in optimising conception remains to be tested in prospective studies. [65]

Keefe first promoted direct visualisation of the cervix in the 1960s, but later determined that self-palpation was more accurate. Some women continue to use a speculum to examine their own cervix and its secretions. The *Beautiful Cervix Project* (www.beautifulcervix.com) is an online gallery containing numerous serial photographs taken by women for personal interest, FA or health reasons. This resource provides a useful teaching aid, but there is no research to validate whether direct visualisation of the cervix can accurately define the limits of the fertile time.

SELF-ASSESSMENT QUESTIONS

Answers are at the end of the chapter.

1 Describe the cervix of a woman (with an anteverted uterus) at the infertile time.
2 Describe the cervix of a woman (with an anteverted uterus) through the fertile time.
3 How are the limits of the fertile time identified using cervical changes alone?
4 What might make you suspect that a woman has a retroverted uterus? How would you explain this to her?
5 Would you recommend cervical palpation as a single-indicator method?

EFFECTIVENESS OF CERVIX AS A SINGLE INDICATOR

There is a dearth of research on cervical changes in non-pregnant women. Some studies have correlated changes in the cervix with other observed indicators and objective markers (page 143). There have been no effectiveness studies using the cervix as a single indicator, therefore this cannot be recommended as a stand-alone method.

WHO MAY BENEFIT FROM CERVICAL CHANGES?

Many women use cervical changes in conjunction with other fertility indicators to provide a highly effective method of family planning. Cervical changes may be of particular value to postpartum women (when LAM criteria can no longer be met) and during the peri-menopausal years. Cervical changes can also provide vital information when cervical secretions are not reliable, e.g. diaphragm users and some women with very long cycles. The cervix is often the least-affected sign when other indicators are disrupted (for example by illness or medication). Every woman should freely choose whether or not she wants to check her cervix. There is no evidence to suggest that the effectiveness of the method will be compromised without cervical palpation. Calendar-based calculations to determine the start of the fertile time are highly effective for women of normal fertility (page 155).

ANSWERS TO SELF-ASSESSMENT QUESTIONS

1 The cervix will be low, firm and closed. It may also feel quite long and tilted towards one of the vaginal walls. There will be no secretions at the os.
2 The cervix will be high, soft and open and flowing with secretions. It may feel short and stubby and be centrally positioned in the vagina.
3 The fertile time starts at the first sign of fertility – i.e. when the cervix shows the first sign of moving higher, becoming softer, more open or straighter. The fertile time ends when the cervix has returned to low, firm, closed and tilted and remained so for three days.
4 One might suspect a woman has a retroverted uterus if she describes her cervix as soft and open yet low; or firm and closed yet high. Her descriptions may be inaccurate due to inexperience, but if it is confirmed that she has a retroverted uterus (which is mobile) she can be reassured that this is normal for about 20% of women and is no cause for concern.
5 Cervical palpation should not be recommended as a single-indicator method as there have been no effectiveness studies. It should always be used in conjunction with temperature and secretions (with a calendar calculation to identify the start of the fertile time). Cervical palpation can provide a very effective double-check – for example, if a woman is unable to identify secretions – but there must always be at least two indicators to identify the start and end of the fertile time.

CALENDAR CALCULATIONS

7

Fourth indicator

All calendar-based methods are based purely on menstrual cycle length. They aim to predict the fertile time based on the assumption that the forthcoming cycle will be similar in length to past menstrual cycles. The independent discoveries, by Ogino and Knaus, of the relationship between ovulation and the *next* period was pivotal in the development of physiological methods (see timeline on page 14). The Calendar/Rhythm Method, however, proved to be both unreliable and unacceptably restrictive for most couples, contributing to the long-standing bad reputation of FAMs.

CRITERIA FOR USE OF CALENDAR-BASED METHODS

A calendar-based method may be useful to those women who do not wish to observe their subjective indicators and couples who do not have access to other methods of family planning. Personalised calendar calculations, as described here, should not be confused with the simplified SDM, which uses a fixed fertile time, hence may be more suited to women who have literacy or language difficulties (page 187).

To use a calendar-based method a woman must have a clearly documented record of her menstrual history (paper or electronic) as perceptions can be highly inaccurate. Women often falsely describe their cycles as "regular" or "once a month" and tend to show a preference for even numbers or multiples of five when describing cycle length.

Suitability for use

Calendar-based methods are suitable for women in the following circumstances only:

- cycle lengths of 23–35 days;
- a clearly documented history of the previous 12 consecutive menstrual cycles; or
- regular cycles – i.e. variation of seven days or less. If a woman has irregular cycles (varying by eight days or more) she should not use a calendar-based method until she has recorded 12 consecutive cycles with a variation of seven days or less.

Contraindications to use

Calendar-based methods are *not* suitable for women in the following circumstances:

- poorly documented evidence or guess work of past cycle length
- cycle lengths outside the range 23–35 days, or
- irregular cycles (variation of eight days or more); or

- at times of expected irregularity such as
  - in the first few years after the menarche,
  - postpartum (for at least one year),
  - after stopping hormonal contraception (for at least one year), or
  - during the peri-menopausal years; or
- where a high level of effectiveness is required

CALENDAR CALCULATIONS

Calendar calculations are based on accurate information about:

- the timing of ovulation before the *next* period;
- the lifespan of sperm under the most favourable conditions;
- the lifespan of the egg; and
- the probability of when ovulation will occur in the current cycle.

There was a divergence of opinion about some of the physiological details in the development of the Calendar/Rhythm Method. Some calculations were based on Ogino's rules and others on Knaus's, but over time the subtleties of the different methods have been lost.

Timing of ovulation before *next* period

Knaus, a physiologist, stated categorically that the time from ovulation to the next period was always 14 days; but Ogino, a gynaecologist, gave a wider variation of 12–16 days. The accepted length for the normal luteal phase is now 10–16 days (page 72).

Lifespan of sperm under most favourable conditions

Knaus believed that sperm survival was a maximum of 48 hours whereas Ogino suggested three days and possibly up to eight. Most calculations for the Calendar/Rhythm Method were based on a 72-hour survival – but sperm survival depends on the conditions in the female genital tract which will vary between women and from one cycle to the next. The currently accepted upper limit for sperm survival is seven days (page 42).

Lifespan of egg

When calculating the original formula for the Calendar/Rhythm Method, 12–24 hours was allowed for the fertilisable lifespan of the egg. The upper limit for the potential fertilisable lifespan of the egg is now considered to be 48 hours – a maximum of 24 hours for one egg plus 24 hours for the possibility of a second ovulation (page 53).

Probability of when ovulation will occur in current cycle

The variation of cycle lengths for an individual woman is greater than is generally thought – anticipated cycle length remains the most variable factor. Marshall showed that the accuracy of predicting the length of future menstrual cycles increases with the amount of data, reaching 90% when the length of 12 cycles is known. [378] The variability of cycles is defined as the difference between the longest and shortest cycle over a year. Ogino's original rules restricted use of the Calendar/Rhythm Method to women with a cycle length variation of up to 10 days. Tietze suggested that women should not use this method if they had a variation of more than eight days (page 73). [579]

It is the random occurrence of a long or short cycle in an otherwise regular menstrual history which is likely to be problematic for women using calendar calculations. The majority of women who have apparently "regular" cycles are likely to occasionally experience long or short cycles – this is a normal physiological phenomenon. The occurrence of cycles outside the regular pattern explains the majority of unintended pregnancies in women who rely on calendar-based calculations alone.

A study of more than 2,000 women in the US and Canada showed that only about 30% would potentially be suitable to use a calendar-based method alone. Nearly 90% of women aged 15–19 had more than eight days of variability. The 30–34 age group showed the most consistent cycle lengths but still 60% varied by more than eight days. Women with cycles showing more than eight days of variation have very poor effectiveness with calendar-based methods. [84] [62] A total of 2,355 sets of at least 13 consecutive temperature charts from Marshall's database showed that 42% of women had a cycle length variation of more than seven days: this is outside the current recommended limits for the use of a calendar-based method. [99] [102]

Developing the formulae

The calculation to define the start of the fertile time is based on the earliest possible ovulation before the next period, plus sperm survival time. The calculation to define the end of the fertile time is based on the latest possible ovulation before the next period, plus egg survival time. The original formula for the Calendar/Rhythm Method was calculated by identifying the shortest and longest cycles over the preceding six (preferably 12) cycles. The first fertile day was considered to be the shortest cycle minus 18 days, according to Ogino, and the shortest cycle minus 17 according to Knaus. The last fertile day was the longest cycle minus 11 days. The current more conservative formulae use the figures 20 and 10, which offer the simplicity of subtracting multiples of 10.

HOW TO DETERMINE LIMITS OF THE FERTILE TIME

Calculations to identify the fertile time are based on information about **the length of the past 12 consecutive menstrual cycles.** To determine the shortest and longest cycle, identify the first and last fertile day respectively.

Table 7.1 Activity: calculate the fertile time based on the shortest and longest cycle for each series of 12 charts by applying the *S minus 20* and *L minus 10* rules (answers on page 155)

	Length of last 12 menstrual cycles												*First fertile day*	*Last fertile day*
Cycles	*1*	*2*	*3*	*4*	*5*	*6*	*7*	*8*	*9*	*10*	*11*	*12*		
Woman A	29	30	27	27	31	29	28	29	30	28	28	30		
Woman B	26	25	27	25	26	30	25	27	28	30	27	25		
Woman C	30	30	25	24	28	27	27	26	30	27	25	34		
Woman D	29	30	28	28	27	28	29	29	33	27	28	29		
Woman E	30	28	28	27	29	30	28	31	29	28	30	36		

For example: If a woman has cycle lengths of 31, 27, 31, 30, 27, 29, 30, 27, 31, 26, 30 and 29 days, her shortest cycle (*S*) is 26 days and her longest cycle (*L*) is 31 days. The range of 26–31 days is within normal limits for regular cycles (seven days or less) so the calculation can be applied. The cycle range is also within the recommended 23–35 days for use of a calendar-based method.

- Shortest cycle (S) – 20 = first fertile day (FFD)
- Longest cycle (L) –10 = last fertile day (LFD)

In this example, 26 – 20 = 6 (first fertile day) and 31 – 10 = 21 (last fertile day). The fertile time includes the whole of the first and the last fertile days, so the fertile time extends from day 6 to day 21 inclusive (day and night). Calculations are updated at the end of each cycle using the information from *the most recent 12 cycles.*

Note: The wider the variation in cycle length, the more abstinence is required.

Calendar calculations as a guide for planning pregnancy

A woman (and her partner) may find it helpful to be aware of the variability of the potential fertile time when trying to conceive. Too much focus on trying to identify ovulation and the time of maximum fertility can damage the sexual relationship. The calculations *S minus 20* and *L minus 10* generally over-estimate the fertile time whilst the secretions more accurately identify the actual fertile time. Discussions about the potential fertile time often help to explain why pregnancies occur at "unexpected" times.

EFFECTIVENESS OF CALENDAR/RHYTHM METHOD

It is difficult to assess the effectiveness of the Calendar/Rhythm Method based on past studies due to failure to document the calendar rules, lack of standardised teaching, lack of information about the couple's understanding of the method and failure to document how couples broke the rules. [316] [57] Properly conducted clinical trials of the Calendar/Rhythm Method are required to scientifically establish its effectiveness.

Kambic's review of the effectiveness of calendar-based methods identified eight studies published between 1940 and 1989. The overall failure rates averaged approximately 20%, ranging from 5% to 47%. Table 7.2 shows the five studies (using various calculations) which provided enough information to estimate the 12-month Pearl Index. This meta-analysis resulted in a conservatively estimated Pearl Index of 18.5 ± 1.8 and a less conservative estimate of 15.0 ± 4.0, which is almost as effective as other natural methods. [316]

Table 7.2 Effectiveness of the Calendar/Rhythm Method (adapted from Kambic and Lamprecht 1996) [316]

Author and date	*Calendar rule*	*Participants*	*Months*	*Pregnancy rate %*
Fleck (1940)	S – 19, L – 9	207	1,655	17.4
Tietze (1951)	S – 19, L – 9	409	7,269	14.4
Dunn (1956)	S – 21, L – 7	156	4,687	5.8
Jarmillo-Gomez (1968a)	Not stated	701	3,802	47.0
Dicker (1989)	S – 17, L – 12	64	1,388	5.2

Marshall compared Tietze's study, which used standardised teaching, with a survey of Calendar/Rhythm Method users who had accessed their information from whatever source they could. The couples who had not received proper teaching had a pregnancy rate of 38% compared with Tietze's 14%. [579] [385] Calendar-based methods are certainly better than no contraceptive method, whereby 80–90% of women would be expected to conceive in one year. [256]

Bonnar studied 19 couples who received standardised teaching of the Calendar/Rhythm Method over two one-hour sessions. Couples were instructed about the menstrual cycle, the limits of the fertile time and the calculations *S minus 20* and *L minus 10*. There were no pregnancies during the seven-cycle follow-up, however, the real study focus was the couple's sexual behaviour during the fertile time (which averaged 16 days per cycle). Women with the most regular cycles had fewer days of abstinence: for example, women with a three-day cycle variation had 12–14 days of abstinence. Bonnar's findings showed that about 50% of the couples reported different forms of non-coital sexual activity during the fertile time (particularly oral sex and mutual masturbation), about 30% avoided genital contact completely and 20% used condoms in some cycles. [57]

ANSWERS TO ACTIVITY (TABLE 7.1)

- **A:** Shortest cycle (*S*) is 27 days and longest cycle (*L*) is 31 days. 27 – 20 = 7 and 31 – 10 = 21. The first fertile day is day 7 and the last fertile day is day 21 (potentially fertile from days 7 to 21 inclusive).
- **B:** *S* = 25 and *L* = 30. The first fertile day is day 5 and the last fertile day is day 20.
- **C:** Up until her 11th cycle, *S* = 24 and *L* = 30 days, so she would be fertile from days 4–20. However, cycle 12 (most recent) is longer (34 days). As she now has a 10-day variation in cycle length, this excludes her from using the Calendar/Rhythm Method until she re-establishes cycles with a variation of seven days or less.
- **D:** *S* = 27 and *L* = 33. Fertile time days 7–23 inclusive.
- **E:** Cycles range from 27–31 days until her most recent cycle (cycle 12), which is 36 days. This is outside the recommended range of 23–35 days so precludes her from continuing with a calendar-based method until cycle lengths are re-established.

CALCULATIONS TO IDENTIFY START OF FERTILE TIME

Calendar-based methods are not recommended as a single-indicator method for couples who require a high degree of effectiveness, however, a calendar calculation plays a key role in combined-indicator methods. The longest-cycle calculation (*L minus 10*) is relevant only for couples using calendar calculations as a single-indicator method. If combining indicators, temperature and secretions are a more reliable way to identify the *end* of the fertile time. The real value of the calendar calculation is to identify the *start* of the fertile time as a double-check with secretions (and optional cervical changes). FAMs are more effective when a calculation is used, but this requires accurate information about past cycle lengths. The importance of written (or electronic) diary records cannot be overstated as a woman's perception of her cycle length is notoriously inaccurate.

S minus 20 rule

If a woman knows her last 12 cycle lengths she can use the *S minus 20 rule:* **shortest cycle (S) – 20 = first fertile day.**

This needs to be recalculated after each cycle to take account of the most recent cycle length, while dropping the first cycle used in the calculation.

If a woman does *not* know her last 12 cycle lengths, she needs to record 12 cycles to establish her shortest cycle, but in the interim she can apply the *Day 6 rule.*

Day 6 rule

The Day 6 rule is of value during the learning phase while information on cycle length is being collected.

- Cycle 1: This is a learning cycle only. Assume the whole cycle is potentially fertile.
- Cycles 2 and 3: Need to establish if the woman has very short cycles. Unprotected intercourse is limited to the late infertile time (using a combination of temperature and secretions). There is no early infertile time.
- Cycles 4–12: Provided the first three cycles are 26 days or longer, intercourse is safe until day 5 with the fertile time starting on day 6. This is the *Day 6 rule*: **day 6 is the first fertile day** provided cycles are 26 days or longer.
- From cycle 13: The woman has now recorded 12 cycles, so she can start using the *S minus 20 rule*. The calculation is always made on the most recent 12 cycle lengths.
- Short cycles: If cycles 1–3 are shorter than 26 days, there is no early infertile time in cycles 4–12. Unprotected intercourse must be restricted to the late infertile time. If cycles continue to be short, the restrictions remain.

Risk of pregnancy on days 1–7. Wilcox showed that the risk of pregnancy between days 1–3 of the cycle was negligible. By day 7 there was an almost 2% pregnancy risk – the concept of the fertile time starting on day 6 is therefore acceptable to most couples. [630]

Earliest temperature rise minus 7

After a woman has completed 12 cycles of charting, she is considered an experienced user and can use her temperature readings to give a more personalised and accurate estimate of the start of the fertile time (replacing the *S minus 20 rule*). This calculation was developed by Döring in the mid-1950s (hence it is sometimes referred to as the *Döring rule*). He originally used *minus* 6 but later added an extra day: from the most recent 12 cycles, identify the earliest temperature rise and subtract seven days to identify the first fertile day: earliest temperature rise – 7 = first fertile day.

For example, if, in the past year, a woman has recorded her first high temperature on days 14, 14, 16, 15, 16, 15, 16, 14, 15, 16, 14 and 14, her earliest temperature rise is day 14 (14 – 7 = 7) so day 7 would be her first fertile day. If in subsequent cycles, a temperature rise occurs on an earlier day, the calculation is adjusted accordingly. The calculation is always based on information form the most recent 12 cycles.

The "stop bar"

A calculation generally gives the earliest indication of the start of the fertile time, however a woman should always be vigilant for any change in secretions or cervical changes which may precede the day given by the calculation. A short vertical bar, the "stop bar", can be drawn on the chart to show the start of the fertile time based on the *Day 6 rule, S minus 20*, or *earliest temperature rise minus 7*. Couples need to understand that if they

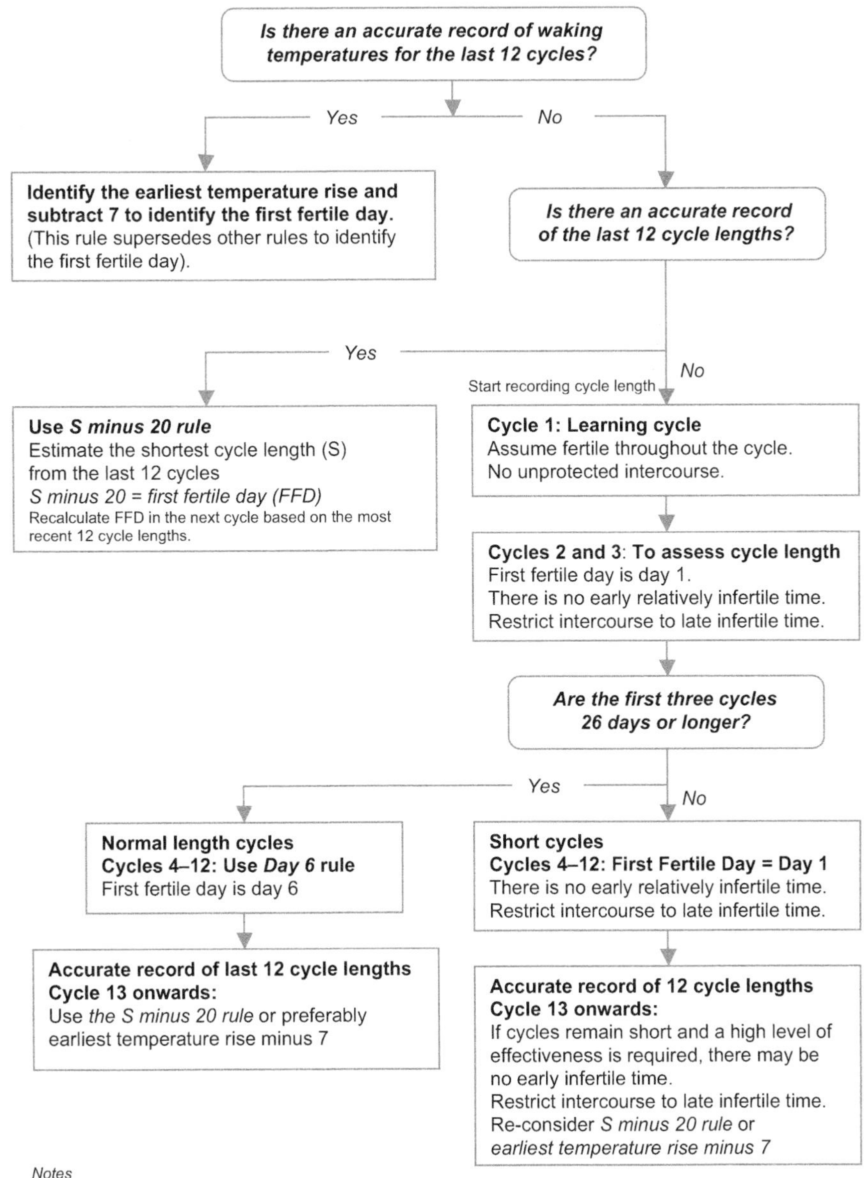

Figure 7.1 Calculations to identify the first fertile day (FFD)

continue to have unprotected intercourse after the day designated by the stop bar they are at increasing risk of pregnancy. Figure 7.1 shows an algorithm to identify the first fertile day by different calculations based on cycle length or earliest temperature rise. The fertile time starts at the *earliest* sign of change, whether from the secretions, cervix or calculation– whichever comes first.

Value of the stop bar

Flynn compared the reliability of women's subjective assessment of the fertile time with urinary gonadotrophins and serial ultrasound. The day after maximum follicular growth was the marker for ovulation (day 0) with the probable fertile time estimated from five days before to one day after ovulation. The start of the fertile time was determined by the calculation *S minus 19* or the first appearance of secretions, whichever came *first*. Using the calculation, two of the 23 cycles fell within the fertile time (by ultrasound) whereas relying on the first appearance of secretions, six cycles fell within the objective fertile time. Flynn reported one conception resulting from intercourse 5 days before ovulation, which resulted in a term pregnancy. The woman recorded the intercourse day (day 5) as a dry day and ignored the *S minus 19 rule*. Had she used the calendar calculation, intercourse would have been avoided seven days before ovulation, so Flynn reasonably assumed that the pregnancy might have been avoided. This confirmed the current teaching of using the first sign of change whether by calculation or secretions. [178] *S minus 20* provides a yet more conservative estimate of the start of the fertile time.

SELF-ASSESSMENT QUESTIONS

Answers are at the end of the chapter.

1 Jill and Ben want a natural method, but Jill does not want to record her fertility indicators. She is keen to use the Calendar/Rhythm Method and accepts its effectiveness. Jill's smartphone app shows her last 12 cycle lengths as 27, 29, 28, 29, 30, 27, 31, 32, 29, 28, 27, 30. How would you advise her about her potential fertile time. Any provisos?
2 Describe the *S minus 20 rule*. Are there any provisos for using this as part of a combined-indicator method?
3 Describe the *Day 6 rule* and in what circumstances it can be applied. How would you explain the risk of pregnancy from intercourse in the first five days of the cycle?
4 Describe the calculation based on temperature readings to define the start of the fertile time.

Correlating all indicators on combined chart

Figure 7.2 shows a combined indicator chart correlating changes in temperature, secretions, cervix and a calculation. The shortest cycle (based on the last 12 cycles) is 28 days. The calculation *S minus 20* indicates day 8 is the first fertile day (note vertical stop bar between days 7 and 8). On day 8 there are no secretions and the cervix has not started to change, but the fertile time starts at the earliest sign – in this case, the calculation. The cervix starts to soften on day 9 and the cervical secretions are first observed on day 10. Peak day is day 15 (the last day of most fertile secretions). The temperature rises to the higher level on day 15. Note the count of three high temperatures in small italic numbers with the third temperature at least 0.2 deg.C above the six low readings. As the first high temperature is on the same day as peak, it is necessary to count an extra day to ensure that there are three high temperatures *after* peak day (note the adjusted readings 1, 2, 3 after peak). The fertile time starts on day 8 and lasts until day 18 inclusive. Note the pattern of intercourse: there is no reason to restrict intercourse to non-consecutive evenings in the early dry days if using a calculation. Intercourse in the late infertile time is unrestricted until the start of the next period.

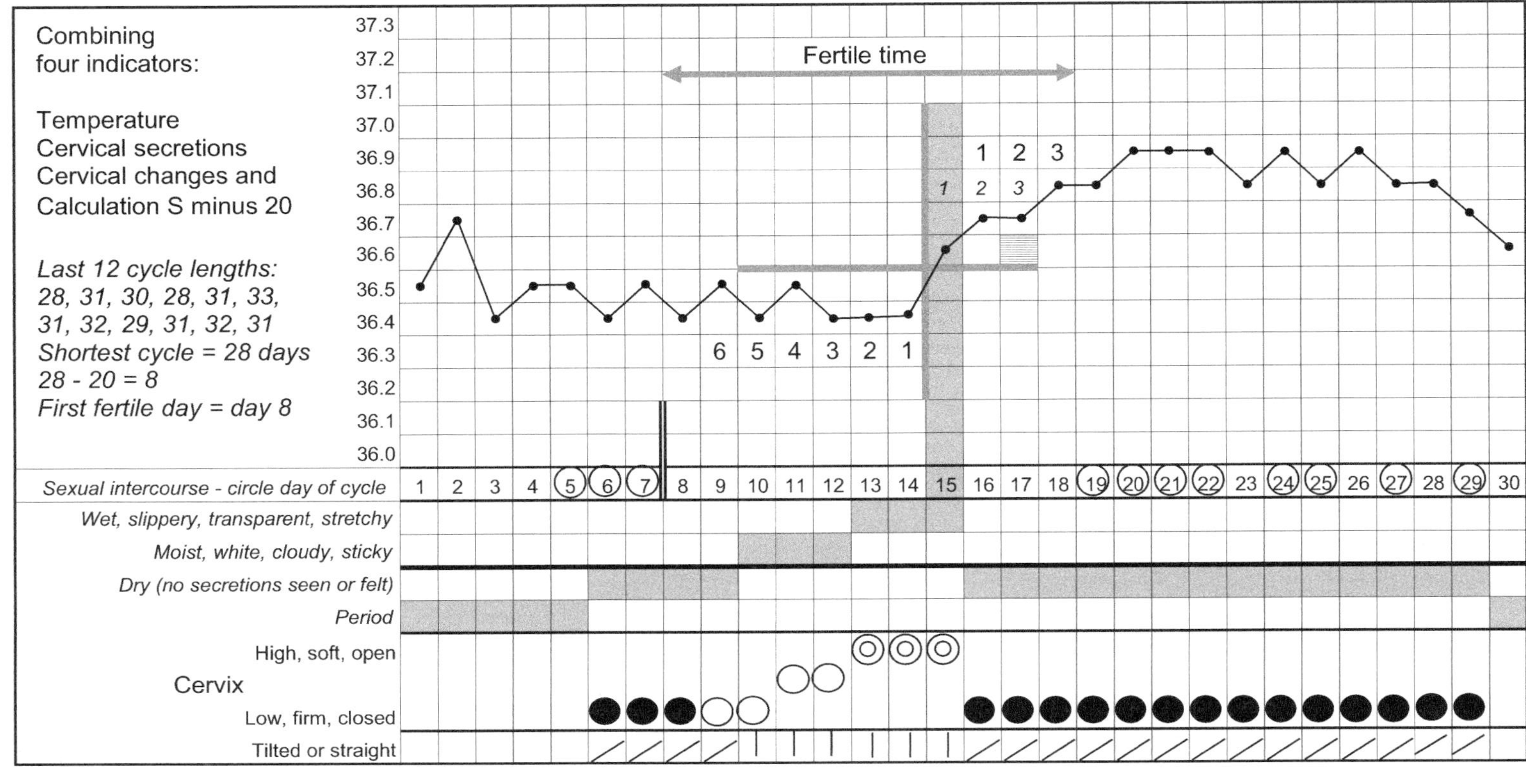

Figure 7.2 Combining temperature, secretions, cervix and *S minus 20* calculation

ACTIVITY CHART-BUILDING EXERCISE (CONTINUED FROM PAGE 148)

Step 4 Adding calculation stop bar based on shortest cycle information

Jo has kept a diary record of her cycle lengths for two years. Her cycle lengths over the last year have been 30, 27, 28, 31, 27, 29, 30, 28, 29, 27, 30 and 28 days.

1 From this information, calculate her shortest cycle. Indicate this in the shortest cycle length box (top left of chart).
2 Use the *S minus 20* rule to identify the first fertile day (add to designated box on chart).
3 Add a vertical stop bar to show the first fertile day by the *S minus 20* rule.
4 Jo had unprotected intercourse on days 5, 20, 21, 22, 24, 25, 26, 28 and 29. Circle the appropriate days.

Activity to be continued on page 182.

ANSWERS TO SELF-ASSESSMENT QUESTIONS

1 Jill's shortest cycle is 27 days and her longest cycle is 32 days. This is within the recommended range for the Calendar/Rhythm Method (23–35 days). She has a cycle length variation of five days, which means the method is suitable. Using the calculation *S minus 20* and *L minus 10*, her first fertile day is day 7 and her last fertile day is day 22. This is a lengthy time of abstinence, so it would be important to discuss how manageable this would be for both partners. She should continue to record her cycle length and readjust the calculations after each cycle to account for a longer or shorter cycle length. If her cycles become irregular (varying by eight days or more) or she has a cycle of less than 23 days or more than 35 days, the Calendar/Rhythm Method will be less reliable and she may need to consider another method.
2 S –20 = first fertile day. The woman needs to base her calculations on an accurate record of her last 12 cycle lengths. Her first fertile day will be based on the *S minus 20 rule* or the first change from dryness (or first change from a low, firm, closed cervix) whichever comes *first*. A stop bar is drawn on the chart to indicate the start of the fertile time.
3 Day 6 is the first fertile day. This is applicable to women who have a record of at least the last three cycle lengths, which must all be 26 days or longer. Research shows that the pregnancy rate in the first three days of the cycle is negligible, increasing to less than 2% by day 7. [630]
4 A woman who has recorded her temperature for the last 12 cycles can identify the earliest temperature rise (first high temperature) in the last year and subtract 7 to identify the start of the fertile time. The calculation is always made on the most recent 12 cycles.

MINOR INDICATORS OF FERTILITY

8

The four major indicators of fertility are temperature, secretions, cervical changes and calendar calculations. The minor indicators are the other recognizable physiological and psychological changes related to fluctuations in estrogen and progesterone. These vary from woman to woman and from one cycle to the next. Common signs and symptoms include abdominal pain, abdominal bloating, breast changes, mood changes and fluctuations in libido. Less common are lower backache, skin changes, vulval swelling and inter-menstrual bleeding. A woman can be helped to manage her symptoms if she records them on her chart and recognises their hormonal nature. Some signs and symptoms may be consistent in an individual but research shows that they are the least reliable indicators of fertility.

OVULATION PAIN

"Mid-cycle" abdominal pain occurs in ovulatory cycles, either regularly or occasionally, in up to 50% of women at some time during their reproductive life. Mittelschmerz varies in intensity and duration. The pain is normally localised in the right or left iliac fossa, although some women describe central abdominal pain. The pain may radiate into the groin, the vagina or the labia. Its characteristic nature means that many women recognise the significance of this pain, but its timing is varied. Many women with normal ovulatory cycles experience no pain.

Mittelschmerz may be mild and cramp-like or more acute and painful. It may have a sudden or gradual onset often increasing in intensity before subsiding. The pain, which may last from a few hours up to about five days (typically 12–24 hours), usually occurs on the side of ovulation. Some studies have documented a greater incidence of right-sided pain while others have reported no difference reporting random occurrence in successive cycles. [376] [439] [601]

The cause of the pain is unclear. It may be caused by the distended follicle putting pressure on surrounding structures, peritoneal irritation from blood and fluid from the ruptured follicle [262], or peristaltic contractions of the Fallopian tube. Pain in the right iliac fossa may be of particular concern as it can mimic appendicitis. [146]

The relationship between mittelschmerz and ovulation is variable. Krohn first reported, in the 1940s, on the case of a young woman who recorded a close correlation between temperature and mittelschmerz for over a four-year time-span. [337] In Vollman's study of 621 women (over 20,000 temperature charts) 45% of the women noted pain in 17% of the cycles. Vollman observed that the pain usually preceded the temperature rise by one or two days, but advised that its sporadic nature precluded it from being a reliable indicator of fertility. [601]

A number of studies have correlated mittelschmerz with objective markers of ovulation. O'Herlihy showed that the majority of women (26 out of 34) experienced mittelschmerz on the same day as the LH peak. In one woman the pain may have coincided with ovulation (by ultrasound) but in all the other women the pain preceded follicular rupture by 24–48 hours. Speculating on the possible cause of the pain, O'Herlihy noted that on the day of the pain the mean follicular diameter was 19.3 ± 2.2 mm. Whilst this is a considerable increase in size, cysts may be considerably bigger in anovulatory cycles and not cause pain. There was, however, a strong correlation between mittelschmerz and LH, which is known to increase contractility of smooth muscle. [439]

Abdominal pain has been shown to be more closely associated with ovulation than backache, abdominal bloating, and inter-menstrual bleeding, but this still showed a wide variation compared with ovulation by hormonal markers. [282] Depares confirmed that, compared with the major indicators of fertility, abdominal pain was the least sensitive marker occurring from two days before to two days after ovulation. [118] Gnoth's study showed a wider variation: although more than 30% of women reported mittelschmerz on the day of ovulation (by ultrasound), the pain varied from six days before to two days after ovulation [230] (see figure 10.1 in chapter 10).

Note: Women may wish to note abdominal pain on the chart as confirmation of the major indicators, but should recognise its variability. Any severe or prolonged abdominal pain requires investigation to exclude other causes such as an ovarian cyst or appendicitis.

CASE STUDY FORGET THE PAIN – JUST DO IT

Gillian, a healthy 32-year-old, had been trying to conceive for more than a year, targeting sex around day 14. She had regular cycles of 33–35 days. On discussing her likely fertile time, it emerged that a day or so after the baby-making sex she often felt "a bit rubbish" due to a pain in her side, usually the right side. It started as a vague pain but became increasingly noticeable, reaching a crescendo after four or five days and then disappearing. The pain felt worse in the evenings and she generally took herself off to bed with a hot water bottle. Gillian conceived on the first cycle she had sex despite the pain and went on to have three healthy children.

BREAST CHANGES

Breast tissue is sensitive to changes in estrogen and progesterone. Boys and girls have equally sensitive breasts before puberty, whereas afterwards sensitivity is higher amongst girls. The breasts are normally most sensitive at or just before a period. Some women notice tenderness or a tingling sensation, particularly around the nipples, which may be related to higher estrogen around the time of ovulation. Hilgers found post-ovulatory breast tenderness was the most common of all inter-menstrual symptoms, but it was not directly related to the level of progesterone. [282]

Breast temperature (influenced by changes in blood flow) is higher in the luteal phase and shows a circadian rhythm being at its lowest in the morning and highest in the evening, but these changes are not sufficiently distinct to be used as indicators of fertility.

The most obvious change for the majority of women is the progesterone-related increase in breast size due to fluid retention. This is experienced as breast fullness or heaviness but the exact timing in relation to ovulation is not precise. Breast volume has been measured using different techniques including plaster casts, water displacement (kneeling with one breast in a bowl of water), ultrasound and magnetic resonance imaging. Drife reported increases in breast volume (water displacement method) by up to 20% during the luteal phase (between 9 and 17 days before the next period) with a total change in volume during ovulatory cycles by as much as 100 ml. [134]

Increased breast size during the luteal phase may be sufficient for a woman to need two sets of bras going up a cup-size premenstrually, which highlights the importance of education about well-fitting bras. Press reports of poor-fitting under-wire bras restricting lymph drainage and increasing the risk of breast cancer are not supported by a population-based case-control study among post-menopausal women. [82] Cyclic breast changes are interesting and can be noted on the chart but they are too varied to be of any practical significance as indicators of fertility. All women should be encouraged to be breast aware and report any signs that could indicate breast disease (page 218).

PREMENSTRUAL SYMPTOMS

Most women who are having normal ovulatory cycles experience some degree of cyclic symptoms during the luteal phase that disappear around the start of the period. These may include breast changes, abdominal bloating, carbohydrate craving, headaches, irritability, tearfulness, aggression, lack of concentration, clumsiness and loss of confidence. Negative cyclical symptoms appear to be directly related to ovulation and the development of the corpus luteum. The most commonly reported premenstrual symptoms include fluid retention, changes in appetite plus changes in mood and libido.

Fluid retention and abdominal bloating Symptoms such as fluid retention and abdominal bloating are highly subjective. In a study of 62 healthy normal-weight women who recorded menstrual diaries and temperature changes, fluid retention was found to be at its highest on the first day of the period and lowest in the mid-follicular phase. It then increased again just before ovulation and continued through the luteal phase. There was no significant difference between ovulatory and anovulatory cycles; however, there were very few anovulatory cycles so this observation may not be valid. The researchers concluded that women's self-reported fluid retention is unlikely to be due to progesterone. [612]

Food intake Appetite and food intake are known to vary during the menstrual cycle being at its lowest around ovulation and its highest premenstrually. This may be associated with lower mood and depression due to reduced serotonin levels. Carbohydrate cravings are more common and alcohol intake is higher premenstrually particularly for women with premenstrual syndrome. [37] [71] [31] [147] [70]

Changes in mood and libido Many women report feelings of well-being and increased sexual interest during the follicular phase and around ovulation but a more depressed mood, with tiredness and irritability, in the luteal phase and premenstrually. This may cause problems for couples avoiding pregnancy if the time the woman feels at her best and desires sex coincides with the fertile time. Women's changes in libido across the menstrual cycle are varied (page 48).

A number of studies have looked at women's mood. Henderson confirmed the peak in positive mood at or about the time of ovulation and negative mood at or about the time of menstruation, but this was only pronounced in women who rated themselves as "sufferers" of premenstrual discomfort and not in those who rated themselves as experiencing very mild discomfort. [275]

In a one-year study of ovulation, exercise and bone change, 62 healthy women (average age 34) recorded temperature and mood diaries scoring their level of anxiety, depression and anger/frustration. Temperature charts showed that out of 739 cycles 72% were biphasic (presumed ovulatory), 25% had a short luteal phase and 3% were monophasic (presumed anovulatory). Minor cyclic mood changes were present in both ovulatory and anovulatory cycles. In anovulatory cycles, mood tended to be more variable but less negative. Mood scores did not differ based on the hormone level or luteal phase length. Harvey concluded that patterns and mechanisms of mood change in symptomatic women appeared to be amplifications of normal experiences. [269]

A systematic review of mood in relation to the menstrual cycle challenged the widespread belief of negative mood premenstrually. Forty-seven relevant studies were identified:

- 18 found no association between mood and any phase of the menstrual cycle;
- 18 found negative mood was associated with the premenstrual phase and another phase of the cycle;

- seven found that negative mood was associated with the premenstrual phase only; and
- four found an association between negative mood and a non-premenstrual phase.

The researchers concluded that when taken together these studies failed to provide clear evidence in support of the existence of a specific premenstrual negative mood syndrome in the general population. [511]

Approximately 5% of women experience severe symptoms (premenstrual syndrome), including anxiety and depression, which may require medical management (page 205).

INTER-MENSTRUAL SPOTTING AND LIGHT BLEEDING

Some women notice spotting, light bleeding, or red, pink or brown blood-tinged secretions around peak day. This may be due to the effect on the endometrium of a rapid drop in estrogen levels around ovulation. This normally occurs while the temperature is still at the low level, or just as it is rising to the higher level. The bleeding may indicate peak fertility and should not be confused with a true period, which occurs about 14 days after the temperature rise. Any inter-menstrual bleeding requires investigation by speculum examination, swabs, cervical screening and pelvic ultrasound to exclude trauma, infection, cervical and pelvic pathology. Provided no cause is found, a woman can be reassured that this may be due to hormonal changes related to ovulation.

RECORDING MINOR INDICATORS ON THE CHART

A woman may wish to record minor indicators on her chart but must understand that these provide supplementary information only. They *cannot* be relied upon to give any indication of ovulation or the limits of the fertile time.

The chart shown in figure 8.1 is from Mandy, a 29-year-old experienced user (with chart 21). She has limited her observations to the necessary part of the cycle, starting from the end of her period until she has established that the fertile time has ended. The fertile time starts on day 7 – she calculated this based on her earliest temperature rise over the last 12 cycles. Her first cervical change is on day 8 and first sign of secretions is on day 9, hence her earliest temperature rise calculation gave the earliest indication of the start of the fertile time. Mandy's peak day is on day 15 followed by a temperature rise on day 17. Her third high temperature is only 0.1 deg.C above the six low readings, so she waits for a fourth high temperature which is above the coverline. All high temperatures are after peak day, so her fertile time has ended. Mandy also notes that her cervix has returned to its low, firm, closed state and remained closed for three days – this gives her extra security that the fertile time has ended and she and her partner can confidently resume intercourse. Mandy has noted on her chart that the temperature spike on day 12 may have been disturbed due to alcohol the night before. There is only one spike in the six low temperatures, so this can safely be ignored. Note Mandy's observation of abdominal pain two days before her rise in temperature. She also notes marked breast fullness for several days before the start of her period. The fertile time lasts from day 7 to 20 inclusive.

Note: New users should always record temperatures (and secretions) through the entire cycle; this helps to consolidate learning and determine a usual coverline. When a woman has charted for one year, provided she has cycles of 26 days or longer, she may choose to restrict her observations and not start recording her indicators until the end of her period. A woman who has short cycles will need to record through her period, or she may miss the start of the fertile time.

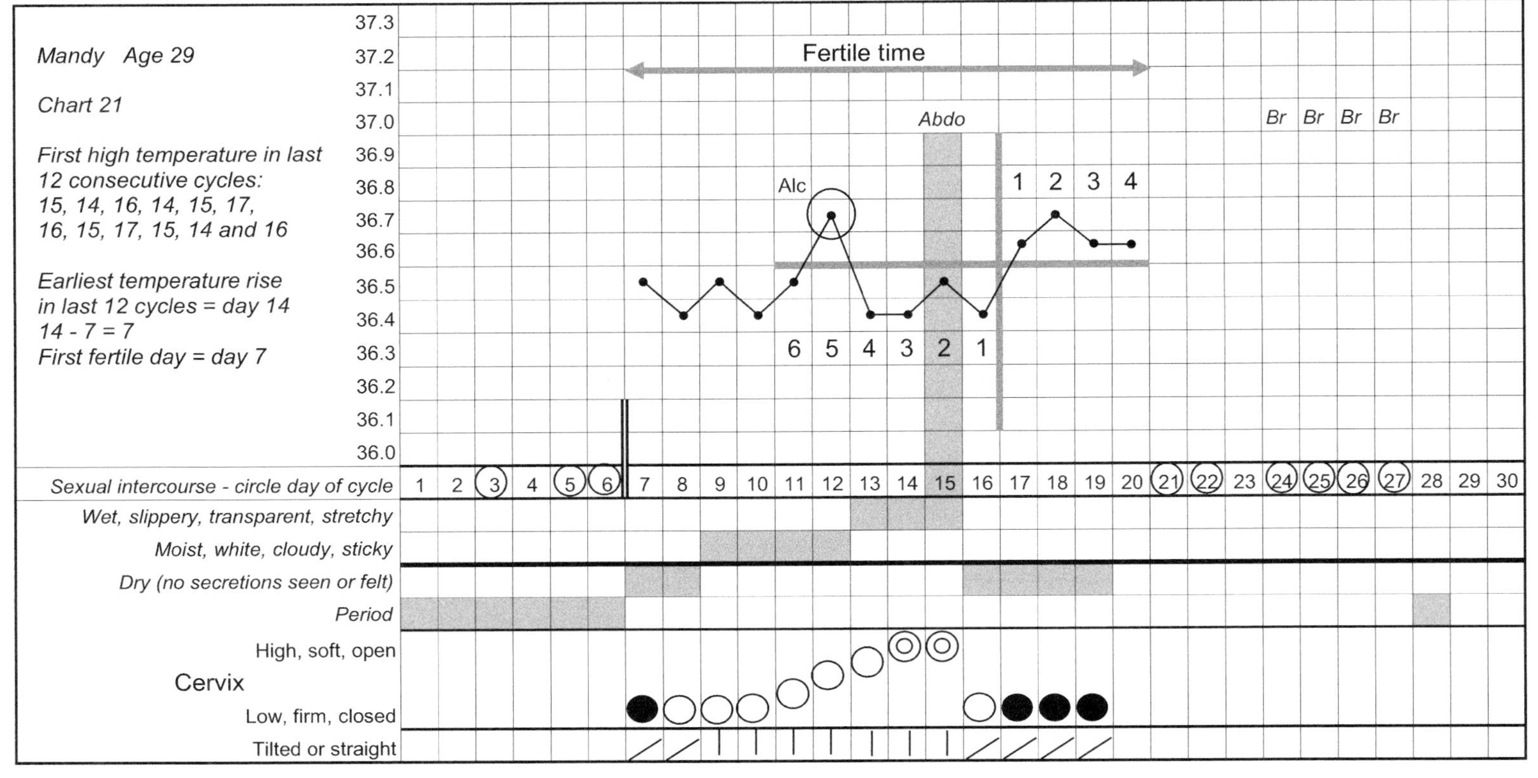

Figure 8.1 Combined indicator chart showing correlation between all indicators. Note the limited observations of an experienced user.

9 HOME TEST KITS AND MONITORS

> Eventually, many a woman in our affluent society may conclude that the determination of when and whether she is ovulating should be a routine item of personal health information to which she is entitled as a matter of course.
>
> (Carl Djerassi, "Fertility awareness: jet-age rhythm method?") [125]

Carl Djerassi is probably best known for his contribution to the development of the contraceptive pill. In 1990 he commented on the crisis in contraceptive research and development owing to the withdrawal of many large pharmaceutical companies and suggested it was time to take a fresh look at FAMs. Djerassi highlighted the advances in analytical biochemistry making it possible to use simple colour-change systems to reflect urinary hormone changes. He suggested that dedicating serious scientific efforts to improving FAMs would make political and ethical sense. Djerassi could see the relevance of direct hormone monitoring for all women – for general health awareness, avoiding pregnancy or optimising conception for subfertile couples with the benefit of analysing hormones directly to avoid confusion with disturbances such as travel.

The first home test kit available to the public was Brown's Ovarian Monitor, which measured urinary metabolites of estrogen and progesterone. The monitor showed a close correlation with laboratory testing (and provided a useful research tool) but the women required careful supervision to meet laboratory standards and the Ovarian Monitor was not practical as a simple home test. [66] [53] The Ovarian Monitor had the distinct advantage of the progesterone marker to confirm ovulation.

Currently available home test kits and devices aim to identify the fertile time by using either direct markers (urinary LH or estrone-3-glucoronide plus LH) or indirect markers (temperature, sodium chloride in saliva and electrical resistance in saliva or cervical secretions). These technologies are intended as stand-alone methods but they can be used in conjunction with observed indicators. Relatively few products have been subject to rigorous testing and independent trials. It is concerning that women use these devices for contraceptive purposes yet products can be released onto the market without effectiveness studies and there are no clear international guidelines for testing and verification.

OVULATION PREDICTOR KITS (OPKS)

OPKs are based on the detection of a rise in urinary LH – the best marker for predicting *imminent* ovulation. [618] [97] They predict ovulation within two days of the serum LH surge in more than 90% of cases. [254] The LH surge, which triggers ovulation, is detectable in urine as a positive test for one or two days. Ovulation normally follows the LH surge within 24–36 hours. There are a number of brands which are widely marketed toward women wishing to achieve a pregnancy. Testing normally begins around day 6 and continues daily for 5 to 9 days or until there is a positive result. Some tests show a darkened line; the newer digital tests, which show a smiley face, are easier to read. Ovulation predictor kits have both advantages and disadvantages:

- They predict the two days of maximum fertility only.
- They may give false positives (in > 7% of cycles). [395]
- They may give false negatives – the surge may occur within the 24-hour testing window.
- The LH peak may occur after ovulation (in > 25% of ovulatory cycles). [513]
- Persistently positive results may indicate an elevated LH (possibly PCOS).
- They are *not* suitable for women with PCOS (with an elevated LH).
- They are *not* suitable for women avoiding pregnancy as a stand-alone method.
- They do not provide proof of ovulation (page 54).

Women's experiences of OPKs Women commonly use OPKs to optimise their chances of conception, but there have been suggestions that timed intercourse causes stress. Tiplady studied two groups: the first were given OPKs and advised to follow the manufacturer's instructions; the control group were asked to have intercourse every two to three days as recommended by NICE guidelines. There was no difference between the two groups in the validated stress questionnaires or the biomarkers (urinary LH and cortisol). [580] Some women using OPKs reported negative experiences including increased pressure between partners, sex becoming mechanical, becoming obsessive about testing (with prolonged use) and anxiety about conception delays. However, they also reported similar negative experiences when trying to conceive without using the tests. Women appreciated an improved understanding of their cycle, reassurance about ovulation and intercourse timing, plus a sense of joint involvement and removing the stress associated with guesswork. Further studies are needed on male partners and amongst a subfertile population. [311]

OPKs to confirm subjective indicators OPKs may provide an additional marker for women using FAMs to avoid pregnancy. There are times when some indicators may not be reliable: for example, temperature may not be feasible during night shift work. An OPK provides a double-check for the *end* of the fertile time. Leiva reported on the use of OPKs by 23 women having difficulty identifying the end of the fertile time. The LH kits identified 100% of the luteal phases, whereas temperature and secretions identified only 87% (using serum progesterone as the objective marker). Leiva concluded that these kits may offer an adjunct for women who wish to have an additional check, but more research is needed. [351]

The need to identify a higher number of fertile days Tests which are based solely on LH typically identify the day of ovulation and the day before. The full fertile time (based on urinary hormones) lasts six days, with a 10% chance of pregnancy from intercourse five days preceding ovulation. [631] Couples who wait to have sex until an LH test shows positive are therefore missing opportunities and may paradoxically be limiting their chances of conception. Some of the newer tests analyse both LH and E3G, typically identifying four fertile days, whilst maintaining the simplicity of a dipstick-only test.

CLEARBLUE FERTILITY MONITOR

The Clearblue fertility monitor (previously known as Clearplan Easy) consists of a hand-held monitor and disposable urine sticks which analyse both LH and E3G. It is designed for couples planning pregnancy, giving predictions of low, high and peak fertility. The monitor is based on the same technology as Persona, the contraceptive monitor. [557] It tracks and stores information, typically identifying around six fertile days. When the monitor's performance was compared with ultrasound and serum LH in 53 healthy women (150 cycles), 91% of cycles showed an LH surge on the monitor (confirmed as ovulatory by ultrasound). One anovulatory cycle was detected by the monitor (no LH surge). Behre supported the use of the monitor by women planning pregnancy and saw the potential for its use in fertility management. [40] A study of 635 women showed an increased pregnancy within two cycles with use of the monitor (23% self-reported pregnancy rate compared with 14% in the control group). This demonstrated that, for normal fertile women, knowledge of the wider fertile window and optimising sex timing significantly increased the chance of conception within two cycles. Women were much more likely to conceive if they had been trying for less than six months. [504]

PERSONA (CONTRACEPTIVE MONITOR)

Persona, released in the UK in 1996, was the first personal hormone monitoring system designed for women avoiding pregnancy. It consists of a small hand-held electronic monitor and disposable dual-hormone urine test sticks. The monitor indicates fertile days with a red light and infertile days with a green light. Currently the original Persona monitor is available in the UK, whilst a similar product the Clearblue Contraceptive Monitor is available in other parts of Europe.

Scientific background and effectiveness Persona was the culmination of years of extensive research (supported by WHO) into personal hormone monitoring. It uses E3G to identify the start of the fertile time [98] and LH to indicate imminent ovulation. [618] [97] [393]

An independent European prospective study of 710 women with regular cycles (23–35 days) using Persona alone showed a method pregnancy rate of 12.1%. Analysis of the primary causes of these pregnancies showed that the system had given insufficient warning of ovulation in cycles 4–13 because the original algorithm did not allow sufficient time for sperm survival. The algorithm was modified accordingly. The method pregnancy rate when used with abstinence was then re-calculated as 6.2%. [56] Trussell argued that Bonnar's calculation of the estimated method failure rate was too low. He examined the differences in their approaches and the complexities of making estimates based on intercourse patterns with red light days carrying higher risks of pregnancy than green light days. [585]

Profile of Persona users A questionnaire survey in the Netherlands of 137 Persona users found that "Persona woman" was typically in a committed relationship, highly educated and with above-average income. She wanted a contraceptive method with no side effects, and said she desired children in the future. For nearly 30% of women, getting to know their body and understanding the menstrual cycle was seen as one of the biggest advantages of the device. Many reported that Persona changed the way they viewed their cycle and their desire for children. One in four women were using the monitor to plan pregnancy. [305]

Correlation of observed indicators with Persona Persona is designed as a stand-alone device but it can used in conjunction with other indicators. It may be particularly helpful to new users: some stop using the device once they have gained confidence in their observed indicators whilst others continue charting both or continue with Persona alone.

Figure 9.1 shows the correlation of indicators. This is a 27-day cycle from a new user (chart number 4). Her shortest cycle in the last year is 26 days (*S minus 20* = day 6). Persona asks for its first test (as standard) on day 6. The first cervical change (softness) is on day 9. This is also the first day that Persona indicates fertility. The first secretions are not observed until day 10. Peak is on day 15 followed by a temperature rise on day 16. The third high temperature is a minimum of 0.2 deg.C above the six low temperatures, indicating the end of the fertile time on day 18 (third high temperature after peak). Note that the last fertile day according to Persona is day 17 (one day earlier). The fertile time by Persona is from day 9 to 17 inclusive, whereas the more conservative estimate given by the observed indicators is from day 6 to 18 inclusive. Persona will generally give a shorter fertile time but it is only about 94% effective compared with 98% for observed indicators. Note the Persona symbols: T indicates a test day (yellow

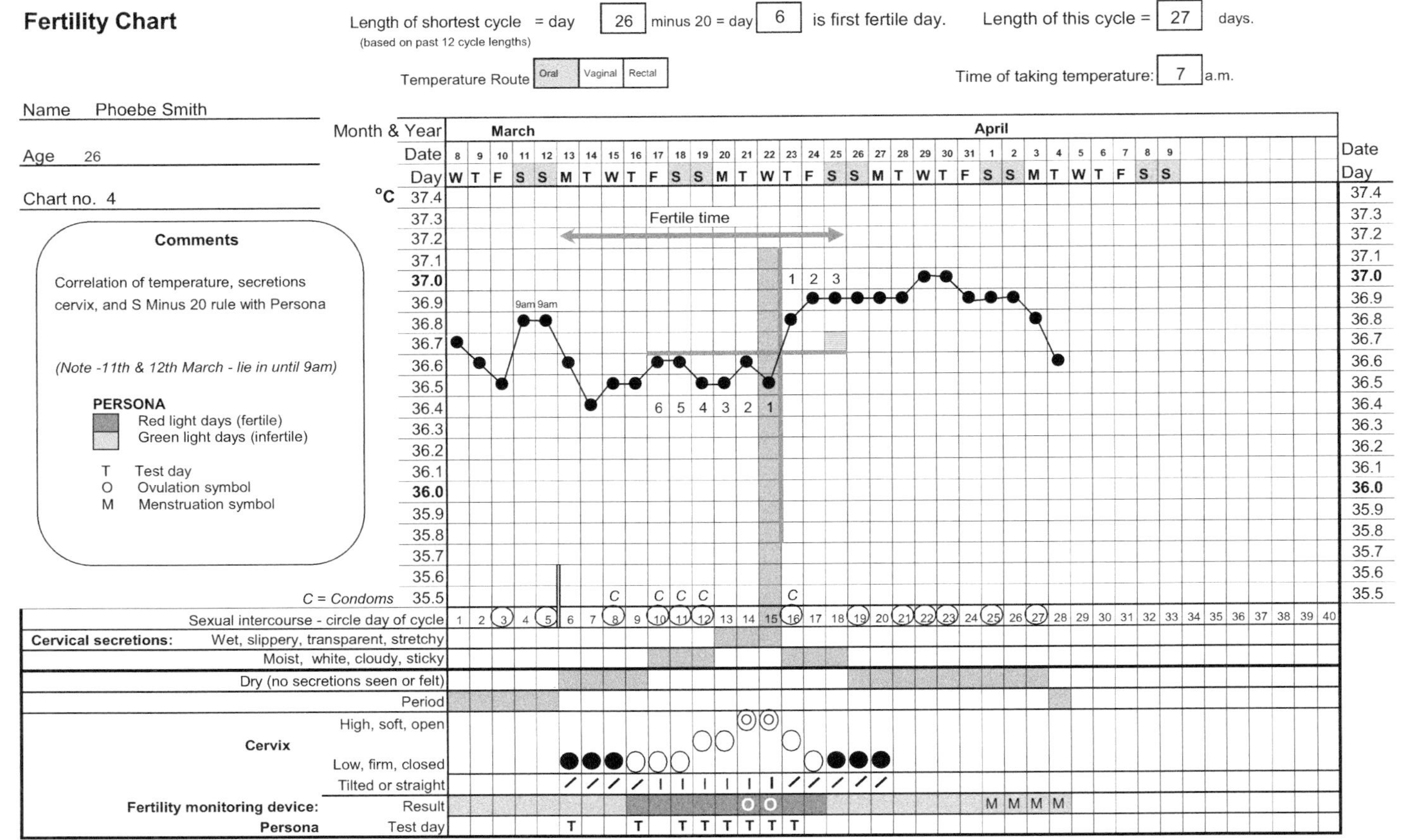

Figure 9.1 Correlation of temperature, secretions, cervix and *S minus 20* rule with Persona. Protected intercourse marked with a “C” (condoms).

light). Days 1–8 inclusive are green-light days (infertile). Day 9 is the start of the red-light days (fertile) – the monitor has detected a rise in E3G. Days 9–17 inclusive are red-light days. Note the "O" symbols on days 14 and 15 – days the LH surge is detected. Day 18 onwards shows green-light days. From day 25 onwards, the "M" symbol shows that menstruation is imminent. The couple have used condoms consistently from days 6–18, marking the chart with a "C". They appear to be using the method correctly with no risk-taking.

COMPUTERISED THERMOMETERS

A number of devices combine an electronic thermometer with a small computer which analyses information about waking temperature with cycle length calculations to indicate the fertile and infertile times. These thermometers allow input of intercourse information and some allow for other indicators such as secretions and urinary LH.

Lady-comp is targeted at women avoiding pregnancy. Freundl's retrospective study of 648 women (10,275 months of use) found that the device was well-accepted by women and their partners. The average number of fertile days identified by the monitor was 14. The correct use rate was 0.7% by Pearl Index (the figure used on the website). The typical use rate by life table analysis was 5.3% after one year, 6.8% after two years and 8.2% after three years of use. [202] (See the section on contraceptive effectiveness in chapter 14 for more on typical use rates.) Lady-comp Baby is a similar device but it has a built-in sex selection feature aimed at women planning pregnancy – there is no reliable evidence to support claims for determining the sex of the child.

Cyclotest 2 is aimed at women avoiding pregnancy. Freundl compared the fertile time identified by 207 women using combined indicators with that according to Cyclotest. The algorithm led to a dangerous reduction in the fertile time in only two out of 207 cycles (0.96%). However, the device requested more abstinence than was necessary at the end of the fertile time in about 12% of cycles. Freundl recommended more research on detecting the end of the fertile time. [199] Cyclotest Baby is aimed at women trying to conceive, although the manufacturers state it can also be used for contraceptive purposes.

CONTINUOUS TEMPERATURE MONITORING

It is feasible that continuous temperature monitoring (day and night) may give more reliable readings than a single waking temperature and may even detect subtle preovulatory changes (see "dip" before the rise: page 103).

The Duofertility device measures temperature through an axillary sensor (an adhesive patch worn continuously). The sensor detects thousands of measurements every day which are analysed to show the most representative nocturnal temperature. The hand-held reader indicates days with the maximum chance of conception. Data is transferred via the Internet to a central consultancy service, which encourages women to input information on secretions, cycle length and LH (and to have intercourse two to three times per week). The manufacturers described a retrospective analysis of the first 500 couples who used the monitor, resulting in an average clinical pregnancy rate of 39% after 12 months of use. [77] A pilot study compared the accuracy of the monitor with ultrasound in eight subfertile women with regular cycles, normal ovarian morphology and normal hormonal profiles. The women used the monitor for one cycle and used OPKs to determine the LH surge and the timing of ultrasound. Duofertility identified ovulation within one day of the ultrasound marker in all cycles. There were no anovulatory cycles, hence the need for a larger study to include women with irregular and anovulatory cycles. [510] **The device requires independent testing to justify its cost.**

Ovusense consists of a thermal sensor and a reader. The sensor is placed in the vagina at night and records core temperature every five minutes overnight. The device analyses the readings to identify the temperature nadir. It personalises information and aims to predict the next ovulation based on past cycle data. When Ovusense readings were compared with oral temperatures (using digital thermometers) in 19 women (81 cycles), core temperatures were more accurate than oral temperatures when compared with ultrasound. [449] The algorithm predicted ovulation one day in advance in 89% of cycles. The nadir occurred on average three days before ovulation so allowed a prediction of ovulation a short time ahead. Ovulation was confirmed after three days. [448]

Temperature-based devices may offer an advantage for some women – for example those with PCOS who have elevated LH levels – but **there is no evidence to suggest that this level of accuracy is of more practical benefit than an inexpensive digital thermometer (and frequent intercourse).**

SALIVARY FERNING TESTS

Saliva testing devices use a small plastic microscope to detect ferning as a sign of ovulation. Kits such as Fertile Focus, Saliva Biotester and Fertility Scope are widely available at low-cost via the Internet, but there is conflicting data about their effectiveness and a literature review was unable to find data on specific brands. [63] Saliva, an easily accessible bodily fluid, has long been considered as a potential indicator because salivary estradiol levels reflect serum levels through the menstrual cycle. [159] Saliva, like cervical secretions, shows changes in viscosity, spinnbarkeit and crystallisation. [297] This characteristic ferning was first reported in cervical secretions in the late 1950s (page 62).

Barbato reported on the value of salivary ferning in 32 women (using the PG/53 pocket microscope). Salivary ferning correlated with observed indicators in 28 women. Ferning started 1–2 days before the first appearance of cervical secretions and lasted a mean of 6.2 days. Ferning was observed on average 7.2 days before the first high temperature but was uninterpretable in four cycles. [27] Guida's study of 40 healthy women reported that LH correlated 100% with ovulation (by ultrasound diagnosis), cervical secretions showed a 48% correlation, temperature a 30% correlation and salivary ferning a 36% correlation. However, 59% of the results from salivary ferning were uninterpretable. [255] Berardono demonstrated that salivary ferning was present during the *entire* menstrual cycle and was observed in pre-pubertal girls, pregnant women, post-menopausal women and men. [44] Braat found similar results. Seventeen women used the mini-microscope, which showed a sensitivity of 53%, and 13 women used a normal light microscope, which had a sensitivity of 86%. The test was repeated in 10 post-menopausal women and 10 men. Eight out of 10 post-menopausal women tested positive and all of the men tested positive for signs of ovulation. **The salivary ferning test is unreliable and its use should be discouraged.** [61]

ELECTRICAL RESISTANCE IN SALIVA AND VAGINAL SECRETIONS

Attempts have been made to measure the electrical resistance of saliva and vaginal secretions which reflect the changing concentrations of sodium and potassium during the menstrual cycle. Ovacue consists of a hand-held monitor with two probes: an oral probe to identify the start of the fertile time and a vaginal probe to identify the end of the fertile time. Ovacue is a computerised version of the Cue monitor; Ovacue Mobile consists of an app for a mobile phone with adapters for the probes. Freundl compared the Cue readings with the fertile time (by ultrasound and LH) in 13 women (16 cycles). The first fertile day was accurately detected in 14 cycles but in two cycles the monitor signal was less than five days before ovulation. The last fertile day was correctly identified by the monitor in 10 cycles but in six it indicated the end of the fertile time when objective markers showed the woman was still fertile. Cue missed the signal for the fertile time in two cycles. Freundl suggested at the time that the monitor, with its existing algorithm, could not be recommended for avoiding pregnancy but suggested the signals were useful and the algorithm should be improved. [196] Reports on the findings of other studies using the Cue monitor, however, confirmed that **salivary electrical resistance is of no use in predicting ovulation.** [201]

THE LURE OF SUCCESS STORIES

Home test kits which purport to increase chances of conception are seductive and the Internet is full of success stories from women attributing their pregnancy to a particular technology. Women frequently spend large sums of money on unnecessary or useless products which are later abandoned, whilst men often resent the regimented sex dictated by these gadgets. A number of home kits have online forums and consultancy services to provide support on the use of these devices and general advice on optimising chances of conception. There is no standardised preconception information and the quality and reliability of these services is not known, however. Under these conditions, pregnancies cannot be attributed to a specific device.

REVIEW OF HOME KITS TO OPTIMISE CONCEPTION

A team from Johns Hopkins university reviewed products available for women who are trying to conceive in what they described as "a billion-dollar industry that continues to grow". They conducted literature searches and used focused communications with manufacturers to determine the usefulness and validity of existing products. **Some products (based on direct hormone monitoring) have been thoroughly tested and offer value in fertility management, but others (including electronic thermometers, salivary ferning and electrical resistance devices) lack enough practical application to be recommended as a valuable adjunct to medical management.** [63] Table 9.1 summarises these technologies with approximate costs for one year's use. The observed indicators are included for comparison.

Quality index to evaluate home kits and devices

Freundl and his team from the University of Dusseldorf developed a quality index score to evaluate fertility monitors prior to full prospective clinical trials. The days predicted as fertile by the monitors were compared with the fertile time by ultrasound and urinary LH. Freundl concluded that a score lower than 0.5 identified a monitor with accuracy in identifying the fertile time that was sufficient to warrant prospective clinical trials: this included Persona and computerised thermometers such as Ladycomp/Babycomp, Bioself 2000 and Cyclotest 2 plus. Devices with a score lower than 0.5 identified a monitor with accuracy that was not sufficient to warrant prospective clinical trials: this included all saliva testing devices (PG 53, PC 2000 and Maybe Baby). The team recommended that saliva testing devices should not be offered to women. [203]

Evaluating devices

Freundl proposed that technologies for identifying the fertile time should be assessed first by efficacy finding studies followed, where appropriate, by effectiveness studies. An *efficacy finding study* compares the fertile time detected by the device to another established and reliable

Table 9.1 Home kits of use in fertility management to identify the fertile time (adapted from Stanford 2002 [563] and Brezina 2011 [63])

Method or device	*Mechanism*	*Fertile days identified*	*Approx. cost for one year*[1]	*Advantages*	*Disadvantages*
Urinary LH kits, e.g. Clearblue or First Response	Identifies LH surge when ovulation is imminent	Two days only	Total: £276 (£23/mth)	Identifies ovulation precisely Widely available Easy to use Can be used intermittently	Days identified may not be the days with the highest probability of pregnancy Costly if used long-term
Urine test sticks with dual hormone indicators, e.g. Clearblue Digital	Identifies rise in urinary E3G and the LH surge	Typically predicts four fertile days (high and peak fertility)	Total: £324 £27/mth)	Identifies more fertile days using simple dipstick technology Easy to use Can be used intermittently	Costly if used long-term
Direct hormone monitoring: Clearblue Fertility Monitor	Identifies rise in urinary E3G and the LH surge	Prospectively identifies the complete fertile time (notes the peak fertile days)	Total: £338 Monitor £140 + Refill tests £18/mth	Easy to use Accurate	Cost may be prohibitive Cycle range 21–42 days
Direct hormone monitoring: Persona (Contraceptive)	Identifies rise in urinary E3G and LH surge	Prospectively identifies the complete fertile time	Total: £219 Monitor £65 + Refill tests £14/mth	Easy to use 94% effective (in avoiding pregnancy)	High cost Cycle range 23–35 days
Electronic thermometer, e.g. Lady-comp or Cyclotest [2]	Identifies temperature rise following ovulation Combined with calculation, cervical secretions and LH	Identifies complete fertile time	£200 – £490	Allows for input of data on cervical secretions, LH, and intercourse. Information easily managed.	Offers little advantage over simple digital thermometer and combined indicators High cost Conflicting data Specific brand data not found by literature review

(*Continued*)

Table 9.1 (Continued)

Method or device	*Mechanism*	*Fertile days identified*	*Approx. cost for one year*[1]	*Advantages*	*Disadvantages*
Continuous temperature monitoring[3] consisting of thermal sensor and reader	Duofertility[3] Adhesive patch worn under the arm takes thousands of readings	Identifies ovulation within one day of objective ovulation by ultrasound	£250 – £900	Report gives feedback on cycle Other indicators encouraged	Skin patch worn continuously High cost No proven benefit over inexpensive digital thermometer Lacks research
	Ovusense[3] Vaginal sensor worn overnight monitors temperature every five minutes	Predicts ovulation one day in advance Confirms ovulation	£295 + replacement sensor after one year	Fertility consultancy includes feedback on cycle data Other indicators encouraged	Overnight vaginal sensor may not be acceptable High cost No proven benefit over inexpensive digital thermometer Lacks research
Salivary ferning kits e.g. Fertile Focus, Fertility Scope, Saliva Biotester	Detects crystallisation due to effect of sodium chloride on mucin	Identifies most fertile time	£15 — £50	Relatively inexpensive	Conflicting data Ferning seen in post-menopausal women and men Specific brand data not found by literature review Not recommended

Electrical resistance monitor, e.g. Ovacue	Measures electrolyte changes in saliva and cervical secretions using oral and vaginal sensors	Predicts ovulation up to seven days in advance	Ovacue: £240 Ovacue mobile: £130 (£60 for new sensor)	Can be used by women with irregular cycles	High cost Not widely available Conflicting data Vaginal sensor may not be acceptable
Observed indicators					
Calendar calculation S–20 and L–10	Estimates fertile time based on shortest and longest cycle in last 12 cycles	Identifies complete fertile time	Free	No or low cost to user[2] Easy to use	Over-estimates the fertile time Takes time to teach
Waking temperature	Identifies temperature rise following ovulation	Confirms ovulation only	Digital (Boots or Omron) £10 – £15 Geotherm galinstan £13	Low cost[2] Digital thermometers can be prescribed Easy to use	Does not predict the fertile time Daily temperatures may be cumbersome
Cervical secretions: self-observation	Identifies changes in cervical secretions which reflect hormonal changes and optimum conditions for sperm survival	Start of fertile time and days of maximum fertility	Free	Accessible and free Increases reproductive health awareness Good predictor of pregnancy probability	Subjective Some women find difficulty observing changes Takes time to teach

1 Costs based on first year use of the method. Monitors which use urine test sticks include tests for the first cycle.
2 Costs for observation-based methods are free to the user in NHS clinics, but may incur teaching charges in some settings.
3 Continuous temperature monitoring was first introduced in 2009. These devices were not included in Stanford or Brezina's literature reviews.

reference method (observed indicators, LH or ultrasound). This confirms that the device helps to identify the fertile time (method performance) but it does not confirm that the device proves useful to avoid pregnancy (user performance). An *effectiveness study* determines the accuracy of the device either using abstinence or barriers during the fertile time defined by the device. This determines the correct and typical use pregnancy rates.

Freundl reported on 65 women who, following a learning phase, tested two home kits. The test cycles used LH and ultrasound as objective markers. The number of false negative and positive results were analysed.

- False negative: the device indicates "not fertile" during the time designated fertile by objective markers.
- False positive: the device indicates "fertile" at a non-fertile time designated by objective markers.

Devices and methods for contraceptive purposes varied widely. The best results were obtained by FAMs using a combination of observed indicators. They were followed by electronic thermometers and Persona. Salivary ferning devices were not recommended. The fertile time identified by combined indicators was longer than that shown by devices, but it is recognised that this is over-estimated by observed indicators. Freundl concluded that no device has a method effectiveness comparable to the guidelines used in the European prospective study. [189] Only Persona and Bioself (which has now ceased operations) have been tested in prospective effectiveness studies. Well-designed studies are needed on all bought devices and any technologies which are marketed without a sound scientific basis cannot be recommended. [201]

ONLINE CHARTING SYSTEMS AND FERTILITY APPS

Online charting systems and apps for mobile phones or tablets offer a convenient way to record and store fertility information, but this rapidly expanding market is unregulated and lacks quality assurance. Potential users currently have to guess which apps have the most scientific credibility. The most reliable apps for planning or avoiding pregnancy are not necessarily the ones with the best user interface or the most convincing marketing hype, yet some of the most popular apps have each been downloaded over a million times. Some apps are simple menstrual cycle trackers, but others allow for the input of one or more fertility indicators. Many apps provide computerised interpretations of charts indicating the fertile and infertile times of the cycle with access to online communities.

One Web-based software application, Fertility Friend (FF), which is aimed at women planning pregnancy, allows registered users to submit charts to an online forum for comments (see www.fertilityfriend.com). Computerised chart analysis purports to identify ovulation and the fertile days to optimise intercourse timing. A randomised trial of 1,238 women planning pregnancy assigned half of the women to FF. There was little evidence of an increased pregnancy rate in the FF group; however, women who had been trying to conceive for five to six cycles at study entry conceived more quickly. [634]

The use of apps to avoid pregnancy is of most concern. In theory, apps based on the guidelines from the European prospective study [189] could offer an effective method but there have been no effectiveness studies to test this approach. The majority of fertility apps are not founded on evidence-based FAMs. Most apps are simple menstrual-cycle tracking apps. Some require payment or subscription, but others are free (the accuracy of fee-based apps is unknown).

A systematic evaluation of free apps initially identified more than 1,000 such apps; 108 were considered to fulfil the study criteria (allowed input of three full menstrual cycles, contained no erroneous health information and gave no gender predictions based on conception dates). Only 20 free English-language apps allowed for accurate menstrual cycle tracking based on average cycle lengths (this included Glow, Clue and Period Tracker). The researchers concluded that most of the free menstrual cycle tracking apps are inaccurate, contain misleading health information or do not function. They commented on their concerns about mobile technologies in relation to privacy and security issues recommending that women should only enter personal information that they would share with third parties. [411]

One fertility app has been widely-publicised as being more effective than the pill. Natural Cycles was calculated to have a Pearl Index of 0.5 with correct use but a CPR (life-table analysis) of 7.5 with typical use. The most conservative estimate was 9.8% when factoring in the high drop-out rate. The retrospective nature of this study may not give an accurate representation and it should be noted that the study was carried out (and funded) by the Swedish manufacturer. In order to make comparisons with other contraceptive methods a prospective randomised trial is required. [45]

A US team have developed a tool to evaluate fertility apps which are designed for avoiding pregnancy and claiming to use evidence-based FAMs (with various indicators). A standardised data set of seven cycles (real cycle data) was used to determine the apps' accuracy in identifying the fertile time. Of the 30 apps which predicted fertile days, only six had either a perfect score on accuracy or no false positive days (fertile days classified as infertile). The top scorers included Ovulation Mentor, Sympto.org, iCycleBeads, LilyPro, LadyCycle and myNFP.net. Natural Cycles was rated 15th and the lowest scorer was Glow. Of the apps which did not predict fertile days, Kindara (which incorporates a thermometer synchronised by Bluetooth) was rated third. For a list of apps excluded from the study and a rating of fertility apps marketed to avoid pregnancy see www.FACTSaboutFertility.org. [135]

It is most challenging for health professionals to be able to give any indication regarding which fertility apps to use. Some apps have similar names, name changes are not uncommon and research is unable to keep up with the pace of technology. **With the currently available evidence fertility apps cannot be recommended for avoiding pregnancy.**

FUTURE DEVELOPMENTS

Electronic devices of some form are likely to be the future for FAMs. Devices need to be acceptable, low-cost and easy-to-use. They should provide an accurate assessment of fertility (including confirmation of ovulation) with a high level of effectiveness but minimum time of abstinence.

Sensiplan

Freundl and colleagues are researching a tracking system algorithm based on Sensiplan, their evaluated teaching programme and guidelines (page 240). This temperature-based system with additional observed indicators is being developed for use on mobile phones. Freundl and colleagues compared 364 cycles from 51 women with a computer programme based on the Triggs tracking system. The two methods gave total agreement in 82% of cycles and differed by one day in 18% of cycles. There are questions about how the software will handle temperature disturbances, but efficacy-finding studies will assess the appropriateness with effectiveness studies to follow. The software identifies a downward trend in temperature before the characteristic rise so may be able to determine the end of the fertile time as the cycle unfolds; however, the practical use of this feature may be limited because couples who are avoiding pregnancy still need to wait for the third high temperature. [200] **If Sensiplan proves to be an effective tool this will be the first such device to have been through the appropriate research stages.**

Direct hormone monitoring

Direct hormone monitoring devices (such as Persona or the Clearblue fertility monitor) offer the most promising technologies because they are less affected by day-to-day disturbances, but there is currently no home kit which confirms ovulation. Brown's Ovarian Monitor measured progesterone metabolites but the technology was not suitable for home use. Ecochard recently compared urinary PDG with ultrasonography and found PDG to be a highly accurate marker of ovulation and the end of the fertile time, hence the theoretical basis now exists for the development of a urine dipstick which confirms ovulation. [149]

COMBINING INDICATORS

10

Combining the indicators of fertility provides the most accurate assessment of the fertile time and therefore the most effective natural method for avoiding pregnancy. This chapter assumes knowledge of the major indicators (chapters 4–7) plus the minor indicators and test kits (chapters 8 and 9).

DEVELOPMENT OF COMBINED INDICATOR APPROACH

Attempts to identify the fertile time date back to around 1,000 BC with Hindu teaching on married life describing the first 16 days of the cycle as "the natural season of woman". Calendar calculations were developed for practical use in the 1920s with changes in temperature and secretions following in the 1950s and 1960s (see timeline on page 14). By the 1970s it was almost universally accepted that combining the indicators increased the effectiveness of FAMs to avoid pregnancy. These combined methods have variously been described as:

- calculothermic, combining a calendar calculation to identify the start of the fertile time with temperature to identify the end of the fertile time (a single-check method); [288]
- mucothermic, combining cervical secretions to identify the start of the fertile time with temperature to identify the end of the fertile time (single-check); [381]
- double-check, or using a cross-check of two indicators for the start and end of the fertile time, e.g. calculation and secretions for the start of the fertile time and temperature and secretions for the end of the fertile time [577] (*Note:* Paul Thyma, who described double-check, was the pen name used by Reverend Jan Mucharski, who documented the history of physiological methods); and [416]
- sympto-thermal, a combination of temperature with a range of other symptoms (cervical secretions, changes in the cervix, minor indicators and calendar calculations) with a double-check of at least two indicators. [506]

EXAMPLES OF COMBINED INDICATOR CHARTS

A combined indicator approach should be encouraged for avoiding pregnancy. At least two indicators (double-check) must be used at both the start and end of the fertile time for maximum effectiveness. Examples of combined indicator charts using different combinations of indicators (some single-check and others double-check) are given on pages 127, 147, 159, 165 and 169, building up from two indicators (temperature and secretions) through to combining all indicators (including minor indicators and Persona).

INTERPRETING A COMBINED CHART

When interpreting a chart, it is important to use a structured step-by-step approach to ensure all parameters are considered and the relevant information is collected:

1. Record the name and age of the woman.
2. Chart number: is she a new user (charting for < 1 year) or an experienced user (> 1 year)?
3. What is the length of the current cycle?
4. Does she have a record of her last 12 cycle lengths? Y/N
   - If yes, what is the length of her shortest cycle (S)?
   - If no, then she should start recording her cycle lengths.
5. Was there a temperature rise in the last cycle? Y/N
   - If yes, then the period is a "true period" and is *relatively* infertile.
   - If no, then the bleed may be associated with ovulation and is potentially fertile.
6. Interpret the temperature chart:
   - Identify the temperature rise by applying the coverline and the *3 over 6 rule.*
   - Identify the last fertile day ensuring that the third high temperature is at least 0.2 deg.C above the preceding six low readings.
7. Interpret the pattern of cervical secretions:
   - Identify the start of secretions (change from dryness).
   - Check the description in the appropriate boxes.
   - Identify the peak day (last day showing most fertile characteristics).
   - Extend the shading on peak day upwards to see the correlation between the secretions and temperature.
   - Double-check the secretions with temperatures, ensuring that there are three high temperatures *after* peak day.
8. Interpret the changes in the cervix (optional):
   - Low, firm, closed, tilted cervix indicates infertile.
   - High, soft, open, straight cervix indicates fertile.
   - Consider how the cervical changes correlate with the other indicators of fertility.
9. If there is a record of the last 12 cycle lengths, to identify the first fertile day apply the calculation *S minus 20* rule.
10. If there is no record of the last 12 cycle lengths, advise the client as follows:
    - In cycle 1, avoid unprotected sex and consider the entire cycle to be potentially fertile.
    - In cycles 2 and 3, there is no early relatively infertile time. Restrict intercourse to the late infertile time.
    - If the first three cycles are 26 days or longer, then for cycles 4–12 use the *Day 6 rule.*
    - If any of the first three cycles are less than 26 days, there is no early relatively infertile time. Continue to monitor cycle length, but restrict intercourse to the late infertile time for pregnancy avoidance.
    - Use the *S minus 20 rule* when sufficient cycle length information is available.
11. If a woman has recorded 12 charts, identify the earliest temperature rise and subtract seven days to identify the first fertile day: *Earliest temperature rise –7 = first fertile day.* This supersedes the *S minus 20 rule.*
12. Consider other factors which may affect the chart (e.g. alcohol, sleep disturbance, changes in temperature-taking time, stress, illness or medication).
13. Apply the guidelines for planning or avoiding pregnancy (summarised on page 227) checking client understanding and motivation.
    - Planning pregnancy: consider intercourse targeting, impact on couple relationship and any concerns about delayed conception.
    - Avoiding pregnancy: check level of effectiveness required and motivation of both partners.

14 Use a horizontal arrow to indicate the start and end of the fertile time based on all the available information.
15 Add any relevant teaching points to the chart to increase client learning.

The chart summary sheet (appendix D) can be used as a checklist for teaching purposes and is especially helpful for new clients.

CHOOSING COMBINATION OF INDICATORS

Women can choose whichever indicators they feel appropriate but should understand the range of effectiveness provided by single- or combined-indicator methods and the use of a single- or double-check at the start and end of the fertile time. The choice of indicators and the level of effectiveness required will vary depending on the couple's motivation and whether they are spacing or limiting pregnancies (page 234). Although in general most women can use FAMs, there are times when irregular cycles create difficulties such as after hormonal contraception, postpartum and peri-menopausally (page 362).

New users

Couples who are avoiding pregnancy are usually taught a combination of indicators. The majority of women start off with temperature because this is easily taught and provides an objective indicator. Cervical secretions, changes in the cervix and calculations then follow. Teaching normally works best at approximately monthly intervals to allow time for the user to build up her knowledge and gain confidence in her observations (suggested teaching schedule: page 363).

Couples who are planning pregnancy can rely on cervical secretions alone. Although some women may wish to record temperatures for a short time, this is not normally necessary. In most cases there no reason for women to check their cervix or use kits or devices (teaching: page 360).

Experienced users

A woman who has recorded her indicators for one year is considered an experienced user. She will have had time to build up a personal record of cycle length, her pattern of secretions, her usual coverline and her earliest temperature rise. This allows her to introduce more personalised calculations to increase the effectiveness and possibly reduce the number of days when abstinence (or barriers) are required.

Some experienced users are keen to limit the number of days they record symptoms. For example, provided a woman has cycles of 26 days or longer there is no need to start taking temperatures while dryness persists (and the cervix stays in its infertile state). The *S minus 20 rule*, or preferably the *earliest temperature rise minus 7*, provides a good guide for when to start recording temperatures. Temperatures must then be recorded consistently until the end of the fertile time. If a woman has short cycles, she may need to take her temperature from day 1 to ensure that she has sufficient temperatures to use the *3 over 6 rule*. The end of the fertile time is established by a combination of temperature and secretions (third high temperature after peak day, ensuring that the third temperature is at least 0.2 deg.C above the six low readings). There is no benefit in continuing to record secretions or cervical changes as this is both unnecessary and confusing (see the chart from an experienced user in figure 8.1, chapter 8)

A woman who has recorded her indicators for a year is likely to have experienced common disturbances such as alcohol, disrupted sleep and factors such as stress, illness and medication, so will begin to understand the effect this can have on the chart.

Most women find one or more indicator which is consistent for them. Some will choose to stop temperature recording completely and rely on secretions and possibly cervical changes. Shift workers may find it particularly difficult to incorporate temperature so be more reliant on other indicators. They may be ideally suited to incorporating direct hormone monitoring such as Persona. Other women may find difficulty with observing cervical secretions and be more reliant on calendar-based calculations with temperature. The indicators are flexible, provided they give sufficient confirmation of the limits of the fertile time. Couples need to understand that the most effective combination of indicators is provided by the guidelines described on page 227.

ACTIVITY CHART-BUILDING EXERCISE (CONTINUED FROM PAGE 160)

Step 5 Interpreting the combined chart

1 Note any disturbances on the chart.
2 Use the *3 over 6 rule* to identify the temperature rise.
3 Identify the end of the fertile time by temperature.
4 Interpret the pattern of secretions.
5 Identify peak day and emphasise it by extending the shading upwards.
6 Check the correlation between the secretions and temperature.
7 Using all the information, use the most conservative estimate to identify the fertile time (see the guidelines for avoiding pregnancy on page 227).
8 Compare your interpretation with the completed chart (figure 10.3).

MAINTAINING RECORDS OF CYCLE CHARACTERISTICS

A woman should keep a record of her cycles in any way that suits her, either on paper or electronically. Many women keep detailed notes on their charts which provides valuable long-term information. The key characteristics to note are shown in table 10.1. The information from the last 12 cycles is used to maintain an ongoing record of cycle length (to identify the shortest cycle). The ongoing record of the first high temperature allows the user to identify her earliest temperature rise. At the end of each cycle the first fertile day (for the next cycle) is recalculated and the stop bar is added to the new chart.

The example in table 10.1 shows the record of a new user (starting with cycle 1). She has identified her shortest cycle from diary records so can use the *S minus 20 rule*. Note that cycle 3 is only 26 days long. This is shorter than her existing shortest cycle (of 27 days) so her new calculation determines that her fertile time now starts on day 6. This user is recording the first day she observes any cervical secretions. If this day precedes the day identified by the calculation, then this is the start of the fertile time. She is also noting her first high temperature so that she can calculate her earliest temperature rise when she has completed 12 charts. The peak day information is useful to see how this correlates with the first high temperature. Some authorities have also used calculations based on peak day to identify the *start* of the fertile time: identify the earliest peak day (in the last 12 cycles) and subtract eight to identify the first fertile day *(peak day −8 = first fertile day)*. This can be helpful if there is no temperature record, but its efficacy has not been tested. The first cervical change can act as an extra indicator to identify the start of the fertile time, but this new user has not yet learnt to check her cervix.

Table 10.1 Example of ongoing record of menstrual cycle characteristics

Period	*Cycle no.*	*Cycle length*			*Cervical secretions*		*Waking temperature*			*Cervix (optional)*
Date of first day of period	Cycle no.	Length of cycle	Shortest cycle	S – 20	First day	Peak day	First high temp	Earliest T. rise	Earliest T. rise – 7	First cervical change
02.10.14	1	29	27	7	8	14	15	Not known	Not known	N/A
31.10.14	2	30	27	7	7	13	15	Not known	Not known	N/A
30.11.14	3	26	26	6	7	12	13	Not known	Not known	N/A
26.12.14	4									

Note: All calculations should be based on information from the most recent 12 menstrual cycles.

CORRELATION BETWEEN SUBJECTIVE AND OBJECTIVE MARKERS

Gnoth reported on the correlation between a woman's subjective indicators and objective markers of ovulation. [230] [234] Forty-nine women contributed a total of 87 cycles, observing changes in temperature, secretions, cervical changes and mid-cycle pain. This was compared with daily urinary LH and trans-vaginal ultrasound.

Figure 10.1 shows the correlation between the markers, as described here:

- For most women, ovulation occurred between peak day and the temperature rise (first high temperature), hence the temperature rise confirmed ovulation.
- The temperature rise occurred on or within two days *after* the objective marker in 81% of cycles and *before* ovulation in 11% of cycles.
- Peak day occurred within one day of the objective marker in 82% of cycles and after ovulation in 21% of cycles (as shown by Guida [255]).
- Cervical changes provided an accurate marker, but this was not an acceptable indicator for some women.
- Mid-cycle pain was the most variable indicator (which confirms other ultrasound studies such as Despares [118]).

Figure 10.2 shows the possible scenarios for the relationship between peak day and the temperature rise in comparison with the objective markers, as noted here:

- Peak day occurred one or two days *before* the temperature rise (scenarios A and B) or on the same day as the rise (scenario C) in 89% of cycles.
- There was a *delay* between peak and the temperature rise, with the peak day occurring three to five days *before* the temperature rise, (scenario D) in some cycles – a phenomenon which has been observed in some women with "unexplained" infertility.
- Peak day occurred *after* the temperature rise (scenario E) in some cycles – an important detail when applying guidelines to avoid pregnancy.

The findings from the European multi-centre study showed similar results to Gnoth's. Peak day generally preceded the temperature rise, but it was noted to be a highly subjective indicator.

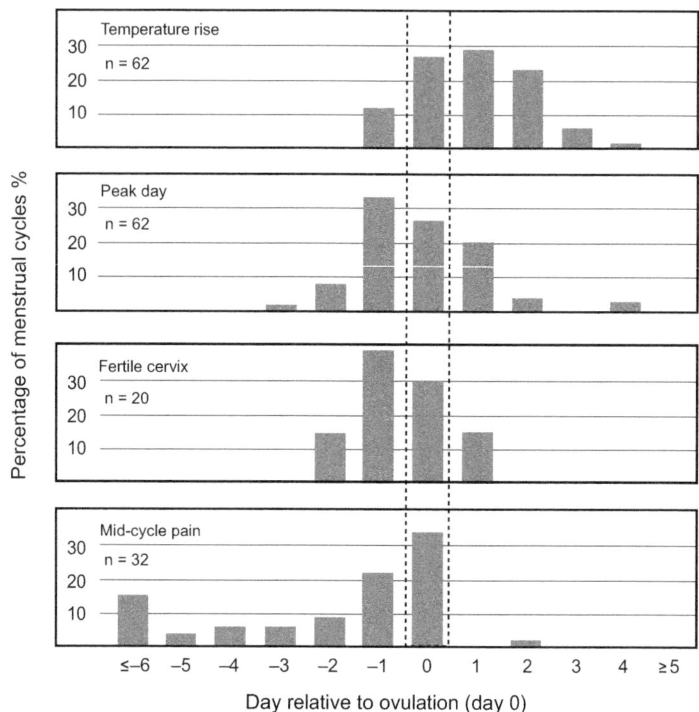

Figure 10.1 Correlation between subjective indicators and objective markers of ovulation (adapted from Gnoth 2002) [234]

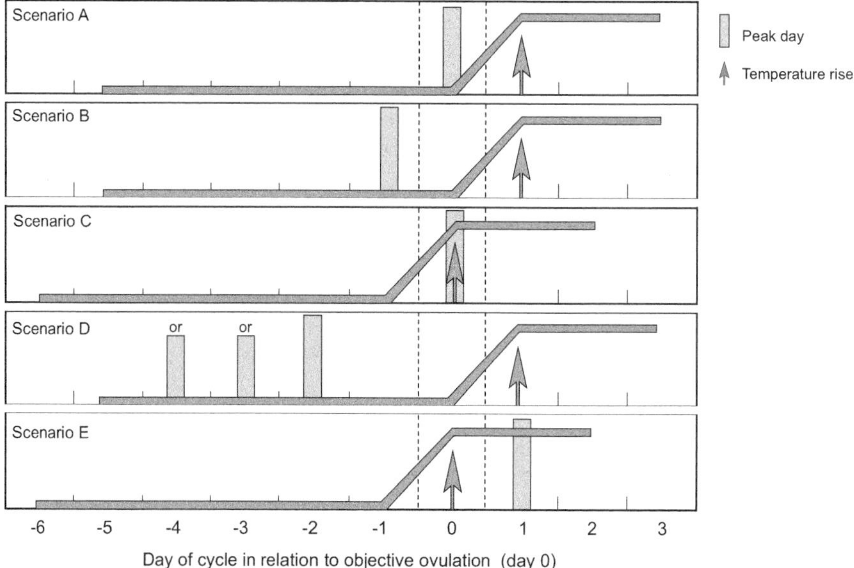

Figure 10.2 Relationship between peak day and temperature rise compared with objective markers of ovulation (adapted from Gnoth 2002) [234]

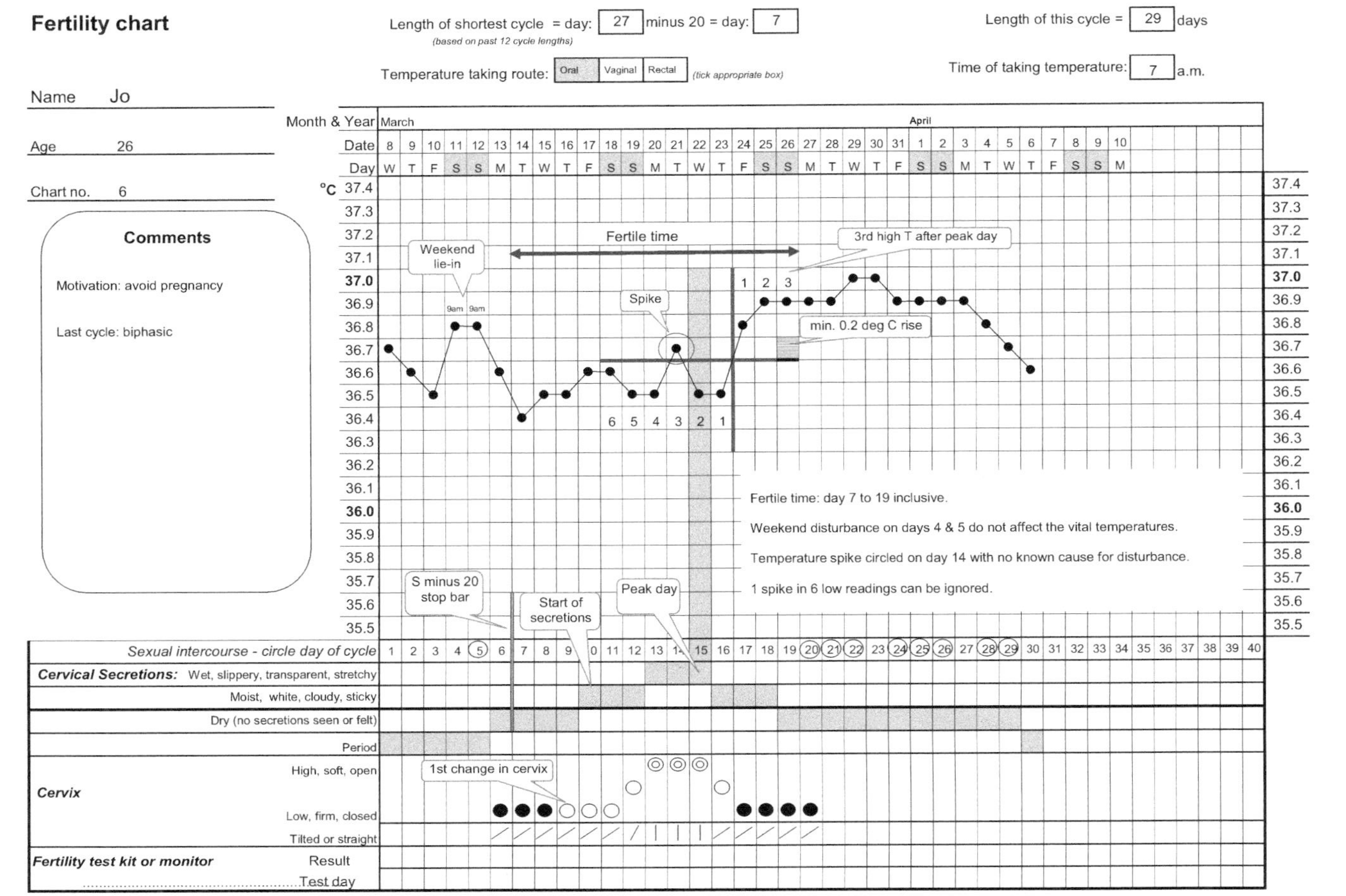

Figure 10.3 Chart-building exercise: interpreted chart

Temperature was more objective, although it was easily affected by disturbances. Peak day preceded the last low temperature by an average of 0.3 days: i.e. peak preceded the temperature *rise* (first high temperature) by an average of 1.3 days. [101] The relationship between peak day and the temperature rise is most significant when determining the end of the fertile time. If peak occurs on the same day as the temperature rise, or after the rise, then to avoid pregnancy the couple must wait until there have been three high temperatures *after* peak day (see figure 7.2 in chapter 7).

ACTIVITY CHART-BUILDING EXERCISE (CONTINUED FROM PAGE 182)

Step 6 Self-assessment of the completed chart (see figure 10.3)

The interpretation of the chart should be demonstrated clearly on the chart itself. A chart summary sheet (appendix D) can be used to provide client feedback.

Jo is 26 years old, of normal fertility. This is her sixth chart. Her last cycle was biphasic so this is a "true period". This is a 29-day cycle.

First fertile day

Jo's shortest cycle over the last 12 cycles was 27 days, so by *S minus 20* calculation this gives day 7 as her first fertile day. Jo's first secretions are recorded on day 10. The first change in cervix occurs a day earlier on day 9 (softer), so the earliest change is shown by the *S minus 20 rule.* Her first fertile day is day 7 (note stop bar).

Last fertile day

Jo's peak day occurs on day 15. Her first high temperature is day 17. Her third high temperature (day 19) is a minimum of 0.2 deg.C above the six low readings. All three high temperatures are after peak so the last fertile day is day 19.

Jo is fertile from day 7–19 inclusive (note arrow)

She has used her combined indicators correctly and not recorded any unprotected sex or risk-taking during her fertile time.

SIMPLIFIED METHODS

In the 1990s IRH at Georgetown University identified the need for (and developed) simplified methods of family planning for use in both developing and developed countries. The time commitment, cost and relative complexity of modern FAMs make it difficult to reach large numbers of users, diverse ethnic groups and low-literacy populations – hence simple, feasible, accurate approaches are a welcome addition to method choice. Simplified methods include the SDM, a calendar-based fixed formula; and the TDM, a simple approach to observing cervical secretions. Although these methods are less effective for avoiding pregnancy than using a combined indicator approach, they may be highly appropriate for family spacing. SDM and TDM are easy to teach and learn, thereby increasing access to, and use of, FAMs in areas of limited resources. These are often areas which also have high unmet need for family planning – defined as a high percentage of fecund, sexually active women who do not want a child, but are not using contraception. All FAMs help to address unmet family planning needs, but SDM and TDM may have particular significance.

STANDARD DAYS METHOD (SDM)

SDM offers an easier alternative to the Calendar/Rhythm Method by using a fixed formula. **For women with cycle lengths of 26–32 days, the fertile time is from day 8 until day 19.** SDM can help pregnancy avoidance by avoiding unprotected sex on days 8–19, or can help pregnancy planning by targeting intercourse between days 8–19.

Science behind SDM

SDM was derived from analysing a large dataset from a WHO multi-centre study [616] and estimating the theoretical probability of pregnancy on different days of the cycle. **According to the SDM algorithm, women with cycle lengths of 26–32 days usually ovulate between days 13 and 17.** Avoiding unprotected sex between days 8 and 19 allows sufficient time for the lifespan of the gametes. In cycles shorter than 26 days or longer than 32 days, SDM still provides some protection against pregnancy, but with shorter cycles sperm may still be viable and with longer cycles the egg may still be viable, so the pregnancy rate will be higher. [346] [162] [10]

CycleBeads

CycleBeads is a mnemonic device to help a woman identify her fertile days, track cycle lengths and communicate this information to her partner. To use CycleBeads, a woman simply moves a small black rubber ring over a series of 32 colour-coded beads representing each of the 32 possible days of the menstrual cycle (the longest cycle within the criteria for use). The beads are

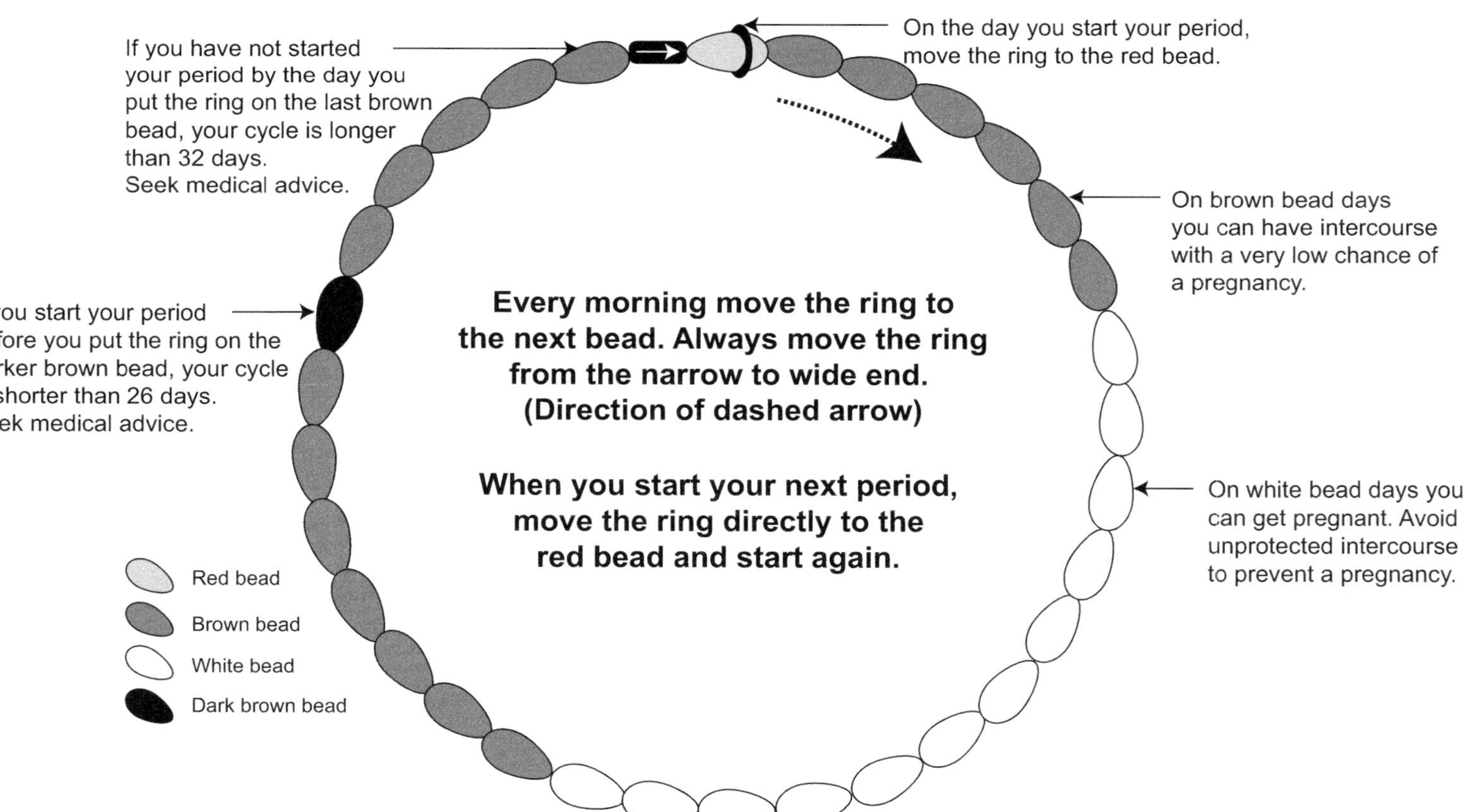
If you have not started
your period by the day you
put the ring on the last brown
bead, your cycle is longer
than 32 days.
Seek medical advice.
On the day you start your period,
move the ring to the red bead.
If you start your period
before you put the ring on the
darker brown bead, your cycle
is shorter than 26 days.
Seek medical advice.
On brown bead days
you can have intercourse
with a very low chance of
a pregnancy.
Every morning move the ring to
the next bead. Always move the ring
from the narrow to wide end.
(Direction of dashed arrow)
When you start your next period,
move the ring directly to the
red bead and start again.
On white bead days you
can get pregnant. Avoid
unprotected intercourse
to prevent a pregnancy.
Red bead
Brown bead
White bead
Dark brown bead

Figure 11.1 CycleBeads and instructions for use (adapted from Arevalo 2002) [12]

narrower at one end than the other. A single red bead represents day 1, the first day of cycle. There then follows six brown beads representing days 2–7, 12 white beads representing days 8–19 and 13 brown beads representing days 20–32. A small black bead with a white arrow shows the direction to move the rubber ring. The brown bead representing day 27 is darker brown (to warn of a short cycle).

Instructions for use

On the first day of the period, the woman moves the rubber ring to the single red bead. Then every morning she moves it to the next bead, always moving it from the narrow end to the wide end of the bead in the direction of the arrow. Brown bead days (and the red bead day) are infertile days with a very low chance of pregnancy. White bead days are fertile days when there is a high chance of pregnancy.

Identifying shorter or longer cycles If the woman's period starts before she puts the ring on the dark brown bead, her cycle is shorter than 26 days. Similarly if her period has not started by the day after she puts the ring on the last brown bead, her cycle is longer than 32 days. If a woman has two cycles outside the range of 26–32 days in any one year, then she cannot use the method. If she is switching from hormonal contraception she cannot use SDM for the first three cycles after discontinuation because the first cycle is not a reliable indicator of future cycle lengths. [14]

CycleTel

CycleBeads was developed in necklace form, but is now distributed in electronic formats including text-based and Web-based services. CycleTel is a Georgetown University initiative in India, where nearly 36 million women aged 20–34 want to avoid pregnancy but don't have an effective, affordable and accessible method. The proliferation of mobile phones offers new opportunities: CycleTel now alerts women to their fertile days (8–19) via Short Message Service (SMS).

CycleBeads online and iCycleBeads smartphone app

An online version of CycleBeads and a smartphone app provide a virtual representation of CycleBeads showing users where they are in the menstrual cycle and the likelihood of pregnancy. Email alerts inform each user whether she is on a fertile or infertile day and when she is likely to start her next period, plus send a reminder to enter the start date of her period. CycleBeads online monitors the cycle range and alerts the woman if a cycle is outside the range of 26–32 days.

The iCycleBeads smartphone app enables women to use SDM by tracking cycles on a smartphone or tablet. This works in the same way as CycleBeads online by monitoring cycle length with alerts for the day of the cycle and the fertility status. CycleBeads is available in all formats at www.cyclebeads.com.

Adapting SDM to community need

CycleBeads is a good visual tool. The simple concept of the fixed fertile days 8–19 has a potential for use in any environment, provided a woman keeps a record of her cycle lengths and has a personal reminder of where she is in her cycle. This can be done on a calendar, a piece of paper or other ways of counting between 1 and 32. The memory aid needs to be appropriate for the setting. For example, a community-based participatory project in Gambia, facilitated by Cecilia Pyper (FertilityUK) and Felix Kuchler (Swiss Solidarity), uses locally available materials to represent the days of the menstrual cycle: red stones, dry sticks and green leaves.

Effectiveness of SDM

A prospective multi-centre efficacy trial of SDM was conducted in Bolivia, Peru and the Philippines. The study participants, 478 women aged 18–39 years (4,035 cycles), had self-reported cycle lengths of 26–32 days and wished to delay pregnancy for at least one year. Couples used the method correctly in 97% of cycles, with unprotected intercourse occurring between days 8–19 in only 3% of cycles. The method failure rate (correct use) was 4.8% with a typical-use failure rate of 12%. [12] Although this is relatively high, the fundamental message about days 8–19 has a significant impact on pregnancy rate compared with the 80–90% probability of conception in one year for young couples who use no family planning method.

Integrating SDM into services

IRH gives 10 reasons to integrate SDM into family planning programmes.

1. Current methods do not meet the needs of all women: 222 million women in developing countries want to avoid pregnancy but are not using a modern family planning method. One in four women in Sub-Saharan Africa cite the main reasons for not using family planning as: fear of side effects (24%); opposition by partner, self or other influential person (23%); and infrequent intercourse, e.g. partner away from home (17%).
2. SDM addresses women's concerns and helps fill a critical gap in programmes. Most women who choose SDM do so because it is free from side effects. SDM identifies the fertile days so couples can avoid unprotected sex or negotiate condom use. It encourages couple communication and overcomes many religious and cultural concerns.
3. When used correctly and consistently, which most users do, SDM is 95% effective, which compares favourably with other short-acting methods.
4. Adding SDM to the method mix expands choice, increases contraceptive prevalence and reduces unmet need. Contraceptive use increased from 24% to 41% in four years by introducing SDM in a community-based reproductive health project in India, and from 45% to 58% in a two-year pilot study in El Salvador aimed at involving men by integrating family planning into water and sanitation activities.
5. SDM brings new users to family planning. The majority of SDM users in India, Peru and Rwanda had never used family planning before.
6. SDM is easy and inexpensive to integrate into programmes. Studies in Guatemala, India, and Rwanda found that SDM was more cost-effective than other birth-spacing methods, including condoms and oral contraceptives. Users, instructors and service providers can be trained in as little as two hours.
7. Pharmacists, community groups or faith-based institutions can be trained to provide SDM instruction whilst referring to health professionals for other methods.
8. Mobile phones extend the reach of SDM because it is compatible with both voice and text messaging.
9. SDM involves men and helps couples to communicate about sex and fertility. Visual information provided by CycleBeads encourages condom use on fertile days.
10. SDM helps to empower women. In a study in Guatemala, after six months of SDM use, women reported a significant increase in their ability to care for their health, refuse unwanted sex and communicate with their partners.

SDM may help to address health inequalities and unmet need amongst minority ethnic groups in the UK, particularly where language barriers exist. It can be incorporated into general practice, contraception and sexual health services, obstetrics and gynaecology, and midwifery practice. [306] [225]

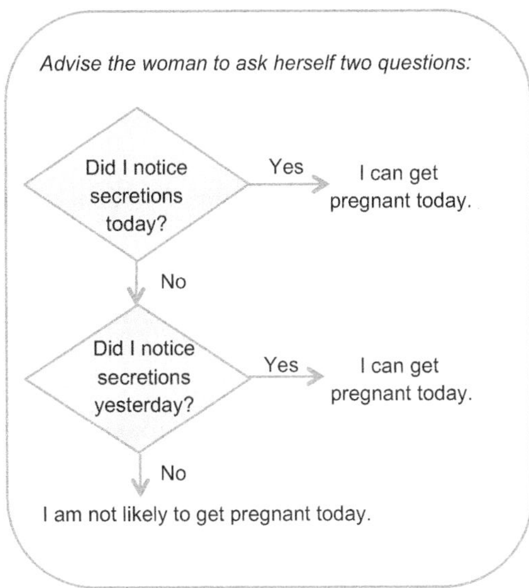
Advise the woman to ask herself two questions:
Did I notice secretions today?
Yes
I can get pregnant today.
No
Did I notice secretions yesterday?
Yes
I can get pregnant today.
No
I am not likely to get pregnant today.

Figure 11.2 TwoDay Method algorithm (adapted from Arevalo 2004 [11])

Pilot studies around the world through health ministries, FPAs and community development organisations have shown that SDM appeals to a broad range of women. Men and women report high levels of satisfaction with the method, using abstinence or condoms during the fertile time. Instruction typically takes no more time than allocated in most family planning settings and the cross-study first-year failure rate of 14.1% is similar to typical-use rates in the SDM efficacy trial. [246] SDM requires the involvement of both partners. It offers a natural entry point to discuss inter-personal and reproductive health issues with potential users, including STIs, the use of condoms, partner communication and intimate partner violence. [365]

SDM is now offered in more than 30 countries, with international agencies including WHO and the International Planned Parenthood Federation (IPPF) recognising it as a method of choice. USAID have looked at the time and cost of integrating SDM into large-scale family planning programmes as part of routine service delivery in Guatemala, India and Rwanda. These programmes are cost-effective, but issues around cost are complex. [593] IRH provides guidance on integrating SDM into family planning services at http://standarddaysmethod.org. [302]

TWODAY METHOD (TDM)

Georgetown University have developed the TDM as a simpler way to use cervical secretions as a single indicator method. The TwoDay algorithm is based on the presence or absence of secretions and is easier to teach and learn than the Ovulation Method. TDM is suitable for couples who prefer a simplified method and accept its effectiveness. [544]

Instructions for using TDM

The woman is taught to monitor her secretions either by the sensation of wetness at the vulva, by observing underwear, or by wiping the vulva and observing the secretions on toilet paper. She is advised to consider "secretions" as *anything* that she perceives to be coming from her vagina, except for menstrual bleeding or seminal fluid. *All secretions* are considered signs of fertility irrespective of the amount, colour or consistency.

Observations are made during the afternoon and evening (not before noon). Focus groups have indicated that most couples have intercourse in the late evening or early morning, so monitoring at these times avoids confusion between seminal fluid and cervical secretions. A woman should understand that the secretions might look or feel different on different days of the cycle; the amount will vary; and once the secretions start, they will be continuous for a number of days.

Every evening, apart from during her period, the woman notes on a calendar or other memory aid what she saw or felt that afternoon or evening. The woman should ask herself two questions:

- Did I notice secretions *today*?
- Did I notice secretions *yesterday*?

If she answers "yes" to either question she is probably fertile and needs to avoid unprotected intercourse if she wishes to avoid pregnancy. If she does not notice secretions on either day, she is unlikely to be fertile (figure 11.2).

Duration of secretions

The normal duration of cervical secretions is between four and 12 days.

Less than four days If a woman observes fewer than four consecutive days of secretions, it is possible that she is unable to identify all the days when secretions are present, therefore she may be at increased risk of pregnancy from intercourse on a day she perceives as dry. It is possible that some women with very few days of secretions have ovulatory problems. The effectiveness of TDM is not known in these circumstances.

More than 12 days If a woman observes secretions for more than 12 consecutive days, she should consult a health professional to consider the possibility of a vaginal infection or a hormonal imbalance such as PCOS. Women who have many days of secretions may find the method unacceptable due to the prolonged abstinence or use of condoms.

Science behind TDM

TDM was based on a theoretical model using several data sources: the WHO multi-centre study of the Ovulation Method (7,592 cycles) [616]; the North Carolina data on the probability of conception on different days relative to ovulation, with consideration for the clinical pregnancy rate (> 6 weeks gestation) [631] [632]; and research on the timing of peak day relative to ovulation based on hormonal assays. [281] An analysis was also made on 183 charts contributed by women using either the Ovulation Method or Sympto-thermal Method from three different NFP programmes.

Three types of information were used to estimate the probability of pregnancy from intercourse on various days of the cycle. The TDM algorithm was applied to the potential fertile time from eight days before peak day to three days after peak. This recognises that the fertile time starts five days before ovulation and ends on the day of ovulation, but peak day can occur from three days before, to three days after ovulation.

- In the days before peak day, the TDM algorithm identified the same fertile days as the Ovulation Method. In the days after peak, the TDM algorithm determined that the first and second post-peak days were fertile in 55% of cycles, while the third post-peak day was identified as fertile in 11% of cycles. By the fifth post-peak day, 94% of cycles were infertile.

Overall, the TDM algorithm identified some days as fertile which would not be likely to be fertile, but the time requiring abstinence or condom use averaged 9 days compared with 9.7 days for the Ovulation Method. In 85% of cycles, secretions were observed for 4–12 days. This was considered the normal duration. TDM was as effective as the Billings Ovulation Method, but simpler, more acceptable and with fewer days considered potentially fertile.

A secondary analysis of the data on cervical secretions from a European fecundability study [141] assessed the relationship between the days predicted to be potentially fertile by TDM and the day-specific probabilities of pregnancy based on 434 conception cycles. The days around ovulation that had the highest fecundability were the days most likely to be classified as fertile by the TDM algorithm. In addition, intercourse on a particular day in the fertile time was twice as likely to result in a pregnancy if cervical secretions were present on that day or the day before. TDM therefore effectively identifies the fertile days of the cycle and predicts days with a high pregnancy rate. The researchers concluded that the theoretical probability of pregnancy in a given cycle is very low for women who are aware of secretions during the fertile time and abstain from intercourse accordingly, but if a woman does not perceive secretions on a day which is fertile, then pregnancy can occur. [544]

Length of fertile time with TDM

TDM may require more abstinence or condom use than the average 9–10 days as it is not uncommon for women to notice secretions in the late luteal phase. Women who are using a more sophisticated method of observing cervical secretions use peak day (last day showing the most fertile characteristics) as a reference point to confirm the end of the fertile time and would be assured that any premenstrual secretions could be disregarded. With TDM, premenstrual secretions related to hormonal fluctuations are indistinguishable so must be regarded as potentially fertile.

Effectiveness of TDM

The effectiveness of TDM was studied prospectively in 450 women of reproductive age in five culturally diverse sites in Guatemala, Peru and the Philippines. Participants were 18–39 years, of proven fertility and living with a partner (total 3,928 cycles). Women who were still partially breastfeeding were admitted to the study only if they had at least three cycles (four periods) postpartum.

At the end of the first cycle of TDM use, 96% of participants reported that they had no problem identifying the presence or absence of secretions. Only 2% of women reported difficulties by the third cycle. The WHO study on the Ovulation Method, by comparison, found that 93% of women charted an interpretable pattern of secretions at the end of the first cycle and 97% by the end of the third cycle.

Study participants were asked to avoid intercourse on days TDM identified as fertile, but to report if they did have intercourse and used a back-up method (condoms or withdrawal). Women reported as follows:

- In 93% of cycles: no intercourse during the days TDM identified as fertile.
- In 3% of cycles: intercourse with a back-up method on fertile days.
- In 4% of cycles: unprotected intercourse on a fertile day (in some cycles couples had both protected and unprotected sex on days identified as fertile).

The average number of intercourse days per cycle was 5.6 days. One in four couples had unprotected intercourse on potentially fertile days, but not habitually. The majority of women (70%) who completed at least six cycles of use reported no intercourse on fertile days. Only 1% of couples had unprotected intercourse in more than one in four cycles. Unprotected sex decreased over time, from nearly 10% in the first cycle of use to less than 1% by cycle 13.

The first-year pregnancy rates for TDM were as follows:

- 3.5% with correct use (pregnancies and cycles with no intercourse on identified fertile days);
- 6.3% when a backup method (condoms or withdrawal) was used on fertile days; and
- 13.7% with typical use (including all cycles and all pregnancies in the analysis).

Nearly half of the pregnancies occurred in the first three cycles of use. This may have been because either the secretions were not adequate markers of fertility for some women or because more learning time was needed – including learning how to modify sexual behaviour to accommodate the fertile time. The efficacy of the TDM compares well with the WHO multi-centre trial [616] of the Ovulation Method, which had a typical use failure rate of 19.6%. [11]

PREDICTING CORRECT USE OF SIMPLIFIED METHODS

FAMs are highly user-dependent. If health professionals are able to identify those couples who are most likely to have unprotected sex on fertile days, they can be appropriately counselled. Georgetown University examined quantitative and qualitative data from the SDM and TDM efficacy studies in which 928 women contributed up to 13 cycles of method use. The studies found that 23% of women had unprotected intercourse on fertile days in at least one cycle and many said their husbands insisted. In addition, couples with reservations about the method, concerns about fertility or lack of partner co-operation were less consistent users.

Couple communication improved with method use: the incidence of unprotected intercourse decreased for both methods, with more marked improvement for TDM. Stress associated with poverty was seen to adversely affect correct use. Although the researchers found no clear profile of user for whom these methods would be inappropriate, they found a number of determinants of correct use:

- older age and higher educational level;
- partner co-operation and his level of satisfaction with the method;
- strong intention to avoid pregnancy; and
- couples with a good understanding of the method.

Researchers also found that couples in committed relationships used condoms more correctly and consistently. Routine is important for any method which requires daily action. The fixed fertile time of SDM (days 8–19) means that couples knew what to expect, had a visual reminder with CycleBeads and could plan accordingly; whereas with TDM the fertile time was subjective and less predictable.

Programmes offering simplified methods should both instruct clients and help them to learn negotiating skills. Women need to understand the consequences of intercourse on fertile days. Practitioners should involve men to encourage couple communication, adherence and correct method use; alternatively, the woman should be provided with written information to share with her partner. [547]

SIMPLIFIED METHODS FOR POSTPARTUM WOMEN

All women require an effective postpartum family planning method. LAM is the method of choice for breastfeeding women who are less than six months postpartum, amenorrhoeic and fully, or nearly fully, breastfeeding (page 271) – but it requires a high commitment to breastfeeding. Women who are only partially breastfeeding their babies or entirely bottle-feeding do not fulfil these criteria.

The first few menstrual cycles postpartum present challenges for FAMs as they are usually irregular – often with delayed ovulation and short luteal phases. Researchers at IRH studied the pattern of returning fertility in an existing dataset of 73 breastfeeding women starting six weeks postpartum until they had at least two potentially fertile cycles. They defined "normal fertility" as cycles with adequate levels of urinary estrogens and pregnanediol glucuronide plus a luteal phase length of at least 10 days from the estrogen peak to the day before the next period.

SDM is not appropriate during the first few cycles postpartum because it requires cycle lengths of 26–32 days. However, by the fourth cycle postpartum about a quarter of the women had appropriate cycle lengths to use the SDM fixed formula: *fixed fertile time = days 8–19*. The TDM is more appropriate for postpartum women and is effective even from the first postpartum cycle as it does not require regular cycles. However, TDM may require lengthy abstinence (or barriers) as breastfeeding women often observe many days of secretions, related to fluctuating hormone levels, especially during weaning. [13] Women who are spacing pregnancies may be well-suited to a simplified method.

A Bridge to SDM

Georgetown University developed a "Bridge" for postpartum women that is usable from the first period after delivery. The Bridge is used as follows:

- **First cycle postpartum:** the fertile time starts on day 11 and lasts until the first day of the next period.
- **Second and subsequent cycles:** the fertile time starts on day 8 and ends on day 24.
- **When cycle lengths are within 26–32 days,** the fertile time reverts to the usual SDM formula: fixed *fertile time = days 8–19*. [546]

The efficacy of the Bridge was tested on 157 postpartum women (aged 18–39 years) with a nine-month follow-up. All the women had experienced at least one period since delivery and had a baby of at least two months old; 11.2% of the women experienced an unintended pregnancy over a six-month interval. Provided the guidelines are followed consistently, the Bridge can offer significant protection from pregnancy for postpartum women who are not yet eligible to use SDM. The researchers noted the difficulties of the lengthy abstinence required, particularly in the first cycle, and suggested modifications to the method so that the usual SDM formula (days 8–19) is resumed in the third postpartum cycle. The efficacy of this revised protocol has not yet been tested. [546]

USE OF SIMPLIFIED METHODS IN LIMITED-RESOURCE SETTINGS

Simplified methods have been well-researched and provide increased contraceptive choice. For women who have cycles of 26–32 days, SDM may be the ideal choice. Women whose cycles are outside this range may be ideally suited to TDM. In the TDM efficacy study, 73% of cycles were within the range of 26–32 days, with 8% of cycles shorter and 19% longer, making SDM a realistic choice for most women. TDM does not require literacy or numeracy, and the majority of women are able to learn to recognise the presence or absence of secretions. Education should be appropriate to the community setting: for example, demonstrating cervical secretions with the use of shea butter (ivory-coloured fat from the nut of the African shea tree) or okra (ladies' fingers), which has a slimy, mucilaginous nature when the seed pods are cooked. The short time taken to teach simplified methods and their ease-of-use make them ideal for limited-resource settings.

12 FACTORS AFFECTING THE MENSTRUAL CYCLE

Any disturbance or change from normal routine could affect the indicators of fertility or disrupt the menstrual cycle. A disturbance can vary in its effects from disrupting a single temperature reading to affecting the menstrual cycle in its entirety. Each woman's response to disturbances will vary. Women should be encouraged to note any disturbances on the chart, either in the comments box or next to the affected reading. A number of common disturbances affect specific indicators: for example, alcohol is likely to cause a raised temperature and antihistamines will dry cervical secretions. These factors are discussed fully in the relevant chapter covering the specific fertility indicator, with a summary on page 224. **Disrupted charts may not be interpretable. If the guidelines cannot be applied, the chart should be clearly marked** "uninterpretable" (figure 12.5). A couple who are avoiding pregnancy should be advised to consider themselves potentially fertile until the situation becomes clear. There are some circumstances where FAMs cannot be relied upon – either because a medical condition makes it impossible to accurately interpret the fertility indicators or because pregnancy is strongly contraindicated (for example, during chemotherapy) – see restrictions on the use of FAMs for avoiding pregnancy on page 362.

CIRCADIAN RHYTHM: SLEEP/WAKE CYCLE AND EFFECTS OF LIGHT

Many physiological processes work on a circadian rhythm, a 24-hour cycle governed by the in-built circadian clock which is synchronised with the Earth's rotation. Some hormones are influenced by the circadian clock: for example, prolactin is produced in greatest quantities an hour after sleep, whereas testosterone is at its maximum in the morning. The circadian clock influences sleep and wakefulness, the urinary and digestive systems, body temperature, heart rate, blood pressure, co-ordination, muscle strength and alertness. Factors such as ambient temperature, meal times, exercise and stress influence this rhythm. The circadian rhythm is significant for women using temperature as an indicator of fertility.

Melatonin, the hormone of sleep/darkness, is the principal hormone associated with the circadian clock and the regulation of the sleep/wake cycle. It is produced by the pineal gland, a small endocrine gland situated behind the eyes in the centre of the brain. Photo-sensitive cells in the retina send signals about light intensity back to the pineal gland via the hypothalamus. Melatonin is stimulated by darkness and inhibited by light, so the longer the darkness the more melatonin; with the highest levels released between midnight and 04:00.

Melatonin modulates the menstrual cycle via the HPO-axis. It is found in preovulatory follicles and may affect estrogen production. Abnormal melatonin levels have been linked to health problems, including PCOS, exercise or malnutrition-induced hypothalamic amenorrhoea [5] and severe premenstrual syndrome (PMS). [453]

A systematic review confirmed the relationship between light exposure, melatonin secretion and the menstrual cycle. Women with endocrinological conditions such as PCOS or with psychopathology such as bipolar disorder seem to be more greatly influenced by light-dark exposure, but more research is needed. [35]

A study conducted in a Russian winter observed the effect of light on the hormone profiles and menstrual cycle characteristics of 22 women. Women who had slightly long menstrual cycles (30–38 days) used light boxes in the follicular phase. Exposure to bright light stimulated the secretion of FSH, LH and prolactin; shortened cycle length; promoted follicular growth; and increased the rate of ovulation (as a result of faster follicle maturation). These results are not generalisable to women with normal-length cycles, very long or irregular cycles, or to other geographical locations with more bright light. [111]

In the US, DeFelice observed the effect of light on the menstrual cycle and the cervical secretions. She found a link, for some women, between additional light at night and cyclic irregularities. DeFelice advised the use of black-out blinds and the elimination of light sources such as digital clocks and phone chargers as a simple first step for women to help regulate cycle length and normalise the pattern of secretions. [116] Women using FAMs need to consider the possible influence of sleep disruption, changes to the sleeping environment, the level of darkness in the room and disruption to the sleep/wake cycle. This includes the impact of factors such as shift work and long-distance travel across time zones.

Effect of daylight saving time

Daylight saving involves moving the clocks forward during the summer months to benefit from more light in the evening. British Summer Time (BST) starts at 01:00 Greenwich Mean Time (GMT) on the last Sunday of March and ends at 01:00 GMT on the last Sunday of October. BST is one hour ahead of GMT, so clocks go forward in spring and back in autumn.

This subtle time change affects temperature readings for some women. If the change occurs after the fertile time, then there is no need to do anything. Some women notice that their temperature is at a marginally different level for a few days while their body adjusts, but this is of no practical significance. If the clocks will be changing during the early part of the cycle, then it may help to make minor adjustments. The time change has the same overall effect as taking the temperature an hour earlier in the spring (so temperatures may be slightly lower) and an hour later in the autumn (so temperatures may be marginally higher than normal).

A recommendation by US women's health educator Toni Weschler [610] is to adjust the waking time slightly around the time-change weekend to smooth the difference. Figure 12.1 shows time adjustments for a woman whose usual waking time is 07:00. Within three days, the usual waking time is re-established. Women who use a combination of indicators should check carefully to ensure that the other indicators correlate.

Travel across time zones

Holidays and travel can be stressful, possibly resulting in cycle disruption which includes delayed or suppressed ovulation. Any travel which involves crossing time zones is particularly stressful as this disrupts the circadian rhythm, making waking temperatures unreliable. Weschler suggests treating time zones in the same way as daylight saving. For example, if a woman is travelling in the US from West to East (three-hour time difference) the effect would be like taking the temperature three hours earlier than usual; conversely, travelling from East to West would be like taking the temperature three hours later. The impact of the time change is likely to last for about one day for every time zone crossed – similar to the impact of jet lag. A woman can try to compensate for time changes but at such a time of uncertainty she must ensure that the other indicators correlate. If the disruption occurs around the fertile time the chart may be uninterpretable.

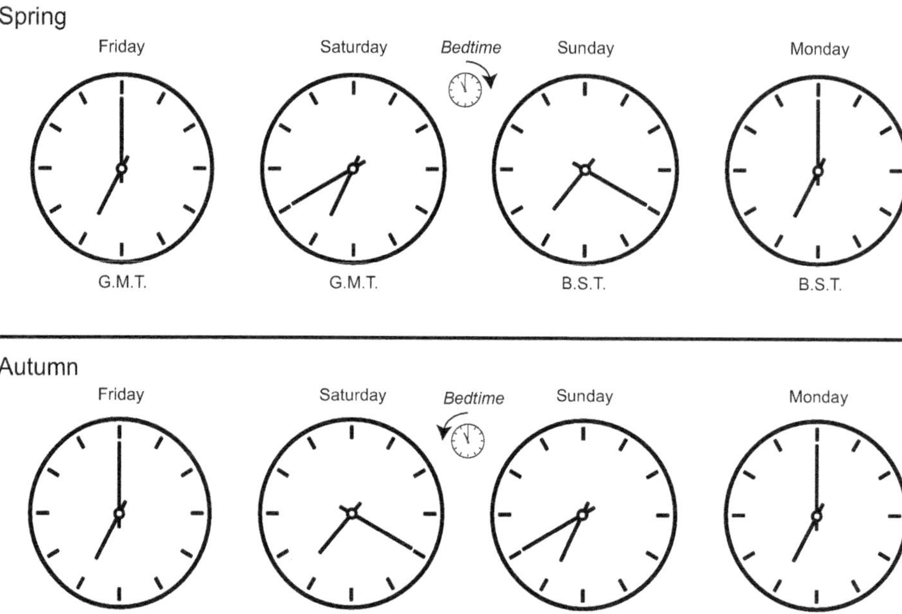

Figure 12.1 Adjusting waking time to accommodate daylight saving (Adapted from Weschler [610])

Shift work

Shift work is stressful. It results in disturbed sleep and often less sleep than usual. In addition, it takes longer to fall asleep. Shift work affects all bodily systems, but particularly the sleep/wake cycle, the digestive and reproductive systems. A number of studies have researched the effect of shift work on the menstrual cycle, particularly involving nurses working night shifts. Cyclic disturbance is common with shift work. This may be related to disruption in the circadian rhythm through disordered sleep or changes in melatonin production affecting the reproductive hormones. Shift work affects the menstrual cycle for most women and in different ways:

- Cyclic irregularities are experienced by more than 50% of nurses working night shifts. This may be a marker of shift work intolerance. [344]
- A study of pharmaceutical workers in Tehran found a higher frequency of menstrual disorders in shift workers compared with non-shift workers. Shift workers had significantly increased prolactin levels, which may contribute to changes in cycle length, ovulation suppression, and the length and amount of bleeding. FSH, LH and thyroid stimulating hormone (TSH) were not significantly different between the shift and non-shift workers. [15]
- Cyclic changes are primarily caused by changes in the follicular phase, resulting in lengthening of the follicular phase and delayed ovulation. [15]
- Inadequate luteal phases are more common in nurses working rotating shifts compared to nurses with fixed day or night shifts. [272]
- Sixty percent of nurses (with regular cycles) working fixed night shifts had cycles of less than 25 days, which was significantly shorter than nurses on other shifts. [15]

- Nurses on rotating shifts for more than 20 months had a higher percentage of irregular cycles and more cycles of fewer than 21 days or more than 40 days. The percentage of cycles outside the normal range increased the longer the nurses were on rotating shifts. [15]
- Cyclic irregularity and painful periods were more common in nurses working rotating shifts for more than seven years. [15]
- Menstrual disorders were more frequent among workers with high work stress and low job satisfaction. [15]
- Epidemiological studies of female shift workers show increased rates of reproductive abnormalities and adverse pregnancy outcomes. It is not known whether this is due to circadian disruption or other factors associated with shift work. It has been shown (in mice) that repeated changes in the light-dark cycle disrupts the circadian rhythm and reduces pregnancy rates. This may have implications for women who do shift work and are trying to conceive. [569]
- Long-term night shift work may be associated with an increased risk of breast cancer. [252]

Practical aspects of charting for shift workers

Shift work presents challenges for observing fertility indicators, particularly temperature. Women who work a combination of "early" or "late" shifts may manage to adjust temperatures using the rule of 0.1 deg.C for every hour later in bed (page 97), but night shifts can be more problematic. Some night workers will get consistent readings by taking their temperature at the same time of day regardless of its relation to sleep, but it is more normal for women to take their temperature after their longest sleep (after at least three hours of rest).

Any woman who works shifts must anticipate changes in her menstrual cycle and the indicators of fertility (similar to stress cycles). Cycles may be varied in length. There may be a delayed temperature rise, short luteal phase or a monophasic pattern. In short cycles there may be no early relatively infertile time. Cervical secretions may be interrupted, or they may show more than one peak day (figures 12.2 and 12.3).

A combination of indicators must be used. Cervical changes can play a key role because they are less affected by the circadian rhythm. Urinary LH tests can provide a back-up to help identify the end of the fertile time or, provided cycle length permits, direct hormone monitoring such as Persona can be useful to confirm the observed indicators.

STRESS

Exposure to severe stress adversely affects female reproduction. [173] Any stressful event or time of life is likely to disrupt menstrual cycles to some extent. Stress is perceived as an emergency situation: in Sapolsky's words, "if the lion's on your tail, two steps behind you, worry about ovulating or growing antlers or making sperm some other time." [523]

The physiology of stress is complex and not completely understood, but the adrenal glands, situated above the kidneys, play a key role. The inner part (medulla) produces adrenaline and nor-adrenaline in response to stimulation from the sympathetic nervous system – the "fight or flight" response to stress – and the outer layer (cortex) produces cortisol. Increased cortisol levels affect the functioning of the hypothalamus, which in turn affects pituitary output of FSH and LH and hence ovarian function.

Physical or emotional stress may significantly increase the production of prolactin (the breastfeeding hormone). High levels of prolactin suppress GnRH with an ensuing suppressant effect on the ovaries. Normal prolactin levels are lower than 400 mU/L, but transient concentrations of double the upper limit of normal are common at times of stress. Prolactin levels greater than 3000 mU/L suggest the presence of a pituitary adenoma and require investigation (page 212). [354]

Stressors including occupational stress

Stressors are situations which create a demand for performance or require adjustments to new demands – this includes situations such as starting university, which is shown to increase the risk of long cycles. [265] However, the response to stress is varied.

Many women blame stress, particularly work stress, for a variety of changes in their menstrual cycle. Similarly, women who are struggling to conceive often believe that work stress is a contributing factor to delayed conception – yet perceived stress does not necessarily match up with stress biomarkers. [369]

A US study which used urinary estrogen and progesterone to confirm ovulation found that women in stressful jobs (high demand but low control) had more than twice the risk of short cycles (< 25 days) compared with women not working in stressful jobs. They found no strong association between work stress and long cycles (> 35 days), long follicular phases (> 23 days), short luteal phases (< 10 days), monophasic cycles, or long periods (> 7 days). [171] However, nurses who worked in high-stress units and perceived their work was stressful had an increased risk of long cycles, short luteal phases and monophasic cycles. [272]

Flight attendants showed an increased incidence of amenorrhoea possibly linked to the disrupted circadian rhythm and its inhibiting effect on LH secretion. Normal fertile cycles were also disrupted when the circadian rhythm was disturbed: for example, in rapid transition through time zones. [501]

Hairdressers have a higher frequency of short, long or irregular cycles and intermenstrual bleeding plus an increased risk of subfertility compared to office workers and shop assistants. It is speculated that chemicals in salons could be responsible, but more research is needed. [512]

Intensive athletic training, or any form of intensive exercise, adversely affects the menstrual cycle. This includes delayed menarche in ballet dancers and gymnasts plus shortened luteal phases and secondary amenorrhoea associated with high training loads and competitive stress. [501] Anovulation and amenorrhoea is most common in women involved in endurance sports such as long-distance running, but is also found in dancers, gymnasts, swimmers and cyclists, predominantly due to low weight and low body fat percentage.

Resistance to stress

A woman's resistance to stress varies throughout the menstrual cycle. It is at its lowest during the luteal phase because a successful pregnancy requires that the woman's immune system is moderated to avoid rejection. The embryo is effectively a foreign body formed from proteins from the woman and her partner – it is genetically and immunologically different. In order to protect sperm and embryos from attack, the immune system dampens down around ovulation and during the luteal phase. This normal physiological response can be observed by fluctuations in the level and activity of white blood cells, including natural killer cells and T lymphocytes (T cells). [457] [350] [571] This moderated immune response in the luteal phase may explain the lowered resistance to stress or disease and why some medical conditions are exacerbated during the luteal phase and menstruation (page 219).

Effects of stress on chart

At times of stress, cycles can move unpredictably from fertile to infertile cycle types – that is, from a full ovulatory cycle through to complete cessation of ovulation and amenorrhoea and back again. This is a normal physiological response to stress (see continuum on page 85). [67]

The duration of stress also affects cycle characteristics. Rhesus monkeys subjected to short-term stress remained ovulatory, but monkeys subjected to longer-term stress showed reduced progesterone and LPD, particularly when the stress was initiated in the follicular phase. Longer-term stress continued to produce detrimental effects on the menstrual cycle following the removal of stress: post-stress cycles showed reduced LH secretion, suggesting continuing disturbance of the HPO-axis. [638]

Possible changes to normal fertile cycles Stress affects the cycle in a variety of ways dependent on the type of stress and its duration, the timing in the menstrual cycle and the woman's response and adaptation to stress. Anticipate the following changes:

- delayed temperature rise;
- interrupted pattern of cervical secretions;
- double or multiple peak days;
- short or deficient luteal phases; or
- monophasic cycles.

Women using FAMs to avoid pregnancy should use a combination of indicators and wait for the temperature rise. Unintended pregnancies occur when couples tire of waiting for the rise and assume the cycle to be monophasic: this can be determined only retrospectively (page 110). Charts showing a delayed temperature rise, short luteal phase and monophasic cycle are shown in chapter 4, in figures 4.8, 4.11, and 4.12 respectively.

Interrupted pattern of secretions If stress occurs in the early part of the cycle, then the pattern of secretions may be disrupted. There may be an intermittent return to dryness before building up to peak day. Ovulation may be delayed until the stress is over or the woman's body adapts. In some situations, there will be no ovulation and the chart will be monophasic with either dryness throughout or an interrupted pattern of secretions.

Figure 12.2 shows a 24-day cycle from a woman under stress as she starts a new job. Note the interrupted pattern of secretions. The secretions start on day 8 and then, instead of building up to peak day, there is a return to dryness on day 11, before building up again to peak day on day 17. Peak day coincides with the first high temperature, so note the readjustment of the *count of three*. Days 7 and 13 are circled to show temperature spikes (due to alcohol and a lie-in respectively). The fertile time starts on day 8 (first sign of secretions) and ends on day 20 (third high temperature after peak day). The work stress may have caused the interrupted pattern of secretions, delayed temperature rise and short luteal phase. The intermittent days of dryness (days 11 and 12) are fertile. Once the fertile time has started, it continues until the temperature rise and cervical secretions confirm the end of the fertile time.

Double peak Some women may experience more than one peak day, particularly when under stress. This is observed as a build-up to peak followed by a return to dryness or sticky secretions, then a return to wetter, transparent, stretchy secretions a few days later. If a double peak occurs, the temperature rise will be delayed until after the second peak day. Multiple peaks may occur due to fluctuating levels of estrogen (unsuccessful attempts at ovulation) and the temperature rise is delayed until after the final "true" peak. It is vital for women avoiding pregnancy to wait for the temperature rise to confirm ovulation.

Figure 12.3 shows a 29-day cycle from a woman under stress during a house move. The *S minus 20* rule gives day 7 as the first fertile day. The secretions start on day 8 and build up to peak day on day 12 (last day of wet, transparent, stretchy secretions), but the temperature rise is delayed. There are further wet secretions on days 17 and 18, with the true peak on day 18, as this is followed by the temperature rise on day 20. The fertile time lasts from day 7 to 22 inclusive. If this woman had been relying on her cervical secretions as a single indicator, she may have resumed intercourse on day 16 (fourth day post peak) with a risk of unintended pregnancy. This chart clearly demonstrates the need for a combined indicator approach and the advantage of a double-check at the start and end of the fertile time.

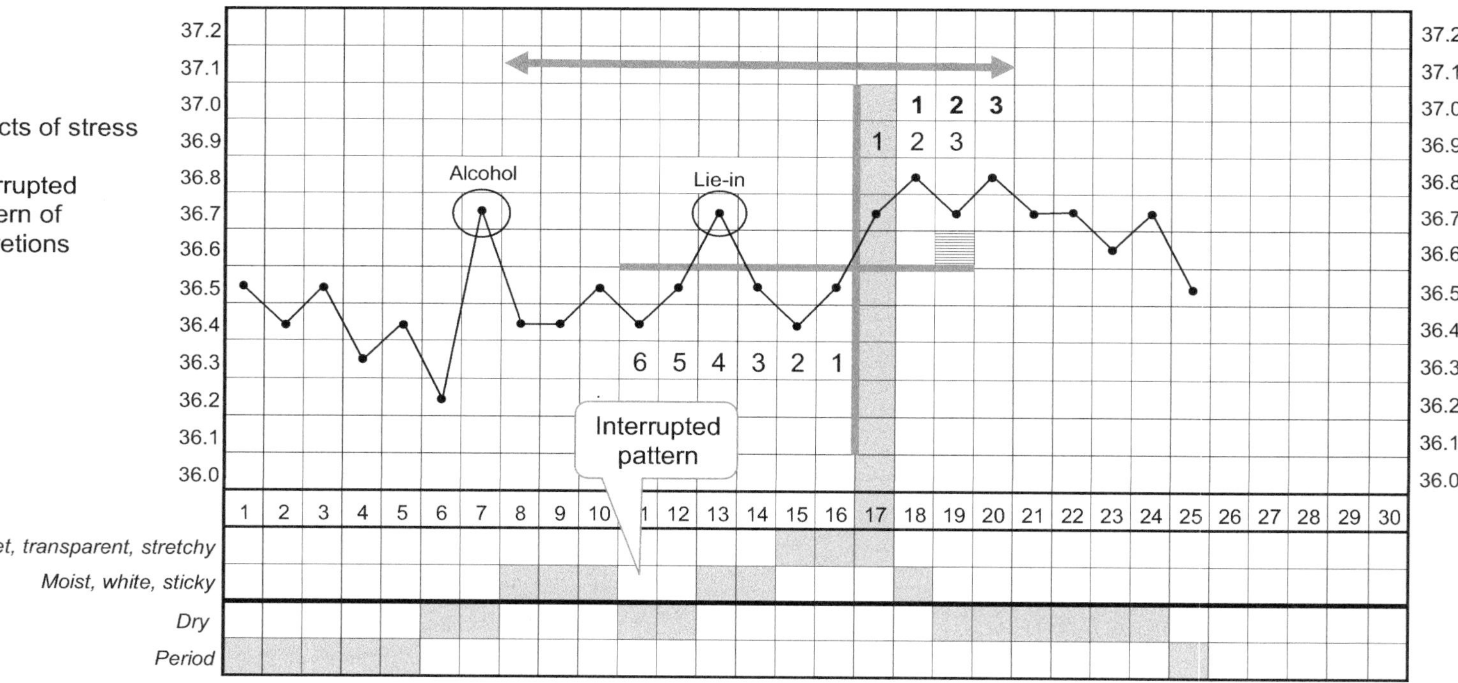

Figure 12.2 Interrupted pattern of secretions. Once the secretions have started, any return to dryness is considered fertile.

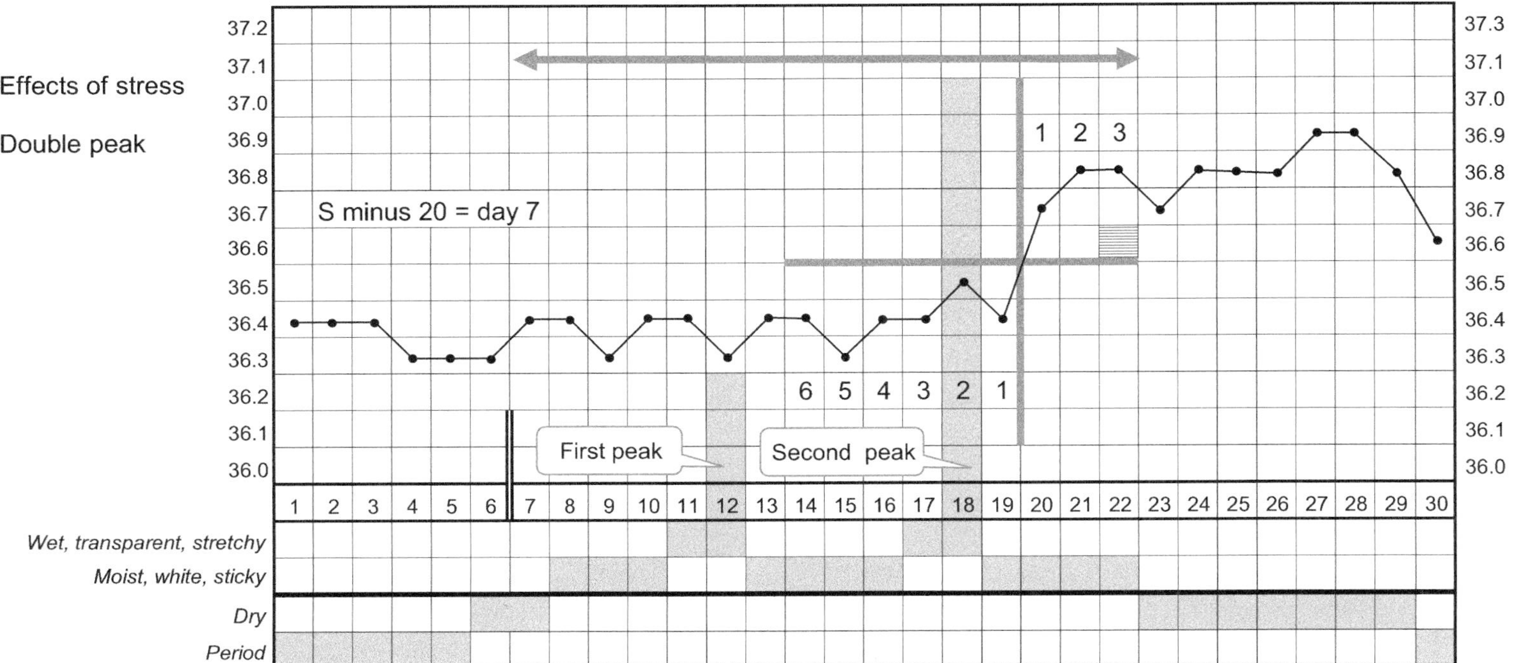

Figure 12.3 Double peak – possibly caused by stress. The first peak day is on day 12, but the temperature rise is delayed until after the second peak day on day 18.

Extreme stress and amenorrhoea In situations of extreme stress such as bereavement, major accident or serious illness, ovulation may be delayed or suppressed for many months. The temperature may remain monophasic and periods may stop completely. There may be a continuing pattern of dryness or unchanging pattern of secretions throughout. Any intervals of increased ovarian activity will be reflected by intermittent patches of the more fertile-type secretions which may or may not build up to a peak day (followed by ovulation). It is more common with prolonged amenorrhoea for menstruation to return prior to ovulation and normal fertile cycles, but it is still possible for ovulation to precede the return of menstruation: the woman cannot assume that she is infertile throughout this time.

High risk of pregnancy from intercourse at times of stress

Trussel's analysis of the WHO study of the Ovulation Method showed that there was a very high risk of pregnancy related to intercourse occurring at times of stress. [588] Couples who are using FAMs to avoid pregnancy should be cautioned about the need for extra vigilance at times of stress. Users, including experienced users, may require additional help from their FA specialist to interpret charts, but many charts cannot be interpreted until the stressful situation is over or the woman's body has adapted to the stress.

Impact of stress on chances of pregnancy

Despite the high risk of unintended pregnancy at times of stress, it is shown that psychological distress reduces fertility, particularly in women with long cycles (> 35 days). [285]

Studies using stress biomarkers show that higher levels of stress are associated with a longer time to pregnancy and an increased risk of infertility. A study of the cumulative effect of "real life" stress in a rural Mayan community in Guatemala showed that increased urinary cortisol levels adversely affected gonadotrophin levels and significantly reduced mid-luteal phase progesterone, which reduces the chance of successful implantation. [425]

The Oxford Conception Study showed that stress (high salivary alpha-amylase) significantly reduced the probability of conception in the first cycle of attempting pregnancy, but salivary cortisol levels were not linked to fecundity. This suggested an effect through the sympathetic medullar pathway. [360]

US data from the LIFE study (Longitudinal Investigation of Fertility and the Environment) confirmed the link between salivary alpha-amylase (not cortisol) and reduced fertility and showed double the risk of infertility among the women with the highest alpha-amylase levels. It was not determined whether stress levels increased over time for the women who continued to fail to conceive. [367]

WEIGHT, BODY MASS INDEX AND BODY FAT PERCENTAGE

Body weight has significant effects on the menstrual cycle in addition to its effects on health, cardiovascular disease and diabetes. Body mass index (BMI) is a simple calculation used to define normal weight, underweight, overweight and levels of obesity. BMI is calculated by dividing body weight (in kilograms) by height (in metres) squared. The BMI chart illustrated in appendix F shows the ideal BMI range (20–25 kg/m^2) for good health and optimum reproductive function. Women who have a normal BMI have the highest percentage of regular ovulatory cycles: this is of relevance whether women are planning or avoiding pregnancy. The further outside the normal range, the stronger the association with risks to fertility and pregnancy (see table 18.2 in chapter 18).

Body weight is important, but it is the percentage of body fat which plays the most significant role in fertility. Body fat is stored in the typical female fat storage areas (breasts, tummy, thighs and bottom). The enzyme aromatase, found primarily in adipose tissue, converts androgens to estrogens (aromatisation). The hormone leptin also has a role. Leptin is released by fat cells. When fat stores are high, leptin levels are high and appetite is suppressed. High leptin levels stimulate pituitary release of FSH and LH, maintaining ovarian function (and improving bone formation). When fat levels are low (as in anorexia nervosa) leptin levels are low, FSH and LH are not released in a pulsatile manner and there is insufficient estrogen to stimulate the feedback necessary for ovulation. In women of reproductive age, about a third of the circulating estrogen comes from body fat, whilst in post-menopausal women all of the estrogen comes from the adrenals and body fat.

Overweight Women who are overweight (BMI 25–30) or obese (BMI 30+) with a high body fat percentage are more likely to be subfertile. If a woman has an excess of body fat there is more aromatase to convert androgens and the serum estrogen levels increase. This extra-ovarian source of estrogen disrupts ovulation.

Underweight Women who are underweight (BMI < 20), with a low body fat percentage and high lean:fat ratio, whether due to calorie restriction or over-exercise, have reduced estrogen production and storage capacity hence low circulating levels of estrogen. About 50% of underweight women will have menstrual irregularities, ovarian dysfunction and delayed conception. Women who are seriously underweight are more likely to become anovulatory and amenorrhoeic (page 330).

Eating disorders are serious mental health issues. They include anorexia, bulimia and binge eating disorder. These affect individuals physically, psychologically and socially. Further information is available from Beat (beating eating disorders) at www.b-eat.co.uk.

WOMEN'S HEALTH PROBLEMS

Some key women's health issues are discussed here from the perspective of their effect on both fertility and the indicators of fertility. More comprehensive coverage of women's health is shown in the reading list in appendix H.

Premenstrual syndrome (PMS)

PMS is defined as a condition which manifests with distressing physical, behavioural and psychological symptoms in the absence of organic or underlying psychiatric disease. It regularly recurs during the luteal phase of each menstrual cycle and either disappears or significantly regresses by the end of menstruation. The precise cause of PMS is unknown but cyclical ovarian activity and the effect of estradiol and progesterone on the neurotransmitters serotonin and gamma-aminobutyric acid (GABA) seem to be key factors.

The degree and severity of PMS symptoms can vary significantly from woman to woman. The symptoms associated with premenstrual *syndrome* can be distinguished from normal physiological premenstrual symptoms (described on page 163) because they cause significant impairment to daily activity. PMS is categorised as mild, moderate or severe with severe PMS and its most severe form premenstrual dysphoric disorder affecting between 3% to 30% of women. See RCOG guidance on the management of PMS. [484]

Diagnosis of PMS

Women who record their fertility indicators frequently note symptoms of PMS and the severity of such symptoms. Symptoms can begin in the early, mid or late luteal phase. Daily fertility charting enables a prospective record of PMS symptoms, but a more detailed symptom diary such as the Daily Record of Severity of Problems provides a more accurate diagnostic tool. [154]

Waking temperature in women with PMS PMS is triggered by hormonal events following ovulation. There is no clear evidence of a hormonal abnormality with PMS but symptoms are related to ovarian production of progesterone. [480] It follows that women with PMS may have some disturbance to waking temperatures. A study which compared the nocturnal temperatures of PMS sufferers with a control group reported that all the women had biphasic cycles, but the women with PMS had significantly higher nocturnal temperatures across the entire menstrual cycle. [535] Women with PMS may therefore have higher than normal waking temperatures. Some women show a wider day-to-day temperature variation in the luteal phase. This swinging temperature may be indicative of progesterone disturbance.

Abnormal reproductive tract bleeding

Between the menarche and the menopause, a woman will have about 400 menstrual periods, during which time she will experience normal cyclic changes but she may also experience abnormal symptoms including changes in the frequency, regularity, duration or amount of flow, spotting between periods or after intercourse. Normal menstrual bleeding is bleeding that occurs after an ovulatory cycle every 21 to 35 days, lasts three to seven days and is not excessive. Normal periods should not cause severe pain or include the passage of identifiable clots; however, the limits for normal menstrual parameters are still being debated internationally (page 77). [417] FAM users may be more alert to abnormal or irregular bleeding, with clearly documented charts allowing a more accurate assessment of the bleeding pattern and its relationship to presumed ovulation.

Abnormal bleeding comes from many parts of the reproductive tract, not necessarily the uterus, hence the term "abnormal reproductive tract bleeding" (not abnormal uterine bleeding). An initial step in the assessment of abnormal bleeding is to confirm whether ovulation is occurring. Clearly documented charts can aid diagnosis with a biphasic temperature curve being highly indicative of ovulation. [387]

Ovulatory bleeding Bleeding in an ovulatory cycle occurs as a result of progesterone withdrawal – a "true period", recognised by a temperature rise 10–16 days earlier. Women who have regular, but heavy, bleeding are likely to be ovulating with associated abdominal cramps and premenstrual symptoms. The most common causes of ovulatory bleeding are pregnancy-related conditions including miscarriage or threatened miscarriage and ectopic pregnancy.

Anovulatory bleeding In an anovulatory cycle, the ovaries produce enough estrogen to stimulate endometrial growth and bleeding occurs due to estrogen withdrawal; this is often referred to as "dysfunctional uterine bleeding". Women with ovulatory disorders are more likely to have irregular, painless bleeding with a variable blood loss which is often heavy (and may be prolonged) but may be infrequent and light. Two distinct groups of women are most affected: adolescent girls in the first 18 months after the menarche and women approaching the menopause. In adolescents the abnormal bleeding is related to the immaturity of the HPO-axis; whereas in pre-menopausal women irregular bleeding is due to reduced estrogen production and is often accompanied by hot flushes, vaginal dryness and mood swings.

Anovulatory bleeding may be related to hormonal disruption caused by obesity, PCOS, crash dieting, excessive exercise, severe stress or thyroid problems. Women with recurrent anovulatory cycles may be at a higher risk of anaemia, loss of bone density and endometrial hyperplasia (which may lead to endometrial cancer). This always requires investigation. [259] Women who do not want to conceive, but are having repeated monophasic cycles may require treatment such as cyclic progesterone or hormonal contraception to protect the endometrium and prevent bone loss. Women who are trying to conceive may require ovulation induction or other forms of assisted fertility.

Couples who are using FAMs to avoid pregnancy must understand that a bleed which is not preceded by a temperature rise is not a true period, hence caution is needed in applying the guidelines (page 227).

Inter-menstrual and post-coital bleeding

Inter-menstrual bleeding is vaginal bleeding occurring at any time of the cycle other than during menstruation or after intercourse; whereas post-coital bleeding occurs immediately after intercourse but is unrelated to menstruation. Inter-menstrual and post-coital bleeding are generally due to a structural problem or inflammatory process, with cervical ectropion being a common cause of post-coital bleeding due to the friable nature of the cervix. *Any* abnormal bleeding must be investigated to exclude the possibility of chlamydia or other STIs.

For a few women, spotting or light bleeding around peak day may be physiologically normal. Provided this has been thoroughly investigated and no cause found, a woman can be reassured that this is linked to hormonal fluctuations around ovulation and is normal for her, but she must attend for regular cervical screening and report any changes.

Premenstrual spotting

Premenstrual spotting describes very light bleeding for a day or more before the period (bright red bleed) starts. This has been linked to LPD, endometriosis and polyps (benign growths arising on a stalk from mucus membrane). Spotting may be particularly relevant for women who are planning pregnancy (page 347). Women frequently express concerns about premenstrual spotting in relation to LPD, but out of 32 women diagnosed with LPD, only two had premenstrual spotting (one of whom had endometriosis). [608]

A recent study showed that endometriosis was significantly more prevalent in subfertile women who reported premenstrual spotting for at least two days compared to women with no spotting (89% compared with 26%). Premenstrual spotting may therefore be a better predictor of endometriosis than painful periods or pain at intercourse. [274]

Heavy menstrual bleeding

Menstrual loss is both hard to estimate and highly subjective. Normal loss is 5–80 ml, with more than 80 ml considered excessive. The NICE guidelines on heavy menstrual bleeding highlight the importance of the patient's perspectives:

> For clinical purposes, heavy menstrual bleeding should be defined as excessive menstrual blood loss which interferes with the woman's physical, emotional, social and material quality of life, and which can occur alone or in combination with other symptoms. Any interventions should aim to improve quality of life measures. [426]

Investigation of abnormal bleeding

Abnormal bleeding should be fully investigated to exclude pathology including chlamydia, genital warts, cervical ectropion, vaginitis, cervicitis, endometriosis, fibroids, cervical or endometrial polyps, thyroid dysfunction, clotting disorders, endometrial hyperplasia or gynaecological cancers including endometrial and cervical cancer. Women should be encouraged to attend for regular cervical screening and to report any changes promptly.

Abnormal bleeding and its effect on cervical secretions

Any abnormal bleeding can mask the normal pattern of cervical secretions, hence creating difficulties for women using this indicator. Some women may be able to distinguish their pattern of secretions during spotting or light bleeding, but heavy prolonged bleeding may mask the occurrence of early dry days and the first sign of secretions. Couples who are avoiding pregnancy should either use a calendar-based calculation to determine the start of the fertile time or restrict intercourse to the late infertile time. Following treatment for a condition causing prolonged bleeding (such as myomectomy for fibroids) the shorter duration of bleeding should lead to noticeably more early dry days.

Infrequent and absent menstruation

Vaginal bleeding may be normal menstrual bleeding but abnormal in terms of its frequency. Infrequent menstruation (cycles > 38 days), also referred to as oligomenorrhoea, and absent menstruation (amenorrhoea) may have a pathological cause and require investigation.

Amenorrhoea is classified as primary or secondary. Primary amenorrhoea is the failure to start menstruating by 16 years of age (in a girl with normal secondary sex characteristics). Secondary amenorrhoea is the absence of menstruation for more than six months in a woman who had a normal menarche. Amenorrhoea is a normal physiological state for women before the menarche, during pregnancy, during lactation and after the menopause. Amenorrhoea at other times is a symptom of an underlying abnormality.

The main causes of infrequent and absent periods are: PCOS (most common cause), premature ovarian insufficiency (formerly premature ovarian failure), hypothalamic disorders including weight-related amenorrhoea, hyperprolactinaemia, thyroid disease, uterine causes e.g. Asherman's syndrome (adhesions obliterating the uterine cavity) and severe generalised illnesses such as leukaemia. Abnormalities of menstrual frequency and associated ovulation disorders are a significant cause of fertility delays (page 349).

Ovarian cysts

An ovarian cyst is an abnormal fluid-filled structure that develops within the ovary – a common finding during a routine ultrasound scan. Most cysts are simple functional cysts which develop from ovarian follicles during the normal course of the menstrual cycle. The less common pathological cysts, which originate from other ovarian tissue, are normally benign but may become malignant particularly in post-menopausal women. Trans-vaginal ultrasound is required to diagnose a cyst with follow-up scans to monitor progress.

Functional cysts

Functional cysts are simple cysts which develop from ovarian follicles during either the follicular or luteal phase. Most functional cysts are asymptomatic and disappear without treatment within about three months.

Follicular cyst A follicular cyst is an enlarged unruptured Graafian follicle which continues to secrete fluid into its cavity. The follicle is termed a cyst when it enlarges to more than 20 mm. A follicular cyst is usually less than 50 mm and is normally on one side or the other. The cyst may secrete estrogen, sometimes in quite large amounts, or it may be inactive. Women who undergo ovulation induction may have multiple follicular cysts. Persistent cysts may require aspiration. A follicular cyst affects the menstrual cycle and fertility indicators to varying degrees depending on its size and associated estrogen levels. The fertility chart may indicate:

- normal length, long or short cycles;
- an increased number of days with fertile-type secretions with delayed peak day; or
- monophasic cycles.

Menstruation may be normal or heavy. (Bleeding is potentially fertile if not preceded by a temperature rise 10–16 days earlier.)

Luteinised unruptured follicle (LUF) LUF syndrome describes a situation where, following the LH surge, the dominant follicle fails to rupture but still undergoes luteinisation, continues to grow and may reach 40 mm. The luteal phase and progesterone production are normal, but pregnancy is not possible as there was no ovulation. LUF syndrome may be a significant cause of subfertility.

Corpus luteum cyst A corpus luteum cyst arises in a cycle where ovulation occurs and the corpus luteum develops, but instead of degenerating it continues to grow forming a fluid- or blood-filled cyst measuring up to 60 mm. A corpus luteum cyst continues to produce progesterone for its duration.

The fertility chart may indicate a normal pre-ovulatory phase with build-up of cervical secretions to peak day followed by the temperature rise. If there is no conception, the high temperature phase may be prolonged for 20 days or more, delaying the next period, although a pregnancy test will remain negative. If conception occurs, a pregnancy test would indicate positive after 20 raised temperatures.

A corpus luteum cyst of pregnancy normally resolves spontaneously by about 16 weeks of gestation. If it ruptures or causes ovarian torsion it may produce signs and symptoms similar to those of an ectopic pregnancy and be a risk to the woman and her pregnancy.

Pathological cysts

Pathological cysts include dermoid cysts (benign teratomas), cystadenomas and endometriomas ("chocolate" cysts), which are deposits of endometriotic tissue in the ovary. These cysts are caused by abnormal cell growth unrelated to the menstrual cycle and may occur at any life-stage. Although normally benign, they may become malignant.

Symptoms of an ovarian cyst

An ovarian cyst is often asymptomatic, however, it may become intensely painful if it becomes very large and causes pressure on adjacent structures, bleeds into itself (haemorrhagic cyst), ruptures into the peritoneal cavity or causes ovarian torsion (twisting). Symptoms include abdominal bloating or swelling, intermittent spotting or light bleeding, pain during intercourse or bowel movements, constant dull pelvic pain, and sudden severe pelvic pain with associated nausea and vomiting (possible torsion or rupture). Ovarian cysts can usually be diagnosed by pelvic ultrasound, but their exact nature may not be apparent until surgery.

Polycystic ovaries and polycystic ovary syndrome

Polycystic ovaries (PCO) and polycystic ovary *syndrome* (PCOS) are distinctly different entities which should not be confused. The term **"polycystic ovaries"** describes a common finding on ultrasound showing 12 or more follicles with a diameter of 2–8 mm in either ovary. The follicles are normally situated around the periphery of the ovary, giving the appearance of a "string of pearls". Polycystic ovaries alone are not likely to have an adverse impact on fertility although women with PCO may later develop the full syndrome. About 25% of women in the general population have polycystic ovaries.

Polycystic ovary ***syndrome*** is an endocrine disorder which tends to run in families. It is a long-term disease characterised in the earlier reproductive years by irregular periods and infertility and in the later years by glucose intolerance, cardiovascular disease and type 2 diabetes. [23] Less than 10% of women of reproductive age have PCOS, but it is the commonest cause of irregular cycles and ovulatory dysfunction hence is of most relevance for women who are trying to conceive. About 15% of women with PCOS have hyperprolactinaemia, of which about 50% have a micro-adenoma. PCOS is also associated with autoimmune thyroid disease.

Symptoms and diagnostic features Symptoms associated with PCOS include irregular cycles (or amenorrhoea), ovulatory dysfunction, hirsuitism, oily skin, acne, alopecia (hair loss on scalp) and depression. Although obesity is associated with PCOS, less than half of the women with PCOS are overweight. There is however an increased rate of eating disorders (including bulimia) in these women.

At least two out of three features are required for the diagnosis of PCOS (Rotterdam criteria): [158]

- menstrual disturbance (irregular or absent ovulation);
- clinical and/or biochemical signs of hyperandrogenism (acne, hirsuitism, raised testosterone); and
- polycystic ovary morphology.

Multiple ovarian follicles are thus not essential for the diagnosis of PCOS.

Women who have amenorrhoea or infrequent periods are at an increased risk of endometrial hyperplasia (overgrowth of endometrial tissue), which may lead to endometrial cancer. RCOG guidelines recommend treatment with progestogens to induce a withdrawal bleed at least every three to four months. The first-line treatment for women with PCOS who wish to avoid pregnancy is COCs. [498]

Diet and weight BMI has the strongest correlation with PCOS status, with every BMI increment increasing risk. Consistent loss of intra-abdominal fat is associated with resumption of ovulation. A systematic review showed that weight loss through reduced calorie intake improved PCOS symptoms regardless of dietary composition. Greater weight loss was associated with a diet enriched with monounsaturated fats (nuts and seeds, avocados, peanut butter and olive oil). A diet with a low glycaemic index was linked to improved cycle regularity and improved quality of life. A high-protein diet was linked to improved depression and self-esteem scores. [413] It is uncontroversial that improved diet and regular exercise is the first-line treatment for women with PCOS. [68]

Insulin resistance The majority of women with PCOS have increased insulin resistance – a reduced response to a given amount of insulin. Insulin resistance can occur irrespective of BMI although it correlates with increased abdominal obesity. [23] Metformin, an insulin-sensitising drug, is a common treatment for PCOS with insulin resistance. It may help to balance blood sugars and restore ovulatory function for women with anovulatory infertility, but they should be warned of side effects including nausea, vomiting and gastro-intestinal disturbances. [428] Supplementation with inositol (for example, myo-inositol), a member of the vitamin B complex, improves weight loss, increases insulin sensitivity, improves cyclic regularity and restore ovulatory function. [592] [181]

PCOS and fertility About 50% of women with PCOS have raised LH levels. Raised LH is associated with poor fertilisation, poor embryo development and poor implantation – resulting in reduced chances of conception and increased risk of miscarriage. It is the raised LH, not the polycystic ovary, which causes the fertility problems. In mild PCOS, women have regular ovulatory cycles but it may take longer to conceive; however, the majority of women with PCOS have irregular cycles and ovulatory dysfunction. Women with PCOS are at an increased risk of miscarriage and gestational diabetes.

Cervical secretions in women with PCOS The cervical secretions in women with PCOS differ from those of women with normal ovulatory cycles as a result of different levels of estrogen and progesterone. Studies of the spinnbarkeit effect showed that profuse amounts of transparent secretion were not always associated with ovulation. Some women with PCOS observed persistent (or fluctuating) transparent, stretchy secretions, but secretions were less profuse with decreased elasticity (3–5 cm stretch compared with 10–20 cm for women without PCOS). [95] Studies show abnormalities in the ultrastructure, crystallisation (ferning) and spinnbarkeit of cervical secretions in women with PCOS. The secretions have a tighter mesh structure with smaller gaps which are less conducive to sperm transport. Compared to a control group of women with normal ovulatory cycles showing the typical fern-like pattern, women with PCOS show indefinite crystallisation as well as crystallisation resembling estrogenic and progestogenic secretions. [600] Metformin may help to induce ovulation but may not restore the normal elasticity of the secretions, thus sperm transport remains compromised. [536]

FA to conceive Women with PCOS report varying patterns of secretions throughout the menstrual cycle. Women with long cycles often report intermittent patches of secretions. Charts show similar overall characteristics to those of stress cycles. There may be a build-up to peak day (or multiple peak) followed by a temperature rise (figures 12.2 and 12.3). The luteal phase may be shortened (see figure 4.11 in chapter 4) or the cycle may remain monophasic (see figure 4.12 in chapter 4). Very long cycles (> 3 months) are not uncommon. Women frequently assume that if they observe wetter, transparent secretions, then they must be ovulating but, as already stated, this is not necessarily the case. A biphasic chart may be indicative of ovulation, but a raised mid-luteal phase progesterone or ultrasound observation of the corpus luteum provide more conclusive evidence.

FA to avoid pregnancy Couples who can cope with lengthy times of abstinence (or barriers) may be able to use a combined-indicator method, but caution is needed, because it is more difficult for women with irregular cycles. The pre-ovulatory phase is uncertain due to irregular cycle lengths and the intermittent nature of secretions. Methods which rely on calendar calculations are not suitable and women who have a raised LH cannot use OPKs or fertility monitors. The most effective time for avoiding pregnancy is the post-ovulatory phase, but this may involve a prolonged wait for the temperature rise.

Support for women with PCOS Hormonal problems such as PCOS may have a noticeable psychological impact. Changes in appearance – particularly obesity and hirsuitism – may adversely affect quality of life and decrease sexual satisfaction. The psychosocial aspects are important irrespective of the severity of symptoms or relief gained through treatment. [258] Women who are affected by PCOS can find information and support through the self-help group Verity (www.verity-pcos.org.uk).

Premature ovarian insufficiency (POI)

Premature ovarian insufficiency (POI), previously known as premature ovarian failure (POF), is defined as the cessation of ovarian function (leading to premature menopause) before the age of 40. Diagnosis is confirmed by a very low AMH and antral follicle count with a raised FSH on at least two occasions. There is no consensus on the exact hormonal criteria. An FSH of greater than 25 IU/L is commonly used (with amenorrhoea of > 4 months), but there are no agreed international standards. The longer the duration of amenorrhoea, the lower the ovarian reserve; and the higher the FSH, the greater the risk that the ovarian failure is likely to be permanent. [23] [266] POI affects between 1% and 5% of women. It can occur at any age, even in girls who have not reached the menarche. For many women, POI is unexpected: there is no family history of premature menopause and there are no obvious signs or symptoms preceding the loss of ovarian function. Most women have a normal menstrual history, normal age at menarche and normal fertility prior to diagnosis.

Reproductive ageing in women with POI In most women with normal reproductive ageing, the transition through the menopause follows a predictable pattern. The reduced ovarian reserve (and decreased estrogen) leads to increased FSH output which tries to stimulate the failing ovaries. Ovulation may still occur sporadically until it finally ceases. Menstruation may continue for many months after ovulation has ceased. In women with POI the transition through the menopause is much more variable. Many women diagnosed with POI will spontaneously start menstruating again sometimes after months of amenorrhoea and may still ovulate and conceive naturally, but there is a high chance of miscarriage due to chromosomal abnormalities. It is not known whether ovarian ageing in women with POI differs depending on the cause.

Cyclic changes indicative of declining fertility and POI Women who record fertility indicators may be alert to cyclic changes which could act as a warning sign of POI. This includes changes in the frequency and regularity of periods plus changes in the duration and volume of menstrual loss. A woman may start to notice short cycles (< 24 days), cycles with short luteal phases or monophasic cycles. She may notice an increasing number of dry days and a reduction in the quantity and quality of cervical secretions. Any reported cyclic changes or menopause-related symptoms should be investigated promptly to exclude POI.

Psychological aspects The diagnosis of POI can be life-changing. Women may suffer intense physical symptoms (e.g. hot flushes, night sweats, vaginal dryness) with consequences for psychological and emotional health. Women with POI are at increased risk of long-term conditions including osteoporosis, cardiovascular disease and dementia. Hormonal replacement therapy (HRT) is required until the time of expected natural menopause. Fertility is a key concern: many women will not have completed their family and may not even have started planning pregnancy. They may become anxious or depressed, reporting feelings of sadness, grief, anger and reduced self-esteem. IVF with egg donation may be the only option. Questionnaire surveys conducted amongst women with POI show that they feel inadequately informed about the condition and require more psychological support. [549] Information and support on all aspects of POI is available from The Daisy Network (www.daisynetwork.org.uk).

Hyperprolactinaemia

Prolactin (breastfeeding hormone) is produced by the anterior pituitary. Normal serum prolactin levels are lower than 400 mU/L. A raised prolactin (hyperprolactinaemia), is physiologically normal during pregnancy and lactation but abnormal at other times. The body's physiological response to stress includes raised prolactin levels, with transient levels up to double the normal upper limit. The prolactin level may be slightly raised as a reaction to having blood taken. The levels will vary from day-to-day hence the need to repeat the test before invasive investigations.

Hyperprolactinaemia is associated with **galactorrhoea**, the secretion of breast milk unrelated to breastfeeding. Women (with the exception of breastfeeders) should be encouraged to report any breast leakage as it is *not* normal. Galactorrhoea or symptoms suggestive of hyperprolactinaemia require investigation including blood tests for prolactin, full blood count and thyroid function.

Effects on menstrual cycles and indicators of fertility Hyperprolactinaemia causes ovulatory dysfunction: irregular cycles, infrequent or absent menstruation and LPD. FAM users may be more aware of subtle cyclic changes such as a delayed temperature rise or short luteal phase. Women with short luteal phases caused by hyperprolactinaemia may benefit from Vitex agnus castus (page 348). Women who are trying to conceive may require medication such as bromocriptine to reduce prolactin levels in order to optimise ovulatory function (page 349).

Conditions associated with hyperprolactinaemia Some medical conditions including PCOS and hypothyroidism have associated hyperprolactinaemia. Prolactin may be raised as a side effect of some anti-emetics, anti-psychotics and estrogen-containing oral contraceptives (see appendix G). A prolactin level higher than 3,000 mU/L may indicate hypothalamic or pituitary tumours, most commonly pituitary adenoma. [354]

Thyroid function and dysfunction

The thyroid is a large butterfly-shaped endocrine gland situated in the neck just below the larynx and controlled by the hypothalamic-pituitary axis. TSH from the pituitary stimulates the thyroid to produce large amounts of the pro-hormone thyroxine (T4) and much smaller amounts of the active hormone triiodothyronine (T3). T4 is converted into the more potent T3 when it reaches its target cells all over the body. Thyroid hormone production requires iodine from food sources, predominantly dairy and fish. The hormone levels are kept constant by a negative feedback mechanism which draws on iodine stores within the thyroid.

The main function of the thyroid is to regulate metabolism. An underactive thyroid slows metabolism whilst an overactive thyroid speeds it up. The thyroid plays an important role in fertility whereby TSH works together with FSH and LH (plus growth hormone) in the recruitment phase of the menstrual cycle preparing the next batch of antral follicles for growth. Thyroid hormones are vital for the production of estrogen and progesterone. Thyroid function is particularly important for women who are trying to conceive because a steady supply of thyroxine is required for optimum fetal growth and neurological development. Thyroid function must be stabilised prior to conception with a TSH level of less than 2.5 mIU/l considered optimum for conception.

Between 5% and 30% of subfertile women may have thyroid disease, many of whom will be asymptomatic. A full thyroid profile is required to determine the levels of TSH, T3, T4 and the presence of anti-thyroid antibodies. Women who have anti-thyroid antibodies have an increased risk of unexplained infertility, miscarriage, stillbirth and preterm birth. [23] [253]

Hypothyroidism

Hypothyroidism (myxoedema) is an underactive thyroid. This results in a reduced output of T4 and T3 with subsequent increase in TSH to boost thyroid hormone output. Many women with an underactive thyroid will have some degree of menstrual disturbance, with longer duration and more severe disease resulting in more serious disruption.

Hypothyroidism is frequently associated with hyperprolactinaemia. Raised prolactin levels disrupt the pulsatile secretion of GnRH, resulting in varying degrees of menstrual disturbance and ovulatory dysfunction. Mildly raised prolactin may cause inadequate luteal function and reduced progesterone, whilst higher levels may result in anovulatory cycles, infrequent menstruation or amenorrhoea. Ovulation and conception may still occur with mildly raised prolactin levels, but there is an increased risk of miscarriage, stillbirth and preterm birth.

Symptoms include weight gain and inability to lose weight; constipation; dry, coarse skin; hair loss; intolerance to cold; low body temperature; tiredness; mental sluggishness; depression; goitre; low libido; and menstrual irregularities. Women who are recording fertility indicators may note a variety of cyclic changes dependent on the severity of thyroid disease and the level of prolactin.

Menstrual disturbances include:

- infrequent periods or amenorrhoea (but may be more frequent periods);
- prolonged heavy periods;
- irregular cycles;
- anovulatory cycles (monophasic charts) or short luteal phases; and
- abnormally low waking temperatures.

Treatment with thyroxine gives almost immediate relief from symptoms. It restores prolactin levels, optimises thyroid output and normalises ovarian function. Thyroxine is a lifelong medication which requires adequate monitoring.

Hyperthyroidism

Hyperthyroidism (thyrotoxicosis) is an overactive thyroid. This results in an excess of thyroid hormones T4 and T3 and a decreased level of TSH. The most common cause is Grave's disease, an auto-immune disease which attacks the thyroid. Hyperthyroidism may result in subfertility and an increased risk of miscarriage.

Symptoms include increased appetite, weight loss, diarrhoea, warm moist skin due to increased sweating, hair loss, intolerance to heat, raised body temperature, palpitations, muscle weakness, tremor affecting the hands, goitre, insomnia, anxiety and menstrual irregularities.

Menstrual disturbances include:

- amenorrhoea, frequent (or infrequent) periods;
- irregular cycles;
- very light periods;
- anovulatory cycles (monophasic charts) or short luteal phases; and
- abnormally high waking temperatures.

Women who have an overactive thyroid require anti-thyroid medication (propylthiouracil or carbimazole) to reduce the level of T4 and T3 and stabilise thyroid function.

Cyclic disturbance related to severity of thyroid dysfunction

Some women with thyroid disease will continue to have normal ovulatory cycles. Others, particularly women with a longer duration of untreated thyroid disease, may show a greater degree of menstrual disturbance. A study of more than 2,000 women with various thyroid diseases found that women with severe hypothyroidism had a higher prevalence of menstrual disturbances than mild-moderate cases (35% compared to 10%). Women with severe hyperthyroidism had a higher prevalence of amenorrhoea (2.5%) and very light periods (4%) than those with mild-moderate hyperthyroidism (0.2% and 0.9% respectively). [312]

As with all medical conditions, it is important for a woman to monitor her cycles carefully and to note any changes in general health. Changes in medication should be recorded to ascertain the effect.

Effect of thyroid disease on waking temperature Thyroid disease affects basal metabolic rate (BMR). A low BMR, characteristic of hypothyroidism, may result in low waking temperatures; conversely a high BMR, characteristic of hyperthyroidism, may result in higher temperatures. In 1942 Barnes suggested that temperatures of 36.6 deg.C or below indicated hypothyroidism and temperatures of 36.8 deg.C or above indicated hyperthyroidism. [29] The Barnes test was not widely adopted by the medical profession but some complementary therapists still use it.

The usual coverline for an *oral* temperature taken at 07:30 am is between 36.5 and 36.6 deg.C. The temperature grid on the FertilityUK charts goes from 35.5 to 37.4 deg.C. This means that most women's temperatures would be expected to fit roughly in the mid-range of the chart. An unusually low or high coverline may give a suspicion of thyroid disease, but this is *not* diagnostic. It simply indicates the need to consider thyroid function tests.

Abnormal vaginal discharge

Normal cervical secretions are transparent, opaque or white and odourless. Women who understand their normal pattern of secretions are more alert to changes from the norm. Any change should be investigated to exclude pathological conditions including STIs. A woman who is using FAMs will not be able to observe her cervical secretions while she has an abnormal discharge and should avoid intercourse or use barriers until the completion of any treatment and until her normal pattern of secretions can be observed. Two very common causes of abnormal vaginal discharge are candida and bacterial vaginosis (BV).

Candida Vulvo-vaginal candidiasis, commonly known as "thrush" or "yeast infection", is a fungal infection which thrives in warm, moist conditions – making the vagina an ideal host. Symptoms include a thick, white, cheesy discharge with an inoffensive odour, vulval redness and itching, and sometimes burning on passing urine. Any change in vaginal pH which creates an alkaline medium may precipitate symptoms. Common triggers include tight clothing, nylon underwear, thongs, scented soaps, biological washing powders, stress and trauma to the vaginal mucosa due to vaginal dryness from tampons or insufficient lubrication during intercourse. Some women are sensitive to alterations in vaginal pH from menstrual blood or residual semen. Candida is common amongst women with diabetes, during pregnancy and following antibiotic use. Hormonal fluctuations during the menstrual cycle influence changes in the immune response to candida with the lowered resistance in the luteal phase possibly explaining why symptoms are exacerbated premenstrually. [313] Daily vaginal swabs on women with recurrent episodes of candida show increasing colonisation during the luteal phase preceding the development of symptoms. [606]

Bacterial vaginosis BV is caused by an imbalance of the vaginal flora with a reduction in the protective acidic lactobacilli leading to the growth of gardnerella and/or mycoplasma. There may be a thin greyish white discharge which is often described as an offensive fishy smell, with little or no itching. Vaginal pH is affected by factors including washing products, vaginal douching and residual semen following intercourse.

Importance of an accurate diagnosis Women who have an abnormal vaginal discharge commonly self-diagnose thrush and medicate with bought treatments. Of 95 women who presented for anti-fungal treatment only 34% had candida. Nearly 20% had BV and 14% had normal swabs. Other final diagnoses included trichomonas, irritant dermatitis, atrophic vaginitis, diabetic pruritis and acute salpingitis. Prompt diagnosis and treatment is vital. [176]

Cervical problems

Abnormalities in the cervix may cause palpable changes and observable differences in the pattern of its secretions. All women should be encouraged to attend for routine cervical screening to help detect early precancerous changes. The most common condition which affects cervical secretions is cervical ectropion.

Cervical ectropion

Cervical ectropion (formerly known as "cervical erosion") is a harmless condition of the cervix in which the mucus-secreting columnar epithelium that line the cervical canal protrudes onto the vaginal aspect of the cervix resulting in a reddened (raw-looking) area around the cervical os. This occurs in response to estrogenic changes associated with pregnancy and hormonal contraception. Cervical ectropion may be observed on speculum examination: for example, during cervical screening. The woman should be informed of its presence and asked about any associated symptoms but she can be reassured that it is likely to go away without treatment and that it is *not* linked to cervical cancer.

Although cervical ectropion is often asymptomatic, the area is friable when touched which may result in spotting or bleeding after intercourse. There may be an associated cervicitis with a persistent wet discharge from the exposed cells; however, most women are still able to distinguish the onset and build-up of their normal pattern of cervical secretions. If symptoms become problematic, then treatment may be appropriate.

Treatment and its effects on fertility Colposcopy (binocular microscope with a light source) allows closer examination of the vagina and cervix followed by treatment with diathermy (heat) or cryotherapy (freezing). There may be a heavier, thicker discharge for about two weeks following the procedure after which the cervical secretions usually return to normal. Cervical ectropion itself (or its treatment) does not affect fertility. However, if a couple are trying to conceive and the woman has a persistent wet discharge or bleeding during intercourse this may reduce the desire and opportunities for sex.

Endometriosis

Endometriosis is defined as the presence of endometrial-like tissue outside the uterus which induces a chronic inflammatory reaction. [139] The main route of spread is by retrograde menstruation via the Fallopian tubes leading to endometrial deposits on the ovaries, peritoneal surfaces, bowel or bladder. These deposits bleed (menstruate) in response to cyclic hormonal changes, but as the bleeding cannot escape, the deposits increase in size causing surrounding tissues to become engorged and inflamed with a risk of pelvic adhesions. A single deposit may occur – this is most commonly in the ovary forming an endometrioma also known as an endometriotic cyst or "chocolate cyst".

Endometriosis causes a number of symptoms, depending on its site: painful periods, generalised pelvic pain, lower abdominal pain, back pain, pain on exercise, deep pain on intercourse, or pain on passing urine or bowel movements. Some women complain of general fatigue and sleep disturbance. **Premenstrual spotting lasting more than two days may be a better predictor of endometriosis than painful periods or pain at intercourse.** [274]

Women who are affected by this common condition can get further information and support from Endometriosis UK (www.endometriosis-uk.org).

Waking temperature as a predictor of endometriosis

Limited evidence suggests a characteristic temperature pattern associated with endometriosis which may be related to the inflammatory process. This "valley effect" shows the waking temperature remaining at the higher (post-ovulatory) level during the period (i.e. a late decline) then falling to the lower (pre-ovulatory) level for a few days before rising again following ovulation.

In a US study of the waking temperatures of 20 subfertile women (21–31 years) with laparoscopically diagnosed endometriosis, a total of 168 cycles were recorded:

- 10% of cycles were monophasic (presumed anovulatory);
- 22% of the biphasic cycles had short luteal phases;
- 34% of cycles showed a late decline during menstruation; and
- 65% of cycles showed elevated temperatures and/or spikes in the follicular phase.

The researchers concluded that a late decline has limited diagnostic value but the elevated temperatures with spikes (unrelated to disturbances) may be more indicative of endometriosis. [339]

A German study compared the temperature charts from 18 subfertile women with laparoscopic evidence of endometriosis, with the charts from 16 subfertile controls:

- The late decline in temperature during the early follicular phase was significant.
- A temperature greater than 36.6 deg.C on the first three days of menstruation was associated with pelvic endometriosis.

The researchers concluded that waking temperature is a useful clinical adjunct when endometriosis is suspected. [75]

Although endometriosis may be suspected from symptoms (particularly premenstrual spotting), and possibly from temperature readings, **laparoscopy is the only way to definitively diagnose endometriosis.** ESHRE guidelines provide recommendations on the diagnosis and management of women with endometriosis. [139]

Breast and gynaecological cancers

Breast and gynaecological cancers are significant women's health issues, with early detection improving outcome. As of 2015 the NHS cancer screening programme extends to breast and cervical cancer (plus bowel cancer), but health professionals have opportunities through primary care services to ensure that women are aware of early warning signs and symptoms of disease.

Breast cancer treatment and its effects on fertility

The diagnosis of breast cancer is devastating for any woman, but if she is of reproductive age the potential loss of fertility may be of major concern. Female cancer survivors have pregnancy rates on average 40% lower than the general population, but this depends on the type of cancer: for example, women who survive melanoma or thyroid cancer have pregnancy rates comparable with the general population. Women diagnosed with breast cancer have the lowest chance of subsequent pregnancy – nearly 70% lower than the general population. This is thought to be due to the combination of chemotherapy and prolonged treatment (up to five years) with tamoxifen. It may also be due to a general misconception that pregnancy could stimulate cancer recurrence as it is a hormonally driven disease. [456]

By the time a woman in her mid-reproductive years has completed breast cancer treatment her natural fertility may have ended. Women of reproductive age must be given opportunities to discuss fertility preservation techniques (egg, embryo or ovarian tissue freezing) prior to cancer treatment, but on the understanding that it does not guarantee success.

Tamoxifen and its effect on the menstrual cycle Tamoxifen, a selective estrogen receptor modulator (SERM), reduces breast cancer mortality and the risk of recurrence in women with estrogen-receptor (ER) positive breast cancer. If a woman is taking tamoxifen she should try to avoid exposure to light at night. A study on rats concluded that exposure to dim light at night (the equivalent of faint light from under a door) reduced the night-time production of melatonin and rendered breast cancer resistant to tamoxifen. [113] The bedroom should be sufficiently dark, eliminating light sources such as TV/computer screens, alarm clocks and phone chargers (page 196).

Tamoxifen has varying effects on the menstrual cycle. Some women (particularly younger ones) continue to have regular periods with normal biphasic temperature charts. Others may have a variety of menopausal symptoms and menstrual disturbances, including prolonged or excessive bleeding. Some women may be amenorrhoeic. Tamoxifen, an anti-estrogen, may reduce the duration, quantity and quality of cervical secretions. [539] Despite strong evidence for the advantages of tamoxifen, many women of reproductive age are reluctant to take it due to fertility concerns. [357]

Avoiding pregnancy during breast cancer treatment Pregnancy must be avoided during chemotherapy and until the woman is advised by her oncologist that her risk of recurrence is very low and it is safe to conceive. Women at risk of pregnancy must use effective contraception but estrogen-containing methods are not generally advisable. If a woman refuses any other method and wishes to use FAMs she should use "life or death" rules (page 228) and be closely supervised by an experienced practitioner.

Planning pregnancy after breast cancer treatment Guidelines from the European Society of Medical Oncology recommend that there is no set time-frame when it is considered optimal to allow women to conceive following cancer diagnosis. The timing should consider the time of completion of therapy, the risk of relapse, and the woman's age and ovarian function. Women who wish to interrupt their tamoxifen treatment in order to conceive need to understand that early interruption could have potentially detrimental effects on their breast cancer outcome – there is no data to support the safety of early interruption. Women who willingly risk interrupting tamoxifen after two to three years in order to conceive should be strongly encouraged to resume tamoxifen following delivery. [456] In view of the potential teratogenic effect of tamoxifen, women must stop treatment three months before trying to conceive. [492] Women require individual assessment and support from their oncologist in co-operation with their gynaecologist.

Breast awareness All women should be aware of the normal appearance, shape and consistency of their breast tissue, remembering that it extends into the armpit. There are natural fluctuations in breast size and sensitivity during the menstrual cycle and some women will have quite lumpy breasts premenstrually (page 162). About 90% of breast lumps are not cancerous, but women should report breast changes promptly. Breast Cancer Care provides information for women on breast awareness, benign breast disease and all aspects of breast cancer at www.breastcancercare.org.uk.

The NHS breast screening programme provides free breast screening every three years for all women aged 50 and over. The benefits of mammographic screening in terms of the number of lives saved is greater than any harm from over-diagnosis (see www.cancerscreening.nhs.uk/breastscreen).

Gynaecological cancers

There are five different gynaecological cancers: ovarian, endometrial, cervical, vaginal and vulval. The majority, with the exception of cervical cancer, occur in post-menopausal women, but the incidence of other gynaecological cancers is increasing in younger women. Assisted fertility has been considered as a possible risk factor for breast and gynaecological cancers but the absolute risks are low.

Cervical cancer and link with HPV Virtually all cases of cervical cancer are attributable to one of the HPVs. In the UK, infection with HPV is very common in young people, genital warts being the most common sexually transmitted viral infection. The UK's vaccination programme offers routine vaccination (Gardasil) to girls aged 12–13 and 17–18 to protect against the strains of HPV which cause about 70% of cervical cancers. The vaccination, which is likely to give protection for up to 20 years, does not obviate the need for cervical screening. It will be many years before it is known whether the vaccination programme reduces the incidence of cervical cancer.

Cervical screening Cervical screening (formerly referred to as the "smear" test) involves visualisation of the cervix and removal of a sample of cells from the transformation zone. Cervical cytology may identify "dyskariotic" cells (cells with an abnormal nucleus) which are graded as mild, moderate or severe dyskariosis. Colposcopy permits closer inspection of the cervix and biopsy of the epithelium. Histological analysis of the sample analyses the structure of the squamous epithelial layers to determine how far the dyskariotic cells have progressed. Changes in the outer layers of the cervix (cervical intraepithelial neoplasia) are divided into CIN I, II and III (mild, moderate and severe dysplasia); see www.cancerscreening.nhs.uk.

Treatment for abnormal cells: effects on fertility The most common treatment for abnormal cervical cells is a **LLETZ** procedure (large loop excision of the transformation zone) also known as loop diathermy. LLETZ uses different-sized wire loops, aiming to remove only the affected cells. Histological testing should show evidence that all the affected area has been removed. Loop diathermy should not affect the mucus-secreting cells of the cervical canal, hence the pattern of secretions should be unaffected with no adverse impact on fertility. In rare cases a **cone biopsy** may be needed to surgically excise the affected cells. Removal of a cone-shaped area may reduce the number of mucus-secreting cells, thus diminishing the production of secretions and potentially reducing the chances of conception. Cone biopsy may lead to scarring of the external os and cervical stenosis. It may also weaken the internal os, resulting in an incompetent cervix which may require a cervical stitch during pregnancy to help reduce the chance of preterm delivery.

Symptoms of gynaecological cancers Women should be educated about symptoms suggestive of gynaecological cancers and referred promptly, where necessary, to a specialist gynaecological cancer team. Early symptoms include menstrual irregularities, persistent vaginal discharge (blood-stained or offensive odour), inter-menstrual bleeding, post-coital bleeding and post-menopausal bleeding. For more information on breast and gynaecological cancers see www.cancerresearchuk.org.

MEDICAL CONDITIONS AFFECTED BY THE MENSTRUAL CYCLE

A number of medical conditions are exacerbated at specific times of the menstrual cycle due to the fluctuations in ovarian hormone levels. These include the following.

- **Acne:** many women with acne experience premenstrual flares.
- **Allergies including anaphylaxis:** these are often exacerbated in the luteal and premenstrual phases.
- **Asthma:** forty percent of women with asthma report increased frequency and severity of asthma attacks premenstrually.
- **Auto-immune and immune-related disorders:** Symptoms of disorders such as rheumatoid arthritis, systemic lupus erythematosus and Crohn's disease may vary over the menstrual cycle, with an increase in symptoms during the premenstrual and menstrual phases.
- **Candidiasis:** many women are more prone to vaginal candidiasis premenstrually due to the reduced immune response.
- **Diabetes:** blood sugars may be higher premenstrually and menstrually due to temporary insulin resistance. All women with diabetes (and PCOS with insulin resistance) should aim to keep blood sugars as low as possible within normal limits.
- **Epilepsy:** up to 70% of women with epilepsy have catamenial epilepsy (related to hormonal changes in the cycle). Women experience more seizures immediately before ovulation and just before a period.
- **Irritable bowel syndrome:** increased bloating, abdominal pain and bowel movements are more common during the luteal, premenstrual and menstrual phases.
- **Mental health conditions:** anxiety, panic disorder, obsessive compulsive disorder, bipolar, bulimia and binge eating disorders are often exacerbated premenstrually.
- **Mouth ulcers:** some women get mouth ulcers in the luteal phase or premenstrually when resistance is lower, but generally they are linked to stress.
- **Migraines:** more than 50% of migraines in women occur during menstruation. There is a strong relationship between estrogen withdrawal and migraine. The majority of women with menstrual migraine experience improvement during pregnancy but may experience attacks again postnatally and during breastfeeding.
- **Multiple sclerosis:** Symptoms may be exacerbated in the luteal and premenstrual phases.
- **Peri-menopausal depression:** this is due to a combination of factors, but linked to declining estrogen.
- **Premenstrual syndrome:** mood disorders related to severe PMS are triggered in the luteal phase and normally resolve by the start of menstruation.

- **Raynaud's phenomenon:** sensitivity to cold is altered during the menstrual cycle, with fingers rewarming fastest during menstruation. There may be no significant temperature rise following ovulation. [245]
- **Stress:** acute mental stress in particular plays a part in the aetiology of many diseases. Stress is likely to exacerbate an existing medical condition. Symptoms may be more severe in the late luteal phase due to the lowered immune response.

Chronic medical conditions are complex. Many are associated with adverse effects on fertility and the menstrual cycle or on specific fertility indicators. Some level of disruption should always be expected with any medical condition.

Some conditions, however, may not have an anticipated effect. For example, Sjogren's syndrome, an auto-immune disease, impairs vaginal lubrication (from the Bartholin's glands), plus tears and saliva, but it does not usually affect the cervical secretions. This is because Sjogren's syndrome affects exocrine glands, while cervical secretions originate from glandular epithelium. (There is, however, a strong link between Sjogren's syndrome and thyroid dysfunction, and any associated thyroid issues may affect the overall menstrual cycle). [112]

It is helpful for a woman with a chronic physical or mental health condition to monitor her menstrual cycles to observe whether there is a hormonal influence. This helps with diagnosis and treatment giving her a sense of control over her condition. If hormonal fluctuations are causing distressing symptoms, then some form of ovulation suppression (such as COCs) may be appropriate. [74] [468]

EFFECTS OF ACUTE ILLNESS

The effects of acute illness on the menstrual cycle are varied. Feverish illnesses cause a much higher temperature than the characteristic ovulation rise. If the pyrexia occurs early in the cycle, the temperature may settle to the lower level and the usual temperature rise may be apparent. If the pyrexia occurs around the time of ovulation, the temperature may settle either to the higher level, confirming ovulation, or to the lower level, indicating the suppression of ovulation. This can be difficult to determine as the temperature often takes a few days to settle following illness. New users who are avoiding pregnancy should observe the changes and assume fertility throughout. Experienced users, who know their usual coverline and are using a combination of indicators, may feel confident to rely on other indicators provided they correlate.

Figure 12.4 shows the effect of a viral infection (flu-type symptoms) from days 8–12. This highly experienced user does not have enough low temperatures to apply the *3 over 6 rule*, although she observes that her temperature has settled to her usual low (pre-ovulatory) level by day 13. She relies on the double-check of cervical secretions and cervix and feels reassured as they correlate closely. The fertile time starts on day 7 at the first sign of the cervix softening. The fertile time ends on day 18, three full days after peak day, which coincides with the third day of a low, firm, closed, tilted cervix.

Figure 12.5 shows the effect of a flu-type illness from days 6–12. The woman is taking paracetamol every four to six hours. The dotted line shows her usual coverline (based on her last eight cycles). The viral illness has completely masked a possible temperature rise. In this situation it may have settled to the higher level with the ovulation rise possibly occurring during the time of illness; however, there is insufficient information to interpret the temperature readings. There appears to be a normal pattern of secretions, with peak day on day 12, but it would be most unwise to rely on the secretions as a single indicator during illness. The combination of illness and regular analgesics means that this chart cannot be interpreted. It is clearly marked "Uninterpretable".

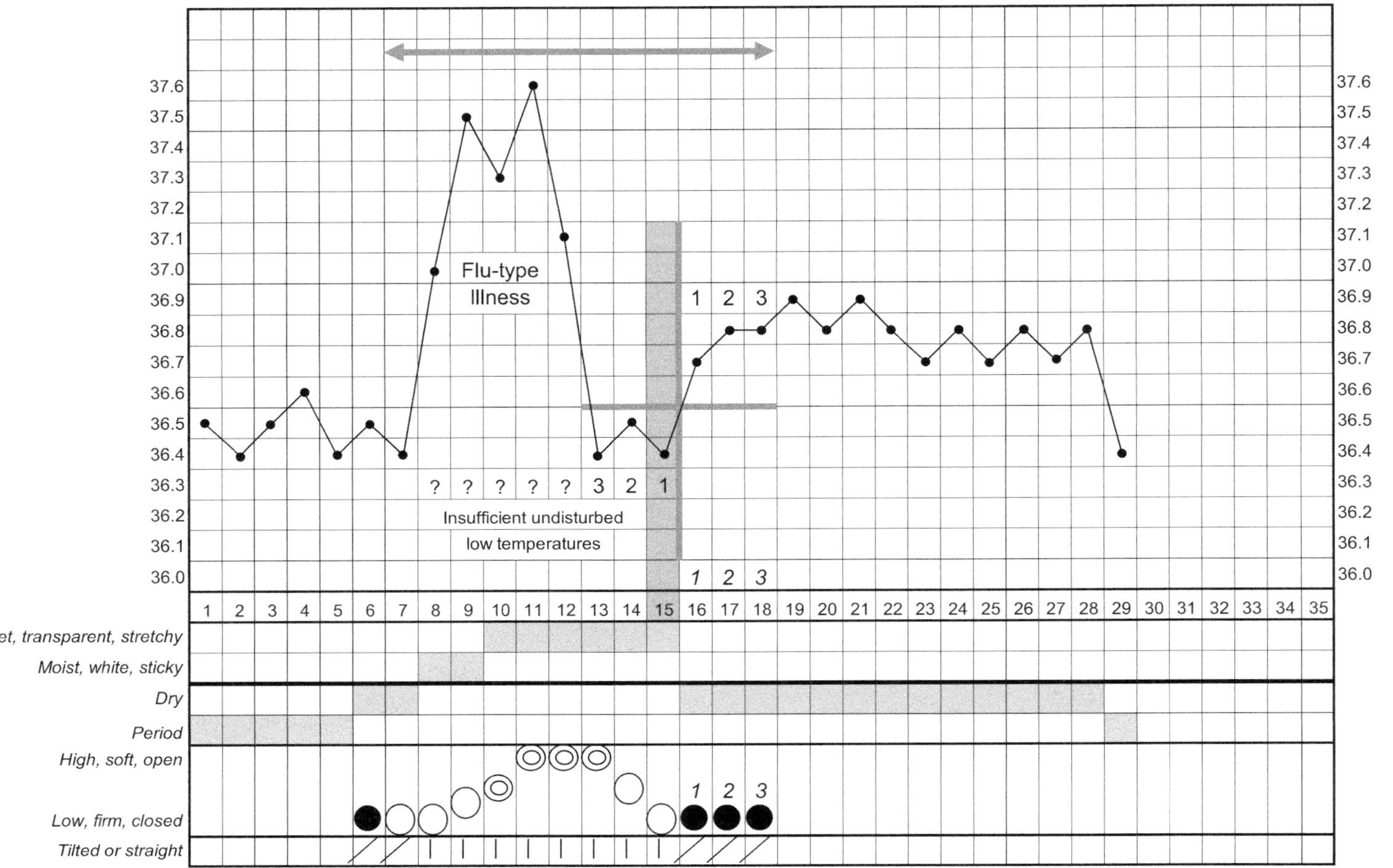

Figure 12.4 Effect of pyrexia before the temperature rise

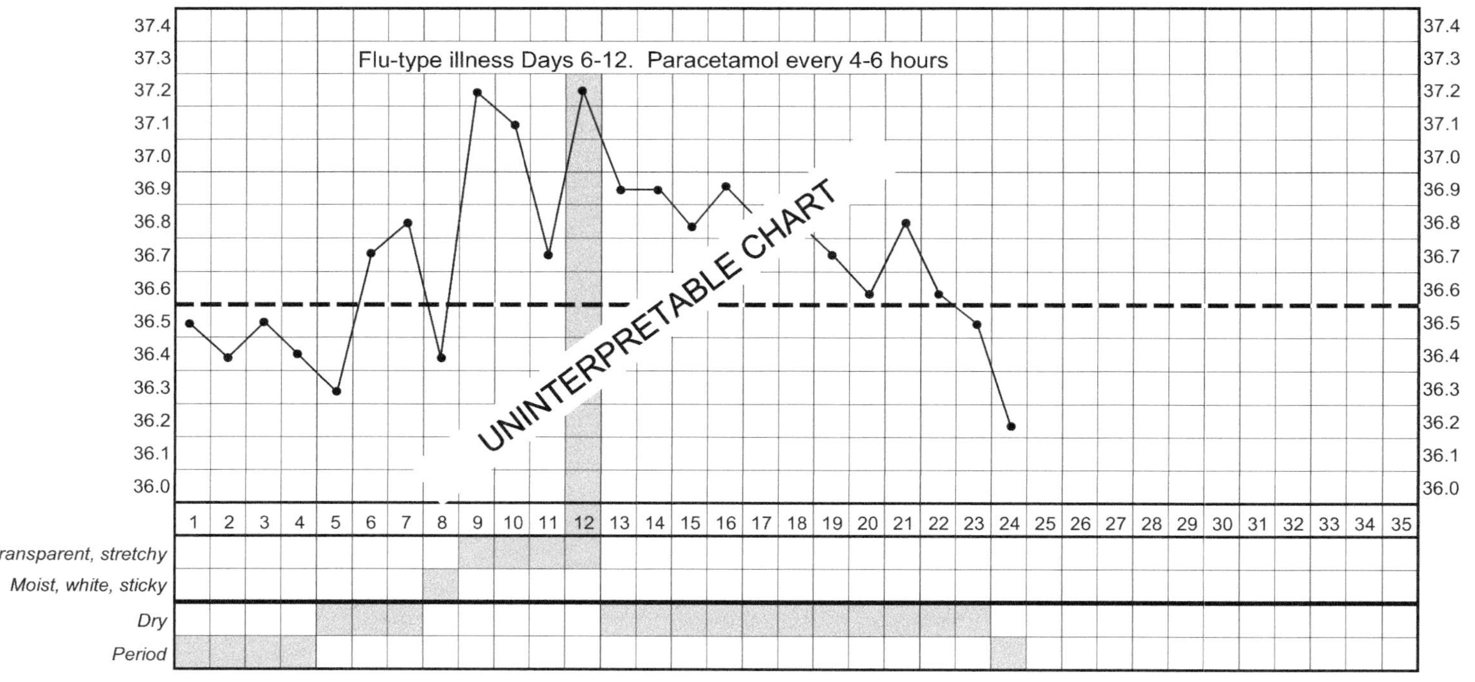

Figure 12.5 Effect of pyrexia around the temperature rise

It can be difficult to distinguish between the effect of illness and any drug being used for symptom relief or to treat the condition. Illness is stressful and carries a high risk of unintended pregnancies due to cycle disruption. It may be safer to abstain completely until the illness is over or to use barrier methods until the position in the cycle becomes clear.

DRUGS AND THEIR EFFECT ON THE MENSTRUAL CYCLE

Information on the effect of drugs on the menstrual cycle is scarce. The impact of drugs will vary for each woman and will depend on the dose and timing within the cycle. Women using FAMs need to carefully observe changes in the fertility indicators and disruption to the cycle. The condition should be carefully evaluated and where appropriate a barrier method offered until the degree of effect has been determined or the drug is no longer being used. A list of drugs and their effect on the menstrual cycle is given in appendix G, but commonly used non-steroidal anti-inflammatory drugs (NSAIDs) are worthy of special note.

Non-steroidal anti-inflammatory drugs (NSAIDs)

NSAIDs are widely used in the treatment of arthritis and other painful inflammatory conditions. Some are available on prescription only and others as bought medications. In addition to gastro-intestinal and cardiovascular risks, NSAIDs can have a significant effect on fertility. Cyclooxygenase-2 (COX-2) selective inhibitors (coxibs such as etoricoxib) are a relatively new type of anti-inflammatory drug which are thought to produce fewer gastrointestinal side effects than the older non-selective NSAIDs (such as aspirin, ibuprofen, diclofenac and mefenamic acid) which many women use on a regular basis.

Prostaglandins and effect of NSAIDs

NSAIDs block the action of prostaglandins, the hormone-like substances that cause inflammation and pain. Prostaglandins are involved in the regulation of body temperature, melatonin synthesis and sleep. They are also involved with the rupture of the ovarian follicle.

Aspirin and ibuprofen have been shown to affect sleep patterns in healthy women. A placebo-controlled study researched the effect of NSAIDs on body temperature and melatonin levels. After a single dose of aspirin or ibuprofen (administered at 11:00 pm) melatonin levels were suppressed and the normal nocturnal decrease in body temperature was not so marked. The differences in body temperature between the NSAID group and the placebo group were apparent within 30 minutes, with the effect lasting for up to four hours. [419] Women should anticipate a possible effect on waking temperature if NSAIDS are taken up to four hours before the normal temperature-taking time. If the temperature is significantly elevated (by pain or inflammation), NSAIDs may have an antipyretic effect, but waking temperature may be normal or relatively higher than expected where there is no associated fever due to the higher nocturnal temperature.

NSAIDs can disrupt ovulation and adversely affect fertilisation and implantation – they have been linked to early miscarriage. When women are taking anti-prostaglandins, the follicles grow around 50% larger, but the dominant follicle fails to rupture and the egg becomes over-mature. Hormone levels are therefore unaffected and the adverse effect of these drugs may not be apparent. Women may show a biphasic temperature pattern, but even if ovulation has occurred the egg may not be fertilisable. The impact will depend on the position in the menstrual cycle, the drug taken and the dosage. **Women who are planning pregnancy should avoid NSAIDs, particularly around the time of ovulation.** Ovulation returns to normal after stopping these drugs. [432]

NSAIDs and LUF syndrome

Women with inflammatory conditions such as rheumatoid arthritis who are on continuous treatment with anti-inflammatories have a high incidence of LUF syndrome. Ultrasound monitoring of 59 cycles found LUF in 36% of cycles compared with 3% in untreated women. Etoricoxib (selective COX-2 inhibitor) was more likely to induce LUF syndrome than aspirin or ibuprofen (nonselective NSAIDs). [402]

INFLUENCE OF LUNAR CYCLES

From time to time women raise the issue of the influence of lunar cycles. It is known that the moon influences the behaviour of insects, fish, birds and laboratory rats, [642] but there is no proven relationship between lunar cycles and menstrual cycles.

In the mid-1950s, Eugen Jonas, a Slovakian doctor asserted that a woman can ovulate twice because she also ovulates during the same phase of the moon as that in which she was born. He suggested that this explains why conceptions happen at "unexpected" times. So, for example, if the woman is born at the time of the full moon, her fertile time during adulthood will coincide with the full moon. Jonas also asserted that the sex of the future child is determined by the position of the moon at the time of conception and claimed 98% reliability for the use of his method. He even had an explanation for non-identical twins of different sexes. Popular books ensued and are still in demand as women continue to be attracted to astrological methods for predicting fertility and the sex of a future child. **There is no scientific evidence for astrological methods of fertility control.** [642]

SUMMARY OF FACTORS WHICH MAY AFFECT CHART

A woman who is using FAMs to avoid pregnancy needs to be vigilant for disturbances or changes from routine which may disrupt the menstrual cycle. Any disturbances should be clearly documented to ascertain their effect. There should be no attempt to interpret the chart unless the rules clearly fit and the relevant guidelines can be applied. Table 12.1 provides a summary of factors which may affect the fertility indicators and the overall menstrual cycle.

Table 12.1 Summary of factors which may affect fertility indicators and the menstrual cycle

Common disturbances	*Factors affecting the menstrual cycle*
Alcohol	Stress
Late night	Anxiety or depression
Disturbed sleep	Rapid weight loss or gain
Oversleeping/lie-in	Strenuous exercise/intensive training
Light exposure at night	Illness acute or chronic
Change in routine such as holidays	Newly diagnosed or pre-existing medical conditions
Travel, particularly air travel and crossing time zones	Drugs, bought or prescribed
Shift work, particularly night shifts	Herbal remedies
Daylight saving/changing the clocks	Abnormal vaginal discharge, including STIs
Change of environment such as house move	Gynaecological conditions (e.g. PCOS)

PART II

Avoiding pregnancy

FAMs FOR WOMEN OF NORMAL FERTILITY

This section focuses on FAMs to avoid pregnancy starting with normal fertility then moving through special fertility circumstances: after contraception, postpartum and approaching the menopause. Most women can use FAMs, irrespective of age or educational level, provided they are properly taught and an assessment is made to ensure that the method is suitable (page 362).

The effectiveness of FAMs depends on key variables:

- Well-trained practitioners delivering quality teaching of an evidence-based method
- The couple's ability to identify the fertile time and follow guidelines consistently
- The couple's ability to modify their sexual behaviour during the fertile time

The major indicators (temperature, secretions, cervix and calendar calculations) are discussed in part 1, with the guidelines for single-indicator methods in chapters 4, 5, 6 and 7, respectively. Most women can be taught to use a combination of indicators with a standardised approach to interpreting the chart using a double-check at the start and end of the fertile time (page 180). The guidelines in this section can be used by most women of normal fertility – they are applicable to both new and experienced users.

GUIDELINES TO AVOID PREGNANCY: COMBINED INDICATORS

Guidelines must be followed consistently and carefully, recognising that the late infertile time (post-ovulatory) is the most effective for avoiding pregnancy.

First cycle The first cycle is a learning cycle only. This allows the woman time to adjust to taking and recording an accurate waking temperature and observing the changes in her secretions. Ideally intercourse should be avoided completely during the first cycle to allow an uninterrupted observation of secretions (page 129).

Second and subsequent cycles The woman needs to establish whether it is likely that she ovulated in her previous cycle. At the start of the period, she asks herself: was there a temperature rise in the previous cycle, 10–16 days before this bleed? If the answer is yes, the bleed is a true period and the guidelines can be applied. If no, she should assume the bleed indicates fertility and avoid unprotected intercourse until the fertile time has ended.

Start of fertile time The first fertile day (FFD) is identified by calendar-based calculations, cervical secretions and changes in the cervix – whichever is the *earliest* indicator (see figure 7.1 in chapter 7). Calendar-based calculations include:

- *S minus 20 rule* (provided there is a record of the last 12 cycle lengths);
- *Day 6 rule* (from fourth cycle provided first three cycles are 26 days or longer); or
- *Earliest temperature rise minus 7* (provided there is a record of the last 12 temperature charts).

When using cervical secretions as an indicator, look for the first sign of *any* cervical secretions. With the cervix (optional), look for the first sign of change from low, firm, closed and tilted (for retroverted uterus, see page 149).

End of fertile time The last fertile day (LFD) is confirmed by temperature, cervical secretions and changes in the cervix. The evening of the third high temperature indicates the end of the fertile time, provided that:

- there are three consecutive undisturbed high temperatures;
- the third high temperature is at least 0.2 deg.C above the six low readings; and
- there are at least six low temperature readings.

When using cervical secretions as an indicator, all high temperatures must be after peak day. The cervix should be low, firm, closed, and tilted for three days. (If temperature and secretions correlate there is no need to wait for the third day of cervical change.)

Summary of guidelines to avoid pregnancy

- FFD = First cervical secretions or relevant calculation – whichever comes *first.*
- LFD = Evening of the third high temperature after peak day.

Note on terminology: The reference points to define the limits of the fertile time are the first and last *fertile* days (start and end of the fertile time). By referring consistently to the *fertile* time, couples who are avoiding pregnancy know when they should avoid intercourse. Note that some texts refer to the last *infertile* day before, and the first *infertile* day after, the fertile time.

Comparative effectiveness of early and late infertile phases

Highly motivated couples who are correctly taught can achieve high levels of effectiveness using both the early and late infertile phases, but there is always a risk of pregnancy from intercourse in the early infertile time due to its unpredictable nature. Women who can distinguish the first changes in secretions in combination with an appropriate calendar-based calculation can confidently have unprotected intercourse in this phase but some women with very short cycles may not have any early infertile days (page 78). Couples who require the highest level of effectiveness may be best advised to restrict intercourse to the late infertile time (post-ovulatory) by waiting until the evening of the third high temperature after peak day.

"Life or death" rules

In situations where pregnancy carries a serious risk to the mother or fetus (for example, during chemotherapy), a couple are best advised to use the most effective suitable contraceptive method or to abstain from intercourse completely. Faculty of Sexual and Reproductive Health Care (FSRH) guidance recommends that women should not rely solely on fertility indicators when using teratogenic drugs. [215]

For couples who will accept FAMs only, the strictest "life or death" rules are needed. Intercourse is restricted to the late infertile time with an added day for safety. The last fertile day is confirmed on the evening of the *fourth* high temperature, provided that all high temperatures are undisturbed and the fourth high temperature is at least 0.2 deg.C above the six low readings. All high temperatures must be *after* peak day. Cervical changes can give added confirmation that the fertile time has ended. In situations where the secretions are not reliable, the couple should wait until after the *fifth* high temperature before assuming infertility. Users – even highly experienced users – should have access to increased follow-up at this time.

MODIFICATION OF SEXUAL BEHAVIOUR

Most women can be taught to identify their fertile time, but the effectiveness of FAMs depends on the couple's ability to avoid unprotected intercourse for its duration. Health professionals must discuss how couples intend to modify their sexual behaviour, which includes discussion around barrier methods or withdrawal. Time and space must be allowed for frank discussions about sexual activity with sensitivity to personal, cultural and religious beliefs (page 365).

Intercourse frequency with FAMs

The WHO multi-centre study of the *Ovulation Method* reported on the degree of satisfaction with intercourse frequency (average required abstinence 15 days). Most couples in Bangalore, Manila and San Miguel were satisfied with intercourse frequency, whereas about 30% of the women and 50% of their partners in Auckland and Dublin would have preferred more intercourse. There were notable discrepancies between centres: for example, participants in the Dublin centre were reluctant to use the early dry days for intercourse so more abstinence was required. The shorter the fertile time, the higher the level of satisfaction with intercourse frequency. [621] The length of abstinence required by a particular method may therefore have a strong influence on user satisfaction.

The intercourse frequency for FAM users may not be very different when compared with other methods, but it is more concentrated at the infertile times. Data from clinical trials of SDM and TDM showed the mean intercourse frequency was similar to that reported by users of other methods. Intercourse frequency increased with progressive cycles of method use, but decreased during menstruation and the days identified as fertile. This was thought to imply a behavioural change as couples gained more experience with their method and communicated more about the fertile days. [545]

Abstinence in NFP

> Abstinence from intercourse is the key to success. Yet those who promote NFP are strangely silent about the effect of abstinence on the couple and their marriage. [383]

Abstinence, an integral part of NFP, means refraining from vaginal sexual intercourse and all genital contact during the fertile time (page 28). Abstinence is what makes NFP an effective method, but it can also make it difficult or unpopular. Some have argued that NFP is *not* "natural" because it requires enforced abstinence for varying times during the cycle. IPPF, for example, refused to use the term "natural" family planning, referring for many years to "periodic abstinence", [299] but more recently to "fertility awareness" (see www.ippf.org).

Abstinence is not restricted to NFP users; it is an accepted part of all relationships – at times of illness, physical separation (such as work travel), or when domestic life dictates that sexual activity would be inappropriate. Individuals continually make decisions about the appropriateness of sexual activity. For most couples, intercourse is the ultimate intimate contact. It is driven by desire, physical proximity and the need for comfort, closeness or physical release. Men and women may use intercourse in different ways: women may need to feel emotionally close to have intercourse whilst men may use it as a route to intimacy. Abstinence from intercourse thus has negative connotations of withholding or being deprived. If sex is taken away, a key source of comfort and self-esteem may be lost, particularly for men, and this presents challenges. Health professionals should never assume that abstinence is either easy or difficult – the only way to assess its impact on the relationship is to encourage couples to talk about it.

Couple's experiences of abstinence

One of the advantages of any FAM is the aspect of the shared method. Couples are empowered to take control of their fertility and this joint responsibility may enhance inter-personal communication. NFP users often describe positive experiences of abstinence with improved communication, increased sexual intimacy, varied sexual techniques and the advantage of preventing sex from becoming "routine". [58] [424] [386] Many couples willingly accept times of abstinence, or "waiting", as part of their relationship [25] but others feel anger and resentment, particularly if pressured into the method – for example, where one partner is more keen for religious (or personal) reasons.

Marshall provided a unique insight into the psychological effects of abstinence from his experience of corresponding with over 10,000 predominantly Catholic couples over 40 years. The majority of these couples were using the *Temperature Method* with an average of 17 days abstinence. Marshall, a "Man of Science", reported that the majority of couples – both men and women – found abstinence difficult. He was harshly criticised by some sections of the Catholic community for breaking the silence about difficulties with abstinence. [383]

Couples' experiences of using NFP in the mid-1950s showed extremes of positivity:

> "I feel quite safe with this method and enjoy the sexual act far more with my husband now, without the dread of perhaps conceiving, and we are more devoted to one another."
>
> "We have tried to keep to these rules with, as I believe, a bad effect on the development of our marriage, our sex relations, my temper and our treatment of our children."
>
> "So where are we 40 years on? We are still together, our friends regard us as a devoted couple and we have three splendid children each two and a half years apart. In fact we are emotionally crippled and live in an affectionate desert where a tentative peck on the cheek when one goes on a journey is an embarrassment, a reassuring hug in times of stress is unthinkable and to hold hands whilst walking on the cliff-top is unthinkable."

Many of these couples had strong religious or ideological reasons for using NFP and frequently persevered despite considerable difficulties. When discussing this research Marshall emphasised the importance of not monitoring "success" simply in terms of contraceptive effectiveness. [384]

A questionnaire survey (revised from the original Marshall and Rowe study) was mailed to 1,400 randomly selected NFP users in the US in 2002 and completed by 334 predominantly middle-class Catholic couples (average age, 40 years). NFP had more positive than negative effects, with 74% reporting a positive effect on the relationship. Positive themes included improved self-knowledge, method success (to plan or avoid pregnancy), enhanced relationships and enriched spirituality. Negative themes included strained sexual interactions (lack of spontaneity, difficulty with abstinence and erectile difficulties resulting from pressure to optimise the infertile time) and relationship problems (anger, frustration and misunderstandings resulting from a partner's unmet sexual needs or women taking sole responsibility for the method). [597]

Length of abstinence using different methods

The length of abstinence is a key factor when considering the acceptability and effectiveness of different FAMs. Prolonged abstinence is more likely to result in risk-taking with subsequent unintended pregnancies or dissatisfaction with the method and a high discontinuation rate. Although the actual physiological fertile time is only six days, the perceived fertile time will always be longer, with its length varying dependent on the woman's menstrual cycle, the selected indicator(s) and the guidelines for use. Single-indicator methods typically involve the longest abstinence. Combined-indicator methods should reduce the abstinence, whilst direct hormone monitoring has the potential to reduce the abstinence still further. The shorter the required abstinence, the higher the method satisfaction – provided that it does not compromise effectiveness.

Average lengths of abstinence using different methods:

- Temperature Method: 17 days [380]
- Ovulation Method: 15–17 days [616] [100]
- Calendar/Rhythm Method: 16 days [100]
- Combined-indicator methods: 13 days for new users but less after the first year of use [189]
- Persona: 14 days for cycles 1–3, then 11 days from cycle 4 as the monitor collects more data [56]
- Standard Days Method: 12 days [10]
- TwoDay Method: 12 days [11]

An online teaching service in the US compared the length of abstinence and intercourse frequency between two FAMs. Both groups used an algorithm which included the *Day 6 rule* for the first six cycles. This was combined either with a fertility monitor (Clearblue) or cervical secretions (page 138). The average estimated fertile time was 13–14 days, with no difference between the two groups when all cycles were included in the analysis. The monitor group required less abstinence and intercourse frequency increased after the first six cycles, which may have contributed to increased satisfaction with the monitor. [164]

Figure 13.1 provides a visual representation of abstinence required by different methods, highlighting the practical difficulties some couples might find with certain methods. This shows the number of days of abstinence required for a woman with regular cycles (27–31 days) in a hypothetical 28-day cycle. This varies from 9 to 17 days depending on the indicator(s) used. Note that the number of days may be shorter than the average based on some FAM studies because the cycle range given in this example is quite narrow – generally the more variable the cycle length, the longer the abstinence.

Outercourse

Abstinence is interpreted in different ways: some couples avoid all forms of sexual activity during the fertile time, but others use barrier methods, withdrawal or various forms of non-coital sexual activity (outercourse). Although strict NFP advocates may emphasise a non-sexual form of abstinence during the fertile time, the vast majority of couples (Catholic and non-Catholic) define abstinence to include other forms of sexual stimulation leading to orgasm. [110] Marshall's questionnaire survey of 502 predominantly Catholic couples using the *Temperature Method* in the 1960s found that 12% of women and 20% of men reached orgasm during times of abstinence. [384]

Outercourse, defined by IPPF as sex play without vaginal intercourse, includes mutual masturbation, oral sex, erotic massage, frottage (body rubbing), fantasy and sex toys. Outercourse allows for reciprocal sexual pleasure and is nearly 100% effective against pregnancy provided that ejaculation takes place away from the vulva. It requires commitment and self-control from both partners, plus good communication.

A study of Calendar/Rhythm Method users in Ireland reported that, whilst about 30% of couples avoided genital contact, 20% used condoms during the fertile time in some cycles. Fifty percent of couples reported using oral sex, mutual masturbation and body rubbing. Twice as many men reported using masturbation compared to women. The motivation for using NFP,

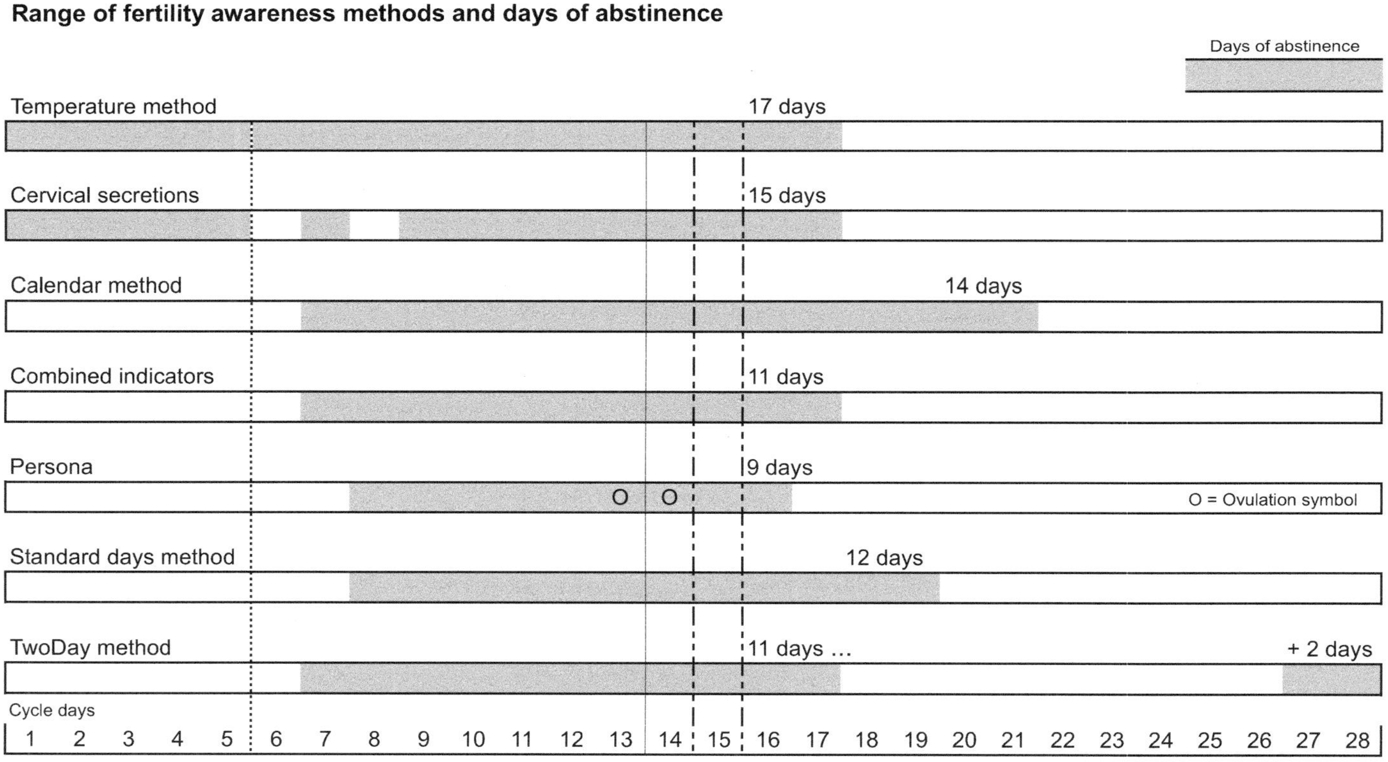

Range of fertility awareness methods and days of abstinence

Days of abstinence

Temperature method 17 days

Cervical secretions 15 days

Calendar method 14 days

Combined indicators 11 days

Persona 9 days O = Ovulation symbol

Standard days method 12 days

TwoDay method 11 days … + 2 days

Cycle days

1 2 3 4 5 6 7 8 9 10 11 12 13 14 15 16 17 18 19 20 21 22 23 24 25 26 27 28

Figure 13.1 Length of abstinence required by different FAMs in a hypothetical 28-day cycle, assuming a cycle range of 27–31 days, five-day period, peak on day 14 and temperature rise on day 15

whether for religious, moral or health reasons, did not appear to affect the rate of outercourse, although the study sample was small. [57]

Barriers during the fertile time

Couples who use barriers during the fertile time (mixed method users) need to understand that there is a high risk of pregnancy if the barrier fails. Effectiveness figures for barriers are based on intercourse at random intervals through the entire menstrual cycle, hence many acts of intercourse would have zero chance of pregnancy (page 246). There have been no effectiveness studies on couples who restrict barrier use to the fertile time, but each act of protected intercourse carries a significant risk of pregnancy if the method fails.

Couples who use barriers during the fertile time require:

- a good understanding of their chosen barrier method;
- careful and consistent use of the method during the fertile time;
- the same level of FA instruction as NFP users;
- the same commitment to charting;
- the same degree of understanding about the limits of the fertile time;
- agreement between both partners about the motivation to avoid pregnancy; and
- an understanding of how spermicide (or vaginal lubricant) affects secretions.

Spermicide and its effect on cervical secretions

The use of spermicide can make the recognition of cervical secretions more difficult, and the same applies to the use of vaginal lubricant. A woman must learn to recognise the characteristic colour, texture and odour of the spermicide, and be able to distinguish this from her own secretions. In practice, this is not normally difficult – particularly if she has recorded her secretions for one cycle before introducing spermicide and she diligently records any protected intercourse. A combined-indicator method which incorporates a calendar-based calculation at the start and temperature at the end of the fertile time helps to counteract any problem with masking secretions. Cervical changes can be extremely useful – particularly for women who use diaphragms or cervical caps. There is no need for condom users to use spermicide, but it should always be used in conjunction with a diaphragm or cervical cap (page 247).

Frequency of barrier use, intelligent use and risk-taking

Many couples (including Catholic couples) state that they wish to use only abstinence during the fertile time, but studies show that barrier use is common. [110] [231] [186] [189] When teaching FAMs, it may therefore be appropriate to offer additional information about barriers.

A German study analysed the sexual behaviour of 300 new FAM users (total 59,000 cycles). Almost 50% routinely combined their FA knowledge with other methods, using barriers at the fertile time in more than 60% of cycles. The other 50% of couples either never used barriers or used them in only about 7% of cycles. The latter group showed a clear decrease in barrier use over time whereas the frequent barrier users (the group who least disliked barriers) continued to combine the advantages of both methods. [231]

Couples can achieve a very high level of effectiveness by intelligent use of FAMs with barriers. Many use barriers on low-risk days, avoid intercourse completely on high-risk days and limit unprotected intercourse to the late infertile time. Some users, particularly beginners, use barriers for every act of intercourse but avoid intercourse completely on high-risk days. It should be noted that many barrier users take occasional risks and have unprotected intercourse at the fertile time. [188]

Withdrawal during the fertile time

Withdrawal is widely used during the fertile time. The issue of whether pre-ejaculatory fluid contains sperm is controversial, but some men may be more likely than others to leak sperm (page 248). Withdrawal may work for experienced couples who have a strong sense of control but if it fails at the fertile time there is a high risk of pregnancy. Couples should be informed that there have been no effectiveness studies on withdrawal limited to the fertile time. In practice, couples can use withdrawal intelligently by restricting it to days they assess to be low risk and avoiding intercourse completely on high-risk days.

Recording sexual activity

Couples who are using FAMs to avoid pregnancy should record all sexual activity on the chart. This is very personal information, but it is the only way to determine whether users understand the guidelines or are taking any risks. Couples who use barrier methods during the fertile time should indicate whether intercourse is protected or unprotected. This can be done by simply adding a letter – for example, "C" for condom, "D" for diaphragm or "W" for withdrawal – although women often record sexual activity (and risk-taking behaviour) with symbols such as smiley faces, stars or exclamation marks (see figure 9.1).

EFFECTIVENESS OF FAMS

FAMs are highly user-dependent methods which rely on couple motivation and day-to-day vigilance. Users who are ambivalent, misinformed, lax or forgetful are at risk of pregnancy. Most couples will get away with a condom mishap or the occasional forgotten pill, but FAMs are most unforgiving of imperfect use. Reports of the effectiveness of FAMs vary widely. Population surveys may not distinguish between different methods, and whether couples are trained or untrained, hence the statistics for experienced users of combined-indicator methods may be masked by those of couples using ad hoc versions of the Calendar/Rhythm Method, or using the term "natural" family planning as a euphemism for no contraception.

Good-quality evidence of effectiveness is lacking. Most FAM studies use an observational design with the observed group only and no comparison group. Lamprecht and Trussell evaluated reports on the effectiveness of FAMs. They described the few well-designed studies and made recommendations for future study designs, but reported that many studies were flawed in design and did not calculate pregnancy rates correctly. [345] Kambic's review discussed data collection, measurement of pregnancy rates and analysis of unintended pregnancies plus the type of study. He demonstrated the increased efficacy of two or more indicators, concluding that (provided the guidelines are followed) FAMs are as effective as barrier methods, with fewer than five pregnancies per 100 women per year. [314]

A Cochrane review which analysed the few randomised controlled trials up to 2007, reported that many studies had methodological weaknesses (problems with recruitment, poor randomisation and high discontinuation rates) and were judged to be of insufficient quality to draw any valid conclusions about effectiveness. [248] When discussing their prospective cohort study, Frank-Herrmann and colleagues [189] commented that randomised controlled trials are rarely used to investigate other family planning methods because most couples have a preference for a particular method and do not wish to be randomised. Additionally, unless comparing different IUDs or hormonal methods, it is not possible to blind couples from the allocated method.

Table 13.1 summarises some of the key FAM studies in chronological order from Marshall's first study of the Temperature Method through to the most recent European study which forms

Table 13.1 Effectiveness of Fertility Awareness Methods

The study	*Description of study*	*Method*	*Start of fertile time*	*End of fertile time*	*Pregnancies % typical use*
Marshall, UK (1968) [380]	Field trial of Temperature Method (n = 502, 8,294 cycles)				
	Intercourse restricted to the late infertile time	Temp.	Day 1	Temperature	6.6
	Intercourse in the early and late infertile times	CT	S minus 19	Temperature	19.3
Döring Germany (1973) [55]	Prospective study of Temperature Method (n = 307, 11,352 cycles – Correct-use pregnancy rate 0.11) Most pregnancies were due to user errors including misinterpretation due to a cold.	Temp	Day 1	Temperature	7.0
Johnston Australia (1978) [307]*	Simultaneous surveys of new users (n = 268, 4595 cycles) The pregnancy rate using cervical secretions only is almost double that of combined indicators. Inclusion of a calculation to define the start of the fertile time made little difference to the pregnancy rate.	OM	Cervical secretions (Billings 1974) [50]	Cervical secretions	26.4
		STM	S –20 or 21 plus secretions	Temperature and secretions	14.3
		STM	Cervical secretions only	Temperature and secretions	13.3
Medina Colombia (1980) [395]*	Comparative randomised study of single and combined indicators: 566 women entered the three-to-five-cycle learning phase; 241 women entered the effectiveness phase. No significant difference in pregnancy rates between the two groups.	OM	Cervical secretions [50]	Cervical secretions	29.2
		STM	Calendar calculation and cervical secretions (Wade 1981) [603]	Temperature and secretions	26.1
Rice (Fairfield study) US (1981) [503]*	Non comparative multi-centre study (1,022, new users 21, 736 cycles). Some centres also taught cervical secretions, but this was not consistent across centres. Note the difference between family spacers and limiters.	STM	S minus 19	Temperature	8.3
	Canadian centre (n = 67): Family Spacers				14.8
	(n = 101) Family Limiters				1.1

(*Continued*)

Table 13.1 (Continued)

The study	*Description of study*	*Method*	*Start of fertile time*	*End of fertile time*	*Pregnancies % typical use*
WHO Multi-centre (1981)*	Non-comparative study among new users. Following a three-cycle learning phase, 725 couples entered the effectiveness phase (7,514 cycles).	OM	Cervical secretions (WHO 1981) [616]	Cervical secretions	19.6
Wade Los Angeles, US (1981) [603]*	Comparative randomised study with new users: 1,247 entered three-to-five-cycle learning phase; 430 entered the effectiveness phase. Note the significantly higher pregnancy rate for OM users.	OM	Cervical secretions (Billings 1974) [50]	Cervical secretions	34.9
		STM	Calendar calculation and cervical secretions (Medina 1980) [399]	Temperature and secretions	16.6
Marshall, UK (1985) [382]	Experienced users charting min. six cycles (n = 108, 2,109 cycles). Of the seven pregnancies, three couples knowingly took a risk and four couples observed the guidelines correctly. No pregnancies amongst the 36 couples who restricted intercourse to the late infertile time.		Cervical secretions and S minus 18	Temperature	3.9
Barbato, Italy (1988) [26]	Prospective effectiveness study (n = 460, 8,140 cycles) Participants had charted six cycles at study entry. - 25 pregnancies amongst family spacers - no pregnancies amongst family limiters - 10 pregnancies related to women's inability to identify change from dryness - 13 pregnancies from sex in the fertile time (12 following intentional departure from the rules)	STM	Cervical secretions and S minus 19	Temperature and secretions	3.6
Clubb, Oxford, UK, (1989) [94]	Cost effectiveness study New users taught with group teaching and audio-visual aids followed by individual sessions.	STM	Cervical secretions and S minus 20	Temperature and secretions	2.7
Thapa, Indonesia (1990) [574]*	Non-randomised comparative study of OM vs. MMM (850 new users). Three-cycle learning phase. MMM resulted in a significantly higher pregnancy rate. Family spacers experienced four times the number of pregnancies compared with family limiters.	OM	Cervical secretions (Billings 1974) [50]	Cervical secretions	2.5
		MMM	Cervical secretions (Dorairaj 1980) [128]	Cervical secretions	10.3

Freundl, Germany (1996) [198]*	Prospective multi-centre trial comparing two variants of STM in European women aged 19–45. Double-check (at least two indicators to identify start and end of the fertile time) is more effective than single check.	STM (double-check)	Calendar calculation and cervical secretions	Temperature, secretions and cervix	2.5
		STM (single-check)	Cervical secretions	Temperature	7.8
Arevalo, US (2002) [12]	Prospective multi-centre trial in Bolivia, Peru and the Philippines (478 women with cycles 26–32 days: 4,035 cycles)	SDM	Day 8	Day 19	12
Arevalo US (2004) [11]	Prospective multi-centre trial in Guatemala, Peru and the Philippines (450 women total, 3,928 cycles)	TDM	First sign of secretions	No secretions yesterday or today	13.7
Frank-Herrmann, Germany (2007) [189]	European prospective study (88% of women < 35 years; 900 users, 17,638 cycles) New users. High-quality training and supervision of teachers and standardised teaching materials. Strict guidelines with average fertile time 13 days for new users (less for experienced users). Discontinuation rate due to method dissatisfaction 9.2% after 13 cycles.	STM	Cervical secretions Day 6 rule or earliest temperature rise minus 7.	Evening of third day after peak. Evening of third high temperature (which must be 0.2 deg.C higher).	1.8
Fehring, US (2013) [170]	Randomised comparative study of electronic monitor vs. cervical secretions using Web-based learning. (667 women but high drop-out rate)	OM	Cervical secretions	Cervical secretions	18.5
		EM	Estrogen	LH + estrogen	7

Key

Temp	Temperature Method
CT	Calculo-thermic Method
STM	Sympto-thermal Method
OM	Ovulation Method
MMM	Modified Mucus Method
SDM	Standard Days Method
TDM	TwoDay Method
EM	Electronic monitor

*Studies identified as well designed by Lamprecht and Trussell (1997) [345]

the basis of the current guidelines. This is not an attempt to make a direct comparison but to use the research to highlight teaching points.

Factors influencing effectiveness

Numerous factors influence the effectiveness of FAMs:

- Choice of fertility indicators (single or combined)
- Different rules for the indicators
- Different parameters for identifying the fertile time (single- or double-check)
- Frequency of intercourse (and documentation of timing: morning or evening)
- Use of barriers or withdrawal during the fertile time and level of risk-taking
- Quality of training and supervision (plus number of practitioners in studies)
- Experience of the teacher and their consultation and teaching skills
- Quality of client teaching (content and standardisation of materials)
- Individual or group teaching and whether one or both partners are taught
- Teaching time and assessment of client autonomy
- Woman's age and fertility status (normal fertility or special fertility circumstances)
- Educational level of users and suitability for use
- New or experienced users (and their classification)
- Couple motivation and level of co-operation from partner
- Type of study – observational, retrospective, prospective, comparative, randomised controlled trials
- Differences in inclusion and exclusion criteria of participants and cycles
- Whether there is a learning phase before recruitment to the effectiveness phase
- Indication of intention to plan or avoid pregnancy (stated at the start of each cycle)
- Methods used to confirm pregnancies (positive pregnancy test or clinical pregnancy)
- Classification of unintended pregnancies – method, teacher or user-related (poor understanding or conscious departure from rules)
- Methods used to calculate pregnancy rates – Pearl Index or cumulative pregnancy rate (CPR) using life-table probabilities
- Methods used to determine discontinuation of study (pregnancy or change of method) [315] [345]

Choice of indicators

Effectiveness is largely influenced by the choice of indicators. FSRH clinical guidance advises that in well-conducted studies, combined-indicator methods are consistently shown to be more effective than single-indicator methods. One-year pregnancy rates for perfect use of combined-indicator methods are comparable to those for perfect use of oral contraceptives: 0.4% and 0.3% for combined indicators and oral contraceptives respectively. The guidance recommends:

> Women wishing to use fertility indicators for contraceptive purposes should receive support and instruction on the method from a trained practitioner and be informed that combining indicators is considered more effective than using single fertility indicators alone. Over 1 year, fewer than 1 in 100 women would be expected to experience a pregnancy with perfect use of the Sympto-thermal Method. [215]

Single vs. combined indicators Table 13.1 shows the difference in typical pregnancy rates between single and combined indicators. Although a Colombian study found no significant difference between cervical secretions alone or combined indicators (29% and 26% respectively), [399] an Australian study reported twice as many pregnancies amongst couples using secretions alone (26% vs. 13%), [307] and a US comparative study reported more than twice as many pregnancies in the secretions-only group (37% vs. 14%). After couples were informed of the difference in effectiveness, almost all of the combined-indicator group continued with the method and most of the single-indicator group learned to combine indicators. [603]

The figures for cervical secretions as a single indicator are similar to the WHO study's 20% pregnancy rate [616] and Fehring's Web-based teaching programme, which showed an 18% pregnancy rate for the group using cervical secretions only (compared with 7% for couples using an electronic monitor). [170] By comparison, SDM and TDM show typical-use pregnancy rates of 12% and 14% respectively. [12] [11]

Variations on rules

The rules for the use of different indicators have evolved over time with improved understanding about the lifetime of gametes plus more objective methods to determine ovulation. Rules about secretions are varied, with some authorities erroneously designating early secretions "infertile". Calculations to identify the first fertile day have moved from *S minus 18* to *S minus 20*. Temperature rules, which initially allowed 0.1 deg.C rise, were changed to ensure that *one* of the three high temperatures was 0.2 deg.C, with the latest evidence confirming the importance of the *third* high temperature.

Restricting intercourse to late infertile time

Couples who are prepared to confine intercourse to the late infertile time (presumed post-ovulatory) can achieve maximum effectiveness. Marshall showed a 1% pregnancy rate with correct use (6% with typical use) for post-ovulatory intercourse only, compared with 19% for intercourse in the pre-and post-ovulatory infertile phases. [380] A similar study by Döring showed a correct-use pregnancy rate of 0.11% when intercourse was restricted to the post-ovulatory phase (7% with typical use, mostly due to user errors). There were no conceptions on or after the third high temperature. [55]

Separate studies by Marshall and Barbato reported no pregnancies amongst couples who restricted intercourse to the post-ovulatory infertile phase. [382] [26] Restricting intercourse until after the fourth high temperature (life or death rules) may be yet more effective, but unnecessary for the majority of couples. The more restrictive the guidelines, the higher the potential effectiveness – but very strict guidelines may encourage couples to take risks.

Combining indicators and use of double-check

With combined indicators, the effectiveness of using both the pre- and post-ovulatory phases is high, provided that at least two indicators are used to identify the start and end of the fertile time (double-check). Barbato's study of experienced users reported two pregnancies occurring after the third post-peak day but before the temperature rise, but there were no pregnancies after the third high temperature. He warned that the high-risk group are women with short-duration or minimal secretions. There were no pregnancies amongst the women who combined secretions with a calculation (*S minus 19*), [26] which concurs with Flynn's ultrasound study in which a term pregnancy resulted from intercourse on a "dry" day when the woman ignored the *S minus 19* rule. [178]

Freundl confirmed that a double-check is more twice as effective as a single check (approx 3% vs. 9%). [195] This reaffirms the importance of identifying the earliest change – whether from secretions or calculation – to identify the start of the fertile time and correlating peak day with the temperature rise to confirm the end of the fertile time. [198]

Basis of current guidelines

The European prospective study (900 women, 17,638 cycles) definitively demonstrated the effectiveness of combined-indicator methods. With correct use, and assuming a 13-cycle year, there were 0.4 unintended pregnancies per 100 women years for couples using abstinence during the fertile time (equivalent to one pregnancy per 3,250 cycles). [189] The typical-use pregnancy rate was 1.8%. This was increased to 7.5% for couples who had unprotected intercourse during the fertile time. This surprisingly low figure was thought to be because many couples were practicing "intelligent risk-taking" – avoiding unprotected sex during the few highly fertile days, and taking risks only at the margins of the fertile time. Couples will still take risks, but women who have accurate fertility knowledge tend to take "intelligent" risks. This fits with Luker's theory of calculated risk-taking, which shows the importance of accurate fertility knowledge (page 6).

The evidence-based guidelines (page 227), developed since the 1980s at the Universities of Dusseldorf and Heidelberg in collaboration with the Malteser Arbeitsgruppe NFP in Cologne, have been adopted by FertilityUK and many other international teaching organisations. In 2011 the methodology was registered under the trademark *Sensiplan*. This was designed for use without any technical devices; however, the German team are now researching a tracking system algorithm that could provide new software for thermometers or smartphones (page 177).

Effectiveness in relation to sexual behaviour

A study which explored the relationship between unintended pregnancies and sexual behaviour found that mixed-method users (FAMs with barriers) still take risks and have unprotected intercourse during the fertile time. In this study, 758 new users recorded a combination of indicators for 14,870 cycles: 54% used abstinence (or barriers in < 3% of cycles), whilst 46% combined FAMs with barriers in more than 50% of cycles. Mixed method users were generally younger and more sexually active.

There was no significant difference in the pregnancy rate with correct use (0.6% for abstinence vs. 0.4% for barriers, mainly condoms). With typical use, pregnancy rates were 9% for couples who had unprotected intercourse in the fertile time, 4% for those who had both protected and unprotected intercourse in the fertile time, and 4% for those who had genital contact (including withdrawal) in the fertile time in every cycle. Only 6% of couples always used the method perfectly (researchers' analysis). Importantly, in almost 2,000 cycles which resulted in eight pregnancies, women thought they had used the method correctly. **Combining indicators is highly effective when either abstinence or protected intercourse is used during the fertile time, but most unforgiving of imperfect use.** [188]

New and experienced practitioners

Effective use of FAMs requires high-quality teaching from suitably trained, professionally competent practitioners. FAM training programmes should use clear teaching protocols, standardised materials and evidence-based guidelines with formal assessment to ensure practitioners are competent to practice. Just as users require monitoring and support until they are autonomous, practitioners require regular updating and ongoing supervision of practice. A Chilean study followed a group of teachers after their initial training course, monitoring their efficiency in their first year's teaching experience and then again a year later. They showed a dramatic improvement in teaching-related failures as they gained experience (pregnancy rates dropped from 17% to 4.7%). [463] This is a stark reminder of the need for quality training and regular supervision, particularly of newly qualified practitioners.

New and experienced users

A new user is generally at an increased risk of pregnancy in the first 6–12 months, although some studies [189] achieve similar effectiveness in the first year (including the first three cycles) as subsequent cycles. This is attributed to high-quality training and supervision using standardised teaching materials. After one year, most women gain experience by charting disruptions such as holidays, illness and stress, and are considered experienced users.

It should be recognised that some studies include new users in effectiveness figures whilst others have a learning phase of between three and six cycles prior to entering the effectiveness phase. Marshall and Barbato's independent studies of experienced users (> 6 months charting) reported typical use pregnancy rates of 3.9% and 3.6% respectively for combined-indicator methods. [382] [26]

Influence of user motivation: spacers and limiters

Effectiveness is highly dependent on user motivation. Many couples use FAMs consistently, but not perfectly. Women who do not understand the method are at risk of unintended pregnancy, as too are women who have a subconscious desire for a child. The effectiveness of any user-dependent method relies on the motivation of both partners, but this is crucial for FAMs. Both partners should be in agreement about their intention to achieve or avoid pregnancy and document this on the chart at the start of each cycle.

The Fairfield multi-centre study (Canada, France, US, Mauritius and Colombia) reported pregnancy rates separately for family spacers (those who plan more children at a later date and are prepared to take risks) and limiters (those who have completed their families). In the Canadian centre, the family spacers had a 14.8% pregnancy rate compared with 1.1% for the conscientious family limiters. The limiters in all five countries consistently showed better effectiveness rates (almost four times that of the family spacers). [503] Thapa reported similar figures, with family spacers experiencing four times the number of pregnancies compared with limiters. [574]

Barbato's study of experienced users reported 25 pregnancies amongst family spacers but none amongst limiters. [26]

A number of factors are predictive of correct use. A key factor is whether the woman feels pressure from her partner for sex at the fertile time (page 194). Wherever possible, men should be actively involved in the learning process as this allows an opportunity to address difficulties with behaviour change and the impact of abstinence on the relationship. [365]

A US study asked 358 women and their male partners, who were using an online teaching programme, to indicate "how much" and "how hard" they wished to avoid pregnancy on a scale of 0 to 10 (motivation scale used by National Survey of Family Growth). Male and female scores were combined in the analysis. There was an 80% greater likelihood of pregnancy with the low-motivation group. [168]

Classification of unintended pregnancies

Although a few pregnancies occur with *correct use* (perfect use of the method and correct application of the guidelines), the majority result from *typical use*. These pregnancies occur due to faulty teaching (or learning), or as a result of conscious departure from the guidelines – that is, intercourse on a fertile day(s) without prior indication of planning pregnancy. In a few situations the reason for the pregnancy may be unresolved. It should be noted that some NFP groups share the philosophy that pregnancies resulting from intercourse in the fertile time are "intentional" pregnancies rather than failures of the method, claiming that NFP can be used to plan as well as avoid pregnancy (page 138). However, most would agree that these pregnancies are either due to problems identifying the fertile time or difficulties with abstinence.

AGEING GAMETES

In the early 1980s there were unconfirmed epidemiological studies suggesting a possible increased risk of miscarriage and chromosomal abnormalities, specifically Down's syndrome, associated with the use of FAMs. When an unintended pregnancy occurs it is more likely to result from intercourse at the limits of the fertile time, hence from either an ageing sperm or egg. Animal studies have demonstrated that delayed fertilisation increases the risk of chromosomal abnormalities, but the rate varies between species.

In their chapter on "Contraception and congenital malformations" Phillips and Simpson discuss the incontrovertible link between maternal age – not the frequency or timing of intercourse – and the risk of miscarriage and major chromosomal abnormalities, including Down's syndrome. They comment that conclusions following numerous studies on ageing gametes are reassuring: there was no significant difference in the rates of miscarriage, low birth weight or preterm birth among women using FAMs who had unintended pregnancies compared with women who had intended pregnancies. Studies in live-borns resulting from these populations show no evidence of an increased anomaly rate. [467]

ADVANTAGES AND DISADVANTAGES OF FAMS

FAMs offer advantages to women at all stages of reproductive life, but may have a particular appeal to women who are in a committed relationship, planning pregnancy in the near future or spacing their family. A number of studies have looked at women's interest in FAMs and their perception of the associated benefits and challenges (page 362), but the reality of the method becomes clear only with use. Table 13.2 lists some of the recognised advantages and disadvantages of FAMs.

Table 13.2 Advantages and disadvantages of Fertility Awareness Methods

Advantages	*Disadvantages*
No chemical agents or physical devices	Takes time to learn: three to six cycles
Free from side effects	Some women find charting difficult
Efficient when well-taught and motivated	Some couples find abstinence difficult
Low cost for methods based on observation	Requires the commitment of both partners
Not dependent on medical personnel after initial instruction.	More difficult at times of stress or hormonal change
Promotes education and bodily awareness	No protection against STIs
Encourages couple communication and shared responsibility	Cannot be used without co-operation of partner
Acceptable to many with ethical, cultural or religious concerns, not only Catholics	Unforgiving of imperfect use, rule-breaking or risk-taking
Can be used with barrier methods if acceptable	Fertility monitoring devices are expensive
Can be used to plan or avoid pregnancy	Many fertility devices and apps have not had reliable clinical trials
No adverse effects on future fertility	Access to high-quality teaching services is patchy

CONTRACEPTION AND RETURNING FERTILITY

14

This chapter discusses contraceptive choice and how FA knowledge helps couples to understand their options. It explores the action of different methods, how they interrupt fertility, the time for return of normal fertility and the use of FAMs after discontinuing the method. For wider aspects of contraception and sexual health, including instructions for use, contraceptive counselling, informed consent, prescribing issues and eligibility criteria see further reading and professional associations (appendix H), particularly Belfield [41], Guillebaud [256] and Everett [161], plus the Faculty of Sexual and Reproductive Health Care (www. srh.org).

CLASSIFICATION OF CONTRACEPTIVE METHODS

Contraceptive methods are classified by the United Nations as either *modern* or *traditional*:

- Modern methods include hormonal contraception, intrauterine contraception, barrier methods and sterilisation (emergency contraception is currently not included).
- Traditional methods include FAMs (reported as rhythm) withdrawal, prolonged abstinence, breastfeeding, LAM, douching and folk methods. [423]

WHO have highlighted inconsistencies in the use of the terms *modern* and *traditional*. For example: some agencies classify modern FAMs (temperature, combined indicators, SDM, TDM and LAM) as modern methods, leaving only rhythm and withdrawal as traditional methods. WHO are currently reviewing the classification systems specifically to classify modern FAMs appropriately and integrate emergency contraception. Standard classification would help to improve data collection, analysis and reporting of contraceptive use. [636]

CONTRACEPTIVE CHOICE

When choosing a contraceptive method, a woman should be given accurate information about the *full* range of methods (including FAMs). She needs to understand how the method works, its advantages and disadvantages (major risks and minor side effects), its efficacy and the expected return of fertility after discontinuation – only then can she give valid consent. Consideration must be given for a woman's age, her medical history, plans for future pregnancy and any family history of premature menopause (pages 326 and 328). Methods which act by ovarian suppression may have a particularly negative effect in women who already have compromised ovarian function. [270]

Contraceptive methods include the following.

- Hormonal methods
  - combined estrogen and progestogen methods, including oral contraceptive pills, transdermal patch and vaginal ring; and
  - progestogen-only methods, including progestogen-only pills, depot injections, subdermal implants and levonorgestrel-releasing intrauterine systems (LNG-IUS);
- Non-hormonal methods:
  - intrauterine methods such as copper-containing IUDs (long-acting method);
  - barrier methods such as male and female condoms, diaphragms, caps and spermicide;
  - FAMs; and
  - withdrawal method.
- Post-coital methods (emergency contraception):
  - hormonal progestogens, and
  - copper IUDs.

Contraceptive methods are defined as short- or long-acting. Long-acting reversible contraceptive (LARC) methods require administration less than once per cycle or month: this includes copper-containing IUDs, progestogen-only injections, implants and LNG-IUS. All other methods, which require more frequent administration, are considered short-acting.

Hormonal methods have a major suppressant effect on fertility, hence the use of FAMs after their discontinuation merits a separate chapter (see chapter 15). Non-hormonal methods have minimal impact on the cycle and the indicators of fertility. Many factors determine method choice but, provided an individual is medically eligible to use a particular method, he or she should be free to choose the method which is most acceptable. [209] Health professionals must be sensitive to cultural and religious beliefs. Some individuals may object to methods such as intrauterine contraception, hormonal methods or emergency contraception. Although their primary action may be to prevent ovulation (pre-fertilisation effects), their secondary action may block implantation (post-fertilisation).

CONTRACEPTIVE USE THROUGH REPRODUCTIVE LIFE

A couple's needs for family planning change through reproductive life, hence the corresponding change of method. Contraceptive needs can be divided into stages:

1. Puberty to marriage (or committed relationship)
2. Marriage (or committed relationship) to birth of first child
3. Postpartum and breastfeeding
4. Family spacing after breastfeeding
5. After the (probable) last child
6. Family complete and children growing up
7. Peri-menopausal

The most appropriate contraceptive method will depend on individual and social need, lifestyle, level of sexual activity, risk of STIs, degree of efficacy required, anticipated short or long-term use of the method, concerns about health risks, toleration of side effects, potential risks to future fertility or the desire for permanent infertility. Effectiveness may be of paramount importance at some stages (for example stages 1, 6 and 7) whereas at other stages couples may have a more relaxed approach. The highest proportion of FAM users, for example, are at stages 2, 3 and 4 – in committed relationships, breastfeeding or spacing their families. A change of sexual partner, at any stage of reproductive life, frequently results in a change of method as contraceptive needs change.

PREGNANCY RATES AFTER CONTRACEPTIVE USE

The evidence for the return of fertility after contraception is reassuring. Mansour's literature review reported one-year pregnancy rates after method discontinuation:

- Oral contraceptives or the LNG-IUS: 79–96%
- Contraceptive injections (only two studies): 73–83%
- Contraceptive implants: 77–86% (with one study reporting < 50%)
- Copper IUDs: 71–91%

These rates are broadly similar to those reported following discontinuation of barriers or no contraceptive method. Importantly, there was no evidence of increased pregnancy complications or adverse fetal outcomes after stopping any of the reversible methods. [373]

INTRAUTERINE DEVICE (IUD)

The IUD is a non-hormonal form of intrauterine contraception. All modern types of IUD contain copper, and most have an inert plastic frame (often T-shaped). The device is medically inserted via the cervical canal to fit into the uterine cavity, leaving one or two fine threads protruding from the cervical os into the top of the vagina. Depending on the type of device, an IUD can remain in place for up to 10 years. The woman checks the threads periodically to ensure the device remains correctly positioned. FSRH guidance provides recommendations and good-practice points on the use of intrauterine contraception currently available in the UK. [216]

Modes of action

The main actions of the IUD are pre-fertilisation, but it also has post-fertilisation effects. The IUD:

- incapacitates sperm, as copper is toxic to sperm, eggs and embryos;
- acts as a foreign body in that the inert plastic produces an inflammatory response in the endometrium plus uterine and tubal fluid impeding sperm transport and fertilisation;
- alters the endometrium biochemically, preventing implantation; and
- may shorten the luteal phase, reducing the chance of implantation.

An IUD may not be appropriate if a woman has religious or ethical reasons for avoiding a method which may occasionally prevent the implantation of a blastocyst.

Effects of IUD on the cycle

A study which compared the menstrual cycles and daily hormone profiles of 30 women using copper IUDs with those of 15 normally menstruating women reported that the rate of ovulation, peak estradiol and LH levels were not significantly different between the two groups, but estradiol and progesterone levels were higher during menstruation in IUD users. There was no difference in total cycle length, but the follicular phase was longer and the luteal phase was shorter in IUD users. Thus although an IUD does not affect ovarian function, the ovarian hormone production and endometrial events become asynchronous. [163]

Fertility awareness with IUD in situ

A woman can be taught to use FAMs with her IUD in situ – this provides effective contraceptive protection during the learning phase. An IUD user may be ideally suited to cervical self-examination as an additional indicator. While the IUD is in situ:

- menstrual abnormalities are common (this includes spotting/light bleeding or heavier, prolonged bleeding, especially in the first three to six months of IUD use);
- the waking temperature may indicate a delayed rise and/or shorter luteal phase; and
- there may be few or no dry days, but a continuous pattern of moistness, possibly due to local irritation from the IUD threads (mild cervicitis).

As a woman observes the changes in her secretions and gains confidence in identifying the fertile time, she may naturally start to avoid intercourse on fertile days. Most women feel ready to have the IUD removed within three to six cycles.

FAMs following IUD removal

After the IUD is removed, fertility indicators may show:

- periods becoming noticeably shorter and lighter;
- total cycle length unchanged;
- a short luteal phase in at least the first cycle; and
- an increase in the number of dry days.

Fertility return is normally immediate (FAM guidelines for normal fertility: page 227).

BARRIER METHODS

Barrier methods include any contraceptive method which uses a physical barrier to prevent sperm from reaching the egg. These comprise male and female condoms plus diaphragms and cervical caps (with spermicide). FSRH guidance provides recommendations and good practice points on the use of barrier methods. [214] As barriers act only as a physical block to sperm, fertility is expected to return immediately on discontinuation.

Male condoms The male condom is a disposable thin sheath which covers the erect penis and physically prevents semen from entering the vagina. When used consistently and correctly condoms are 98% effective (typical use: 82%; see table 14.1). Condoms have the advantage for mixed-method users in that they do not interfere with the observation of secretions. It is *not* recommended to use more than one condom simultaneously (or to combine the use of a male condom with a female condom or diaphragm) because it increases the friction, making them more liable to tear. It is no longer recommended to use additional spermicide with condoms.

Female condoms The female condom is a disposable sheath with two soft rings – a wider outer ring attached to the open end and a separate narrower inner ring at the closed end. The two sides of the inner ring are squeezed together for insertion into the vagina. The inner ring helps to keep the condom in the vagina and the outer ring helps to keep the open end of the condom at the vulva. Female condoms are 95% effective with correct use and 79% effective with typical use. They are used without spermicide so do not interfere with the observation of secretions.

Diaphragms and cervical caps The diaphragm is a soft dome-shaped device with a flexible metal spring reinforcing its rim. It is inserted into the vagina by squeezing the two sides together and positioned to occlude the cervix. It is held in place by the spring tension of the rim and the vaginal muscles, with the front of the diaphragm resting behind the pubic bone. Cervical caps are smaller devices which fit snugly over the cervix. It is not possible to get a perfect fit with diaphragms or caps (and the vagina changes shape during intercourse) so they should *always* be used with spermicide. The barrier acts as a spermicide reservoir, providing a back-up mechanism to kill sperm which escape around the edges of the device. Mixed method users should take note of the characteristics of the spermicide to help distinguish changes in cervical secretions (page 233).

Spermicides

Spermicides are chemical substances used vaginally to immobilise sperm. They are available in the forms of gels, creams, foams, films or pessaries. Most spermicides contain the active ingredient nonoxynol-9 (N-9) – a surfactant that disrupts cell membranes. Spermicides should only be used in conjunction with a diaphragm or cervical cap. They should not be used alone due to their low effectiveness. [249] N-9 was originally thought to offer some protection against STIs including HIV; however, repeated and frequent use is associated with an increased risk of genital lesions, which potentially increases the risk of HIV acquisition. Any woman who experiences vaginal irritation or soreness should discontinue use of spermicide. Women should be warned that there is no good evidence to support the use of "natural" spermicides such as lemon juice, vinegar or Coca-Cola. [214]

Lubricants

Many couples use vaginal lubricants to overcome vaginal dryness/discomfort during intercourse, or purely to increase sexual pleasure. Lubricants may be oil-, water- or silicone-based. Oil-based lubricants – such as petroleum jelly, baby oil or massage oils – can damage both standard latex condoms and newer brands made from polyisoprene or lamb intestine, increasing the risk of condom breakage. Water- or silicone-based lubricants can safely be used with barrier contraception but, with the possible exception of couples who experience condom breakage, there is insufficient evidence to routinely advise their use. [214] Lubricants may mask changes in secretions (see glass of water test shown in chapter 5, table 5.1) Couples who are trying to conceive may be wise to avoid some lubricants because of the damaging effects on sperm (see table 18.2 in chapter 18).

Increasing FA knowledge for barrier users Barrier users frequently do not readily identify themselves to health professionals, but they often lack accurate information about the fertile time and take uneducated risks. There is therefore a case for increasing fertility knowledge for *all* barrier users. Those who wish to have unprotected intercourse, and are not at risk of STIs, must learn to identify the limits of the fertile time as accurately as couples who use NFP with abstinence (page 233).

WITHDRAWAL METHOD

Withdrawal method (coitus interruptus) allows vaginal intercourse until ejaculation is imminent, at which time the man withdraws his penis and ejaculates away from the woman's genital area. The man relies on sensation to determine when he is about to ejaculate, so effectiveness is highly dependent on his awareness, compliance and ability to withdraw before any sperm are released. As with barrier users, couples who use this method may benefit from increased FA knowledge (page 234).

Does pre-ejaculatory fluid contain sperm?

It is widely reported that pre-ejaculatory fluid contains sperm, thus making withdrawal very risky. Pre-ejaculatory fluid itself, which originates from the Cowper's gland, does not contain sperm; however, as the pre-ejaculate leaves the urethra it may flush out sperm from a previous ejaculation, which could result in pregnancy. This gives rise to the advice: "If a man urinates between ejaculations before having sex again, it will help clear the urethra of sperm and may increase the effectiveness of withdrawal." [452] Although it makes practical sense, there is no clear evidence to support this assertion. Indeed, a review of the literature on all aspects of withdrawal method commented on the paucity of research on the use and effectiveness of withdrawal. [508]

The research is conflicting. A study of 12 men with normal semen analyses provided samples of pre-ejaculatory fluid on at least two different occasions. The study included normal healthy volunteers, men with premature ejaculation, and men who produced excessive fluid during foreplay. None of the samples contained sperm. The researchers concluded that pre-ejaculatory fluid secreted during sexual stimulation did not contain sperm and therefore cannot be responsible for pregnancies. [646]

In another study (27 men), the pre-ejaculatory fluid samples from 11 men (41%) contained sperm, with 10 men's samples showing motile sperm. The men produced fluid on up to five separate occasions and sperm were found in either all or none of the samples. One limitation of this study was the lack of confirmatory testing to ensure that the samples were pre-ejaculate. Nearly half of the men either had pre-ejaculate that contained sperm or were unable to accurately identify when ejaculation was imminent. Although the actual numbers of sperm in the pre-ejaculate were low, the presence of motile sperm implied a pregnancy risk. Some men may be less likely to leak sperm in pre-ejaculatory fluid and may therefore be more effective users of withdrawal. Importantly in this study, prior to providing samples the men had urinated several time since their last ejaculation. [329]

Effectiveness

Figures from the US suggest that withdrawal method is 96% effective with correct use, implying withdrawal before ejaculation every time, and 78% effective with typical use. [586]

If a couple are using withdrawal effectively, it may be inappropriate to advise them to discontinue the method. Experienced older couples, with a trusting relationship and good self-control, may be ideally suited to withdrawal provided that they are both satisfied with the method; but young inexperienced, highly fertile couples may be at significantly higher risk of unintended pregnancy. [204]

A survey of young American women (aged 15–24) compared women who used withdrawal to those who used other methods of contraception only; 31% of women used withdrawal during the four-year study. Of the withdrawal users, 21% experienced an unintended pregnancy compared with 13% who used other methods only. Withdrawal users were 7% more likely to have used emergency contraception. Single women were 15% more likely to use withdrawal than married women. This group might be encouraged to consider a more effective contraceptive method. [136]

EMERGENCY CONTRACEPTION (EC)

EC also known as post-coital contraception (or, inappropriately, the "morning after pill"), is designed to prevent pregnancy after a single act of unprotected intercourse or contraceptive failure. It works by preventing fertilisation or implantation, depending on the position in the cycle. There are three different types of emergency contraception: two different forms of emergency pills (which must be taken within three or five days of unprotected intercourse) or a copper IUD which can be fitted up to five days after unprotected intercourse or within five days of the earliest estimated date of ovulation. See FSRH Clinical Guidance on Emergency Contraception for recommendations to guide clinical practice. [211]

Determining the risk of conception

Determining a woman's risk of conception is complex. It depends on the timing of all episodes of unprotected intercourse in the current cycle, the timing of ovulation, the age and fertility of both partners, and whether contraception has been used correctly.

Most women are not aware of their ovulation day but they usually know the day their period started. Wilcox [630] estimated the probability of conception on each day of the cycle allowing for variability in the day of ovulation. The probability of conception with *one completely random act of intercourse* was 3.1%. The probability of conception following intercourse on different days of the cycle was as follows.

- On days 1–3 there is negligible risk.
- By day 7 there is nearly 2% risk, rising to a peak of nearly 9% on day 13.
- From day 14 onwards the probability of conception declines, but remains at around 1% as late as day 40 and beyond.

The figures may seem relatively low, but this is for *one* intercourse act only and the probability of conception is generally calculated on multiple acts. The 1% ongoing risk is low but significant because some women who *think* they are premenstrual may still not have ovulated if they are having a long cycle. [630]

Discrepancies between self-reported cycle day and hormonal profiles There may be significant discrepancies between self-reported cycle day and hormonal profiles, hence calculating the risk of pregnancy from cycle day only may, in some cases, not give an accurate assessment of pregnancy risk. In a study of 94 women consulting about EC, less than half were certain of their LMP date. Although the majority of women could accurately recall intercourse timing, 60% had had unprotected sex more than once in the cycle, and 22% had urinary pregnanediol concentrations that were inconsistent with their estimated cycle day. [566] If a woman has an accurate record of her cycle lengths, the calculations *S minus 20* and *L minus 10* can help to determine the outer limits of the fertile time. Provided the unprotected intercourse is outside the fertile time, it may be feasible to reassure her that EC is unnecessary. However, Wilcox advised that for a woman who needs maximum protection from pregnancy, emergency contraception may be appropriate even with intercourse beyond the time she expects her next period. [630]

FAMs after emergency contraception

FAM users who have unprotected intercourse, or experience barrier failure, during the fertile time may access EC recognising that they are at substantial risk of pregnancy. If hormonal methods are used, a woman may experience some ongoing cycle disruption, similar to other hormonal methods of contraception, but this is usually minimal. If a woman is requiring EC on a number of occasions, an assessment should be made as to whether the couple are suited to FAMs or whether another contraceptive method may be more appropriate.

Contraceptive or abortifacient?

Many individuals have deeply held beliefs about where life begins which may be at odds with the medical definition. Until the 1950s, the definition of conception and the start of pregnancy was the time of *fertilisation* (fusion of egg and sperm) – a definition which is still used by some dictionaries and a viewpoint held by many with strong religious convictions. The definition has been challenged by the medical establishment, with the revised medical definition stating that conception occurs at *implantation*. Methods which block implantation such as EC are legally accepted as a form of contraception (working against conception).

Conception starts with fertilisation but the process takes six to seven days and is not complete until the blastocyst has implanted in the endometrium. Any intervention after implantation is regarded as abortifacient. EC, which is given within three to five days of unprotected intercourse is legally, medically and ethically considered to have contraceptive effects. A pregnancy is not recognised to exist until there is "carriage", which logically says that no contraceptive method can cause "miscarriage". In 2002 a UK Judicial Review of emergency contraception confirmed the Government's position that a pregnancy begins at implantation (not fertilisation). The High Court ruled that EC methods work before implantation and are therefore contraceptive not abortifacient. [126]

Some individuals may object on moral or religious grounds to *any* method which prevents conception by interfering in any way with the sperm meeting the egg. Even the term *contraception* may be difficult for some because this implies working against conception; whereas *family planning* may not have the same connotations as it can also be used for planning pregnancy.

SELF-ASSESSMENT QUESTIONS

Answers are at the end of the chapter.

1 A 30-year-old woman is learning FAMs while her IUD is in situ. She plans to keep it in place until charting confidently and then to conceive in about two years. At her first follow-up she is concerned because she has only eight high temperatures. Is this normal? How would you advise her about longer-term plans for conception?
2 Identify the active ingredient in most spermicides and describe any concerns related to its use.
3 A woman seeks advice about emergency contraception. She had one episode of unprotected intercourse 12 hours ago (the second day of her period). In the last year she has recorded cycle lengths of: 29, 28, 31, 26, 29, 31, 28, 27, 30, 28, 28 and 29 days. How would you advise her about her pregnancy risk?
4 How would you explain the effectiveness of male condoms?

CONTRACEPTIVE EFFECTIVENESS

The reliability of a contraceptive method depends on its inherent effectiveness when used under ideal conditions (perfect or correct use) and the ability of couples to use the method correctly (typical use). Even if a method is relatively ineffective, this has to be considered in relation to the risk of pregnancy if no method is used, which will vary dependent on a woman's age. A sexually active woman under 40 has an 80–90% risk of pregnancy in one year; a 40- year-old woman has a 40–50% risk; a 45-year-old has a 10–20% risk; and a 50-year-old has an estimated 0–5% risk of pregnancy in one year (if she is still menstruating). [256]

Hierarchy of contraceptive effectiveness

Table 14.1 shows the percentage of women experiencing an unintended pregnancy during the first year with typical and perfect use of each method (compared with no method). [586] A systematic review confirmed the hierarchy of contraceptive effectiveness in descending order: female sterilisation, LARCs (LNG-IUS and implants), copper IUDs, short-acting hormonal methods (injectables, oral contraceptives, the patch and vaginal ring), barrier methods and FAMs. Mansour commented on the high level of effectiveness afforded by LAM and the wide typical-use rate with FAMs. [374] The UK summary was broadly consistent with Trussell's 2004 data from the US.

Table 14.1 Percentage of women experiencing an unintended pregnancy during the first year with typical and perfect use of each method of contraception (adapted from Trussell in Hatcher 2011) [586]

Method	*Typical use*	*Perfect use*
Male sterilisation	0.15	0.10
Female sterilisation	0.5	0.5
Contraceptive implant (Implanon)	0.05	0.05
Intrauterine system (Mirena)	0.2	0.2
Intrauterine device (copper T)	0.8	0.6
Depo-Provera	6	0.2
NuvaRing	9	0.3
Evra patch	9	0.3
Combined pill and progestogen-only pill	9	0.3
Diaphragm	12	6
Male condom	18	2
Female condom	21	5
Withdrawal	22	4
FAMs	24	
Sympto-thermal Method		0.4
Ovulation Method		3
TDM		4
SDM		5
Spermicide alone	28	18
No method (woman under 40 years)	85	

Presenting information on contraceptive effectiveness

Consumers need to understand the risk of pregnancy and the effectiveness of their chosen method both with correct and typical use. RCOG guidance [485] on how best to present risk advises that tables with categories communicate relative effectiveness better than numeric tables. However, women grossly over-estimate pregnancy risk unless they are shown tables with numbers, so a combination of both methods is best. Pregnancy risk should be both negatively and positively framed: for example, Persona has a failure rate (negative framing) of 6 in 100 vs. the chance of successful contraception (positive framing) of 94 in 100. The actual number of people affected (frequencies) is more meaningful than percentages: for example, if 100 women use Persona correctly for one year, six would be expected to become pregnant. This means that 94 women out of 100 would successfully use the method to avoid pregnancy.

Visual aids may help to facilitate communication about risk because images are a powerful learning tool for some people. Figure 14.1 uses a simple 10 × 10 grid representing the effectiveness of Persona compared to the risk of pregnancy if no method is used. Discussion about pregnancy risk should be clearly documented in a woman's notes.

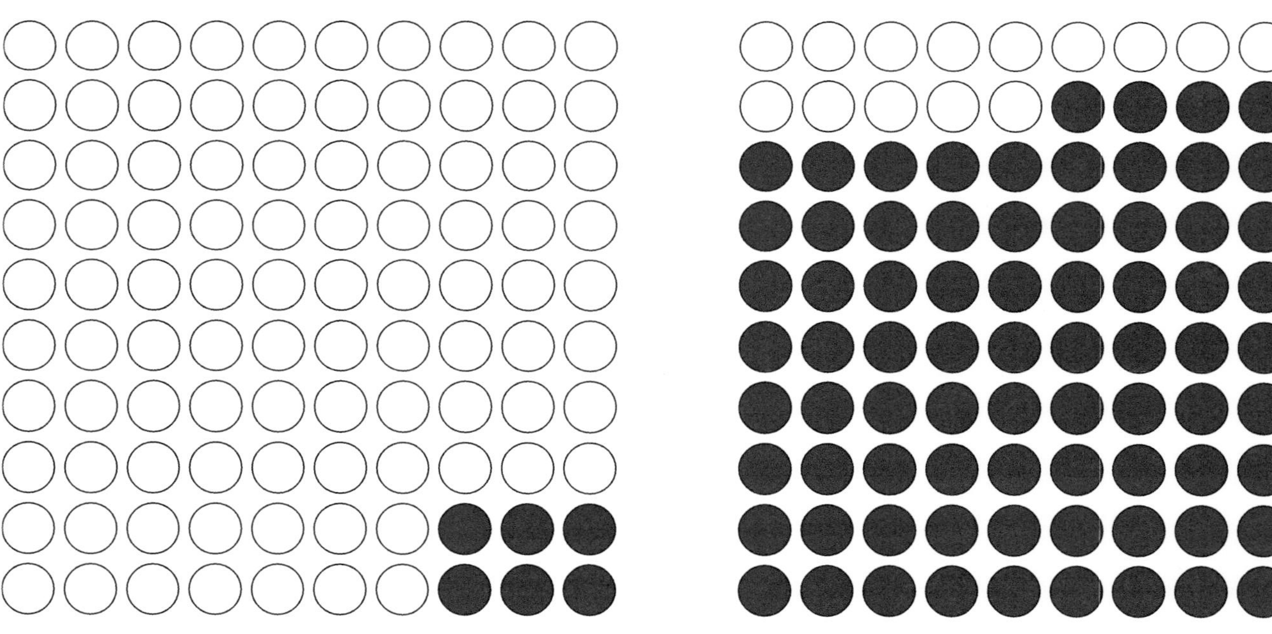

94% effective
About 6 women out of 100 will get pregnant within one year if they use Persona according to instructions.
About 85 women out of 100 will get pregnant within one year if no contraceptive method is used.

Figure 14.1 Comparison of the effectiveness of Persona vs. no contraceptive method. Persona is 94% effective (94 white dots) – that means that six women out of 100 will get pregnant in one year if used according to instructions. By comparison, 85 women out of 100 (85 black dots) would be expected to get pregnant if no method was used. [586]

A Cochrane review of different strategies for communicating contraceptive effectiveness concluded that interventions could not be compared because most reports did not provide specifics about how effectiveness was presented. [359]

CONTRACEPTIVE RISK-TAKING

Everyday life involves calculated risk, but some people take more risks than others. Couples who choose highly user-dependent methods such as FAMs, barriers and withdrawal, are at a high risk of pregnancy if the method is not used consistently. Women who have a basic understanding of FA can make a more accurate assessment of their chances of conception on a given day of the cycle (page 6).

ABORTION

Abortion is an emotive topic which polarises opinions, the controversy being between the woman's rights over her own body and the embryo's right to life. In Great Britain (England, Scotland and Wales) abortion is governed by the Abortion Act of 1967, [286] which was amended by the Human Fertilisation and Embryology Authority (HFEA) in 1990. [278] Abortion is legal if two doctors decide in good faith that, in relation to a particular pregnancy, one or more of the grounds specified in the Abortion Act are met. More than 98% of induced abortions in Britain are undertaken because of risk to the mental or physical health of the woman or her children. RCOG guidelines on the care of women requesting induced abortion aim to ensure that all women have access to a service of uniformly high quality. [490]

Ovulation after abortion The average time to ovulation after abortion is three weeks (with first menstruation at four to six weeks). Around 85% of women ovulate prior to their first period. The anti-progesterone mifepristone does not appear to have a lasting effect on ovarian function. [530] There is little difference in the return of ovulation between medical and surgical abortion. One study found a mean time to ovulation of 24 days (range 16–32) in the medical group compared with 29 days (range 16–37) in the surgical group (not statistically significant). [567]

FAMs after abortion Extreme caution is required with women who choose to use FAMs after abortion. Women should not rely on calendar-based calculations until they have had at least one period. The cervical secretions may be disrupted and the temperature rise may be delayed possibly with a short luteal phase (or absent). Intercourse should be restricted to the late infertile time until the situation becomes clear.

Psychological effects For most women, the decision to have an abortion is not easy, and the experience is stressful and probably unpleasant. Most women will experience a range of emotions around the time of the decision and the abortion procedure; however, only a minority experience long-term feelings of sadness, guilt and regret. Women with an unintended pregnancy are no more or less likely to suffer adverse psychological consequences whether they have an abortion or continue with the pregnancy and have the baby, but those with a past history of mental health problems are at increased risk of further problems after an unintended pregnancy – whatever the outcome [490] (see Rowlands' [517] comprehensive review of abortion).

ANSWERS TO SELF-ASSESSMENT QUESTIONS

1 A short luteal phase is commonly seen in IUD users – this back-up action reduces the chance of implantation. There would only be cause for concern if there continued to be fewer than 10 raised temperatures after the IUD has been removed.
2 Nonoxynol-9 was previously thought to offer protection against STIs, including HIV. However, repeated and frequent use is associated with an increased risk of genital lesions which potentially increases the risk of HIV acquisition.
3 There is about a 3% chance of pregnancy from one completely random act of intercourse, but the chance of pregnancy on days 1–3 of the cycle is negligible. Her shortest cycle is 26 days and her longest cycle is 31 days. Her potential fertile time is from day 6 to day 21 inclusive. She has an accurate record of cycle lengths and can be reassured that her chance of conception is extremely low. The choice would still be hers dependent on the potential impact of an unintended pregnancy.
4 Male condoms are 98% effective when used consistently and correctly. With typical use they are 82% effective (i.e. up to 18 women out of 100 experience an unintended pregnancy in the first year of use).

FAMs AFTER HORMONAL CONTRACEPTION

This chapter provides an overview of hormonal contraception from the perspective of its effects on the menstrual cycle, the indicators of fertility and the return of normal ovulatory cycles. For details of products, risk factors, non-contraceptive benefits, efficacy and prescribing issues, see works by Guillebaud [256] and Belfield [41]. Method-specific guidance can be found at the FSRH website (www.fsrh.org).

COMBINED ESTROGEN AND PROGESTOGEN METHODS

Combined hormonal contraception includes pills, patches and rings. Each work on a 28-day cycle: hormones for 21 days followed by a seven-day break (or seven days of placebo pills).

- Combined oral contraceptive pill (COCs):
  - Conventional regimen, taken for 21 days with a seven-day break (pill-free week), include monophasic pills (fixed dose) and phasic pills (variable dose).
  - Everyday pills have no pill-free week (packs contain 21 active and seven placebo pills).
- Combined transdermal patch: a new patch is applied weekly for three weeks followed by a patch-free week.
- Combined vaginal ring: a ring is inserted into the vagina and left in place for three weeks followed by a ring-free week.

Hormone withdrawal bleed or continuous regimen: Women should be informed that the bleed experienced during the hormone-free interval is due to the withdrawal of hormones – it is *not* a true period. Women who prefer not to have a withdrawal bleed can take COCs continuously. Breakthrough bleeding is common, particularly after a few months, but this varies between women.

Mechanism of action

Combined methods act via the HPO-axis to:

- suppress the development and maturation of ovarian follicles (reduce FSH levels);
- prevent ovulation (suppress the LH surge);
- produce thick barrier-type mucus at the cervix (prevent sperm penetration); and
- suppress the development of the endometrium (reduce the chance of implantation).

These multiple actions provide highly effective contraception, with similar efficacy rates for all combined methods (see table 14.1).

Bleeding associated with combined methods Combined methods generally provide the most regular pattern of bleeding, although some users experience irregular bleeding. Hormone withdrawal bleeds during the pill-free interval are lighter and less painful than normal menstrual periods. Women feel reassured by these monthly bleeds, but in some situations they can mask an underlying problem: for example, a woman who is seriously underweight will not get warning signs given by infrequent or absent periods and may be falsely reassured by regular "periods".

PROGESTOGEN-ONLY METHODS

Progestogen-only methods include the following.

- Progestogen-only pills (POPs) are taken daily at a consistent time with no breaks (no pill-free week):
  - Traditional POPs must be taken within three hours (i.e. within 27 hours since the last pill was taken).
  - Desogestrel POPs must be taken within 12 hours (i.e. within 36 hours since the last pill was taken). [217]
- Injectables, including intramuscular (IM) or subcutaneous (SC):
  - Depot medroxyprogesterone acetate (DMPA) is effective for 12 weeks, or (by self-injection)13 weeks.
  - Norethisterone enanthate (NET-EN) is effective for eight weeks. [213]
- Implants: flexible rod inserted subcutaneously (up to three years) [212]
- Intrauterine system: LNG-IUS (three–five years) [216]

Mechanism of action

Progestogen-only methods have a similar mechanism of action to combined methods, however they rely more heavily on their effect on cervical mucus – creating an impenetrable barrier to sperm. Progestogen-only methods suppress the development of the endometrium, and some disrupt the HPO-axis suppressing ovulation.

Level of ovarian suppression with progestogen-only methods The level of ovarian suppression varies between methods and over time:

- Traditional POPs suppress ovulation in about 50% of cycles.
- Desogestrel POPs suppress ovulation in up to 97% of cycles.
- Injectables suppress ovulation in 100% of cycles.
- Implants suppress ovulation in 100% of cycles for the first two years, but there are rare occurrences of ovulation by the third year of use.
- The LNG-IUS has little effect on the HPO-axis and ovulation is suppressed in less than 25% of cycles.

The majority of women using the LNG-IUS will therefore continue to ovulate. Similarly, a high percentage of women on POPs (particularly three-hour pills) continue to ovulate – hence the risk of pregnancy with delayed pills once the blocking effect of cervical mucus is lost.

Bleeding associated with progestogen-only methods Traditional POPs are most commonly associated with frequent and irregular bleeding, although some women have prolonged bleeding and others may be amenorrhoeic. With desogestrel POPs, most women have infrequent bleeding or amenorrhoea, some have regular bleeding or spotting, and a few have frequent bleeding. Some may have prolonged bleeding or spotting.

The majority of women using LARCs become amenorrhoeic with increased duration of use. Amenorrhoea, infrequent bleeding, spotting or prolonged bleeding are common with DMPA injectables, with a trend towards reduced bleeding and amenorrhoea with increased duration of use. The most common pattern with implants is infrequent bleeding or amenorrhoea, but some women have prolonged or frequent bleeding. Most women using the LNG-IUS have amenorrhoea or infrequent bleeding with lighter, less painful bleeds.

It should not be assumed that abnormal bleeding is related to hormonal contraception, particularly for women with prolonged, heavy bleeding or bleeding following amenorrhoea. Consider screening for STIs, cervical cytology and gynaecological pathology.

RETURN OF FERTILITY AFTER HORMONAL CONTRACEPTION

After discontinuing modern hormonal methods there is an almost immediate return to normal ovulatory cycles for most women, with pregnancy rates at one year similar to those for women not using hormonal methods (page 245). Despite this, women still have concerns: a German survey of 1,000 women (aged 14–44) reported that 27% expected fertility to be reduced after discontinuing oral contraceptives (OCs), 52% anticipated no change and 3% expected it to be higher. [625] Women who have ovulatory problems following hormonal contraception are most likely to have had pre-existing factors.

The changing types, amounts and combinations of hormones must be considered when analysing research findings, which means that early epidemiological studies may not be relevant to today's products. Contraceptive pills of the 1960s had significantly higher hormone levels than today's. One brand on the market in 1962 contained more estrogen in one day than is now given in a week, and almost the same daily dose of progestogen as is now given in a complete pack of pills. Concerns about long-term use are not related to the contraceptive itself, rather that the longer a woman uses a method the older she gets: advanced age is the critical factor. [256]

The time taken for fertility to return varies dependent on the type of hormonal contraception:

- Conventional combined methods: the European Active Surveillance Study on OCs (EURAS-OC), which included almost 60,000 users across seven European countries, confirmed that the type of pill, duration of use and parity had no major influence on pregnancy rate. Twenty-one percent conceived on the first cycle and 79% had conceived by one year – this is comparable to women who have not taken OCs. [109]
- Continuous regimen: concerns have been raised about amenorrhoea after continuous regimens. A US study showed pregnancy rates of 57% and 86% at three and 13 months respectively, suggesting there is no fertility delay. [30]
- Traditional POPs: observational studies have reported no fertility delays. [217]
- Desogestrel POPs: no significant delay: average 17.2 days (range 7–30) to first ovulation. [217]
- Injectables: fertility delays are common. Although some women will ovulate within six months of the last injection, it may take up to one year for the majority (irrespective of duration of use). There is no significant difference in CPR two years after discontinuation, [213] but women may prefer to switch to an appropriate short-acting method if they are planning pregnancy in the near future.
- Implants: fertility is likely to return immediately following removal. [212]
- LNG-IUS: few data exist, but the evidence suggests that there is no delay once the device is removed. [216]

Fertility delays are minimal or absent on discontinuation of all modern hormonal methods apart from injectables. Women who are switching from hormonal methods to FAMs should be managed by a specialist practitioner (appendix H.3) and must consistently follow the guidelines to maintain the contraceptive effect (page 259).

"Post-pill" amenorrhoea

Reports of "post-pill" amenorrhoea may fuel women's concerns about infertility related to hormonal methods. COCs are commonly indicated in young women with irregular periods. There is a higher incidence of ovulatory problems in women who are older at menarche, underweight, or obese, and with a history of irregular cycles in adolescence. As cyclic irregularities frequently recur after discontinuation, subfertility may be falsely attributed to hormonal use. Epidemiological studies show that amenorrhoea is equally common amongst women not using hormonal methods with around 2% of the general population reporting more than six months of amenorrhoea (particularly women under 24). [256] [625]

Post-pill amenorrhoea (secondary amenorrhoea of more than six months duration following discontinuation of COCs) is not associated with any particular preparation or, in most studies, with the duration of use. Guillebaud has proposed that the term should be abolished because, by assuming amenorrhoea is related to COC use, there is a risk of delaying diagnosis of potentially serious medical conditions. [256]

Rebound fertility after hormonal contraception

There are many anecdotes about *rebound* fertility after hormonal contraception. There is evidence of a higher pregnancy rate with IVF following one month on the combined pill, [218] but this does not necessarily hold true for natural conception. It is most probable that OC use neither positively nor negatively affects age-appropriate chances of natural conception. [109]

CYCLE CHARACTERISTICS AFTER HORMONAL CONTRACEPTION

Hormonal contraception has a profound effect on the menstrual cycle and the indicators of fertility. The most pronounced changes are seen following injectables, but some level of disruption should be anticipated after all hormonal methods.

Vaginal bleeding The altered bleeding pattern reverts to normal over time. Women who have had absent or infrequent bleeds start to menstruate more regularly. Prolonged or shortened flow normalises, and heavy or light flow returns to normal bright red loss, often accompanied by abdominal cramping. Women who have become accustomed to amenorrhoea or infrequent, short, light, pain-free periods may be alarmed by longer, heavier, redder more painful periods – yet these are likely to indicate normal menstruation. A bleed is only a true period, indicative of an ovulatory cycle, if it follows 10–16 days after a temperature rise.

Cycle length Total cycle length after discontinuing hormonal methods may be slightly longer, with some cycles longer than 35 days. This is attributable to longer follicular phases. The luteal phase may be shorter (possibly due to disturbed follicular maturation). Some women will have normal cycle length variation, but others may have increased variability. The first cycle after discontinuing hormonal methods is *not* a reliable indicator of future cycle lengths, therefore women should not rely on fertility monitors or calendar-based calculations for the first three cycles. [14]

Temperature Temperature curves will be varied. A woman may have normal biphasic cycles with an adequate luteal phase, a delayed rise, short luteal phase or monophasic cycles. Some women may observe persistently high (but false) readings unrelated to ovulation. The coverline may be higher than normal, particularly in the first cycle after discontinuation. To minimise errors when interpreting the rise, aim to include more than six low temperatures by using the coverline technique (see page 101 and figure 15.2).

Cervical secretions The progestogenic effect on the mucus at the cervix causes varying degrees of disruption to the secretions. There may be more days of dryness or reduced-quality secretions, with no wetter, transparent, stretchy secretions particularly in the first few cycles. Some women notice a continual watery or milky pattern with a heavier flow of secretions. The build-up to peak may be interrupted. There may be a delayed or multiple peak. It may take up to six cycles or longer for the return of optimum secretions and for a close correlation between peak day and temperature rise.

A German prospective study compared the cycle characteristics of 175 OC users (3,048 cycles) with a control group of 284 women who had never used OCs (6,251 cycles). The mean duration of pill use (predominantly monophasic pills) was 3.5 years. For 58% of women, the first post-pill cycle was a normal fertile cycle. Only 10% of first post-pill cycles were monophasic. Major cycle disturbances were more frequent up to cycle 7. There was a significantly higher percentage of long cycles (> 35 days) up to cycle 9 with nearly 2% of women reporting cycles longer than 90 days. Cycles showed a prolonged pre-ovulation phase resulting in a delayed peak day and temperature rise. There were significantly more cycles with short luteal phases (< 10 raised temperatures). Cycle disturbances after OCs were reversible, but the time of regeneration took up to nine months. [232]

A US study similarly reported significant differences in the cycle characteristics of recent OC users for the first six cycles. This included longer cycles (average two days longer) with more cycle length variability. Recent OC users reported a later peak day (particularly in the second cycle) and significantly lower scores for the quality of secretions in cycles 1 and 2 with ongoing reduced scores up to cycle 6. Periods were significantly lighter in the first four post-pill cycles, with shorter, lighter periods lasting up to cycle 6. The researchers commented on the need to replicate these studies using current hormonal preparations with observation beyond six months. [422]

Definitions of cycle characteristics after discontinuing hormonal contraception

Major cycle disturbances are defined as cycle lengths of more than 35 days, luteal phases of less than 10 raised temperatures and monophasic cycles. These, and other subtle disturbances, should be anticipated for up to six cycles and in extreme cases for longer. The beginning of **regular ovulatory cycles** is defined as the first of at least three consecutive cycles with a luteal phase of 10 days or more. [232]

GUIDELINES TO AVOID PREGNANCY AFTER HORMONAL METHODS

These guidelines are for use following discontinuation of any hormonal method.

First cycle

Intercourse must be avoided throughout the first cycle. Even if the first cycle appears bi-phasic, there is no discernible infertile time due the effects of the contraceptive hormones.

Second cycle

Intercourse must be avoided during the early infertile time. Use the coverline technique to identify the temperature rise. Extend the coverline back as far as possible, excluding the first four temperatures during the period. Intercourse can be resumed after the fourth high temperature has been recorded, provided they are all at least 0.2 deg.C above the low temperatures (at least six low temperatures).

Third and subsequent cycles

The late infertile time starts on the evening of the third high temperature, provided that it is at least 0.2 deg.C above the six low temperatures. All high temperatures must be after peak day.

Intercourse is restricted to the late infertile time until regular ovulatory cycles are re-established. When there have been at least three consecutive biphasic cycles with a luteal phase of 10 days or more, intercourse is permitted in the early relatively infertile time using the guidelines for normal fertility (page 227).

Period or bleeding

Intercourse is allowed during a period (up to day 5) from the fourth cycle onwards provided the first three cycles are 26 days or longer and the period is a "true" period (preceding temperature rise 10–16 days earlier).

Calculation based on cycle length

Calculations to identify the first fertile day (*Day 6 rule*, *S –20* and *earliest temperature rise –7*) must be recalculated after discontinuing any hormonal method (see figure 7.1 in chapter 7).

SELF-ASSESSMENT QUESTIONS

Answers are at the end of the chapter.

1 Define long-acting reversible contraceptives (LARCs) and their delivery routes.
2 What advice would you give to a woman about fertility after injectables?
3 List the major cycle disturbances after hormonal contraception.
4 Define the beginning of a regular ovulatory cycle after discontinuation of hormonal contraception.

INTERPRETING CHART AFTER HORMONAL CONTRACEPTION

Women who switch to FAMs should start recording on a normal fertility chart as soon as possible. Couples should be prepared for immediate return of fertility but also be warned that cyclic disruption is common. Women need to understand that cycles can be very long, with ovulation delayed for many weeks. The fertility chart spans 40 days but, in some cases, cycles can go on for longer. Where necessary, charts can be joined so that recordings continue from one chart to the next (figure 15.3).

The three example charts show part of a series after discontinuation of the combined pill. Figure 15.1 shows the first cycle – a 32-day cycle. The temperature rise is delayed but there is an apparent rise on day 25 followed by a short luteal phase. The secretions are consistently sticky white. There is no identifiable infertile time in the first post-pill cycle: assume the entire cycle is potentially fertile.

Figure 15.2 shows the second cycle post-pill – a 25-day cycle with an interrupted pattern of secretions. There are two days of wetter, stretchy secretions, with peak day on day 12 followed by a temperature rise on day 14. The coverline has been extended backwards to the start of the cycle (excluding the first four days). There are four temperatures which are all at least 0.2 deg.C above the low temperatures. Intercourse can be resumed following the *fourth* high temperature after peak (day 17) until the end of the cycle. The luteal phase is of normal length.

Figure 15.3 shows the seventh cycle. This 54-day cycle continues from one chart to another. The temperature spike on day 31 (which protrudes above the coverline) is permitted. A woman

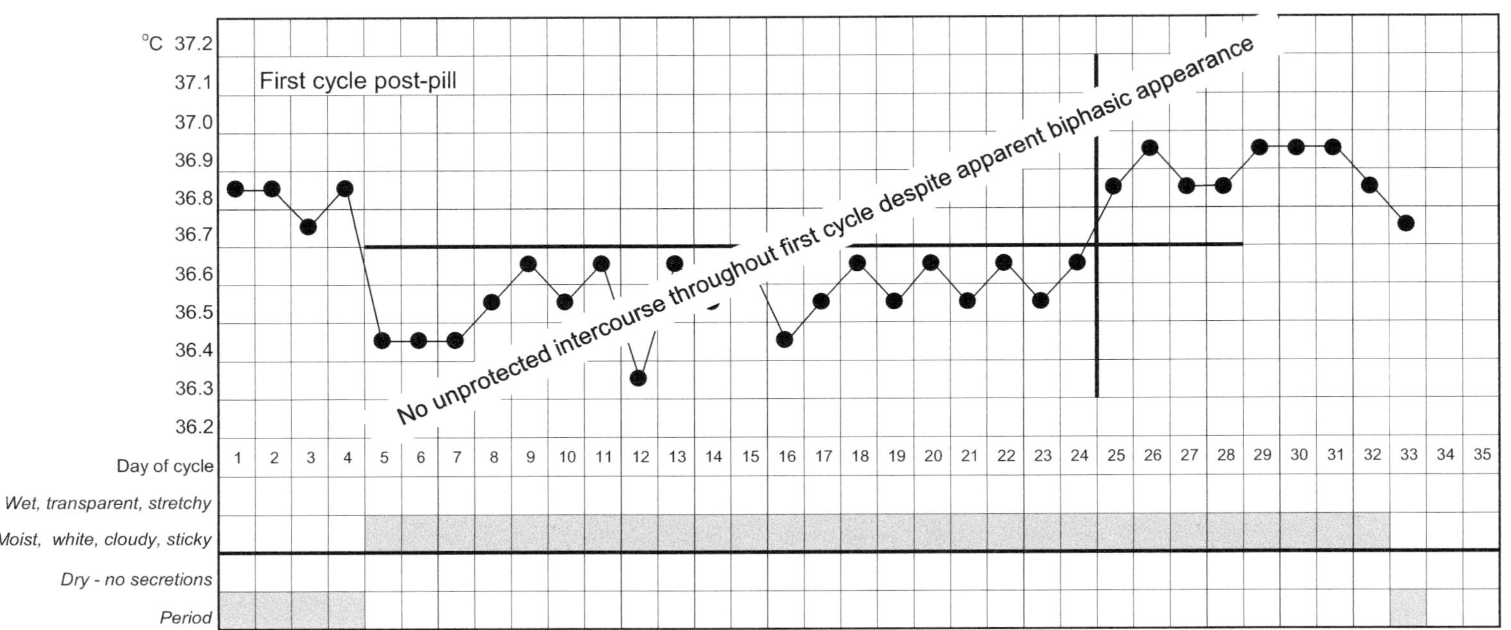

Figure 15.1 First cycle post-pill: there is no identifiable infertile time

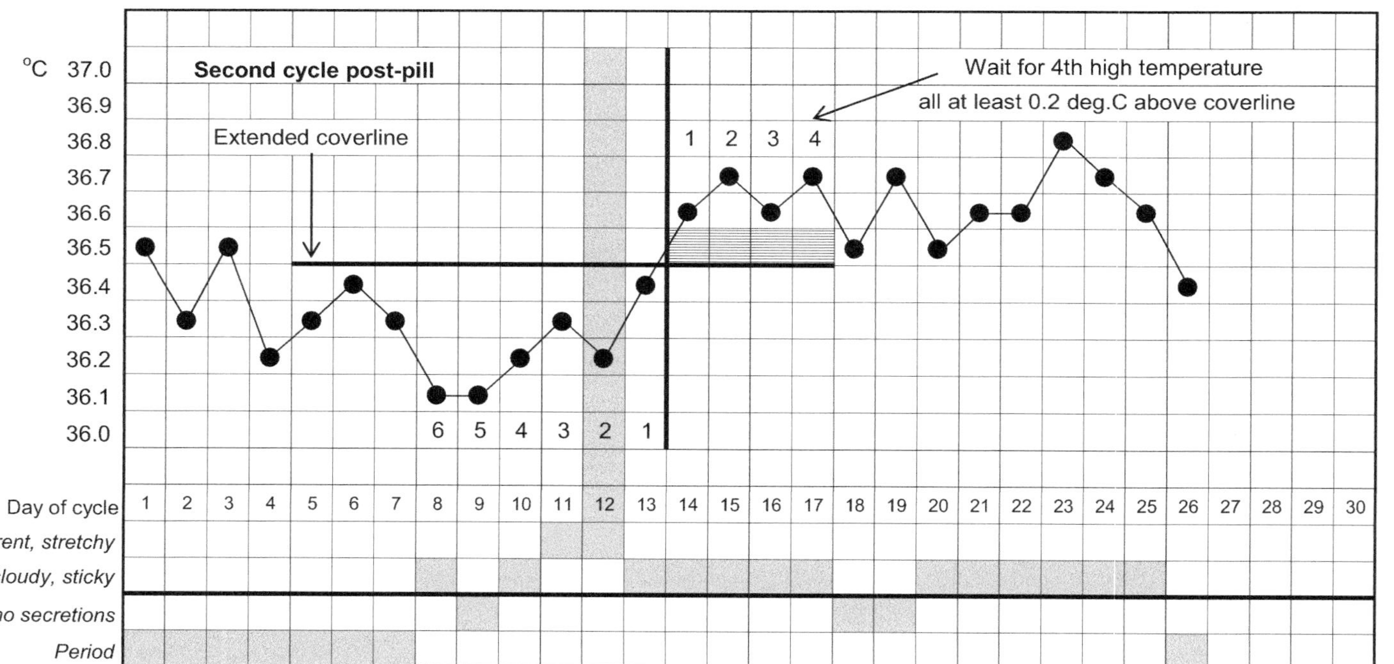

Figure 15.2 Second cycle post-pill: the fertile time ends after the *fourth* high temperature provided they are *all at least 0.2 deg.C* above the low temperatures (and all after peak day): Note the coverline extended back to day 5.

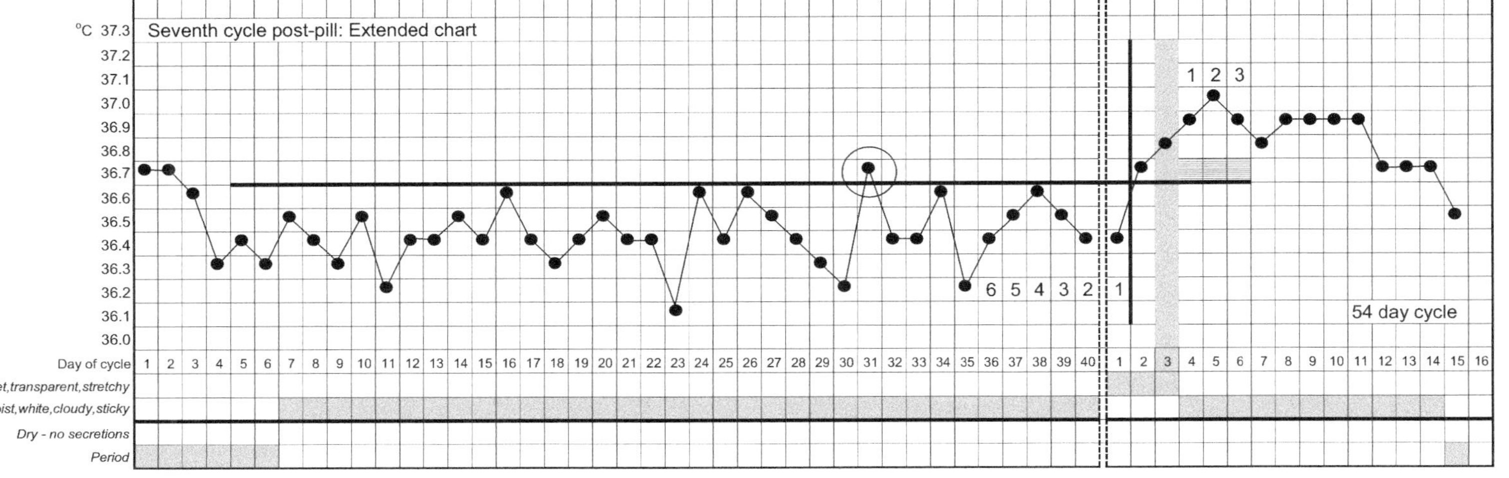

Figure 15.3 A 54-day cycle recorded on seventh post-pill cycle: note the extended chart (cycle days can be changed to run incrementally if easier (i.e. 41–55)

should never give up waiting for the temperature rise – in this case the rise occurs on day 42. There are only three days of wetter, stretchy secretions with peak on day 43 (day following the rise). This couple could assume infertility from day 46 (third high temperature after peak day) until the end of the cycle.

PLANNING PREGNANCY AFTER HORMONAL METHODS

Women can start trying to conceive immediately after discontinuing hormonal methods. Former advice to wait for three months was based on higher hormone doses with the likelihood of irregular cycles after discontinuation and issues with estimating the due date. Low-dose hormonal methods are safe, and pregnancy dating is performed by ultrasound. Provided a woman is immune to rubella and starts taking folic acid, she can start trying immediately.

Effect of hormonal contraception on ovarian reserve

Hormonal contraception suppresses a woman's ovarian reserve. Long and profound suppression of pituitary gonadotrophins is associated with reduced ovarian volume, a reduced number of antral follicles and decreased AMH. Concentrations of AMH are reduced by 13–50% with some evidence of increased suppression with longer-term use. Two months after discontinuing oral contraception AMH levels increase by an average of 30%.

It is recommended that women who want reassurance about their ovarian reserve should wait at least one month after discontinuing hormonal methods, but three months gives a more reliable estimate. It should be recognised that hormonal contraception could mask a severely diminished ovarian reserve. [340]

ANSWERS TO SELF-ASSESSMENT QUESTIONS

1 Contraceptive methods that are administered less frequently than once a month. LARCs include injectables, implants, intrauterine devices (copper IUDs) and intrauterine systems (hormonal IUS).
2 There may be a delay of up to one year (irrespective of duration of use). If this is unacceptable, consider switching to another method. Pregnancy rates by two years are equivalent to non-users.
3 Cycle lengths of more than 35 days, luteal phases of less than 10 raised temperatures and monophasic cycles.
4 The first of at least three consecutive cycles with a luteal phase of 10 days or more.

BREASTFEEDING, LAM AND RETURNING FERTILITY

16

Breastfeeding has many benefits for mother and baby. It provides the baby with complete nutrition, a safe food source and immunological defence against infectious diseases. Breastfeeding strengthens the attachment between mother and baby. The main physiological effect of interest here is the suppression of fertility.

The natural contraceptive effect of breastfeeding has been recognized since 400 BC (see table 1.1 in chapter 1). Traditionally, babies were breastfed from birth and supplements were not introduced until after the milk teeth had erupted at about six months. This temporary reduction in fertility is widely recognized to lengthen intervals between pregnancies in parts of the world where women practise demand-feeding and often breastfeed for two years or more (with no postpartum sexual abstinence and no additional contraception). [470]

A study in the 1980s compared the duration of lactational amenorrhoea and birth interval among Quechua Indians of Peru, Turkana nomads of Kenya and Gainj of Papua New Guinea – societies where infants suckle very frequently for up to two years. Turkana nomads resumed menstruation three months earlier than the Gainj and had the shortest birth intervals. (29 vs. 44 months). This may be due to a combination of early supplementation (butterfat, goats' milk or camels' milk) and differences in suckling patterns due to the unpredictable labour demands of the Turkana pastoral system. [243]

In 1988, in Bellagio (Italy), an international group of scientists reached a consensus about the conditions under which breastfeeding can be used either as a birth spacing method in its own right, or as a means to delay the introduction of other family planning methods:

> The maximum birth spacing effect of breastfeeding is achieved when a mother fully or nearly fully breastfeeds and remains amenorrhoeic (bleeding before the 56th postpartum day being ignored). When these two conditions are fulfilled, breastfeeding provides more than 98% protection from pregnancy in the first six months. At six months, or if menses return, or if breastfeeding ceases to be full or nearly full before the sixth month, the risk of pregnancy increases. [327]

The criteria were subsequently developed into an algorithm with emphasis on the need for another family planning method when any of the three criteria changed – this is LAM. [342]

PHYSIOLOGY OF LACTATION

The breasts

The breasts (mammary glands) are milk-producing tubo-alveolar glands. Each breast is divided into 7–10 glandular lobes radiating out from the nipple. Individual lobes are embedded in fatty tissue, separated by dense layers of connective tissue. Each lobe consists of a single major branch of alveoli with lactiferous (milk) ducts that ends at the nipple. The alveoli are grape-like clusters of glandular tissue containing the milk-secreting (acini) cells. Surrounding the nipple there is a pigmented area, the areola, which contains numerous sebaceous glands (Montgomery's tubercles) to lubricate the nipple during lactation. During pregnancy estrogen and progesterone stimulate the proliferation of the lactiferous ducts and the alveoli in preparation for lactation.

Until recently, anatomical textbooks have been based on Sir Astley Cooper's 19th century dissections, which involved injecting hot wax into the breasts of lactating cadavers. Ultrasound imaging now shows that almost all women have fewer than the commonly cited 15–20 lactiferous ducts. It was previously thought that milk collected in sinuses behind the nipple, but scans have been unable to detect these. The ducts are described as superficial tubular structures with elastic walls capable of significant expansion and compression. There is wide variation in the distribution of glandular and fatty tissue between women, but an individual woman's breasts show relative symmetry. The proportion of glandular and fatty tissue, and the number and size of ducts does not appear to be related to milk production. [479]

Initiation and maintenance of lactation

Lactation and lactational amenorrhoea are controlled by the mammary HPO-axis. The infant's suckling provides the physiological signal that maintains lactation and suppresses fertility. During pregnancy the level of prolactin from the anterior pituitary increases steadily, but the very high levels of placental estrogen suppress lactation. By late pregnancy the breasts start to secrete small amounts of colostrum, a thick yellowish fluid which is rich in proteins, fats and immunoglobulins. Following delivery, and over the next 48 hours, estrogen levels fall dramatically, allowing prolactin to act on the alveoli to initiate and maintain lactation. Colostrum production continues for the first two to three days after delivery, followed by transitional milk, then fully mature breast milk by four to six weeks. Lactation is encouraged by early and frequent suckling, which both increases and maintains the level of prolactin.

As the baby suckles at the breast, he or she stimulates sensory nerves in the areola which transmit messages via the hypothalamus to the anterior pituitary to release prolactin, which in turn causes the alveolar cells to secrete milk – the prolactin reflex (figure 16.1). Each act of

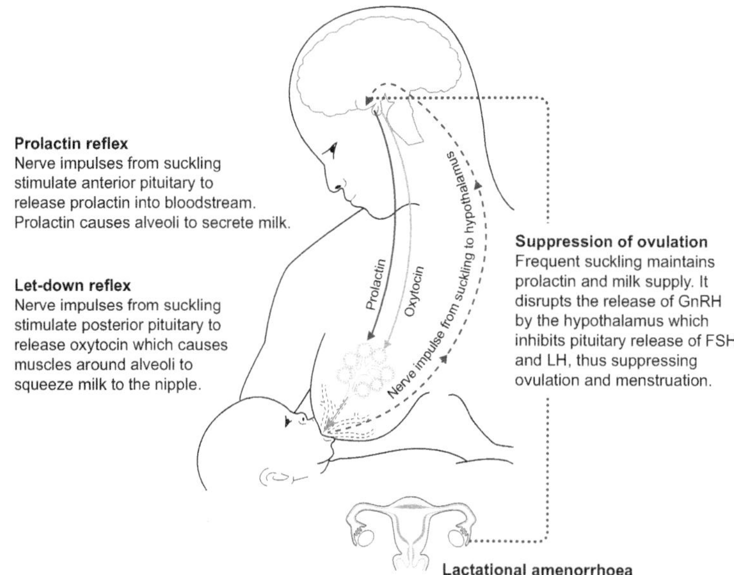

Prolactin reflex
Nerve impulses from suckling stimulate anterior pituitary to release prolactin into bloodstream. Prolactin causes alveoli to secrete milk.
Let-down reflex
Nerve impulses from suckling stimulate posterior pituitary to release oxytocin which causes muscles around alveoli to squeeze milk to the nipple.
Prolactin
Oxytocin
Nerve impulse from suckling to hypothalamus
Suppression of ovulation
Frequent suckling maintains prolactin and milk supply. It disrupts the release of GnRH by the hypothalamus which inhibits pituitary release of FSH and LH, thus suppressing ovulation and menstruation.
Lactational amenorrhoea

Figure 16.1 Hormonal control of breastfeeding and LAM (adapted from Oats 2016) [433]

suckling produces a prolactin spike, but the level falls again within three hours. Suckling opens prolactin receptor sites on the acini to begin milk production. The receptor sites start to close if they are not primed by prolactin, thus endorsing the need for early and frequent breastfeeding to maximise the potential for milk production.

At first, the milk distends the alveoli and small ducts, causing the breasts to become full and tender. Distended veins are visible under the skin and the milk ducts can be felt as tender strings in the breast tissue, but the milk is not yet ejected through the larger ducts to the nipple. During suckling, nerve impulses are transmitted via the hypothalamus to the posterior pituitary stimulating the release of oxytocin (love/bonding hormone). Oxytocin causes the muscles around the alveoli to contract, squeezing milk to the nipple – the milk ejection or "let-down" reflex. Suckling is the main stimulus for this reflex, but it is also a conditioned reflex: the sight or cry of a baby causes milk ejection; whereas embarrassment, pain and stress inhibit the reflex. Frequent suckling is vital both to maintain lactation and suppress ovulation.

BREASTFEEDING PRACTICE

Women who breastfeed frequently and delay the introduction of supplementary feeds remain amenorrhoeic for longer, but to achieve this they must be able to breastfeed successfully. WHO/UNICEF's Baby Friendly Initiative provides recommendations for successful breastfeeding and strategies for its promotion from maternity services through to community support (see www.unicef.org.uk/babyfriendly). [157]

Recommendations for successful breastfeeding practice conducive to LAM:

- Encourage early skin-to-skin contact between mothers and babies. [412]
- Encourage mothers to breastfeed soon after birth.
- Ensure the baby is correctly positioned at the breast.
- Avoid separating mother and baby.
- Encourage unrestricted breastfeeding, day and night.
- Avoid supplementary fluids unless medically indicated.
- Discourage the use of dummies (pacifiers).
- Continue breastfeeding even if the mother or baby becomes ill.
- Encourage full breastfeeding for up to six months.
- After six months, when supplements are introduced, continue to breastfeed for up to one year or more.

Optimal duration of exclusive breastfeeding

WHO's systematic review recommended six months exclusive breastfeeding as optimal, with the introduction of supplementary foods and continued breastfeeding thereafter. [624] A Cochrane review stressed the importance of individual management but concluded that, as a general policy, there are no apparent risks in recommending exclusive breastfeeding for the first six months in both developing and developed countries. Babies who are exclusively breastfed for six months or longer have lower rates of morbidity from gastrointestinal infection, with no deficit in growth. Moreover, the mothers of such babies have more prolonged lactational amenorrhoea. [336]

Prevalence of breastfeeding

FSRH guidance recommends that breastfeeding should be promoted and supported in all populations, but acknowledges that there will be circumstances in which it is not possible due to maternal illness or medication, or because of conditions affecting the new-born. [208] Although more women are now starting to breastfeed and are feeding for longer, the latest Infant Feeding Survey shows that very few mothers follow the government's recommendations, with only around 1% still exclusively breastfeeding at six months. Breastfeeding was most common amongst mothers who were aged 30 plus, from minority ethnic groups, in higher education, in managerial and professional occupations, and living in the least-deprived areas. [293] The opportunity for using breastfeeding as a fertility suppressant is therefore limited to a select group.

PHYSIOLOGY OF PUERPERIUM

The puerperium is the time when the physiological and morphological changes which occurred during pregnancy revert to the non-pregnant state. By convention, this phase lasts for six weeks. The uterus undergoes the most dramatic changes during its involution as it returns to its pre-pregnant size: muscle cells are broken down, proteins are absorbed into the circulation and excreted in urine. Although bleeding before the 56th postpartum day can be ignored for LAM purposes, it is useful to reflect on the typical pattern of vaginal loss following delivery.

Lochia

The lochia is the postpartum blood-stained vaginal discharge. For the first three to five days, lochia is heavy and bright red (contains blood and remains of trophoblastic tissue from the placental site). As the thrombosed vessels become organised, lochia gradually decreases in amount and changes in character, becoming reddish-brown in colour (up to about the 12th day). When most of the endometrium has been covered in epithelium, the lochia changes to yellowish/white lasting up to about six weeks postpartum. Although this is still technically lochia it is perceived by most women as cervical secretions. Occasionally blood clots break and lochia becomes red again for a few days. [433]

Duration of lochia The WHO multinational study of breastfeeding and LAM (4,118 women) compared the duration of lochia to determine the frequency and type of bleeding before day 56. The median duration was 27 days (range 22–34 days) whilst 11% reported persistent lochia for more than 40 days. Lochia usually stops and starts again at least once in breastfeeding women, before it completely stops. Eleven percent of women reported bleeding before day 56 (separated from lochia by at least 14 days). The duration of lochia varied significantly among different study populations. Factors including parity and infant's birth weight may influence the duration of lochia. [623] [622]

End of puerperium bleeding

In some societies an episode of bleeding is anticipated at about 40 days postpartum (sixth week bleed) which is distinctly separate from lochia. This "end-of-puerperium bleeding" which traditionally marks the end of postpartum sexual abstinence was reported by 20% of women in the WHO study. The cause of this bleeding is unknown. [623]

Note: Lochia which is unusually heavy/persistent or has an offensive odour could indicate postpartum infection. Abnormal lochia, perineal/wound pain, abdominal pain, breast pain and febrile illness should be investigated promptly. Untreated genital tract infection, particularly uterine infection (endometritis), could lead to puerperal sepsis and risk of maternal death (see RCOG guidance). [495]

PHYSIOLOGY OF LACTATIONAL AMENORRHOEA

In healthy women, the suckling stimulus signals the suppression of fertility. Frequent suckling disrupts the pulsatile secretion of GnRH from the hypothalamus, which in turn inhibits pituitary release of LH. There will be some circulating FSH which stimulates follicular growth, but estrogen levels remain low and the absence of LH prevents follicular maturation and ovulation. Provided the baby suckles frequently, prolactin levels remain high, thus suppressing ovulation and menstruation (figure 16.1).

Basal prolactin levels have a circadian rhythm, with peak concentrations between midnight and 6:00 am. Breastfeeding induces a significant rise in prolactin: the longer the feed, the higher the prolactin response. Both basal prolactin levels and the prolactin response to suckling diminish with time, starting about two months after delivery. **Breastfeeding at night releases more prolactin than during the daytime, so when the night feed is dropped, fertility is likely to return.** However, women who have comparable breastfeeding patterns may have different basal levels of prolactin and different prolactin responses to suckling. Women who have lower basal and suckling-induced prolactin levels will have shorter intervals of lactational amenorrhoea. [123]

The strength of the suckling stimulus is a unique situation between mother and baby. Although the precise mechanisms whereby suckling affects GnRH secretion remain unknown, exclusive breastfeeding provides a reliable means of birth spacing for the first six to nine months. [396]

RETURN OF FERTILITY IN BREASTFEEDING WOMEN

The return of fertility in breastfeeding women follows a well-defined pattern. In the early stages of breastfeeding, GnRH is almost completely inhibited and there is virtually no ovarian activity. When the frequency and duration of breastfeeding is reduced, the prolactin level falls. Decreased prolactin allows the return of erratic pulsatile secretion of GnRH (with increases in pituitary FSH and LH) which results in some ovarian follicle development and increases in estradiol.

It may take a while before normal ovulatory cycles are restored. Follicle growth may appear normal with selection of a dominant follicle and an increase in estradiol, but there may be either an absence of ovulation or an inadequate corpus luteum. [228] [396] The pattern of ovarian activity follows Brown's continuum – generally seen as amenorrhoea merging into anovulatory cycles, deficient and short luteal phases and finally ovulatory cycles. [67]

Ultrasound studies confirm that the ovaries are not completely inactive during lactational amenorrhoea. Several patterns of follicular development have been observed: multiple follicles, luteinised unruptured follicles, recurrent persistent follicles and delayed ovulation. Both luteinised and persistent unruptured follicles may be accompanied by increased estrogen (and progesterone) and sometimes by long phases of highly fertile-type secretions which are not associated with ovulation. Before the LAM guidelines were in use this caused much anxiety and unnecessary abstinence for couples relying on FAMs. [177]

Although lactation delays menstruation, women can conceive before their first period:

- In the first six months postpartum, although some breastfeeding mothers may ovulate and have a normal length luteal phase before their first menstruation, this is unlikely provided breastfeeding is frequent both day and night. [250]
- After six months postpartum, about 60% of breastfeeding mothers will ovulate before their first period. [250]
- About 60% of women have a short luteal phase preceding their first menstruation after childbirth. [250]
- The abnormal endocrine profile of the first luteal phase offers protection to women within the first six months, but as luteal phases improve women are at increasing risk of pregnancy. [462] [292] [122]
- On average it takes three cycles for full ovulatory function to be restored. Some women will not achieve this status until they have completed weaning. [462] [292] [122]

Factors which may precipitate return of fertility

The following factors may precipitate the return of fertility in breastfeeding mothers:

- less frequent suckling (longer intervals between feeds, particularly at night);
- reduction in total suckling time over 24 hours;
- baby sleeping through the night;
- introduction of supplementary feeds (formula, juice and solids; see page 277);
- separation from baby/returning to work/expressing breast milk;
- anxiety, stress or illness in mother or baby (unlike normal menstrual cycles where stress often delays ovulation, stress may precipitate ovulation); and
- age of baby (fertility will eventually return despite continued breastfeeding).

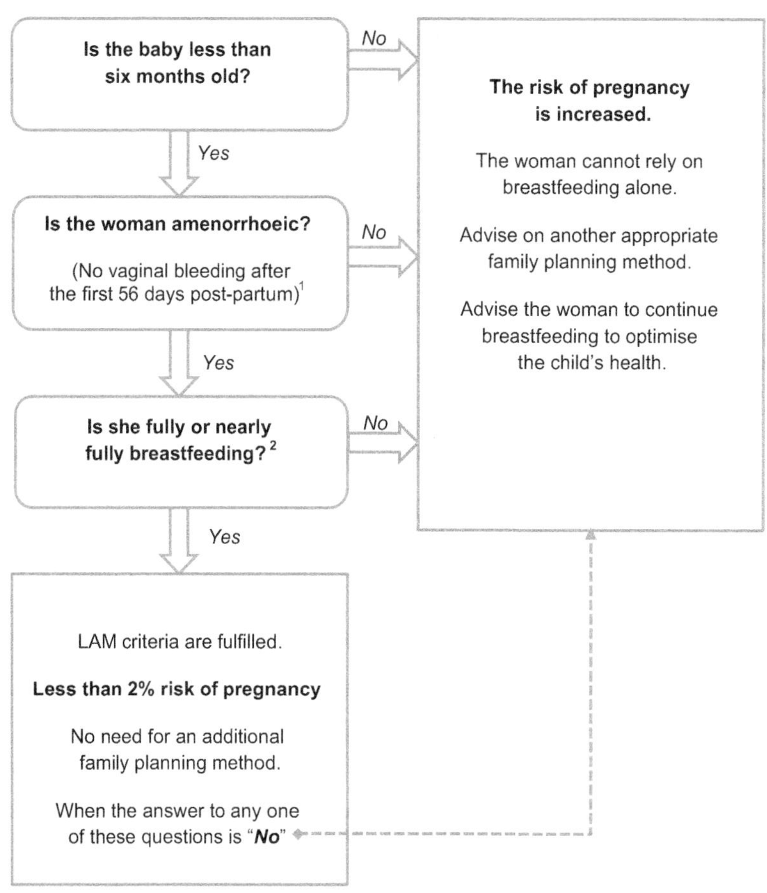

Notes:

1 Bleeding during the first 56 days postpartum is *not* menstruation. It is normal postpartum vaginal loss (lochia): usually bright red for 3–5 days becoming brownish/pink until about day 12 then yellowish/white until about 6 weeks postpartum. Some women have a slight bleed around day 40 postpartum. Lochia which is unusually heavy/persistent or has an offensive odour could indicate postpartum infection.

2 See figure 16.3 for definitions of breastfeeding and its impact on fertility.

Figure 16.2 LAM algorithm showing criteria for use (adapted from Labbok 1994) [342]

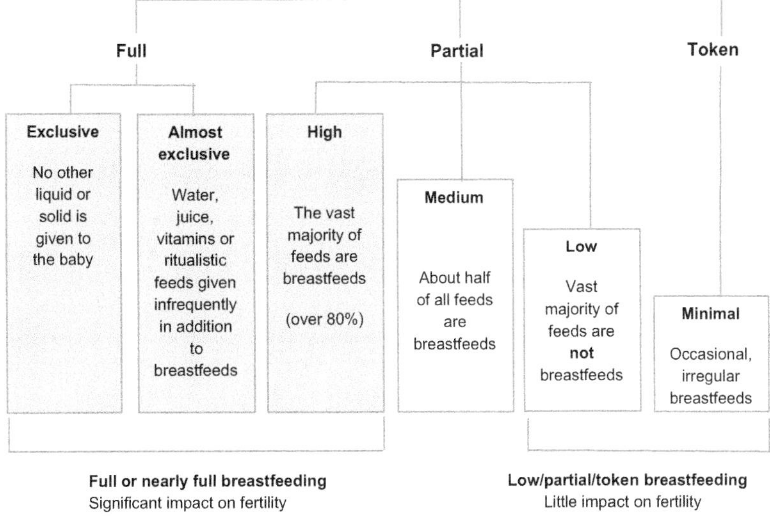

Notes:
Intervals between breastfeeds should not exceed 4 hours during the day or 6 hours at night.
While the high-partial pattern is adequate for fertility suppression, any supplementation or disruption to the breastfeeding pattern, which reduces the amount of suckling, increases the risk of returning fertility.
The use of dummies (pacifiers) should be discouraged.
Expressing breast milk does not have the same fertility-inhibiting effect and reduces the effectiveness of LAM.

Figure 16.3 Definitions of breastfeeding and its impact on fertility (adapted from Labbok 1994) [342]

LACTATIONAL AMENORRHOEA METHOD (LAM)

LAM is a transitional method which is highly effective for postpartum women who plan to breastfeed exclusively for the first six months. It is widely accepted as a FA method that does not require abstinence. [343] LAM is endorsed by FSRH:

- Women may be advised that if they are < 6 months postpartum, amenorrhoeic and fully breastfeeding, LAM is over 98% effective at preventing pregnancy.
- Women using LAM should be advised that the risk of pregnancy is increased if the frequency of breastfeeding decreases (stopping night feeds, supplementary feeding, use of pacifiers/dummies), when menstruation returns or when more than 6 months postpartum. [208] [215]

A woman needs to understand the definitions of amenorrhoea and full breastfeeding (figures 16.2 and 16.3). When any of the three LAM criteria are not met, another family planning method should be started.

Defining first postpartum menstruation

The first postpartum menstruation is defined as:

- any bleeding after day 56 postpartum that is perceived by the woman as a period; or
- at least two consecutive days of bleeding after day 56 postpartum (requiring sanitary protection for at least one day) – whichever come *first*.

Episodes of vaginal bleeding are almost always the consequence of some form of ovarian activity (ovulation, inadequate ovulation or estrogen withdrawal due to collapsed follicle), therefore *any* bleeding must be considered fertile. [326] The woman should begin another method as soon as she notices any bleeding which fits the descriptions. In practice, however, women who have had only one bleed are still likely to have decreased fertility provided that they continue to fully, or nearly fully, breastfeed because the majority of early cycles are anovulatory (or deficient), particularly in the first six months postpartum. [122]

The Human Reproduction Programme rule was developed for the WHO study to confirm the first menstruation (i.e. end of lactational amenorrhoea). The term "menstrual bleeding episode" was used for vaginal bleeding that lasted at least two days and required the use of sanitary protection for at least one day. Any bleeding episodes that occurred within two weeks of the end of lochia were ignored. A bleeding episode was only confirmed (retrospectively) as a *first menstruation* if a second episode (meeting the same criteria) occurred within the next 21–70 days. If a second bleeding episode occurred outside those limits, the first bleed was ignored and the second bleed was defined as the first postpartum menstruation. Only *one* bleeding episode could be discounted. [622] The Human Reproduction Programme rule may be helpful when counselling women who experience a sporadic bleed (most likely anovulatory) during lactational amenorrhoea. It may be safe to ignore a first bleeding episode in this situation, but the woman should understand that although her fertility is still likely to be suppressed, her risk of pregnancy is increased. **Any bleeding after day 56 indicates significantly increased risk of pregnancy.**

Definitions of breastfeeding

The definitions of full, partial and token breastfeeding are shown in figure 16.3. Only full, or nearly full, breastfeeding (with > 80% of feeds being breastfeeds) will have a significant impact on fertility. Note the importance of the intervals between breastfeeds. Any reduction in either the frequency or duration of breastfeeds impacts the contraceptive effect of LAM.

Use of dummies

Breastfeeding acts as both nourishment and comfort for a baby. **Using a dummy as a comforter results in reduced suckling time at the breast and is associated with an earlier return to menstruation.** [296] A study which looked at the effect of dummies on the duration of breastfeeding found that 74% of mothers had started using a dummy by six months. Women who introduced dummies early tended to feed fewer times per day; by 12 weeks these women were more likely to report that breastfeeding was inconvenient and they had insufficient milk supplies. [290]

Effect of expressing breast milk

Women express breast milk for a variety of reasons. It may be vital for mothers with preterm babies who face challenges initiating breastfeeding, but women with healthy term babies may choose to express so that their babies can continue to benefit while someone else is caring for them. Many breastfeeding mothers have responsibilities, including paid work, outside the home. Some rarely or never feed their babies at the breast but exclusively feed them expressed milk. [481] Women who wish to feed their babies expressed breast milk require guidance on safe techniques for its expression and storage to reduce the risk of contamination.

Expressing breast milk does not have the same stimulatory effect as a suckling baby. However, there is evidence that electric pulsatile pumps compare most favourably with natural suckling (both in terms of hormone release and breast milk yield [644]), with simultaneous/double pumping producing a higher yield than sequential pumping. [309] [310] One might speculate that electric pumps would therefore have the strongest suppressant effect on fertility, but further research is needed.

A Chilean study assessed the efficacy of LAM amongst working mothers. Women were taught hand expression to help maintain milk supply while separated from their babies. Almost half of the women managed to breastfeed to six months. Half of the women who were still fully breastfeeding remained amenorrhoeic, while 28% of the women still met the LAM criteria at six months (about half the level found in non-working women). Among working women who were expressing, the pregnancy rate for LAM was 5.2% at six months. [595] This can be compared with 0.45% for non-working women in a similar population. [461] **Women should be informed that the effect of expressing breast milk on the efficacy of LAM is not known but it may be reduced.** [215]

EFFECTIVENESS OF LAM

The effectiveness of LAM is indisputable provided the three criteria are met. After the original Bellagio conference concluded that the risk of pregnancy was less than 2% in the first six months postpartum, a number of studies were conducted to test this opinion. [124] [461] [319] When the experts reviewed the evidence in 1995, they concluded that the consensus had clearly been confirmed. [325] Subsequent studies, in both developed and developing countries, continue to show this very high level of effectiveness. [103] [343] [279] [622] [465] [251] [478]

The WHO study reported cumulative pregnancy rates in the first six months postpartum ranging from 0.9% to 1.2% for women who were fully breastfeeding and amenorrhoeic, with no significant difference between full and partial breastfeeding at either six or 12 months. [622] Labbok reported a 1.5% pregnancy rate at six months and 7.8% at one year for women who continued to rely on breastfeeding alone after six months. [343] Women in Australia, with similar breastfeeding practices to many in the UK (supplementing regularly from around five months), remained amenorrhoeic for over eight months on average, with no pregnancies in the first six months amongst the women who remained amenorrhoeic. [251] **A literature review in 2010 concluded that in the first six months LAM has failure rates between 0.4% to 2.0%,** depending on how lactational amenorrhoea is defined but, **as expected, failure rates are much higher at 12 months (4.4% to 8.8%).** [374]

Recommendations for future research A Cochrane review concluded that fully breastfeeding women who remain amenorrhoeic have a very small risk of becoming pregnant in the first six months after delivery. The reviewers highlighted the importance of definitions being uniform and transparent, suggesting that amenorrhoea should be redefined as "no vaginal blood loss for at least 10 days after postpartum bleeding". They recommended that a control group from the same culture/site is a prerequisite because the length of lactational amenorrhoea in fully breastfeeding women is culture and site specific. [596]

EXTENDING LAM BEYOND SIX MONTHS

The restriction of LAM to the first six months postpartum is conservative. Short estimated the theoretical cumulative probability of conception in a group of Australian breastfeeding mothers (who introduced supplements at an average of five months). Hormonal assays confirmed that all women resumed ovulation while still breastfeeding – confirming that **breastfeeding alone is not an effective contraceptive.** Short estimated that 1.7% of the women would have conceived if meeting the six-month LAM criteria, 7% would have conceived by one year and 13% by two years. The emphasis again was on the need to use other forms of contraception at the first sign of menstruation. [543] A study of breastfeeding mothers in Pakistan reported

Table 16.1 Advantages and disadvantages of Lactational Amenorrhoea Method

Advantages	*Disadvantages*
Highly effective for the first six months postpartum	Requires a high commitment to breastfeeding
Can be used immediately after childbirth	May not fit with demands of a working mother
Universally available/under the woman's control	No protection against STIs including HIV
Requires no medical intervention	Only suitable for women in the first six months postpartum
Requires no drugs or devices	Less suited to women with previous early return of fertility during breastfeeding
Inexpensive	
No religious or moral objections	
Facilitates transition to other methods	
Supports breastfeeding strategies	

a 1.1% pregnancy rate at one year, showing a high degree of contraceptive protection for a full year during lactational amenorrhoea, but *not* after the return of menstruation during breastfeeding. [319]

A programme in Rwanda extended the LAM time-frame to nine months. This was based on Short's theoretical pregnancy rate with recognition of the longer-than-average mean duration of breastfeeding (26 months) and postpartum amenorrhoea (17 months) in Rwandan women. MAMA-9 recommended exclusive breastfeeding for the first six months, after which time women were advised to breastfeed prior to offering supplements. There were no pregnancies amongst the 286 breastfeeding mothers who completed nine months of method use. The mean time until resumption of menstruation was 12.4 months. [103]

Extending LAM to nine months may be acceptable for some women with a strong commitment to breastfeeding, provided that they remain amenorrhoeic. However, women need to understand that there is an **increased risk of pregnancy after six months due to the increasing probability of ovulation with a normal luteal phase prior to the first period.**

WHY DON'T HEALTH PROFESSIONALS PROMOTE LAM?

LAM requires minimal instruction and follow-up and is suited to women's needs in a variety of cultures and health care settings, [465] yet health professionals still lack confidence in its use. The main reasons for not considering LAM include lack of awareness of the method (amongst women and health professionals), belief that there is insufficient breastfeeding in the local population, inadequate information about LAM and concerns about its efficacy. [341] Women need consistent and accurate information from general practitioners, midwives, health visitors, family planning specialists and professional online resources. [447] Local initiatives to produce consumer information and increase awareness of LAM may help to improve knowledge and overcome barriers to its use. [445] [446]

POSTPARTUM FAMILY PLANNING CHOICE

Women need to start using an effective family planning method before they are at risk of another pregnancy. This may be within six weeks of delivery as the general advice for resuming intercourse is as soon as the woman and her partner feel ready. Postpartum family planning aims both to prevent unintended pregnancies and to optimise birth spacing. The choice of method depends on personal beliefs and preferences, cultural practices, level of sexual activity, medical and social factors plus whether the woman is breast- or bottle-feeding (and if breastfeeding, how long she hopes to continue). Consideration must be given for the couple's plans, if any, for further children – to determine whether a short-acting, long-acting or permanent method may be more appropriate. RCOG provides guidance for best practice in postpartum family planning. [500]

LAM as part of method choice

LAM may be an ideal transitional method for a breastfeeding woman who is spacing her family. If a woman is older or subfertile, but desires another child in the future, she may be reluctant to use other methods, whereas a woman who is limiting her family may prefer not to rely on any user-dependent method (see table 16.1 for advantages and disadvantages of LAM). A woman who is using LAM must be ready to start another method while she is still protected by the LAM criteria. In practice this means that she should switch methods when she is preparing to introduce supplementary feeds or approaching six months (or at the first sign of a period), whichever occurs *earliest*. A woman who is switching to FAMs requires the support of an experienced practitioner.

Why use LAM rather than FAMs in the first six months?

LAM is the method of choice for any breastfeeding mother who wishes to use a FA-based method. There is no advantage in using observed indicators while the LAM criteria can be met. Breastfeeding women commonly report intermittent secretions and sometimes prolonged patches of highly fertile-type secretions which are unrelated to fertility (page 269).

An international study compared women's subjective symptoms with urinary metabolites of estrogen and progesterone. The women were all covered by the LAM criteria. Some reports of fertile-type secretions were accurate reflections of underlying ovarian activity and approaching ovulation, but others were deceptive – secretions indicated fertility when in reality there was no estrogen production. The researchers recommended LAM over FAMs for women who meet the criteria. LAM avoids the need to observe indicators for the first six months and avoids unnecessary abstinence or barrier use. The researchers concluded that the risk of pregnancy with LAM is no higher than with observed indicators (and may be lower). [326]

When new breastfeeding mothers in New Zealand were offered the choice between LAM or FAMs, 57% chose LAM because of its simplicity. Forty-nine percent of the LAM users were able to use the method for the full six months, but less than 20% of the FAM users were still fully breastfeeding and amenorrhoeic at six months. None of the LAM users conceived, but there were two pregnancies in the FAMs group. [187]

TRANSITION FROM LAM TO FAMS

Ideally a woman would start to observe her fertility indicators at least two weeks before she anticipates that she will no longer meet the LAM criteria. [334] [474] Although bleeding is the first sign of fertility for many women, some will ovulate before their first period and may have a normal ovulatory cycle, hence risk moving straight from one pregnancy to another.

Combined-indicator methods Studies show that breastfeeding mothers can detect signs of fertility with reasonable accuracy, but only about half of the days that women designated fertile were deemed to be fertile based on hormonal profiles. [324] Fertility indicators can be particularly confusing for a woman who continues to breastfeed after her periods have returned (lactational menses). She is no longer covered by LAM but does not have the reassurance of regular cycles. A study which looked specifically at fertility indicators during the first three cycles after the cessation of lactational amenorrhoea found a lack of correlation between LH and the temperature rise in the first cycle, but improvements in subsequent cycles. Luteal phase lengths were initially deficient but improved over time. [643]

Persona Persona is not recommended for breastfeeding women. A woman should wait until she has had at least two normal periods, with cycle length of 23 – 35 days, before starting the monitor at the beginning of her third period.

Simplified methods Some women may be suited to using either the SDM "Bridge"or the Two Day Method. This may be particularly appropriate for women who are spacing their family, so are planning another child in the future (page 194).

ESTABLISHING THE BIP

During lactation, estrogen levels remain low, sometimes for many weeks or months, before the return of ovulation or the first menstruation. This persistently low estrogen is observed as the BIP – this is *exclusive* to breastfeeding women. The BIP must be established as an unchanging pattern over at least two weeks (figure 16.4).

BIP (secretions)

Some women will experience a continuous pattern of dryness whereas others will experience a continuous moistness. The woman must observe at intervals throughout the day and record an *unchanging* pattern for two full weeks before she can be assured that it is her BIP.

- BIP dryness: This implies a continuous pattern of dry days (infertile). Any secretions must be considered potentially fertile.
- BIP moistness: This implies a continuous pattern of secretions producing a moist sensation. Secretions may feel sticky and appear white/milky. The essential features are the unchanging characteristics. Days established as a BIP of moistness are infertile; similarly, dry days occurring during a BIP of moistness are infertile.

Temperature

The temperature in some breastfeeding women shows greater day-to-day variations (swinging temperature) characteristic of the natural infertility associated with breastfeeding. (figure 16.4).

Cervix

By about 12 weeks postpartum, the cervix will have returned to its non-pregnant state and can then be checked. A woman who has previously been aware of her cervix will notice distinct changes following childbirth, particularly after the first birth. The parous os remains slightly dilated at all times, even when the cervix is in its infertile state. It may take some time to adjust to these changes. The cervix should remain at the same height and position, with the same consistency and degree of dilatation, for two weeks to establish its basic infertile state. Days on which the cervix is low, firm, closed and tilted are infertile. Any change from the infertile state indicates fertility.

RECOGNISING SIGNS OF FERTILITY

Once the woman has established her BIP, any bleeding, change in secretions or the cervix could indicate approaching fertility (figure 16.5).

Bleeding

Any bleeding (after 56 days postpartum) is potentially fertile (page 271).

Cervical secretions

Any change from the BIP of dryness indicates potential fertility: this includes any change from the sensation of dryness (to stickiness/moistness/wetness) or any visible secretions. Any change from the BIP of moistness indicates potential fertility: this includes any change in the quantity, colour or consistency of secretions. Intermittent patches of secretions may reflect increased ovarian activity so must be considered fertile. Many women get anxious about these patches but find (retrospectively) that their first presumed ovulation was accompanied by profuse amounts of wetter secretions. Any secretions which do not conform to the BIP must be considered fertile.

Temperature

Although temperature has no predictive value for women of normal fertility, in some lactating women it may indicate returning fertility. As the ovaries become increasingly active, and estrogen levels rise, the swinging temperature stabilises. It may be at a slightly lower level than the usual coverline in a normal fertile cycle. A Canadian study reported that this levelling occurred in a significant number of women for one or more weeks before the temperature rise. [450] Temperature changes are interesting but cannot be relied on.

Cervix

Any change in the height, position, consistency or dilatation of the cervix indicates fertility. Cervical changes often provide the earliest sign of approaching fertility. The cervix (in a woman with an anteverted uterus) rises higher in the vagina and becomes more centrally positioned, straighter and softer, with an open cervical os. In a woman with a retroverted uterus, the first sign of approaching fertility is when the cervix drops lower, becomes more centrally positioned, softer and more open.

SUPPLEMENTARY FEEDS AND WEANING

The introduction of supplementary feeds – which includes formula, juice and solids (weaning) – is likely to precipitate the return of fertility, so this is a time when a woman needs to be extra vigilant. A study of 27 breastfeeding mothers monitored the effect of supplementary feeds on the suckling pattern and ovarian activity (using hormonal assays). None of the women ovulated during full breastfeeding, but two showed evidence of follicular activity. The introduction of supplements was associated with an abrupt decrease in both the duration and frequency of suckling. The rate at which supplements were introduced influenced not only the suckling frequency and duration, but also the resumption of ovulation. **Ovulation and conception are more common after a sharp decrease in suckling time and frequency.**

> As a general rule, an abrupt/rapid introduction of supplementary feeds or weaning usually results in a rapid return to normal fertility, whereas gradual/slow weaning (prolonged over weeks or months) generally results in a slower return to normal fertility. [291]

If a breastfeeding mother wishes to rely on the infertility associated with lactational amenorrhoea, she must suckle at least five times per day with a total suckling duration of more than 65 minutes per day (> 10 minutes per feed). Any reduction below either of these limits results in a return of fertility. [397] In an Italian study of 40 breastfeeding mothers (using ultrasound as a marker), 20% had their first menstruation before weaning, but none of the women had an adequate luteal phase, whereas 80% had their first menstruation after weaning with 37% showing an adequate luteal phase. [581]

CASE STUDY ABRUPT WEANING

Zoe was breastfeeding at least six times per day. She had to return to work so started introducing formula and solids at 20 weeks and had completely stopped breastfeeding within two weeks. As she reduced her breastfeeds, she was aware of secretions with increasingly fertile characteristics and avoided intercourse. Her temperature rise occurred six days after her last breastfeed and her period started 13 days later.

CASE STUDY GRADUAL WEANING

Liz was giving up to 10 breastfeeds per day. She introduced solids at 16 weeks and planned to wean her baby gradually. She remained amenorrhoeic but observed intermittent patches of secretions. At 26 weeks, when the baby was having three meals per day and five breastfeeds, Liz recorded her first temperature rise followed by an eight-day luteal phase. Her next cycle was 29 days with a nine-day luteal phase, followed by a 32 day cycle with a 13-day luteal phase. Her full fertility was restored by week 36 while still breastfeeding twice a day (20 weeks after starting solids).

RECORDING ON BREASTFEEDING CHART

The breastfeeding mother can record her fertility indicators, feeding pattern and information about her baby on a specialised breastfeeding chart (figure 16.4). The eight-week chart allows time to see a pattern of emerging fertility so is well-suited to a woman who is still amenorrhoeic and may have a lengthy interval approaching her first ovulation or first menstruation. Once the woman has started menstruating again, she can switch to the usual 40-day chart.

Information about baby

The woman should record the following information about her baby on the breastfeeding chart:

- Baby's age in weeks
- Number of breastfeeds (with estimate of total suckling time)
- Longest interval between feeds (over 24 hours)
- Notes on the baby's appetite, alterations in suckling vigour, illness or upsets such as teething or immunisations

Information about mother

The woman should record the following personal information on the breastfeeding chart:

- Waking temperature (note if recording time is affected by night feeds)
- Cervical secretions: BIP of dryness or moistness and any alteration from BIP

- Bleeding episodes (including spotting)
- Cervical changes (can be recorded after 12 weeks postpartum)
- Any disturbances, disruption to routine or change in circumstances (e.g. holiday)
- Illness and drugs (suitable for breastfeeding mothers)
- Breast milk expression and times of separation from the baby

GUIDELINES TO AVOID PREGNANCY DURING BREASTFEEDING

These guidelines apply to women who continue to breastfeed but no longer meet the LAM criteria.

Basic Infertile Pattern

The BIP rules only apply to women who have not yet had their first postpartum period or their first postpartum temperature rise (first presumed ovulation).

- Intercourse should be avoided on any days of bleeding and for the following three days.
- Intercourse is allowed on non-consecutive evenings only during the BIP. The day after intercourse is marked with an "X" as a non-intercourse day.
- Intercourse should be avoided at the first sign of any change from the BIP (by cervical secretions, or cervix), while the fertile signs last and for three days after return to the BIP. (This allows time to ensure that the BIP has been re-established). Intercourse can be resumed on the evening of the fourth day.

Identifying the first temperature rise

In order to identify the first postpartum temperature rise, a horizontal coverline is drawn on the line immediately above the highest of the low-phase temperatures. The coverline should be extended as far back as possible, excluding any disturbances. This allows time to ensure that a swinging temperature has settled. There must be at least six low temperatures. There should be at least four temperatures at the higher level.

Intercourse can be resumed on the evening of the fourth high temperature, provided that all high temperatures are at least 0.2 deg.C above the low readings and all high temperatures are after peak day. The luteal phase may be shorter in the first postpartum cycle.

Subsequent cycles

Once the first postpartum temperature rise has been confirmed the following guidelines apply.

Early relatively infertile time

- Only non-consecutive dry days are relatively infertile with intercourse restricted to evenings.
- Calculations to identify the first fertile day (*Day 6 rule, S minus 20* and *earliest temperature rise minus* 7) must be recalculated following the re-establishment of normal fertile cycles (see figure 7.1 in chapter 7).

Late infertile time

Intercourse can be resumed on the evening of the third high temperatures provided it is at least 0.2 deg.C above the low temperatures and all high temperatures are after peak day.

RECORDING RETURNING FERTILITY ON BREASTFEEDING CHART

Figure 16.4 shows a breastfeeding chart from 26–33 weeks postpartum. The woman has relied on LAM for the first six months. At week 26 she is still fully breastfeeding and amenorrhoeic. She observed her secretions from five months postpartum and has established a BIP of dryness (unchanging > 2 weeks). She is breastfeeding six to eight times per day with a maximum interval of six hours at night. She starts to introduce solids in week 28, gradually reducing the number of breastfeeds while increasing the number of supplements. Her temperature shows wide day-to-day variation and her cervix remains low, firm and closed. After introducing solids, she starts to notice intermittent patches of secretions. She records unprotected intercourse using an "I" ensuring that she marks the following day with an "X". When she notices any moistness/visible secretions that are unrelated to intercourse, she avoids intercourse for those days and for the following three days, ensuring that her BIP of dryness is re-established. She indicates times of potential fertility with a horizontal arrow.

Figure 16.5 shows a chart from the same woman from 34–41 weeks postpartum. The number of breastfeeds are decreasing as she increases solids. The baby is sleeping for longer at night, with intervals of up to 10 hours. She notices the first change in her cervix in week 35. By week 38 her cervix is showing signs of softness which builds up to a high soft open cervix, correlating with a build-up of secretions to peak day in week 40. Her temperature rises to the higher level and she counts four high temperatures that are all at least 0.2 deg.C above the low readings. Intercourse is resumed after the fourth high temperature past peak day. Note that the coverline has been extended backwards to ensure that the temperature has stabilised. In this situation the temperature has provided an extra indicator of approaching fertility, but this pattern is not consistent for all breastfeeding women. Analysing these charts *retrospectively,* it is apparent that some intermittent changes in the cervix and its secretions were unrelated to fertility. With hindsight, much of the abstinence was unnecessary but a woman can act only on the information available at the time.

COMBINING OBSERVATIONS WITH FERTILITY MONITOR

Researchers at Marquette University developed a postpartum protocol that uses a fertility monitor to identify the return of fertility (for a modified version of the Marquette Model, see page 136). The protocol can be used by women who are breast- or bottle-feeding. Users record information on bleeding and secretions; they reset the monitor at 20-day intervals during lactational amenorrhoea and at the start of each period. Of the 198 women who recorded information for one year, there were two unintended pregnancies with correct use and eight with typical use. The researchers concluded that the online protocol may assist a select group of women to avoid pregnancy during the transition to regular cycles. [59]

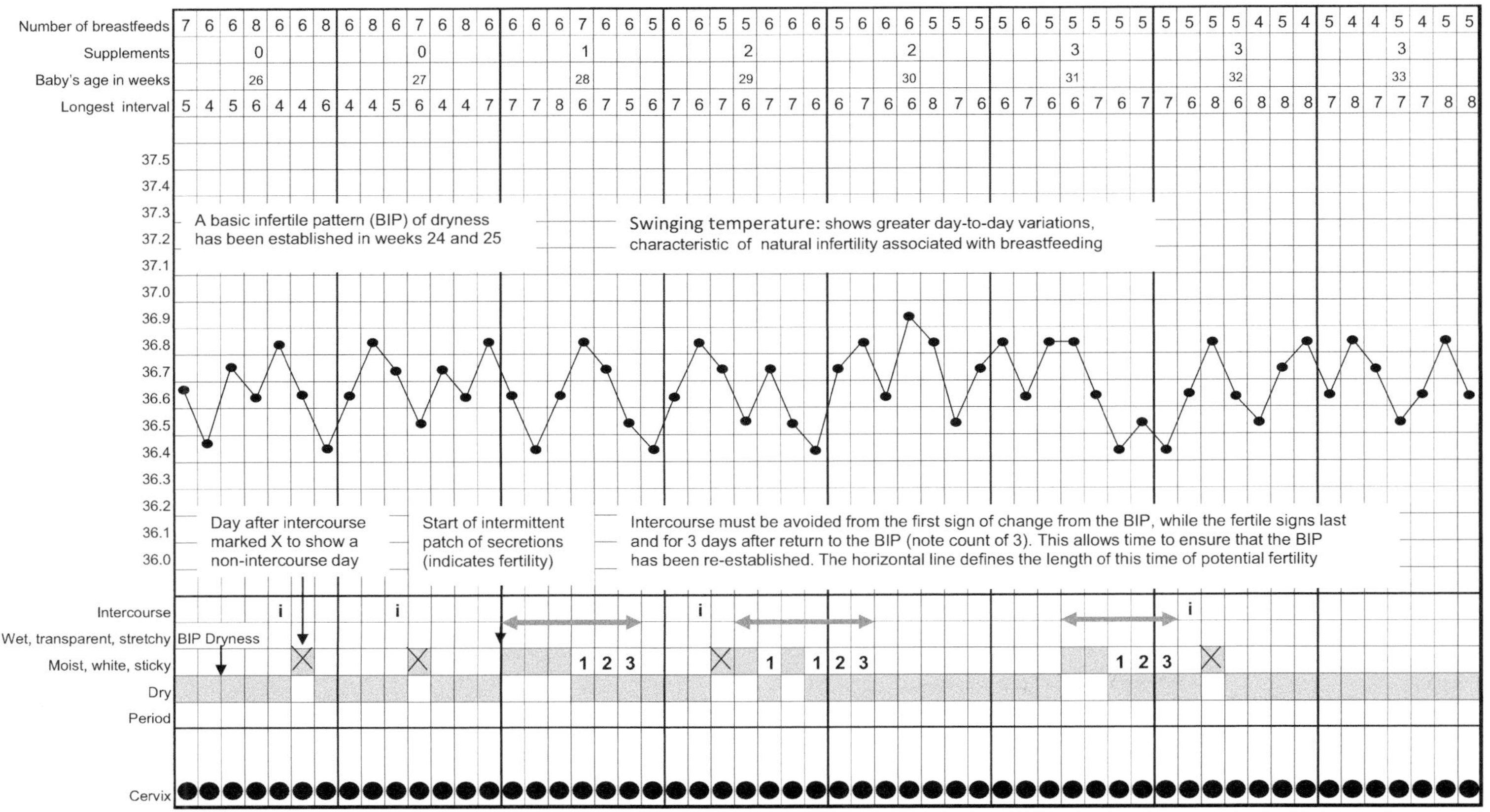

Figure 16.4 Basic infertile pattern during breastfeeding and introduction of solids (the BIP has been established as unchanging from week 24–26)

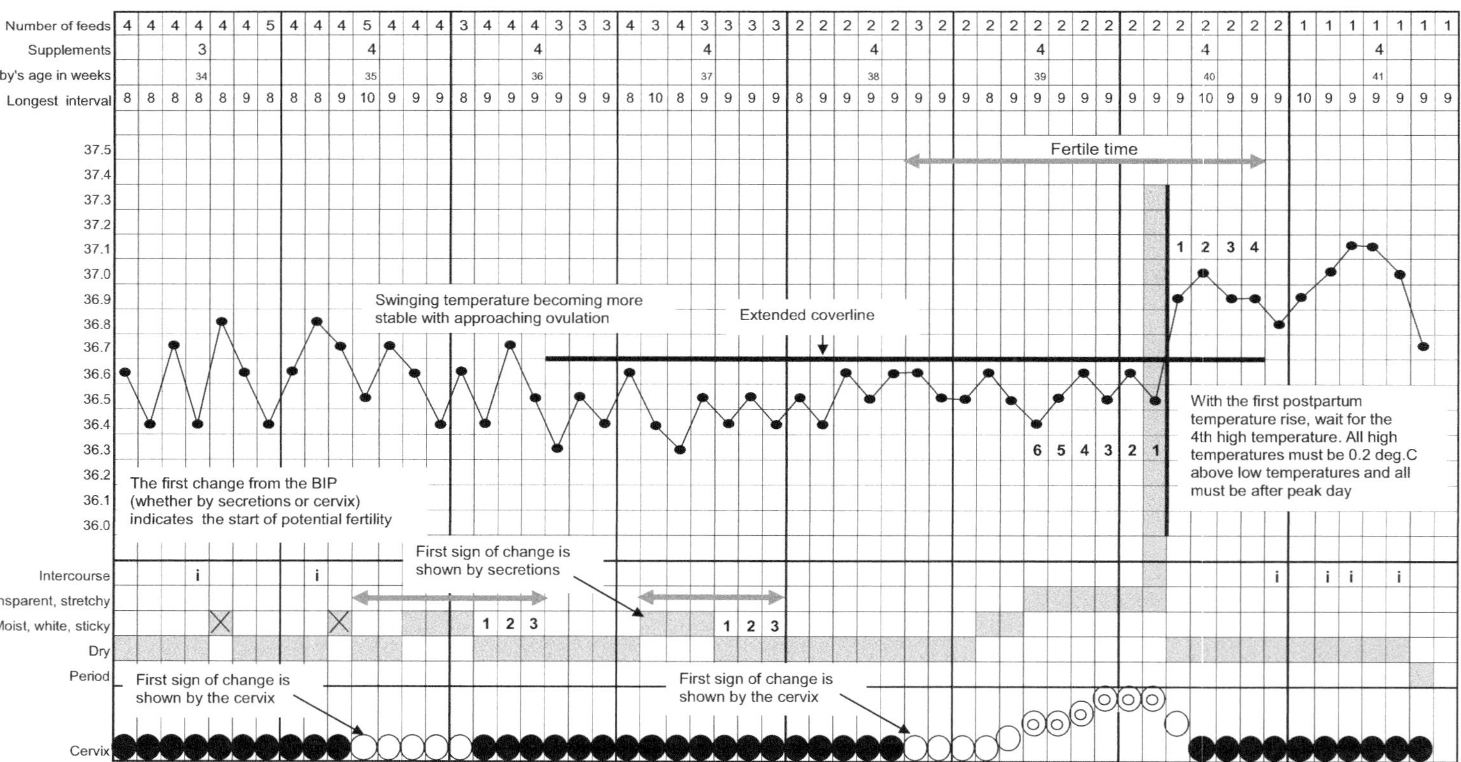

Figure 16.5 Return of fertility during weaning

CASE STUDY RELACTATION

Katie was breastfeeding her second baby, Tom, but struggling with the demands of a toddler. She hoped that introducing formula could allow her partner to share the feeding. Tom took well to the bottle and by 17 weeks he was completely formula-fed. Katie was charting her cycles and recorded fertile-type secretions followed by a temperature rise in week 18. She had her first period in week 20 following a normal length luteal phase. In week 21, Tom developed a viral infection and completely refused the bottle. In desperation, Katie put him to the breast and he started suckling. After over a month since her last breastfeed Katie re-established full breastfeeding. Her fertility was quickly suppressed again and she resumed a BIP of dryness with a swinging temperature.

RETURN OF FERTILITY IN WOMEN WHO DO NOT BREASTFEED

If a woman bottle-feeds her baby from birth, or breastfeeds for less than one month, her prolactin levels decline rapidly, FSH and LH levels increase and ovarian activity returns rapidly. [229] The return of fertility varies but is generally rapid:

- Most women have their first menstruation about six to eight weeks after delivery, but it may be delayed until 10 weeks or longer (menstruation has been reported as early as five weeks).
- Some women will ovulate as early as the fourth week postpartum (although the fertility potential of these very early ovulations is not well established).
- Up to 70% of women will ovulate before their first period and up to 60% of first ovulations are estimated to be potentially fertile.

A new mother who does not breastfeed must understand that she could ovulate within the first month and conceive again before she has her first period. Postpartum contraception must be considered from day 21. [208] [303] In women who have medical suppression of lactation, ovulation may occur as early as day 18. [487]

Howie's study, which compared the return of fertility in bottle- and breastfeeding mothers, reported that the first menstruation occurred at an average of eight weeks in the bottle-feeders compared with 32 weeks in the breastfeeders. First ovulations occurred at an average of 11 and 36 weeks respectively. Regular ovulatory cycles were quickly established, with ovulation occurring in 94% of the bottle-feeding women on the second and subsequent cycles. By comparison in the breastfeeding women the frequency of ovulatory cycles increased progressively but did not return to normal until weaning was complete. [292]

GUIDELINES FOR WOMEN WHO DO NOT BREASTFEED

A woman who wishes to use FAMs should start recording her fertility indicators from two to three weeks postpartum. The following guidelines should be applied:

- In the first cycle, intercourse may be resumed on the evening of the *fourth* high temperature (provided that all high temperatures are at least 0.2 deg.C above the low temperatures), with all high temperatures occurring after peak.

- On the second and subsequent cycles, intercourse can be resumed on the evening of the *third* high temperature (provided the third high temperature is at least 0.2 deg.C above the low temperatures), with all high temperatures occurring after peak day.
- Intercourse can be resumed on non-consecutive dry evenings in the early infertile time from the second cycle onwards.
- The *Day 6 rule, S minus 20* and *earliest temperature rise minus 7* to identify the first fertile day must be recalculated following the re-establishment of normal fertile cycles (see figure 7.1 in chapter 7).

Learning FAMs at times of change is always more difficult and may involve lengthy times of abstinence or barrier use until regular cycles are re-established.

SELF-ASSESSMENT QUESTIONS

Answers are at the end of the chapter.

1 What is the optimal duration of exclusive breastfeeding?
2 What are the three criteria for the use of LAM?
3 Define "fully" and "nearly fully" breastfeeding.
4 Define the first postpartum menstruation.
5 What is the earliest ovulation in women who do not breastfeed?

POSTPARTUM SEXUAL DIFFICULTIES

Although many couples are able to resume a healthy sex life within weeks of delivery, others may still not have resumed intercourse by six months. The main postpartum risk factor for dyspareunia (pain on penetration/during intercourse and/or pain at orgasm) is the extent of the birth injury. In the first three months after delivery, women (particularly primiparous women) commonly report loss of desire, vaginal tightness (or loss of tone), lack of vaginal lubrication and dyspareunia. Sexual difficulties are more commonly reported by women with perineal damage related to episiotomy, particularly following instrumental deliveries (forceps or ventouse), but women who have had C-sections may also experience problems. [33] [208] [69]

Loss of libido, vaginal dryness and painful intercourse is more common in breastfeeding women, possibly due to low levels of estrogen. A water-based lubricant can provide effective relief, but should be used with caution by women who are relying on cervical secretions as an indicator of returning fertility (page 130).

Women's sexuality during breastfeeding is varied. Motherhood can be exhausting – whether breastfeeding and caring for a first baby, or juggling the demands of a boisterous toddler. Fatigue adversely impacts libido, hence many women report that sexual activity occurs only in response to the demands of their partner. Some women, however, report increased libido and may experience sensual or sexual pleasure related to breastfeeding. Although this is rarely talked about, this is completely normal and not something for women to feel anxious or guilty about. [8]

About 1 in 10 women are affected by postnatal depression and may show symptoms of anxiety, depression, fatigue, failure to cope, guilt, low self-confidence and self-esteem (plus low libido). Women who are at risk of postpartum mental health issues need to be identified and assessed early (see RCOG guidance on perinatal mental health [491]).

PLANNING NEXT PREGNANCY

There is strong evidence from large population-based studies that optimal birth spacing is achieved by allowing 18 months or more between pregnancies. Following an inter-birth interval of less than 18 months, babies have a higher risk of being born preterm, of low birth weight or small for gestational age. [542] [117]

Prolonging the duration of breastfeeding optimises birth spacing, but many women are keen to complete their families in a relatively short time. This may be of particular concern for women who are older or have experienced past delays in conceiving. Such women may need to curtail breastfeeding to allow earlier resumption of normal fertility. This can create significant dilemmas for a woman who is considering stopping breastfeeding one child (which she rationalises could be her only child) in an effort to create a sibling. The balance has to be struck between the baby's need for optimum nutrition and comfort, the woman's emotional attachment to breastfeeding, and her anxieties about future fertility. It may not be necessary to completely stop breastfeeding. Some women will regain normal fertility if they significantly reduce the number of breastfeeds, particularly if they stop night feeds; but others will have anovulatory cycles or inadequate luteal phases for several months before full fertility is restored and conception is possible.

CASE STUDY PLANNED PREGNANCY WHILE BREASTFEEDING

Jess was a 39-year-old first-time mother. Her son, Luke, was conceived on her third IVF cycle following years of unexplained infertility. She wanted him to have a sibling and hoped to have a further IVF cycle after he was fully weaned. Jess reduced her breastfeeds from 28 weeks onwards. She had her first period at 30 weeks and another at 34 weeks. She was delighted to see profuse amounts of clear wet secretions in week 36 followed by a temperature rise and then a further rise in week 38. A pregnancy test confirmed conception following timed intercourse while she was still breastfeeding twice a day.

ANSWERS TO SELF-ASSESSMENT QUESTIONS

1. Six months
2. Less than six months postpartum, amenorrhoeic (after the first 56 days) and fully or nearly fully breastfeeding
3. Full breastfeeding means that the mother is giving no other liquid or solids (apart from infrequent water, juice, vitamins or ritualistic feeds). Nearly full breastfeeding means that more than 80% of feeds are breastfeeds.
4. Any bleeding after day 56 postpartum that is perceived by the woman as a period, or at least two consecutive days of bleeding after day 56 postpartum (requiring sanitary protection for at least one day) – whichever comes first
5. The fourth postpartum week

17 FAMs DURING THE PERI-MENOPAUSE

The menopause is a significant life-event marking the end of a woman's reproductive lifespan. For most women the menopause (final menstrual period) occurs between 45 and 55 years (average 51 in the UK) but this varies widely. Up to 5% of women will experience premature ovarian insufficiency (POI) leading to menopause before 40 – these women require special consideration (page 211).

By their mid-40s most women have completed their families and are finding new areas of fulfilment in career, work or further study. Some may have adult offspring and be helping out with grandchildren. An unintended pregnancy at this stage could have significant physical, psychological and social repercussions. Women need to understand the need for continued use of effective contraception despite perceptions of loss of fertility related to advanced age or menstrual irregularities (page 12).

FSRH provides guidance on contraceptive choice for older women, including advice on the age at which contraception can permanently be stopped. [210] The most commonly used methods in women over 40 are sterilisation (either partner), the contraceptive pill, male condoms and intrauterine methods. It is not known how many rely on FAMs because many do not present for health professional advice. FAMs may provide very adequate contraception at a time of declining fertility, [267] but the support of a specialist practitioner is vital – both for new and experienced users. [215]

The NICE menopause guidelines provide a framework for the diagnosis of menopause and peri-menopause, plus the management of menopausal symptoms. The guidelines review the evidence for the long-term benefits and risks of HRT plus the role of non-hormonal, herbal and other therapies such as cognitive behavioural therapy. The guidelines emphasise the importance of individualised management and the referral of women with complex issues to health professionals with expertise in menopause. [429]

Stages of reproductive ageing

The STRAW staging system (developed in 2001 at the Stages of Reproductive Ageing Workshop) defines the stages of reproductive ageing through the menopause. The recommendations were revised and extended in 2011 on the basis of new data on ovarian reserve testing. [554] [266]

Figure 17.1 provides a visual representation of the stages from menarche to menopause. The adult female lifespan is divided into three broad phases: the reproductive years, menopausal transition and post-menopausal years. These phases are sub-divided before and after the menopause (point 0). Despite advances in the understanding of diminishing ovarian reserve (page 326) there are limited data on these markers from normal fertile women, with no agreed international standards. Menstrual cycle characteristics therefore remain the most important criteria.

Late reproductive stage Fecundability starts to decline during the late reproductive years. AMH levels and antral follicle count decrease to a low level (during stage –3b) but the woman

Menarche ↓							Menopause (0) ↓		
Terminology	REPRODUCTIVE YEARS				MENOPAUSAL TRANSITION		POST-MENOPAUSE		
	Early	Peak	Late		Early	Late	Early		Late
					← *Peri-menopause*		→		
Stage	–5	–4	–3b	–3a	–2	–1	+1a | +1b	+1c	+2
Duration of time	*Variable length of time*				*Variable*	1–3 years	2 years (1+1)	3–6 years	Remaining lifespan
Principal criteria *Menstrual cycle characteristics*	Variable at first then becoming regular	Regular cycles	Regular cycles	Subtle changes in menstrual flow and cycle length. Cycles <24 days are typical	Variable length. Persistent difference of 7+ days in length of consecutive cycles	Interval of amenorrhoea of >60 days	Amenorrhoea	Amenorrhoea	Amenorrhoea
Fertility awareness observations (not included in STRAW)	High % monophasic cycles and short luteal phases	Biphasic cycles with adequate luteal phases (optimum)	Mostly normal biphasic cycles with adequate luteal phases	Short luteal phases common. Some monophasic cycles	Increasing percentage of monophasic cycles	High % of monophasic cycles and short luteal phases	Temperature remains consistently monophasic throughout. Stop recording after 1 year	Intermittent patches of secretions but these are infertile	Occasional patches of secretions but these are infertile
Supportive criteria *FSH (cycle day 2–5)* *Anti-mullerian hormone* *Antral follicle count*		Low Normal Normal	Low Low Low	Variable Low Low	↑ Variable Low Low	↑ >25IU/L** Low Low	↑ Variable Low Very low	Stablises Very low Very low	
Descriptive characteristics *Menopausal symptoms*						Vasomotor symptoms likely	Vasomotor symptoms most likely		Increasing urogenital symptoms

Figure 17.1 The stages of reproductive ageing (adapted from STRAW + 10 [266])

continues to have regular cycles and her FSH remains low. Subtle changes then start to occur in menstrual flow and cycle length (stage –3a): this typically includes cycles of less than 24 days. Note that very short or very long cycles are significantly more likely to be anovulatory (page 111).

A woman who is aware of her fertility will be alerted to early cyclic changes. She may record short luteal phases, monophasic cycles, and a shorter duration of secretions with reduced quantity and quality. Figures 4.13 and 4.14 in chapter 4 illustrate the frequency of monophasic cycles by gynaecological age and the age-related distribution of different cycle types. The late reproductive stage lasts for a variable length of time.

Early menopausal transition The early menopausal transition (stage –2) is marked by increased variability in cycle length, defined as a persistent difference of seven days or more in the length of consecutive cycles ("persistent" is defined as recurrence within 10 cycles of the first variable-length cycle). FSH levels start to rise but are variable. Cycles with short luteal phases and monophasic cycles are increasingly common. There may be an increased number of dry days. This phase lasts for a variable length of time.

Late menopausal transition During the late menopausal transition (stage –1) cycles vary increasingly in length with some cycles of 60 days or longer. FSH levels are elevated into the menopausal range and estradiol levels are low. FSH levels greater than 25 IU/L from a random blood test are characteristic of the late menopausal transition (agreed levels for FSH vary dependent on the assay). This stage lasts for one to three years, during which time a woman is likely to notice vasomotor symptoms.

Early post-menopause The early post-menopause phase marks the time when FSH levels continue to increase and estradiol levels continue to decrease for approximately two years after the menopause, after which time they stabilise. Stage +1a marks the end of the year, which confirms that the final menstrual period has occurred (end of peri-menopause). Stage +1b includes the remaining time of rapid change in FSH and estradiol, which is associated with the most likely occurrence of vasomotor symptoms. FSH and estradiol levels then stabilise over the next three to six years (stage +1c).

Late post-menopause The late post-menopause phase (stage +2) is the time when many women experience symptoms related to loss of elasticity and thinning of vaginal and urethral tissue (urogenital atrophy).

Do women move consistently through stages?

Data from the TREMIN study were used to test the STRAW stages and determine whether women move uniformly from pre- to peri- to post-menopause. One hundred women provided annual self-reports of menopausal stage (over 3–12 years) based on their cycle characteristics: "regular", "changing" or "menopausal". The most common pattern fitted with the STRAW stages, but some women moved unpredictably between stages. and others moved directly from regular bleeding to menopause. [372]

Applicability of STRAW staging

STRAW staging is not based on age, but on the time before and after the final menstrual period (similar to the concept of gynaecological age based on the time following the menarche). STRAW staging is therefore applicable to most women irrespective of age, demographic, BMI or lifestyle characteristics such as smoking. However, there are some exceptions: women who have menstrual disturbance due to ovulation disorders (such as PCOS or hypothalamic amenorrhoea), weight-related amenorrhoea, chronic illness or POI may not fit easily into the STRAW criteria.

Definitions

Menopause The stage in a woman's life when she stops menstruating. The menopause (final menstrual period) can be recognised only retrospectively one year later. The menopause marks the end of reproductive life. The associated physical and psychological changes occur because the ovaries stop functioning and no longer produce estrogen and progesterone.

Menopausal women Includes women in peri-menopause and post-menopause.

Menopausal symptoms Includes all symptoms associated with the peri- and post-menopause.

Peri-menopause The time around the menopause starting when ovulation and menstruation become irregular: this ends one year after the final period. The peri-menopause is also referred to as the "menopausal transition" or the "climacteric". This time is usually accompanied by vasomotor symptoms (hot flushes and night sweats).

Pre-menopause The variable number of months or years preceding the menopause, during which time there are changes in menstrual cycle characteristics sometimes accompanied by vasomotor and urogenital symptoms.

Post-menopause The time after menopause has occurred, starting one year after the final menstrual period.

These definitions are in line with NICE guidelines. The term "pre-menopause" in this text implies times of change approaching menopause, but some use it to imply the female reproductive years (i.e. *any* time before the menopause).

PHYSIOLOGY OF REPRODUCTIVE AGEING

The transition from the reproductive years to post-menopausal infertility effectively mirrors the events at puberty and the start of reproductive life. A girl's first period (menarche) is preceded by increasing amounts of estrogen recognisable by the development of the breasts and pubic hair, female fat distribution, and the maturation of the genital tract. The menarche is followed by irregular, anovulatory cycles and cycles with inadequate luteal phases. Over a few years, cycles mature to regular ovulatory cycles with an adequate luteal phase capable of supporting pregnancy – the woman has reached her peak reproductive years.

Towards the end of reproductive life, a woman's ovarian reserve declines rapidly, her ovaries become less responsive to FSH and LH and produce less estrogen. The levels of female sex hormones fluctuate almost daily but over time there is a gradual increase in FSH, then of LH and a fall in levels of estradiol (and inhibin). Menstrual cycles become irregular, luteal phases become inadequate and there are an increasing number of anovulatory cycles. Finally, the ovaries completely fail to respond to increased FSH stimulation, hence ovulation and menstruation permanently cease.

As estrogen levels decline, body fat distribution changes, resulting in an accumulation of fat around the waist, more typical of male fat distribution. The reduced hormonal stimulation of the uterus, breasts and vagina leads to shrinkage of breast tissue, vaginal dryness and thinning of the vaginal walls. When a woman has been amenorrhoeic for one year since her menopause she is considered post-menopausal. The main source of estrogen then becomes the weaker estrone produced by the adrenal glands and body fat. Women who are slightly fatter at the start of the menopausal transition may therefore have less severe symptoms due to their relatively high levels of estrone.

MENOPAUSAL SYMPTOMS

Menopausal symptoms are related to decreased estrogen. By the time a woman reaches post-menopause her estrogen levels will have decreased by about tenfold. The majority of women experience symptoms typically lasting about four years, although about 10% of women experience symptoms for up to 12 years. Women whose menopause is surgically induced (e.g. post-hysterectomy) or chemically induced (e.g. following chemotherapy) may suffer debilitating symptoms related to rapid decrease in estrogen.

The most significant feature of the peri-menopause is menstrual irregularity, but as estrogen receptors are found in the genital tract, breasts, bone, brain and the cardiovascular system, symptoms may be widespread. Menopausal symptoms include:

- vasomotor symptoms, including hot flushes, night sweats and heart palpitations often leading to sleep disturbance and insomnia, tiredness and lethargy;
- musculo-skeletal symptoms such as joint and muscle stiffness and pains;
- accumulation of central body fat, particularly intra-abdominal fat;
- mood changes such as increased anxiety, panic attacks, loss of confidence, low mood, depression, irritability, difficulty concentrating and impaired memory;
- urogenital symptoms, including vaginal dryness, soreness, irritation, itching, urinary frequency, nocturia, urgency and recurrent urinary tract infections; and
- sexual difficulties such as loss of libido, lack of arousal, painful intercourse and difficulties with orgasm.

The occurrence of symptoms in menopausal women should not automatically be assumed to be hormonal: symptoms could be related to stress or pathological conditions such as thyroid disease. Women should be encouraged to report any disturbing symptoms, including abnormal vaginal discharge, breast changes, heavy bleeding/flooding, bleeding between periods, bleeding after intercourse or bleeding after menopause.

Women who have reached post-menopause have an increased risk of metabolic syndrome leading to an increased risk of type 2 diabetes and cardiovascular disease. [582] Post-menopausal women are at increased risk of osteoporosis, breast and gynaecological cancers and dementia. Guidance on all aspects of post-reproductive health is available from the British Menopause Society (www.thebms.org.uk).

PROS AND CONS OF HORMONE REPLACEMENT THERAPY (HRT)

HRT aims to alleviate menopausal symptoms by supplementing the woman's decreased hormone levels with estrogen (and progestogen) in the form of pills, patches, gels or implants. Many women report dramatic improvements in vasomotor and urogenital symptoms plus improvements in libido. HRT protects against osteoporosis and bowel cancer, but increases the risk of breast cancer, ovarian cancer and cardiovascular disease.

The publication of two major studies has increased concerns about the safety of HRT. The Million Women study found a significantly increased risk of breast cancer, the effect being substantially greater for estrogen-progestogen combinations than for other types. [43] These results, and those of the Women's Health Initiative trial, [515] have greatly influenced national policy on HRT. Women need accurate information to make informed choices. NICE offers guidance on starting and stopping HRT, and its long-term benefits and risks. [429] FAMs are not compatible with HRT because it affects the interpretation of fertility indicators. Women must wait three months after stopping HRT before they can rely on FAMs.

COMPLEMENTARY THERAPIES FOR MENOPAUSAL WOMEN

Women who use FAMs are more likely to turn to complementary therapies believing them to be safer and more natural than HRT. Although women's experiences of therapies such as acupuncture and reflexology are often very positive, with anecdotal reports of physical and psychological benefits, there is currently no strong research evidence for their beneficial effects. RCOG guidance on the use of alternatives to HRT highlights concerns that many products are unlicensed, with unproven benefits and limited evidence for their efficacy and safety. [486] The physiological and psychological benefits of Qigong and Tai Chi are, however, of increasing interest for the management of menopausal women. A systematic review showed that both activities help to improve posture, muscle strength, balance, movement and breathing. [304]

CHARACTERISTICS OF PERI-MENOPAUSAL CYCLES

Peri-menopausal cycles follow a typical overall pattern, as described by the STRAW staging system, but different cycle types occur randomly, resulting in a variable sequence of fertile and infertile cycles.

Ovulatory and anovulatory cycles

As estrogen levels decrease and FSH levels increase (in an attempt to stimulate follicle growth) one of two things happen. Either:

- follicles respond and estrogen levels rise, and the LH surge triggers ovulation; or
- follicles fail to respond and estrogen levels remain low with no ovulation.

In the ovulatory cycle the ovaries may respond quickly to high FSH levels, resulting in an early ovulation and a short cycle ending with a heavy, and sometimes prolonged, period. This is a "true period" preceded by a temperature rise 10–16 days earlier – a fertile cycle. In some cycles the higher concentration of FSH may lead to a second ovulation and an increased incidence of dizygotic twins (page 52), but in other cycles the luteal phase may be inadequate (or short), reducing the fertility potential. Conversely, in the anovulatory cycle the lack of response from the ovaries may lead to a long cycle ending with a short hormone-withdrawal bleed and minimal loss.

A study of 36 peri-menopausal women (aged 45–54), which measured urinary E3G and pregnanediol glucuronide through 107 menstrual cycles, reported that about 33% had regular cycles consistent with potential fertility, 19% had cycles consistent with infertility and 48% had a mixture of both cycle types. [179]

Cycle length and variability in pre- and post-ovulatory phases

Towards the end of the reproductive years, subtle changes occur in cycle length and menstrual flow, reflecting significant changes in FSH (and inhibin B). [238] [259] The first sign of change is often a shortening of the cycle (with some cycles < 24 days). Short cycles may be interspersed with average length cycles. Cycles then become more irregular, with variations of more than seven days, followed by much longer cycles, often with intervals of more than 60 days, until menstruation ceases completely (see Treloar's cycle length variations by age in chapter 3, figure 3.11). A re-analysis of Treloar's data showed that the most substantial increase in cycle length did not occur until the year before menopause, at which time the majority of women spent at least 75% of their time in cycles of longer than 40 days. [175]

Cycle length is affected by variations in the length of both the pre- and post-ovulatory phases. As women progress through the menopausal transition, there are an increasing number of cycles with very long pre-ovulatory phases plus cycles with inadequate or short post-ovulatory phases showing decreased luteal phase progesterone. [522]

Temperature

The rise in temperature may occur at the expected time, earlier than anticipated, or following a delay of weeks or months. A bleed may occur with no preceding temperature rise. Users should anticipate a combination of biphasic cycles with adequate luteal phases, cycles with inadequate or short luteal phases and monophasic cycles – occurring in any sequence.

Vaginal bleeding

During the peri-menopause there may be changes both in menstrual volume and duration of loss: periods may be lighter or heavier, of shorter duration or more prolonged. Heavier bleeds may be accompanied by clots. There may be sudden brief or more prolonged episodes of "flooding".

Studies of women in the late menopausal transition (one to three years before menopause) show that, compared with the mid-reproductive years, the average menstrual loss following ovulatory cycles more than doubles (median 69 ml vs. 30 ml). Many women with excessive bleeding have abnormally high estrogen levels and disturbed estrogen secretion. Menstrual loss following ovulatory cycles in the late menopausal transition is significantly heavier than loss following anovulatory cycles (median 69 ml vs. 12 ml). [259] As a general rule:

- if periods are becoming more infrequent, shorter and lighter, there is no cause for concern, but
- if periods are becoming more frequent, prolonged and heavier, this requires investigation (including tests for anaemia; see page 207).

Bleeding is considered a "true period" only if preceded by a temperature rise; any other bleeding may be associated with estrogen activity and increased fertility (page 206). Some women experience intermittent light bleeding/spotting between periods. This is not uncommon during very long cycles (possibly due to hormonal fluctuations), but should always be investigated. Any bleeding which occurs more than one year after the final menstrual period requires investigation.

Cervical secretions

As estrogen levels decline, there is a reduction in the quantity and quality of secretions. Over time, the number of dry days increases and the number of days with any type of secretions decreases. Wetter, transparent, stretchy secretions decrease most noticeably. A woman may experience persistent dryness or only occasional patches of sticky white/yellowish secretions, with minimal (if any) wetter secretions. It may be harder to recognise peak day. If there are no highly fertile-type secretions, peak day is the last day of sticky secretions before the return to dryness.

The build-up of secretions to peak day can be rapid during the peri-menopause. Women who have less than five days warning of peak may be at an increased risk of unintended pregnancy. The majority of menopausal women experience dryness and can identify the first sign of change but occasionally women report a constant pattern of secretions with no dry days. Some authorities identify this as a BIP if it is unchanging for over two weeks (as with breastfeeding mothers), but this is not recommended practice because there may be insufficient warning of peak day.

Cervix

A woman who can confidently identify cervical changes will find this information invaluable during the lengthy pre-ovulatory phases of the peri-menopause. Checking the cervix usually gives the earliest warning of approaching fertility, with the added advantage that secretions taken directly from the os may be detectable at least one day before their appearance at the vulva. To get the most up-to-date assessment of the cervix it can be rechecked shortly before intercourse.

Minor indicators

There may be reduced frequency or complete absence of the minor indicators of fertility, reflecting the decline in ovarian hormone levels. As the number of ovulatory cycles diminishes, women who have previously experienced symptoms such as mittelschmerz, breast changes or abdominal bloating may notice these subside.

Home test kits and monitors

OPKs and fertility monitors which measure urinary hormones are not suitable for menopausal women due to cyclic irregularity and increasingly elevated LH levels. Although LH will not be as high as FSH it may still be elevated above the testing threshold.

A number of home kits measure urinary FSH as a predictor of menopause. These may reassure some women that symptoms are related to menopausal changes, but as FSH levels are highly variable from the late reproductive years onwards these tests cannot give any indication of menopausal status. Even if levels are elevated, women must not stop using contraception on the basis of these kits.

FAMS DURING THE PERI-MENOPAUSE

Women who use FAMs during the peri-menopause require the support of a specialist practitioner. The time from the earliest sign of change until the final menstrual period is varied and unpredictable: some women cease to menstruate abruptly with little warning but others have many years of change during which time close supervision is vital. Although many women feel empowered by an increased understanding of their declining fertility, it can be a challenging time for couples who rely on abstinence. Couples who have previously had concerns about the effectiveness of barriers may now be well-suited to their use in combination with increased confidence about their reduced fertility.

Recording indicators on peri-menopausal chart

The fertility indicators are recorded in the usual way (appendix B). Specialised 16-week charts make it easier to monitor cycle variability over a longer time-span, but the same effect can be created by sticking a series of normal fertility charts together. Women can be encouraged to record menopausal symptoms on the chart to monitor their intensity and impact on well-being but, although symptoms such as hot flushes are related to low estrogens, their presence on a specific day gives no indication of fertility status.

Recognising signs of infertility

The key to successful use of FAMs during the peri-menopause lies not so much in identifying signs of fertility but in positively identifying infertility. If cycles are very short, there may be no early infertile days, but as the menopausal transition progresses and cycles lengthen there may be increasingly lengthy times of pre-ovulatory infertility. Infertility is recognised by the following indicators.

- Cervical secretions: dry days are infertile. Anticipate increasingly long intervals of persistent dryness
- Cervix (anteverted uterus) remains low, firm, closed and tilted.
- Temperature: a monophasic curve is indicative of anovulation.

During the peri-menopause the *Day 6 rule* cannot be applied due to the frequent occurrence of short cycles. Using the *S minus 20 rule*, the first three days of a true period *may* be infertile, provided there have been no cycles shorter than 24 days, but this carries an unknown risk as there is a strong possibility of cycles shortening further.

Recognising signs of fertility

Fertility is recognised by:

- Temperature: biphasic curve with adequate luteal phase
- Vaginal bleeding:
  - True period: bleeding could mask the start of secretions in a short cycle
  - Withdrawal bleed: could be related to ovarian activity and mask secretions
- Cervical secretions: any change from dryness indicates fertility
- Cervix (anteverted uterus): first change from low, firm, closed and tilted

In a woman with a retroverted uterus, the cervix will feel high during times of infertility and drop lower at the first sign of fertility. Other features follow the same changes as an anteverted uterus.

GUIDELINES TO AVOID PREGNANCY DURING PERI-MENOPAUSE

The following guidelines are for use by women during the peri-menopausal years.

Early relatively infertile time

Provided a woman accepts the relative risk of pregnancy associated with the pre-ovulatory phase (early infertile time) she can use the following guidelines:

- Intercourse is permitted on non-consecutive evenings during the early dry days.
- Intercourse should be avoided during any bleeding or spotting.
  - If the bleed is a true period, intercourse should be avoided for its duration but can be resumed on non-consecutive evenings during the early dry days.
  - If the bleed is not preceded by a temperature rise, intercourse should be avoided for the duration of the bleed and for the following three days to establish a return to dryness. Intercourse can be resumed on the fourth evening and thereafter on non-consecutive evenings during the early dry days.
- Intercourse should be avoided at the first sign of fertility (i.e. first change from dryness or first change from an infertile cervix whichever comes earliest) for the duration of the fertile signs and for *three days* after return to dryness (and an infertile cervix). Intercourse can then be resumed on non-consecutive evenings.

Late infertile time

The post-ovulatory phase (late infertile time) is highly effective provided these guidelines are followed:

- Intercourse can be resumed on the evening of the third high temperature after peak day, provided all high temperatures occur after peak day.

- There must be at least six low temperatures, but the coverline should be extended backwards as far as possible, excluding the first four temperatures of the period.
- The third high temperature must be at least 0.2 deg.C above the low temperatures.
- Unrestricted intercourse is permitted until the start of the next period.

SELF-ASSESSMENT QUESTIONS

Answers are at the end of the chapter.

1 Define the menopause.
2 What is the average age of menopause in the UK?
3 Define peri-menopause.
4 Describe a typical pattern of change in cycle length through the peri-menopause.
5 During the late menopausal transition, would you expect menstrual loss to be higher in ovulatory or anovulatory cycles?

Figure 17.2 shows a peri-menopausal chart recorded by a 46-year-old experienced user. The chart spans eight weeks. There was no temperature rise in the previous cycle, hence the bleed could indicate ovarian activity. The horizontal arrow indicates the time when intercourse must be avoided (duration of bleeding plus three days). Intercourse is permitted on non-consecutive evenings, and the following day is marked with a cross. On day 15 the woman observes secretions that are unrelated to intercourse and therefore avoids intercourse on that day and for the following three days. The cervix remains low, firm, closed and tilted until day 23, when it softens – this is the earliest sign of change. The fertile time continues until three high temperatures after peak day on day 31, followed by a short luteal phase. Intercourse is avoided during the period and is resumed on the evening of day 6 when the woman felt confident of dryness and a closed cervix. The cervix softens on day 7, giving the earliest sign of change. The fertile time lasts from day 7 until day 14.

Figure 17.3 shows a series of charts from a 46-year-old woman and the same woman five years later. Note the irregular cycle lengths and the combination of biphasic and monophasic cycles. By 51 she only has one biphasic cycle (in June). This is followed by six months without further signs of ovulation, although she has intermittent bleeds and patches of secretions. She then waits for one year after which she can retrospectively define the December bleed as her final menstrual period. She is now post-menopausal and can assume permanent infertility. She can finally stop all charting.

EFFECTIVENESS OF FAMS DURING PERI-MENOPAUSE

Fertility in menopausal women is dramatically reduced, in comparison with the peak reproductive years, but there will still be many ovulatory cycles where conception is possible. Unprotected intercourse is particularly risky in the pre-ovulatory phase during short cycles because ovulation could occur much earlier than expected. Women in the late reproductive years may therefore be well-advised to restrict intercourse to the post-ovulatory infertile time. As cycles lengthen during the menopausal transition (with some cycles lasting several months), restricting intercourse to the late infertile time may be impractical (and unnecessary). Although the pre-ovulatory phase always carries a pregnancy risk, experienced users may be able to use this time confidently, provided that they have a double-check of secretions and cervical changes.

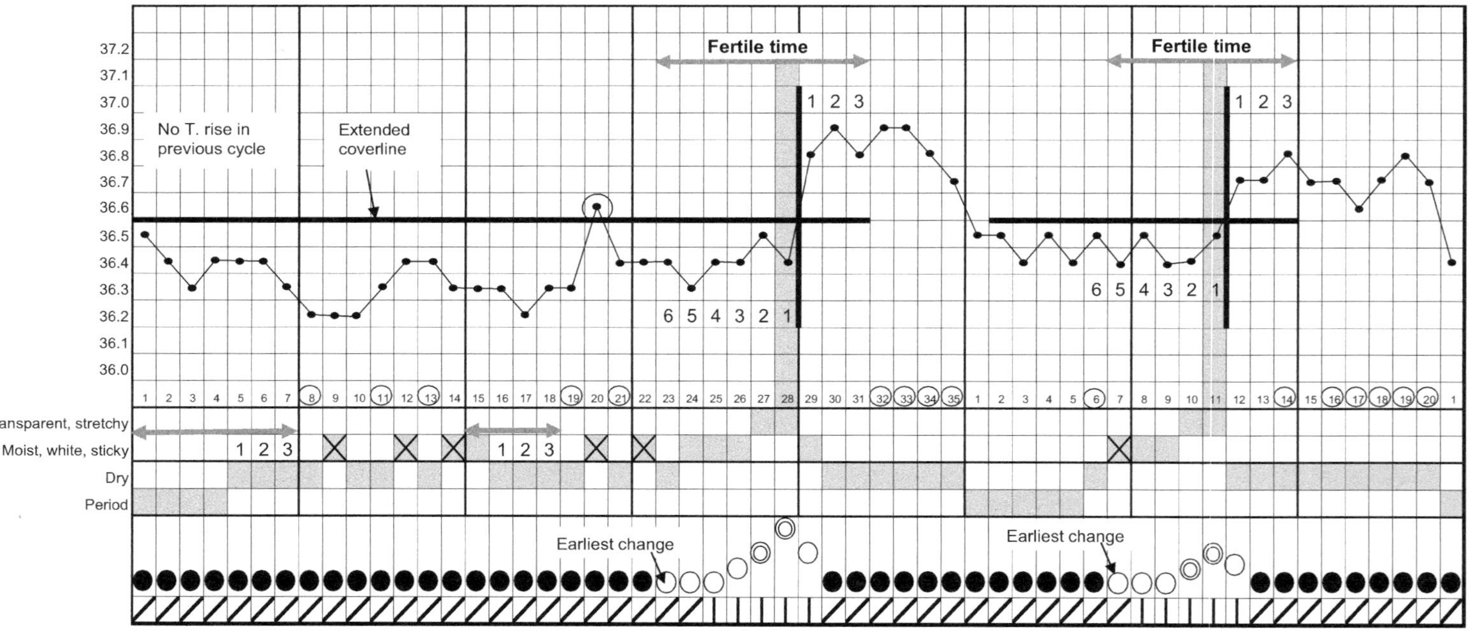

Figure 17.2 Peri-menopausal chart recorded by a 46-year-old experienced user (section of 16-week chart)

Anne Scott aged 46 years January–July

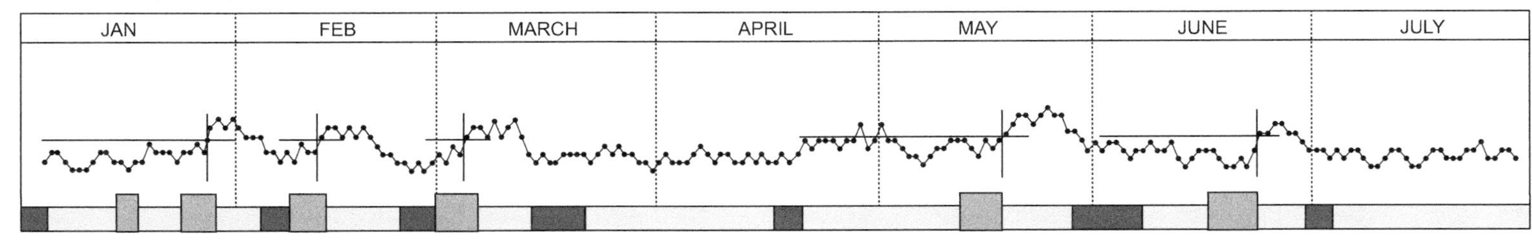

Anne Scott aged 51 years May–December

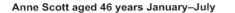

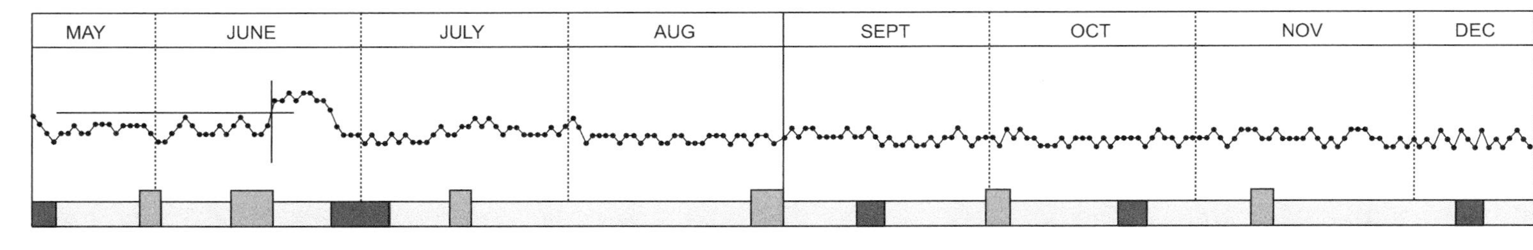

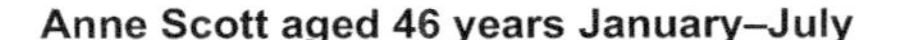

Figure 17.3 Cycles recorded by 46-year-old pre-menopausal woman and the same woman five years later

The menopause guidelines are used successfully in practice but they have not been validated by large prospective studies, hence the effectiveness of FAMs during the peri-menopause remains uncertain.

ANSWERS TO SELF-ASSESSMENT QUESTIONS

1 The menopause is the final menstrual period.
2 It occurs between 45 and 55 years (average age 51 in the UK).
3 The time around the menopause starting when ovulation and menstruation become irregular and ending one year after the final menstrual period
4 The first sign of change is often a shortening of the cycle (with some cycles < 24 days). Short cycles may be interspersed with average length cycles. Cycles then become more irregular with variations of more than seven days, followed by much longer cycles often with intervals of greater than 60 days until menstruation completely ceases.
5 Menstrual loss following ovulatory cycles is significantly heavier than loss following anovulatory cycles during the late menopausal transition.

PART III

Achieving pregnancy

PLANNING PREGNANCY

The words of Freely and Pyper in *Pandora's Clock* as they explored the puzzling gap between the way people talk about family planning in public and the stories to which they admit in private:

> If starting a family means putting your career on hold, cementing your relationship, permanently changing your way of life, in other words turning your world upside down, how does anyone decide the right time, or is risk-taking behaviour a way that many couples get around to having their family? [192]

Decision-making about parenthood is complex. A Scottish study used semi-structured interviews with 13 women and 12 men to explore intentions towards parenthood. The findings were comparable to other similar studies. Decision-making about fertility and parenthood is a process rather than a one-off event, but parenthood is often assumed as a natural course of events. Discussions are a two-stage process: early in the relationship there may be discussion about whether or not each partner wants children, then later the issue of the timing of conception is raised. The first stage of exploring views on parenthood is most important for individuals with strong views because persistent disagreements can lead to relationship breakdown. Individuals who are more highly educated and/or from more affluent backgrounds are more likely to delay parenthood to fulfil educational, travel or leisure pursuits. Marriage is generally not seen as a strict prerequisite for parenthood although many still express a preference for marriage before children. Men are likely to voice concerns about being older fathers in relation to levels of physical activity and fitness. [83]

For the majority of couples, it takes only two things to make a baby: time and opportunities for sex. Many women have unrealistic expectations of a normal time to pregnancy (and may feel pressured by age). The NICE guidelines suggest that

> People who are concerned about their fertility should be informed that over 80% of couples in the general population will conceive within 1 year if the woman is aged under 40 and they do not use contraception and have regular intercourse (every 2 to 3 days). Of those who do not conceive in the first year, about half will do so in the second year (CPR over 90%). [428]

These statistics should be reassuring, but fertility delays are common.

FACTORS ESSENTIAL FOR A HEALTHY PREGNANCY

For natural conception to occur, it requires:

- a chromosomally normal spermatozoon;
- a chromosomally normal egg;
- patent tubes in both the man and woman;

- normal sexual functioning with vaginal intercourse at the fertile time;
- successful fertilisation in the Fallopian tube; and
- successful implantation in a healthy endometrium and ability to carry the pregnancy to term.

This process, which is delicately balanced by the reproductive hormones, can be interrupted or fail at any stage.

FERTILE TIME AND PROBABILITY OF CONCEPTION

Conception can occur from intercourse only during the fertile time – the six-day window that ends on the day of ovulation. [631] Intercourse should be targeted across the entire fertile time, with the day of ovulation and the preceding 24 hours carrying the highest chance of pregnancy (page 80).

Likely occurrence of fertile time

The timing of the six-day fertile window will vary, with its relative position being dependent on the day of ovulation (page 78). Wilcox studied the likely timing of the fertile window in 221 healthy women planning pregnancy. It occurred between days 10 and 17 (the days stated by many clinical guidelines) in only about 30% of women. The fertile time started earlier for most women and much later for others. The earliest ovulation was estimated to have occurred on day 8 and produced a healthy baby. The latest ovulation occurred on day 60. [629] Women with regular 28-day cycles were most likely to be fertile from days 8–15, but the fertile time was highly variable even among those with regular cycles. The women who reported irregular menstrual cycles (16%) tended to ovulate later and at more variable times of the cycle. Figure 18.1 shows the probability of women with regular cycles being in their

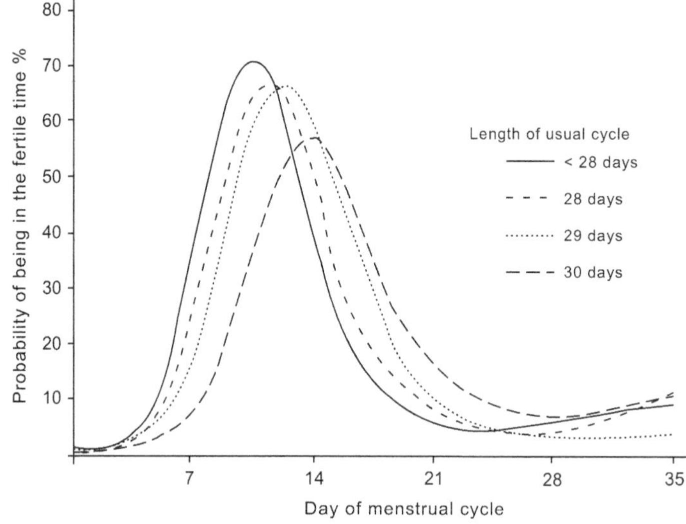

Figure 18.1 Probability of women with regular cycles being in the fertile time grouped by usual cycle length (adapted from Wilcox 2000) [629]

fertile time grouped by their usual cycle length. The fertile time was estimated to have started by the end of the first week in about 30% of the 39 women with cycles of less than 28 days compared with only 7% of the 55 women with cycles of 30 days.

Women's knowledge of day of ovulation and fertile time

Women's knowledge of the day of ovulation and the likely fertile time is generally poor. A study of 330 women who had been trying to conceive for an average of eight months compared the women's perception of their day of ovulation (reported at recruitment) with the estimated day of ovulation using urinary LH. Only 13% correctly estimated their day of ovulation. More than 50% of women believed that they ovulated on day 14 or 15 (because this is what health professionals tell them). However, only 20% ovulated on days 14 or 15: the actual ovulation was on average two days later. Many of these women then conceived with the use of a fertility monitor, which confirmed the value of an accurate prediction of the fertile time. [645]

NICE GUIDELINES ON INTERCOURSE TIMING

NICE guidelines on the frequency and timing of intercourse recommend: "People who are concerned about their fertility should be informed that vaginal sexual intercourse every 2–3 days optimises the chance of pregnancy." [428] The recommendation for intercourse two to three times per week is logical. It aims to encourage couples to have intercourse throughout the menstrual cycle, thus maintaining optimum sperm health and covering the entire fertile time. This approach may work well for some, but it is not practical or possible for others. Ideally pregnancy planning should not interfere with the spontaneity of a couple's sex life, but women frequently claim that their rate of spontaneous sex would not be sufficient to achieve conception. Women are therefore keen to understand more about their fertility to allow them to optimise intercourse timing.

ROLE OF FERTILITY AWARENESS IN PLANNING PREGNANCY

FA education helps couples to optimise intercourse timing, identify factors which may contribute to fertility delays and seek timely medical advice. The secretions provide the best information for timing intercourse to conceive, but other indicators play a role. The fertility indicators (described in detail in earlier chapters) are considered here specifically in relation to their role in planning pregnancy.

Cycle length variability

If the woman has an accurate record of her last 12 cycle lengths, this gives a very broad estimate of the fertile time. The calculations *S minus 20* and *L minus 10* can be used to identify the first and last fertile days (page 153). This helps to reassure couples about the potential window of opportunity when intercourse could result in pregnancy. Within that very wide target time, the secretions will identify the fertile days more precisely.

Cervical secretions

The presence of cervical secretions and the quality of the secretions provide the best prospective markers for planning pregnancy and the best predictors of the chances of conception (page 139). [49] [560]

The following facts about cervical secretions are relevant for pregnancy planning:

- Intercourse on *any* day of secretions could result in pregnancy.
- The days when a woman experiences a wet, slippery sensation (with or without the appearance of transparent, stretchy secretions) reflect rising estrogen levels facilitating sperm survival, storage, and transport. [150]
- The highest chance of conception is from intercourse on peak day (last day of wet, slippery, transparent, stretchy secretions) which coincides closely with ovulation.
- There is a very high chance of conception the day before peak, which often coincides with the day of the most profuse secretions. [242]
- Within the six-day fertile window, the type of secretion observed on the day of intercourse is more predictive than the timing relative to ovulation (based on temperature rise). [49]
- Cycles in which cervical secretions were monitored consistently were significantly more likely to result in pregnancy independent of intercourse frequency or the use of urinary LH kits. [160]
- Ultrasound studies confirm that peak day is a highly sensitive marker of the day of ovulation. [150]

Charting cycle length and cervical secretions

Appendix C includes a blank chart suitable for women planning pregnancy. It provides instructions for charting, an example chart and four blank charts on a single sheet. In the example chart (illustrated in figure 18.2) the first five days are marked as period, then two days of dryness with no secretions seen or felt. Days 8, 9 and 10 are recorded as moist days with white/cloudy, sticky secretions. Days 11, 12 and 13 are recorded as wet days with slippery, transparent, stretchy secretions – the highly fertile days. Day 13 is marked as peak day, recognised retrospectively the following day by a change back to sticky secretions on day 14. This is followed by dryness until the next period. The horizontal arrow shows the fertile time, which starts at the first sign of any secretions and ends three days after peak day (days 8 to 16 inclusive).

In figure 18.2 the woman has cycles ranging from 25–30 days. Using the calculations *S minus 20* and *L minus 10* gives the broadest estimate of the fertile time from days 5 to 20 inclusive – so in a cycle as short as 25 days it would be possible for intercourse from as early as day 5 to result in pregnancy. Likewise, with a cycle as long as 35 days it would be possible for intercourse as late as day 20 to result in pregnancy. This couple are having frequent intercourse and have specifically targeted the days when the cervical secretions show the most fertile characteristics.

A series of three or four such simple charts can be recorded on one sheet (appendix C) to confirm that a woman is experiencing a normal pattern of secretions and that intercourse occurs across the entire fertile time. For many women an awareness of the changes in secretions is all that is required with no need to document the changes, as with the case of the busy academics that follows. If intercourse is well-timed and there is no pregnancy after six months of fertility-focused intercourse, further investigation may be appropriate, depending on the woman's age and medical history.

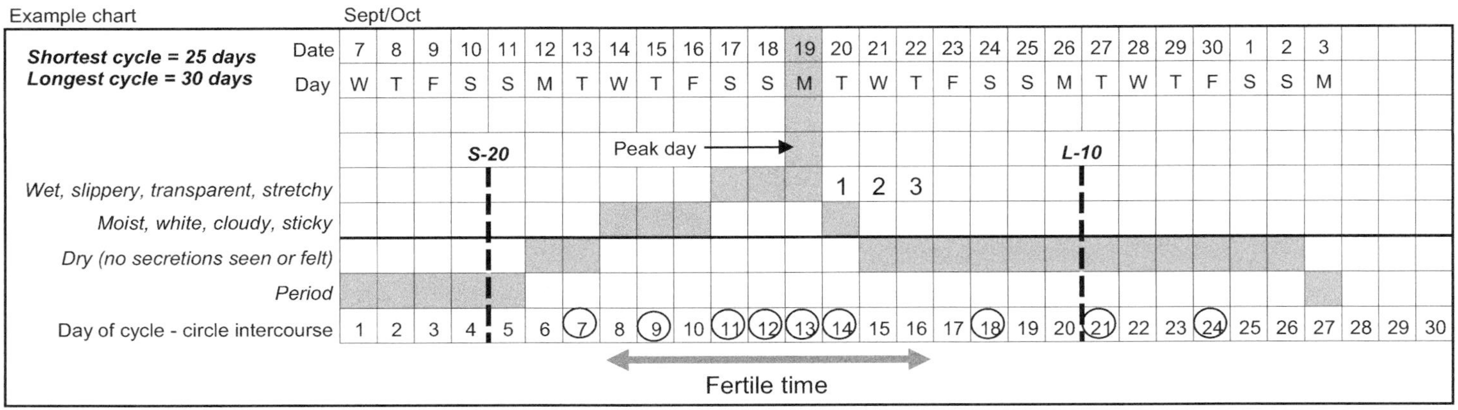

Example chart

Sept/Oct

Shortest cycle = 25 days Longest cycle = 30 days	1	2	3	4	5	6	7	8	9	10	11	12	13	14	15	16	17	18	19	20	21	22	23	24	25	26	27	28	29	30
Date	7	8	9	10	11	12	13	14	15	16	17	18	19	20	21	22	23	24	25	26	27	28	29	30	1	2	3			
Day	W	T	F	S	S	M	T	W	T	F	S	S	M	T	W	T	F	S	S	M	T	W	T	F	S	S	M			
Wet, slippery, transparent, stretchy											▒	▒	▒	1	2	3														
Moist, white, cloudy, sticky								▒	▒	▒				▒																
Dry (no secretions seen or felt)						▒	▒								▒	▒	▒	▒	▒	▒	▒	▒	▒	▒	▒	▒				
Period	▒	▒	▒	▒	▒																						▒			
Day of cycle - circle intercourse	1	2	3	4	5	6	(7)	8	(9)	10	(11)	(12)	(13)	(14)	15	16	17	(18)	19	20	(21)	22	23	(24)	25	26	27	28	29	30

S-20

Peak day →

L-10

Fertile time

Figure 18.2 Chart showing cervical secretions as a single indicator with intercourse timing to optimise chances of conception. Note the cycle range of 25–30 days and the potential width of the fertile time by calculation.

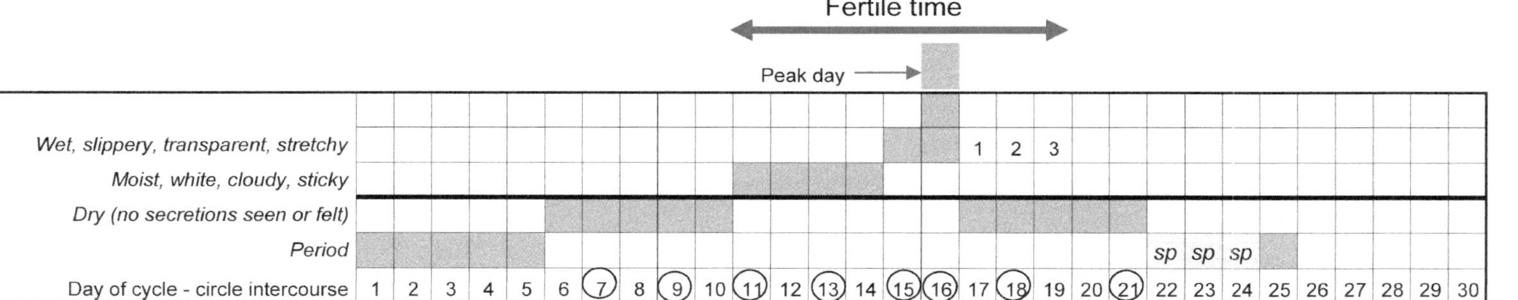

Figure 18.3 Pattern of cervical secretions in a woman planning pregnancy showing short luteal phase and three days of premenstrual spotting

CASE STUDY BUSY ACADEMICS

Anna and Anthony, both young academics, had been trying to conceive for nearly two years. Anna had regular 28-day cycles with no known gynaecological problems. Sex was fitted in around their hectic schedules, which meant it was limited to Saturday nights. Anna was taught about the significance of cervical secretions. A month later at her follow-up she rather dramatically slammed a positive pregnancy test stick onto the desk.

What had changed? Anna had been cycling home when she felt a characteristic wetness. They had sex that night (despite being Thursday) and she conceived.

Note: Questions about sex targeting need to be specific. "Are you having regular sex?" is not enough. This couple were having very "regular" sex (every Saturday night) and Anna's cycles were like clockwork. They could have continued to mistime sex indefinitely.

Charts which document only the changes in secretions are simple to teach and use but, despite their simplicity, they can identify a number of factors which may contribute to fertility delays. For example: figure 18.3 shows a normal build-up of secretions to peak on day 16, but then the period starts on day 25, which is suggestive of a short luteal phase (page 346). The three days of premenstrual spotting could be indicative of endometriosis and may require further investigation (page 207).

Waking temperature

Temperature can be a useful retrospective sign confirming ovulation and conception. It may provide useful diagnostic information. A sustained high temperature for at least 20 days is highly indicative that conception has occurred. [601] [99] Some women notice a second increase in temperature (to around 37 deg.C), giving a triphasic pattern, but it is the sustained high temperature that is diagnostic, not the temperature level (figure 4.10 in chapter 4).

Temperature charts are discouraged by current NICE guidelines: "The use of basal body temperature charts to confirm ovulation does not reliably predict ovulation and is not recommended." [428] It is well-recognised that temperature has no *predictive* value; however, for women experiencing delayed conception, temperature may still have a role (page 309).

If a woman wants to take her temperature for a few cycles, then this can be encouraged. Many women feel empowered by knowing where they are in their cycle and maintaining a level of control; however, this should not be allowed to intrude on the relationship. Studies show that the majority of women describe positive experiences of temperature possibly because they are more actively involved in the investigative process (page 113).

Temperature during pregnancy

A number of women, fascinated by their elevated temperatures following implantation, have continued to record temperatures throughout pregnancy. Some women have reported temperatures staying elevated until the onset of labour and others have observed falling temperatures followed by miscarriage. In a study of six pregnant women in the late 1950s, all women showed elevated temperatures until week 13 or 14. Temperatures then started to drop mid-trimester, with some dropping to the pre-ovulatory level around the 24th week, and one continuing at a sustained higher level until just prior to labour. Benjamin speculated on whether the decreased temperature level (at a time when circulating progesterone would be very high) might be due to the difference in progesterone from the placenta compared with the corpus luteum or whether the higher estrogen levels in later pregnancy caused the decreased temperature. [42] Reports on temperature changes during pregnancy are largely anecdotal and there seems to be no consistent pattern. Fluctuating temperatures are likely to increase anxiety levels, particularly in women with prior pregnancy loss. There is no practical value to be gained from continuing temperature recordings during pregnancy and its use should be discouraged.

Cervical changes

Cervical changes may be a useful additional indicator of the fertile time, but there is generally no need for women planning pregnancy to be checking their cervix. Women who observe only scant amounts of secretions at the vulva may, however, find that secretions are more apparent when checked directly at the cervix.

OPKs and fertility monitors

Ovulation predictor kits do just as their name implies: they *predict* ovulation (by detecting the LH surge). Most kits identify only the two days of maximum fertility whilst others typically identify four fertile days. Many women assume that a positive result or "seeing the smiley face" confirms that they are ovulating. OPKs identify the trigger hormone for ovulation; they do *not* prove its occurrence (page 166).

The Clearblue fertility monitor, which analyses LH and E3G, aims to identify the entire fertile window and typically identifies six fertile days. The monitor provides an accurate assessment of fertility and may be useful for women who are trying to conceive, its main drawback being its cost (page 167). One study has shown that women who use an online charting system in which they learn to identify days of low, high or peak fertility through changes in the secretions, a Clearblue fertility monitor (or both) have a higher chance of pregnancy when intercourse is focused around high and peak fertile days (87% pregnancy rate at one year for high or peak days compared with 5% when intercourse occurred only on low fertility days). [415]

Women with PCOS who have raised LH levels cannot reliably use OPKs or fertility monitors. If a woman reports test results which are either persistently negative or positive this should be investigated.

Electronic thermometers, saliva kits and fertility apps

Electronic thermometers, saliva testing kits and fertility apps are discussed in chapter 9. Many of these technologies, which aim to identify the fertile time, lack evidence to support their use. This is of serious concern for women who use them to avoid pregnancy, but may purely be a waste of money for women planning pregnancy. Fertility apps which purport to identify the fertile time and even the sex of the baby may be a useful way to store cycle data but their accuracy has not been established.

Choice of methods to identify fertile time

Couples need to understand that methods that prospectively identify the fertile time are likely to be more effective than calendar calculations or temperature alone, hence changes in cervical secretions should always be discussed. Table 9.1 in chapter 9 summarises the advantages, disadvantages and cost of different technologies for identifying the fertile time for women planning pregnancy. Some products have been through rigorous testing, but others have no practical use and should not be recommended (page 172). [563] [63]

Preconception consultations provide an ideal opportunity to discuss intercourse frequency and optimal timing to achieve pregnancy. A fine line exists between encouraging a woman to develop an awareness of the signs indicating her fertile time, thus giving her a sense of control over her fertility, and allowing her to become obsessed with meticulous charting or home tests.

CASE STUDY GETTING IT ALL WRONG

Edie had been trying to conceive for more than a year. For the first six months she had been targeting sex around day 14 (the day she thought she ovulated). She then started using OPKs but had difficulty with them. If ever she saw the smiley face and managed to have sex at the "right" time, she felt convinced she must be pregnant so then avoided sex for the rest of the cycle for fear of dislodging the embryo. Her partner was abstaining for up to 12 days in an effort to save up his sperm.

At her first FA consultation Edie was noted to be a very anxious, underweight young woman with irregular cycles of 24–41 days. She had cut out all alcohol, coffee, processed food, wheat and gluten, and replaced dairy with soya. Edie admitted that her relationship was suffering because there was no longer any fun in their life. After discussing her weight and the link with irregular cycles plus explaining about the timing of ovulation, the need for frequent sex and the importance of getting the balance back in their relationship, Edie conceived within two cycles.

Combined chart for achieving pregnancy

Figure 18.4 shows a combined indicator chart in which conception has occurred. The woman's cycles ranged between 26 and 31 days, so it was theoretically possible for her to conceive from intercourse any time between days 6 and 21 (shown by dotted lines). She used her knowledge of secretions to target intercourse more precisely and recognised the most fertile characteristics on days 10, 11 and 12 with peak on day 12. She confirmed her observations with an OPK, which showed positive on days 11 and 12, and her temperature went up to the higher level on day 13. It then showed a second rise on day 21. By day 33 she felt confident that she was pregnant and a positive pregnancy test confirmed her observations.

Fertility chart as diagnostic aid

An accurately recorded fertility chart acts as a useful diagnostic aid, providing information on normal and abnormal function of the menstrual cycle. It also helps to highlight infrequent or poorly targeted intercourse. The fertility chart can be used as a basis to consider the need for further investigation into fertility delays. The following information can be gained from the chart:

- A biphasic chart is indicative of ovulation.
- A raised temperature of 10 days or more suggests the luteal phase is adequate.
- A raised temperature of 20 days or longer is indicative of pregnancy.
- A short luteal phase (less than 10 days) suggests insufficient time for implantation.
- Premenstrual spotting (two days or more) suggests inadequate luteal function or endometriosis.
- A persistently raised temperature during the period and early follicular phase may be indicative of endometriosis [339] [75]

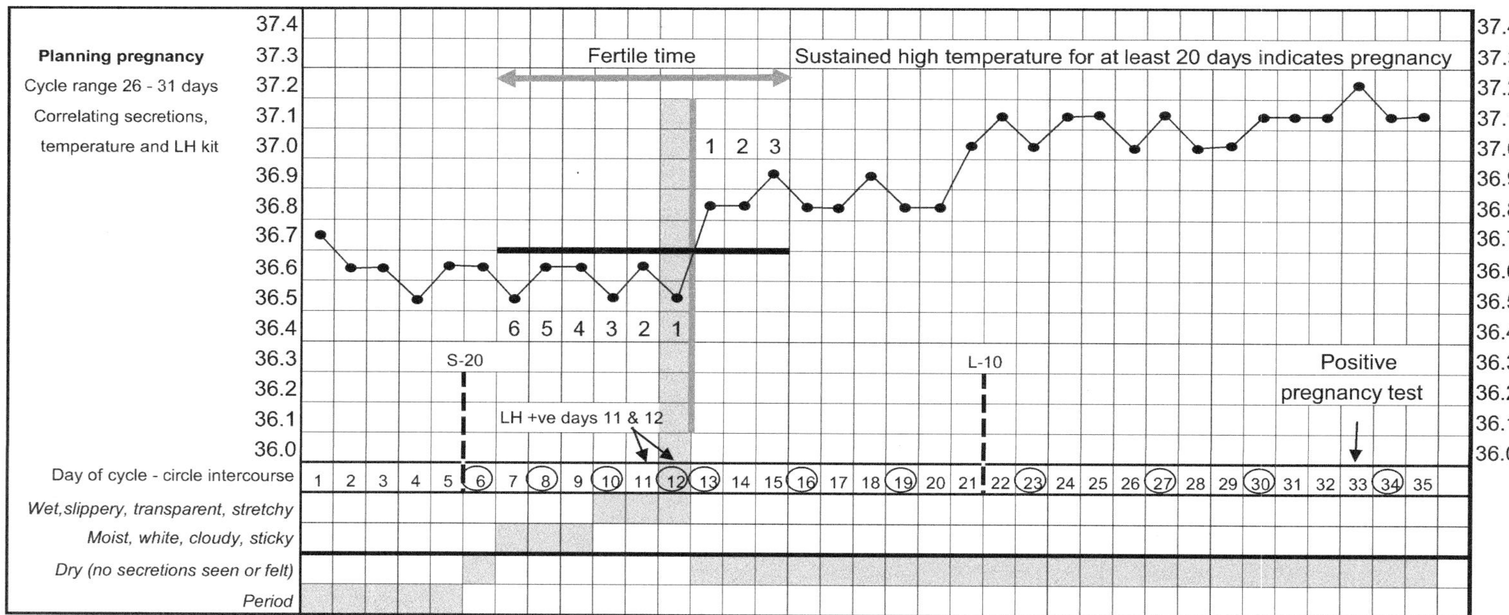

Figure 18.4 Conception cycle showing correlation of cervical secretions, LH and temperature with sustained high temperature of 22 days

- A monophasic chart is indicative of anovulation.
- Cycles of less than 25 days or more than 32 days are more likely to be anovulatory.
- Irregular cycles (varying by eight days or more) may indicate hormonal imbalance such as PCOS.
- Irregular cycles may highlight mis-timing of intercourse.
- Scant secretions or an absence of wetter, transparent, stretchy secretions may indicate reduced chances of conception.

Note: To confirm ovulation, a mid-luteal phase progesterone test can be accurately timed for six days after the temperature rise (seven days after peak). If a woman has *three* consecutive cycles with a short luteal phase or three monophasic cycles, consider further assessment. Any persistent cycle disturbance and any abnormal bleeding should be investigated.

INTERCOURSE FREQUENCY AND CHANCES OF PREGNANCY

For couples who are trying to conceive, sex frequency is probably the most significant factor. The data from Barrett and Marshall, and Schwartz (figure 18.5), clearly demonstrate that couples who have sex most frequently have the highest chance of pregnancy – ranging from around 15% per cycle for couples who only have intercourse weekly to more than 50% for couples having daily intercourse. [34] [532] Contrary to popular belief, too much sex does not weaken sperm. Frequent ejaculation decreases the volume of seminal fluid and the total sperm count, but it improves both sperm motility and DNA, thus enhancing the fertilising capacity of sperm. [437] Couples typically report a similar pattern of intercourse when trying to conceive. After abandoning contraception, most couples report a relaxed, care-free approach with intercourse following their usual pattern or possibly more frequently. After a few months, as anxiety increases, sex often becomes more focused, sometimes with the

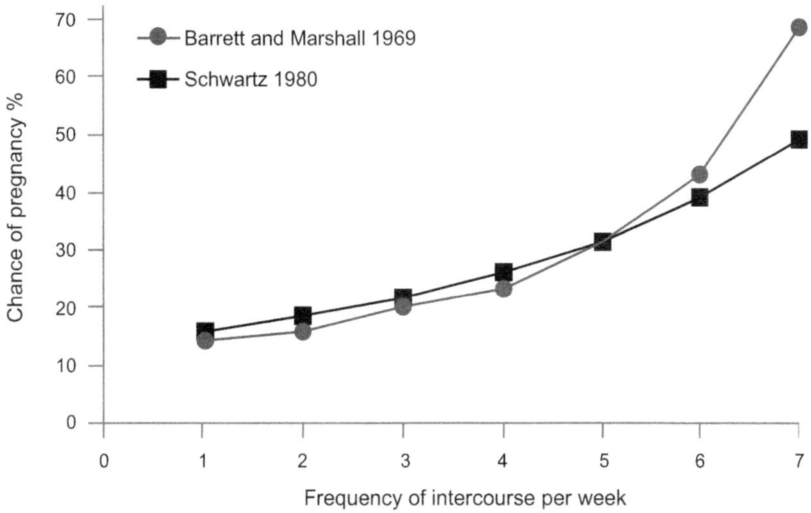

Figure 18.5 Chance of pregnancy in relation to intercourse frequency (adapted from Barrett & Marshall 1969 [34] and Schwartz 1980 [532])

use of OPKs, temperatures and secretions – the "*really* trying" stage. Couples often switch between different approaches: saving up sperm, alternate nights, every night, morning and night or "giving up" altogether.

TIME TO PREGNANCY WITH AND WITHOUT FERTILITY AWARENESS

Many couples trying to conceive find difficulty maintaining the required intercourse frequency. FA education allows intercourse to be timed more precisely, maximising the chance of pregnancy with minimal acts of intercourse. A statistical calculation determined the optimal rules to maximise the chance of pregnancy whilst limiting the number of intercourse days: **time to pregnancy is reduced by assuming fertility from day 7 to 20 inclusive with intercourse timed to the days with the most fertile secretions.** [526]

The evidence for whether FA education reduces time to pregnancy is controversial. Population studies show that approximately 90% of fertile couples conceive within one year of trying (without FA education). A delay of more than a year is therefore usually used to define subfertility. [578] [294] The Walcheren study (719 pregnancies) in the Netherlands showed a CPR of 97% by one year. [551] It is plausible that there is a higher chance of conception in the first few cycles for couples using optimally timed intercourse, but by six months the conception rates with or without targeted intercourse are similar. Table 18.1 summarises studies with and without FA. There are some differences in the study populations, but the outcomes at one year are similar.

In Germany a prospective study of 346 women educated in FA showed 92% conception rate by one year, with most couples conceiving within six cycles. The researchers concurred

Table 18.1 Time to pregnancy with and without fertility awareness education

Study details		*Percentage of pregnancies by month*				
		1	*3*	*6*	*12*	*24*
Population study, (Tietze 1956) [578]		–	50%	75%	> 90%	95%
Population study, Walcheren, Netherlands (Snick 1997) [551]		40%	75%	89%	97%	–
German prospective study, Women trying to conceive with FA education (Gnoth 2003) [233]		38%	68%	81%	92%	–
European prospective fecundability study, with FA education By age category (Dunson 2004) [143]	19–26 years	–	–	–	92%	98%
	27–29 years	–	–	–	87%	95%
	30–34 years	–	–	–	86%	94%
	35–39 years	–	–	–	82%	90%
Parallel randomised trial,with or without education in cervical secretions by CrMS Utah (Stanford 2014) [562]	Control group Sex 2–3 × per week	17%	50%	88%	–	–
	CrMS group Timed intercourse	4%	45%	87%	–	–

with Hilgers' recommendation [283] that with timed intercourse a diagnosis of subfertility can be established in six months, rather than a year, and it may then be appropriate to start initial fertility investigations. [233] The data from the European Fecundability study (782 women educated in FA) showed the impact of female age with 92% CPR by the end of the first year for women in the youngest age group (19–26 years) and 82% for those in the oldest age group (35–39 years). By two years the CPR across all age groups was more than 90% (with 98% of the youngest age group achieving pregnancy Dunson [143] quoted in NICE 2013 [428]).

Snick, who led the Walcheren study, was renowned for actively discouraging interference with couples' sex lives. He commented on the need for well-designed trials to justify teaching FAMs as a way to reduce time to pregnancy, demonstrating that the results from his study were almost identical to studies using FA education. [552]

A recent parallel randomised trial showed that teaching cervical secretions had no significant impact on time to pregnancy. In Stanford's two study groups the control group were advised to have intercourse two to three times per week and the intervention group were taught to observe secretions using the Creighton Model FertilityCare System (CrMS). [562] The researchers were surprised to find no significant impact on time to pregnancy, because in a prior study of couples using CrMS, 76% conceived in the first cycle of documented intercourse in the fertile time and 90% by the third cycle. [283] Stanford's study supports the NICE guidelines on intercourse timing to conceive. [428] The very low conception rates (4%) in the first cycle in Stanford's study is noteworthy. Both groups were instructed to avoid pregnancy in the first cycle – this is routine practice when teaching CrMS (or Billings Method) to allow the woman to learn to distinguish between different types of secretion prior to introducing seminal fluid. Some couples in both groups ignored the instruction and were not willing to wait. The advice to avoid intercourse in the first cycle was a noted weakness in the study and most authorities would agree it is both unnecessary and counterproductive for couples who are planning pregnancy.

Note on religious infertility Mistimed intercourse can cause conception delays for some Orthodox Jewish women. For women who have a short follicular phase or prolonged menstruation, the practice of delaying intercourse until after the ritual cleansing bath (seven days after the end of the period) may cause "religious infertility". Women can ask their rabbi for a special dispensation to have intercourse earlier in the cycle. It is common practice in Israel to delay the LH surge by administering estrogen from day 2 of the cycle until bleeding stops or until two "clean" days. Studies show that ovulation occurs between five and 15 days after stopping estrogen therapy and the conception rate is equivalent to a normal cycle. [639]

PRECONCEPTION HEALTH AND LIFESTYLE FACTORS

Preconception care aims to identify health and lifestyle factors which may adversely affect a woman's reproductive health or the outcome of her pregnancy. Lifestyle factors are defined as the modifiable habits and ways of life that influence general health and fertility – this includes the age at which to start a family and factors such as alcohol, smoking, weight, diet and exercise, all of which can have a significant impact on fertility.

Negative lifestyle factors may have a significant cumulative effect on fertility, reduce success rates with assisted fertility and increase the risk of miscarriage. The time to pregnancy was significantly longer for couples who had more than four negative lifestyle factors: for example, social deprivation, the woman's BMI of more than 25 kg/m^2, the man consuming more than 20 units of alcohol per week, either partner smoking more than 15 cigarettes per day and a caffeine intake of more than six cups per day. [271]

Information and advice on preventative health care and healthy lifestyle should, where possible, be provided three months prior to conception to optimise pregnancy outcome. In the UK, both general practice and contraception and sexual health (CASH) services provide an ideal setting for discussion of family "planning" and the promotion of a healthy lifestyle prior to conception. [538] A Danish study showed that pregnancy planning was associated with a healthier lifestyle, but many women still drank more than the recommended limit of alcohol when trying to conceive and 20% reported binge drinking in early pregnancy. Despite actively planning pregnancy, 50% of all women had not taken folic acid before conception. [16]

Preconception checklist

Consider the following (for both partners unless indicated):

- age (particularly the woman's);
- occupation, occupational hazards and work stress;
- time trying to conceive;
- contraceptive history and time since discontinuing;
- the woman's previous pregnancies, including abortion, miscarriage, ectopic and late pregnancy loss;
- general health, chronic medical conditions, prescribed drugs and past abdominal surgery;
- use of bought drugs, including NSAIDs;
- the woman's gynaecological history and risk factors;
- psychological health and psychiatric risk factors;
- family history of thyroid, gynaecological issues and chronic medical conditions;
- the man's former partners' pregnancies
- the man's known problems or risk factors, such as history of mumps/orchitis or undescended testicle(s); testicular surgery or trauma
- weight, BMI and body fat percentage;
- diet and nutritional health, plus supplementation (particularly folic acid);
- exercise (type and intensity);
- rubella status (provide advice on prevention of infection, including toxoplasmosis);
- cervical screening history for the woman and history of candida, cystitis and STIs (for both partners);
- use of alcohol, smoking, caffeine and illicit drugs;
- stress levels from work, family, social and travel;
- stress management;
- the fertile time and identification of the days of maximum fertility;
- sex targeting, with vaginal sex two to three times per week;
- use of lubricants, including saliva; and
- ask if they are both psychologically ready for a child.

Potential teratogens Women who are planning pregnancy require information and advice on the use of bought and prescription drugs, and women who regularly use illicit drugs need a supervised withdrawal programme. A number of drugs and chemicals are teratogenic resulting in miscarriage or congenital abnormalities. The UK Teratology Information Service (www.uktis.org) and Toxbase (www.toxbase.org) provide information regarding medications, chemicals, illicit drugs and alcohol that may pose a risk in pregnancy.

Table 18.2 provides a list of health and lifestyle factors and their impact on pregnancy, with recommendations to optimise preconception health and the health of the baby.

Table 18.2 Preconception health and lifestyle modifications: interventions and recommendations (adapted from Anderson 2010 [6] Seshadri 2012 [534] and Sharma 2013 [537])

Health and lifestyle factors	*Impact on fertility and pregnancy*	*Preconception recommendations*
Age	A woman's age is possibly the most significant factor (page 86 and 326). A man's fertility declines with age, but less dramatically (page 88).	The optimal time biologically for childbearing is 20–35 years.
Occupation	Occupational stress may impact fertility: this includes shift workers, hairdressers, flight attendants, chefs and athletes (page 200).	
Occupational hazards and environmental exposure	Exposure to chemicals and environmental pollutants have potentially detrimental effects on reproductive health and fetal development, but many of these risks are unproven. Heavy metals, such as lead and mercury, affect the hypothalamic-pituitary gonadal axis. Lead (e.g. in batteries, pipes and lead-based paints) reduces the oxygen-carrying capacity of red blood cells. It reduces sperm quality, causes irregular cycles, miscarriage, stillbirth and pre-term delivery. Mercury (e.g. in thermometers and batteries) disrupts spermatogenesis and fetal development. Welders exposed to toxic metals and gases have reduced sperm motility and morphology. Some chemicals mimic estrogen and disrupt hormonal activity. Endocrine disruptors are found in household cleaning products, pesticides, paints, glues, personal care products, plastics, plus food and drink tin linings. These chemicals have the potential to reduce fertility and increase the risk of miscarriage or fetal loss. Men working with high concentrations of pesticides have reduced semen parameters. High residues of pesticides on fruit and vegetables may also reduce sperm count and morphology. [85]	RCOG recommendations for dealing with potential but unproven risks posed by environmental chemicals include: – Use fresh rather than processed foods. – Reduce use of food/drinks in tinned or plastic containers. – Minimise use of personal care products (cosmetics etc.). – Avoid garden pesticides or fungicides, including fly sprays. – Avoid paint fumes and solvents. – Take over-the-counter analgesics only as necessary. – Do not assume the safety of products labelled "natural" (herbal or otherwise). [497] See the Health and Safety Executive website (www.hse.gov.uk).

(*Continued*)

Table 18.2 (Continued)

Health and lifestyle factors	*Impact on fertility and pregnancy*	*Preconception recommendations*
Chronic medical conditions and prescribed drugs	A woman with a chronic medical condition such as diabetes, epilepsy, thyroid dysfunction, heart defect, allergies or inherited conditions (e.g. sickle cell anaemia) may require a specialist preconception review to consider the potential effect on pregnancy and any modification to prescribed drugs.	Consider the need for early referral for fertility assessment. Consider the need for shared specialist/obs. and gynae. care. Review the use of prescribed drugs. Discuss bought medications such as NSAIDS (page 223).
Existing gynaecological conditions	A woman with a known gynaecological problem such as endometriosis, PCOS or fibroids may require follow-up prior to conception or within six months if there are fertility delays.	(See appendix C.)
Genetic disorders	A couple with an affected child or family history of a genetic disorder may require preconception genetic counselling.	Consider the need for genetic counselling.
Past surgery	Women who have had past abdominal surgery (e.g. appendectomy or ectopic pregnancy) may have impaired fertility. Men who have a varicocele (abnormal dilatation of testicular veins) or history of orchitis (following mumps), testicular injury or testicular surgery (e.g. orchidopexy for testicular maldescent) may have reduced fertility.	Women: Consider risk of tubal damage or pelvic adhesions. Men: Consider the risk of testicular damage.
Psychological health	Pregnancy, birth and the postpartum are challenging psychologically. A woman with a diagnosed psychiatric condition should see her psychiatrist to discuss the proposed pregnancy. Some women will need to change medication or reduce dosage, which requires careful monitoring. A man with mental health problems may require additional psychological support and adjustment to medication.	Discuss any anxieties around pregnancy or childbirth. Consider history of anxiety and/or depression and the risk of postpartum depression. Consider history of eating disorders and body image in relation to pregnancy. Consider existing support and the need for increased services.

Body weight and body fat percentage	Women with a BMI > 25 have significantly reduced fertility plus an increased risk of miscarriage, stillbirth, hypertension, pre-eclampsia, gestational diabetes and thromboembolism. Babies are at risk of being large for gestational age and have an increased risk of congenital abnormalities including neural tube defects, cardiac abnormalities, abdominal wall defects and oro-facial defects. The further outside the ideal BMI range the higher the risks to fertility and pregnancy. Overweight men have reduced testosterone, an increased incidence of erectile dysfunction, reduced sperm concentration and increased DNA damage. Underweight women with a low body fat percentage have an increased risk of ovarian dysfunction, delayed conception, miscarriage, fetal growth restriction and pre-term birth. Underweight men, particularly men with severe weight loss (such as due to illness or anorexia) have reduced sperm concentration.	Advise a woman that the ideal BMI for fertility is 20–25kg/m^2. Weight loss in overweight anovulatory women leads to a return to normal ovulatory function. Couples have a high risk of subfertility if both are obese. Increasing weight in underweight anovulatory women leads to a return to normal ovulatory function. Consider body fat percentage. Women who exercise intensively may be too lean (not necessarily underweight). Advise a healthy diet and exercise to optimise weight. Women who have a history of an eating disorder may need psychological help to achieve a healthy weight.
Exercise	Moderate physical activity is associated with optimum fertility, but excessive exercise (marathon running, long distance cycling) negatively affects energy balance and disrupts the menstrual cycle. Increased frequency, intensity and duration of exercise are linked to decreased female fertility. Women should be cautioned about exercise during pregnancy including the potential for fetal trauma due to loss of balance/being thrown or falling if they participate in exercise such as cycling, horse-riding, or skiing. [483] Moderate physical activity in men is associated with improved sperm count, motility and morphology compared with men who do not exercise or exercise intensively (such as elite sportsmen). Cycling for more than five hours a week reduces total motile sperm count and concentration.	Regular moderate exercise of about 30 minutes per day helps to optimise weight and improve general health. Exercise boosts natural endorphins and helps to reduce stress. Yoga or Pilates help with relaxation and muscle tone, but when pregnant a woman should advise her instructor as some exercises may need to be moderated. Avoid over-heating during exercise if there is a chance of pregnancy. Advise men that moderate physical exercise (at least three times per week for one hour) optimises hormonal levels and semen parameters. Cyclists should wear padded cycle shorts whilst avoiding hard saddles, prolonged time in the saddle and excessive jolting such as mountain biking.
Cervical screening	In the UK all women over 25 are invited for cervical screening on the NHS every three years (>20 in Scotland and Wales). If any abnormal changes are detected, these are more easily treated in a non-pregnant woman.	Advise a woman to ensure her cervical screen is up-to-date and if necessary to repeat prior to conception.

(*Continued*)

Table 18.2 (Continued)

Health and lifestyle factors	*Impact on fertility and pregnancy*	*Preconception recommendations*
Sexual health checks	Untreated STIs such as chlamydia and gonorrhoea cause pelvic inflammatory disease and tubal damage. Early diagnosis and treatment is vital to ensure that fertility is not compromised. Common non-sexually transmissible infections such as candida and BV may mask changes in cervical secretions (see abnormal vaginal discharge on page 214).	Advise women (and men) to get regular sexual health check-ups and to report any symptoms promptly. Self-diagnosis is unreliable and use of over-the-counter products such as anti-fungal treatments may delay appropriate treatment.
Alcohol	Heavy drinking (more than 4.5 units a day) increases the risk of delayed conception, anovulation, miscarriage, luteal phase defect, low birthweight, small for gestational age, pre-term birth and stillbirth. Binge drinking (more than 7.5 units in a single session) may lead to fetal alcohol syndrome or fetal alcohol spectrum disorder (FASD) – a range of abnormalities including damage to facial features, brain, heart and kidneys, plus learning difficulties and behavioural problems. Drinking moderate amounts of alcohol in pregnancy can affect a child's future intelligence. Heavy drinking in men damages sperm production and reduces testosterone which can lead to loss of libido, erectile difficulties, decreased semen volume, sperm count and morphology.	Advise a woman that the safest approach is to avoid alcohol completely before conception and throughout pregnancy. If she chooses to drink, then limit to one to two units once or twice a week around conception and in the first trimester. Men should avoid binge drinking and not exceed three to four units in one day. – See the Drinkaware website (www.drinkaware.co.uk). Signpost women to the patient information leaflet on alcohol and pregnancy. [499]
Smoking	Women who smoke have reduced fertility and delayed time to conception. Smoking disrupts the reproductive hormones and increases the risk of ovarian dysfunction, reduces progesterone levels, and alters endometrial receptiveness to implantation. Smoking may also affect ovum pick-up and transport plus embryo transport thereby increasing the risk of ectopic pregnancy. Smoking in pregnancy affects blood flow through the placenta and increases the risk of miscarriage, pre-term delivery, low birth weight, fetal growth restriction, stillbirth and sudden infant death syndrome. Smoking also increases the risk of congenital defects including heart defects, musculo-skeletal defects, gastro-intestinal defects and attention deficit hyperactivity disorder (ADHD) Men who smoke have decreased sperm count, concentration, motility, morphology and fertilising capacity. Smoking causes oxidative damage to sperm DNA and may increase aneuploidy rates.	Counsel women that smokers have reduced fertility and an earlier menopause (before 45 years). Counsel men and women to stop smoking before conception. Inform men that the concentration of sperm among male smokers is nearly 20% lower than non-smokers. Advise couples that passive smoking can lead to intrauterine growth restriction and lower birth weight. Offer advice on smoking cessation to both partners because a woman is more likely to feel supported and be able to quit if her partner gives up with her. Likewise, a man may be more able to quit if he is doing it for his partner and family. See the Smoke Free website (www.smokefree.nhs.uk).

Caffeine	Caffeine is linked to short cycles and delayed conception (particularly in heavy caffeine drinkers (more than 500 mg per day) but there is no evidence that it has teratogenic effects. There is a possible association between caffeine intake >145 mg/day and miscarriage, fetal death and stillbirth.	There is insufficient evidence to recommend strict caffeine avoidance, but caffeinated drinks should be considered a "treat". Advise a woman to limit caffeine intake to no more than 200 mg caffeine per day (equivalent to two mugs of instant coffee, one mug of filter coffee, two mugs of tea, five cans of cola, two cans of energy drink, or four bars of plain chocolate). Note that some caffeinated drinks contain high levels of sugar which could increase the risk of gestational diabetes. Anyone with a high caffeine intake should reduce it slowly because withdrawal symptoms (headaches, nausea, irritability, disorientation and fatigue) can be severe.
Recreational drugs	Women who use marijuana are at increased risk of irregular cycles, ovulatory problems and delayed conception. It negatively impacts on the tubes and causes placental problems, increasing the risk of stillbirth and low birth weight, plus behavioural and mental health problems in children. Men who frequently use marijuana may have reduced testosterone, a reduced sperm count and motility, decreased sperm capacitation and acrosome reaction. Cocaine reduces testosterone and increases prolactin negatively impacting male fertility. It is associated with miscarriage, preterm birth and growth restriction. Cocaine, amphetamines and ecstasy cause vasoconstriction and are linked to major birth defects including gastroschisis. Heroin is associated with miscarriage, fetal growth restriction, pre-term labour, hyperactivity, severe neonatal withdrawal symptoms and increased risk of infections including HIV, hepatitis B and C. In men, heroin affects sexual function and sperm motility.	Counsel a woman about the effects of recreational drugs on the fetus. Counsel men about the adverse effects of recreational drugs on sperm quality and sexual function. Offer preconception interventions, where possible, to reduce risks to maternal and fetal health. Offer methadone maintenance treatment to women who are dependent on opiates. See the Frank website (www.talktofrank.com).

(*Continued*)

Table 18.2 (Continued)

Health and lifestyle factors	*Impact on fertility and pregnancy*	*Preconception recommendations*
Prolonged heat exposure and testicular temperature	A significant increase in a woman's body temperature during early pregnancy is linked to neural tube defects such as spina bifida. In men, prolonged exposure to heat increases scrotal temperature and adversely affects sperm production.	Advise women who are pregnant or trying to conceive to avoid hot tubs, saunas or steam rooms. Advise men to avoid wearing tight-fitting underwear or jeans, or sitting for prolonged intervals. Advise men that wearing boxers during the day and none to bed improves semen parameters (decreased DNA fragmentation index). [524] Advise men to avoid additional heat from hot baths, saunas, hot tubs or heated car seats. Caution men about long distance driving. [72] Caution men about the posture-related effect of using a laptop on the knees. [541]
Mobile phones	Concerns have been raised about the effect of a mobile phone in a trouser pocket on male fertility due to radio-frequency electromagnetic radiation disrupting sperm production or damaging DNA. However, studies have either radiated sperm in vitro or used questionnaire surveys lacking controls, so epidemiological studies are required. [221]	There is no clear evidence to advise a man against keeping his mobile phone in his trouser pocket.
Vaginal lubricants	Sperm are damaged by oils, water-based lubricants (such as KY jelly) and saliva (in in-vitro studies). [338] [7] [590] Pre-seed does not significantly reduce sperm motility or damage sperm DNA. [4] [598] Rapeseed and baby oils may be considered sperm-friendly because although they cause an initial decline in sperm motility, progressive motility remains high. [521] A study of normal fertile couples showed that over 40% used additional lubricants during procreative sex either occasionally or frequently, but this did not appear to reduce their chances of conception. [564] It is not known if lubricant use reduces chances of conception in subfertile couples.	Additional vaginal lubrication may help with vaginal dryness and discomfort during intercourse. When observed under laboratory conditions, most lubricants (and particularly saliva) are damaging to sperm. Pre-seed does not adversely affect sperm motility or DNA so can be used by couples who are trying to conceive. There is no evidence that any lubricant *increases* the chances of conception. Choice of lubricant may be relevant in fertility practice for trans-vaginal ultrasonography.

Stress	Stress can reduce the daily probability of pregnancy. It increases the risk of irregular cycles, short luteal phases and anovulatory cycles. Long-term chronic stress suppresses the immune system. Work stress (including working more than 32 hours per week) can cause menstrual irregularities and delayed conception. Men who are stressed at work or experiencing stressful life events may have reduced sperm count, motility and morphology.	Advise women to manage the work environment: take a proper lunch break and leave work on time. Exercise (particularly outdoors) is a good stress-buster. Some complementary therapies (such as acupuncture and reflexology) can help with relaxation. Consider the need for support groups, counselling, cognitive behavioural therapy or relationship counselling. (See page 199 for the impact of stress on the menstrual cycle.)
Air travel	Concerns have been expressed about flying when trying to conceive due to atmospheric pressure changes and a slight increase in radiation. There is no evidence that flying is harmful to a normal pregnancy, but there is an increased risk of DVT with long-haul flights in cramped conditions. [496] Women who are pregnant, or trying to conceive, require up-to-date information about risks associated with foreign travel. Women should avoid travelling to areas where vaccinations are required or there is a risk of malaria or other mosquito-borne diseases. Zika virus is of particular concern because microcephaly is linked to Zika infection through maternal/fetal transmission. There are a few cases of sexual transmission.	Most women can fly safely when trying to conceive. The safest time to travel during pregnancy is 14–28 weeks. There is no evidence of increased risk of miscarriage with flying, but women should check with their own doctor and consider whether they are at an increased risk of thrombophilia or other pregnancy complications. Ideally a woman should have an early pregnancy scan before flying to exclude ectopic pregnancy. Women with clotting disorders (such as antiphospholipid syndrome) or recurrent miscarriage may require special precautions or be advised not to fly. For the latest travel information see the National Travel Health Network and Centre (NaTHNaC) at http://travelhealthpro.org.uk/pregnancy/.

(*Continued*)

Table 18.2 (Continued)

Health and lifestyle factors	*Impact on fertility and pregnancy*	*Preconception recommendations*
Folic acid	Supplementation with 400 mcg of folic acid for 3 months before conception and during the first trimester decreases the risk of neural tube defects (NTD), such as spina bifida, by up to 70%. Folic acid also protects against cleft lip and palate. If taken for a year it protects against pre-term delivery.	Advise all women to start taking 400 mcg of folic acid three months prior to conception. Consider increased folic acid (5 mg daily) if a woman has: – previous pregnancy affected by NTD; – NTD herself (or partner or close relative has NTD); – epilepsy and takes anti-epileptic medication; – diabetes; – BMI > 30; or – chronic health condition affecting absorption including coeliac disease, liver disease, kidney disease or sickle cell disease. Advise women to eat foods rich in folate, including dark green leafy vegetables, pulses (peas, beans and lentils) oats, bread and fortified cereals.
Vitamin D	Vitamin D deficiency is linked to polycystic ovarian syndrome, miscarriage, pre-eclampsia and gestational diabetes. It is also linked to subfertility and reduced chance of IVF success. [443] Severe vitamin D deficiency is associated with rickets and convulsions in infants. Sub-optimal levels are linked to sub-optimal bone size and density.	Advise all pregnant and breastfeeding women to take 10 mcg of vitamin D daily. Advise women who are of South Asian, African, Caribbean or Middle Eastern family origin to routinely take 10 mcg of vitamin D daily prior to conception. Advise women who have limited exposure to sunlight, dietary deficiency of vitamin D, or a BMI above 30 to routinely take 10 mcg of vitamin D daily prior to conception. Advise women to get out in the sun for 20 minutes a day without sunscreen. Advise women to eat eggs, oily fish such as herring, mackerel, sardines and fresh tuna plus fortified bread and cereals.

Vitamin A	The corpus luteum contains high levels of beta-carotene (precursor to vitamin A) – this correlates with good progesterone levels. Vitamin A is important for the development of the fetal brain and eyes. Retinol (animal form of vitamin A found in liver and cod liver oil) increases the risk of congenital defects particularly cardiac, brain, and facial defects.	Good dietary sources of vitamin A include eggs (well-cooked) and butter. Carotene-rich foods include yellow, red and orange fruits and vegetables plus dark green leafy vegetables. A multivitamin and mineral supplement must be suitable for pregnancy. Vitamin A must be in the form of beta-carotene (safe vegetable form), not retinol.
Omega 3 fatty acids	The essential fatty acids omega 3 and 6 must come from the diet. The typical western diet has sufficient (often excess) omega 6 from vegetable oils used in processed foods and fried foods, but sub-optimal omega 3's eicosapentaenoic acid (EPA) and docosahexaenoic acid (DHA). EPA supports the heart, immune system and inflammatory response. DHA is a major structural fat in the brain and eyes. Omega 3's are vital for the formation of cell membranes (including egg and sperm cells) and development of the fetal brain and eyes. Omega 3's prevent pre-term delivery and reduces the risk of pre-eclampsia.	Good sources of omega 3 include seafood, oily fish (salmon, fresh tuna, sardines), nuts and seeds, flaxseed and flaxseed oil, rapeseed oil plus fortified eggs and oils. A fish oil supplement should be a reputable brand (ensuring high-quality fish with advanced refining process to prevent contamination with heavy metals). [244] *Note:* Cod liver oil contains EPA and DHA but is high in retinol so unsuited to pregnancy.
Iodine and selenium	Iodine is essential for the production of thyroid hormones. Low iodine levels cause fetal growth restriction and also affect neurological development including a child's IQ. [36] Selenium is a vital trace element for thyroid function with low levels being linked to miscarriage.	Good sources of iodine include sea fish, shellfish, non-organic dairy products and iodised salt. Iodine supplementation for pregnant women may be advisable. Good sources of selenium include brazil nuts, seafood, eggs, garlic, onions, broccoli, mushrooms and asparagus.
Multi-vitamin supplements	Vitamins for preconception and pregnancy should contain 400 mcg of folic acid. This can be taken as folic acid alone or in a preconception multi-vitamin. Vitamin C, a powerful anti-oxidant, protects egg and sperm cells. A multi-vitamin supplement is not a replacement for a healthy balanced diet including fresh fruit and vegetables.	Advise women to keep to recommended limits with vitamins. Vitamins A, D, E and K are fat soluble so can accumulate to dangerous levels, whereas the B vitamins and vitamin C are water soluble so are excreted more easily. Advise women to avoid high doses of vitamin C (>1g per day) as this may reduce cervical secretions.

(*Continued*)

Table 18.2 (Continued)

Infections	*Effects of congenital infection*	*Advice for prevention of infection*
Rubella (German measles)	Rubella, a viral infection, causes a red-pink rash and mild flu-like symptoms. It is now rare in children due to immunisation programmes. If a woman is not immune and contracts rubella during the first 20 weeks of pregnancy it can have serious consequences. Rubella syndrome causes hearing impairment and deafness, eye damage including glaucoma, cataracts, blindness, cardiovascular defects, brain damage including mental retardation, microcephaly, and cerebral palsy.	Advise routine vaccination – measles, mumps and rubella (MMR) in babies. Recommend preconception blood test to confirm the presence of rubella antibodies. Women who are not immune to rubella should be immunised (with MMR vaccine) and avoid pregnancy for a month after vaccination. *Note:* Some women do not seroconvert, hence the importance of checking serum levels *prior to* conception.
Varicella zoster (chickenpox)	Chickenpox, a common childhood illness, causes red itchy spots that blister before dropping off. Chickenpox in pregnancy can be more serious for the woman and cause serious complications for the baby particularly before 28 weeks. Foetal varicella syndrome is rare but causes skin lesions and scarring plus eye damage and neurological defects.	Vaccination is not routinely given in the UK, but is available in many countries. Women who have had chickenpox as a child are not at risk.
Toxoplasmosis	Toxoplasmosis is caused by the parasite Toxoplasma gondii. Most warm-blooded animals including dogs, cats and sheep can be infected. It is transmitted through the environment, food chain or the placenta. Most people who get toxoplasmosis are asymptomatic, but some develop mild flu-like symptoms. Toxoplasmosis during pregnancy can cause miscarriage, stillbirth, eye damage, hydrocephalus, microcephaly, neurological problems, hearing impairment and learning disabilities.	Advise women to avoid handling used cat litter, and to wear gloves when gardening. Wash hands thoroughly after handling pets and food bowls. Wash all soil off fruit and vegetables. Avoid undercooked meat and raw cured meat and wash hands well after handling raw meat.

Listeriosis	Listeria, a bacteria, is found in soil and water plus poultry, sheep and cattle. Listeriosis is mainly spread through contaminated food. Infection with Listeria causes a mild flu-like illness. Listeriosis in pregnancy can cause miscarriage or stillbirth.	Avoid unpasteurised milk and soft ripened cheeses such as Brie, Camembert and blue-veined cheeses. Cooked-chilled food must be adequately reheated. Meat, poultry and seafood should be thoroughly cooked. Avoid contact with sheep at lambing time if pregnant.
Cytomegalovirus	Cytomegalovirus (CMV, a herpes virus) is spread through bodily fluids. Most people are first infected during childhood. It is usually asymptomatic but may cause mild flu-like symptoms. An active CMV infection during pregnancy can be serious. Congenital CMV cause causes petichiae (red or purple spots of 1–2 mm), hepatomegaly, splenomegaly, hepatitis, neurological signs such as microcephaly, chorio-retinitis, neurological problems, deafness and cerebral palsy.	Advise regular hand-washing especially if handling saliva or urine (tissues and nappies) or items used by young children. Avoid kissing young children on the face (kiss on the head). Avoid sharing food, drink and eating utensils with young children.

AGE

Age is an important factor affecting chances of conception, time to pregnancy, and the outcome of pregnancy. The decline in female fertility is of most significance, but male fertility also shows a decline with age and older fathers have an increased risk of passing on genetic mutations (pages 86 and 327).

Woman's age

The majority of women who conceive in their mid-30s will conceive naturally and deliver a healthy baby at term, but the proportion who experience fertility problems, miscarriage or fetal abnormality increases rapidly from the mid-30s onwards. Only about 40% of women who plan to have a child at 40 will achieve it. The reasons women delay childbearing are individual and complex – some may have pursued career goals but many have not met the right man to father their child until later in life or have lost vital fertile years waiting for a partner to commit. Older women have often had challenging life circumstances working against them, as illustrated in Helen's case.

CASE STUDY THE DREAM VERSUS THE REALITY

Helen, a 40-year-old single woman, was contemplating sperm donation. She was struggling to accept the reality of her situation. In her teens Helen had hopes and dreams that by 25 she would be married with a family. Through her 30s she had a relationship with a man who kept promising marriage and children. Helen hung on but finally recognised this would never happen and got out of the relationship after eight years. Within weeks her father was diagnosed with an aggressive cancer and she helped to care for him for the next 18 months. Single and childless at 40 was not part of her life plan.

Most women who are trying to conceive in their late 30s or early 40s are acutely aware of the impact of age on fertility, but others have unrealistic expectations about their chances of a successful pregnancy. Older women (over 35) have an increased risk of gynaecological problems including fibroids, polyps and endometriosis and may require earlier referral for investigation. A diagnosis of "unexplained infertility" is common in women over 35: this is largely due to poor egg quality. A poor-quality egg is less likely to fertilise, but if fertilised is more likely to produce an embryo which is slow to divide and either does not implant or miscarries due to chromosomal abnormalities. A woman over 35 is at increased risk of miscarriage, ectopic pregnancy and stillbirth. She also has a higher chance of pregnancy complications including gestational diabetes, placenta praevia, placental abruption, hypertension and Caesarean section. [493]

Ovarian reserve and ovarian ageing

A woman's chronological age has the most impact on her fertility, but her ovarian reserve also plays a part. Ovarian reserve describes the quantity of eggs remaining in the ovaries at a specific point in time. A woman needs to understand that she is born with all of her eggs (around 2 million) but her reserve is depleting continuously. She may be complimented for looking young, but her ovaries are ageing faster than any other part of her body. At the age she starts her periods (around 12) she has about 400,000 viable eggs left, but she is losing them at a rate of about 1,000 per month. She will ovulate less than 500 eggs in total through her entire reproductive life and her ovaries will stop functioning when the reserve drops to around 1,000 eggs. As the number of eggs decline, the percentage with chromosomal abnormalities increases.

A woman normally has her menopause (final menstrual period) between 45 and 55 years (average 51). However, she has up to 10 years prior to this when she is likely to be permanently infertile due to the normal physiological decline in ovarian function (see figure 3.18 in chapter 3). Some women have an "early menopause" (before 45 years); this is common in smokers. Two key factors

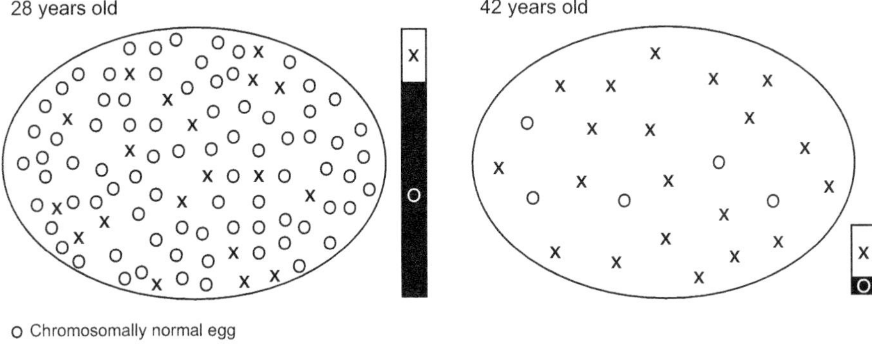

Figure 18.6 The ovarian reserve of a young woman compared with an older woman to show the percentage of chromosomally abnormal eggs

determine a woman's age at menopause: her number of follicles at birth and the rate of attrition. A poor complement of follicles at birth and/or a rapid rate of attrition could result in POI and consequently premature menopause (before 40 years; see page 211).

Figure 18.6 represents a sample of an ovary from a woman in her late 20s compared with a woman in her early 40s. The young woman on the left has a good ovarian reserve. She has a lot of eggs left and a high percentage of chromosomally normal eggs (shown by the open circles). By comparison the older woman on the right has a low ovarian reserve. She has a low number of eggs with a high percentage of chromosomally abnormal eggs (shown by the Xs). During ovarian stimulation, such as for IVF, the ovary on the left would be expected to respond well and produce a good number of chromosomally normal eggs, whereas the ovary on the right would have a poor response to the drugs, few eggs would be collected and a high percentage would be chromosomally abnormal. Aneuploidy is the largest cause of IVF failure and miscarriage.

A variety of tests for ovarian reserve can help couples to make decisions about planning their family, as illustrated in Mia's case, which follows. These tests can determine how the reserve compares with other women of similar age, but their main value is in predicting ovarian response to stimulation during assisted fertility. Ovarian reserve tests will be inaccurate if a woman is taking hormonal contraception due to its suppressant effect on the ovaries (page 264). **There are no tests which can predict how long childbearing can safely be delayed:** chronological age remains the best predictor of chances of conception, both naturally and with all forms of assisted conception (page 344).

CASE STUDY OVARIAN RESERVE

Mia is 30 years old. She has a family history of premature menopause – her mother and grandmother both went through the menopause in their late 30s. Mia's partner of two years is 28. They want children together (ideally at least two), but they are at a crossroads with plans including travelling, a wedding, job change and house move. Mia has read about ovarian reserve tests and is keen to know her fertility status in view of her mother's pattern. Her AMH and antral follicle count (AFC) are found to be very low for her age, which confirms her fears. With this new knowledge they change their priorities and start trying to conceive.

Man's age

Men continue to produce sperm throughout their adult life, but their fertility starts to decline from around 35 years of age (see figure 3.20 in chapter 3). This is due to a decrease in sperm quality and a higher percentage of DNA fragmentation plus genetic mutations, leading to a longer time to pregnancy, increased rate of miscarriage and increased chance of passing on some developmental disabilities and mental health conditions. Children born to men over 45 are at an increased risk of autism, schizophrenia, bipolar disorder, ADHD and achondroplasia. The absolute risks are still low, however, and older fathers may bring social advantages such as more committed relationships and higher incomes which may outweigh the risks. [335]

With advancing years, a man is more likely to have developed a chronic medical condition where either the condition or the treatment may affect his potency or sperm quality. Drugs including narcotics, tranquillisers, some antidepressants and anti-hypertensives may cause erectile dysfunction, or ejaculation difficulties including retrograde ejaculation. Lifestyle factors including alcohol, smoking, illicit drugs, heat, weight, and stress may further adversely impact sperm quality (table 18.2).

Older men may benefit from increased antioxidant intake to counteract sperm DNA damage. Men over 44 with the highest intake of vitamins C and E plus zinc and folate showed levels of sperm DNA damage similar to those of younger men – that is around 20% lower than men of the same age with the lowest antioxidant intake. [529]

Value of fertility awareness for older couples

It may be especially important for older couples to understand their fertility and to optimise their preconception health because adverse lifestyle factors could compound the age factor. The key issue with female age is egg quality but the following factors may reduce chances of conception:

- Irregular cycles: at 35+ a woman may start to experience more irregular cycles and an increased percentage of anovulatory cycles or short luteal phases. Reassure her that during an ovulatory cycle, the fertile time will be of a similar length to that of a younger woman. [145]
- Reduced quantity and quality cervical secretions: an older woman may experience more days of dryness. She may not observe the wetter, slippery, stretchy secretions, in which case her peak day will be the last day of the sticky, white secretion before a return to dryness. Reassure her that it is not necessary to see spinnbarkeit-type secretions; intercourse on days with any secretions carries a chance of pregnancy.
- Sexual difficulties: older couples may struggle with the recommended sex frequency and/or timing. Reassure couples that sexual difficulties are common when trying to conceive – consider whether erectile dysfunction or ejaculation difficulties are impacting chances of conception and whether the couple are using vaginal lubricants which could damage sperm (table 18.2). Consider the need for medication and/or counselling.
- Stress: consider additional pressures such as work stress, complex relationships (for example with ex-partners and responsibilities for other children), support for elderly parents and pressures to produce a grandchild. How can this stress be managed?

When working with an older woman who is planning pregnancy, it is important to acknowledge her age (and that of her partner) and to help her face the reality of her situation. But it is also important to focus on the positive changes that can be made and the ability to regain control of the situation. Women may need psychological help to cope with their sense of failure and to deal with past regrets, including past abortions and relationship breakdown.

When is the right time to start trying?

Young people need to understand the optimal age for childbearing, the physiology behind reproductive ageing and the risks of delaying starting a family (pages 11 and 86).

Figure 18.7 shows a hypothetical timeline spanning forty years – a typical reproductive lifespan from the menarche at the age of 12 to the menopause at 52. Recognising that a woman

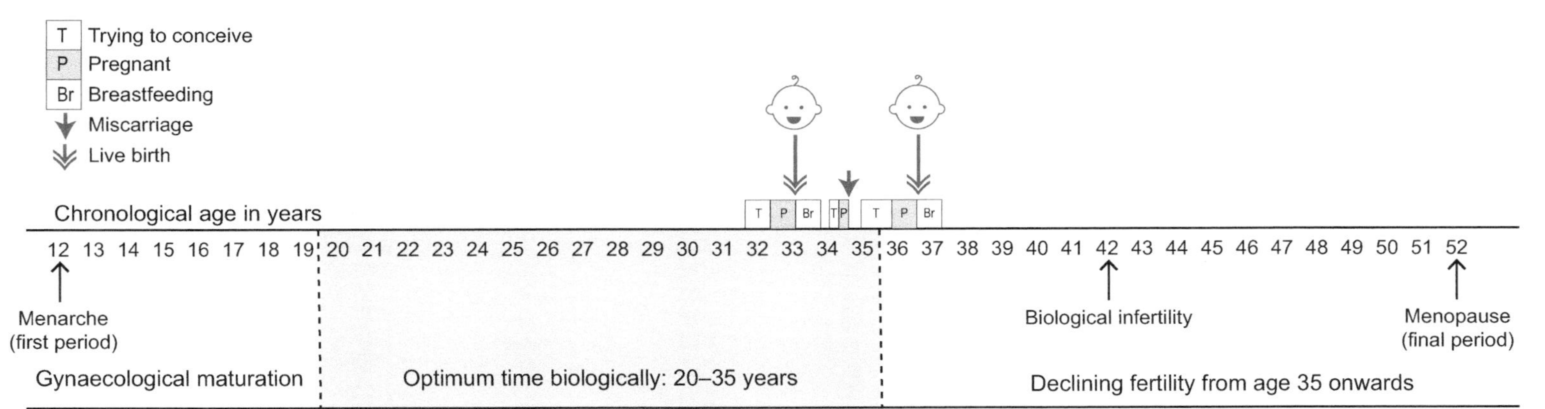

Figure 18.7 Planning ahead: is there a right time to have a baby?

is likely to be infertile for up to 10 years before her menopause, this woman would be infertile from around 42 years of age, with a significant decline in fertility from around 35. Suppose this woman stopped using hormonal contraception on her 32nd birthday. It takes her around nine months to conceive, followed by nine months to carry her pregnancy to term, so she would deliver at 33.5 years. She then breastfeeds for nine months. Her periods may return around six months postnatally at the start of weaning but her full fertility returns at around a year. She now starts trying to conceive again (at 34.5 years) and may conceive fairly quickly this time but have an early miscarriage around her 35th birthday. She feels she needs some time after her miscarriage and starts trying again after three months. This time it takes her a year to conceive and she is becoming increasingly anxious as she was keen to have a close gap between her children. She may start initial fertility investigations, but conceives naturally and delivers her second child around her 37th birthday. This couple have now achieved their desired family size, but some may not be so fortunate.

Health education programmes for young people must aim to improve education about age and fertility with consideration for desired family size (page 359). Scientists at the university of Rotterdam have shown by computer simulation that women who want a 90% chance of having three children without resorting to IVF should start trying to conceive by the age of 23 years (page 12).

WEIGHT, BODY FAT AND FERTILITY

Weight, BMI and body fat percentage are key factors affecting the menstrual cycle (page 204). Normal-weight women are more likely to conceive and carry a pregnancy to term than those who are not of normal weight for their height. Body fat has a vital role in preconception health. The mother's preconception weight and her weight gain during pregnancy is linked to birth weight and the infant's nutritional status (see table 18.2).

Appendix F shows a BMI chart with the shaded zone representing the ideal BMI range for fertility (20–25 kg/m^2). The further outside the ideal range, the stronger the association with risks to fertility and pregnancy.

Managing overweight women

Women who are overweight (BMI 25–30) or obese (BMI 30+) with a high body fat percentage and excess estrogens are more likely to have cyclic disturbances. Excessive weight impacts as follows:

- Obesity may be linked to PCOS and accompanying hormonal disturbance.
- Cycles may be irregular in length, anovulatory or have short luteal phases.
- Overweight and obese women who have delayed ovulation are more likely to have an interrupted pattern of secretions or multiple peak days.
- Some women report profuse amounts of highly estrogenised wet secretions.
- Weight loss significantly improves the percentage of ovulatory cycles and the pregnancy rate in overweight women including those with PCOS.
- As little as a 5% reduction in body weight can restore normal ovulatory cycles. [92] [454] [431]

Too often women who face fertility delays are told to "go away and lose weight" before further investigations are initiated or before starting assisted fertility programmes. This can be very challenging for those who may have psychological and emotional issues related to food, but the fact remains that overweight women have a reduced chance of conception naturally and with all forms of assisted fertility.

Women should be discouraged from using rapid weight loss programmes as this is generally not sustainable and has adverse effects on egg quality. Weight loss programmes which include nutritional advice and exercise programmes plus consideration for the psychological aspects of eating may help to achieve a normal BMI, hence improving general health and optimising fertility with the added benefit of improving levels of self esteem, anxiety and depression. [222] [641]

Managing underweight women

A woman's body requires optimum nutritional levels for regular ovulatory cycles. Underweight women with a low body fat percentage and low estrogen levels have an increased risk of anovulatory cycles and amenorrhoea. The lower the body fat percentage, the higher the chance of amenorrhoea due to complete suppression of the HPO-axis. Women with a body fat composition of less than 22% rarely ovulate. Underweight women often report persistent dryness or scant amounts of reduced quality secretions. Many underweight women will not observe wetter, stretchy secretions. Peak day is then the last day showing the most fertile characteristics before the change back to dryness.

In figure 18.8 both women are 18 years old and 165 cm (5 ft. 5 in.) tall. The woman on the left weighs 57 kg (8 st. 3 lb.), giving her a normal BMI of 21 (body fat percentage: 28%). The woman on the right weighs 47 kg (7 st. 6 lb.), giving her a BMI of 17 (body fat percentage: 19%). The normal-weight woman has a normal body composition with sufficient fat stores in her breasts, tummy, thighs and bottom to maintain normal estrogen levels and regular ovulatory cycles. The underweight woman has a pre-pubertal body composition with a low body fat percentage and low estrogen levels. Reduced GnRH secretion from the hypothalamus has switched off the pituitary release of FSH and LH and suppressed the HPO-axis. She has stopped ovulating and menstruating.

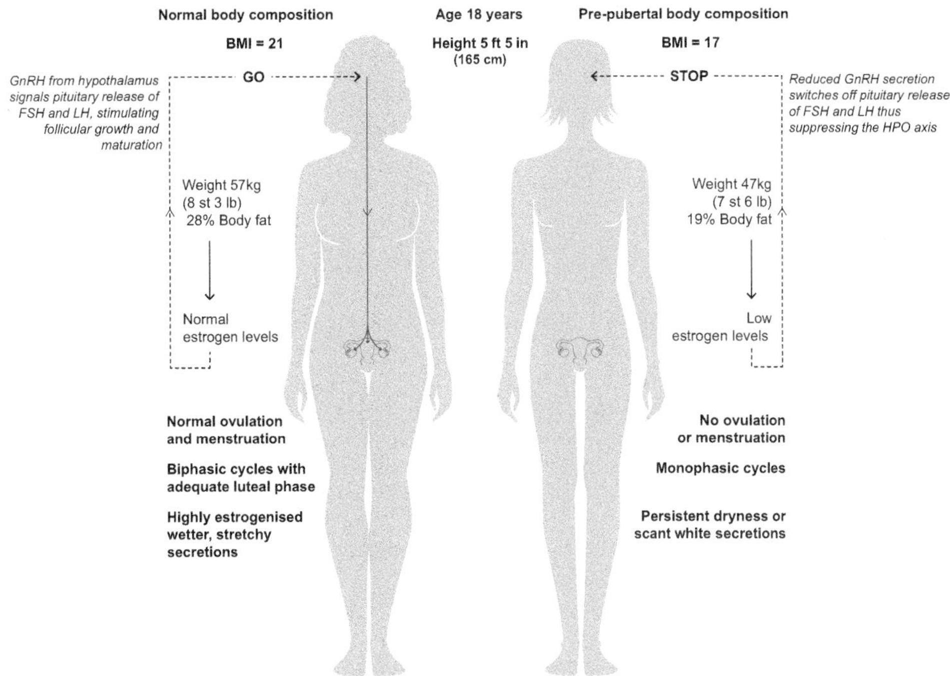

Figure 18.8 Impact of body fat percentage on female fertility (adapted from Frisch 2002) [207]

A woman may resume menstruation with a BMI of 19 (body fat percentage around 23%) – mid-way between the two figures illustrated – but many women will still have a higher percentage of anovulatory cycles or cycles with longer follicular phases (delayed ovulation) and short luteal phases. Women's ovaries respond to weight fluctuations in the same way as any other stressful situation, with cycles moving unpredictably between the different cycle types defined by Brown's continuum until weight and body fat percentage have stabilised and full ovulatory cycles can be maintained (page 85).

For women who are facing delays in conception, optimising weight and body fat percentage is a vital first step before considering any form of ovulation induction. Women who have been severely underweight and then manage to reach a healthy weight (BMI 20+) may find that periods and ovulatory cycles still do not return for several months. This may be due to temporary polycystic ovaries (detectable by ultrasound). Women who have achieved their target weight, but still fail to resume regular ovulatory cycles may require some form of ovulation induction.

CASE STUDY THE IMPORTANCE OF BODY FAT

Amy was initially seen when trying for her first child (BMI: 18.5). She acknowledged that her disrupted cycles and lack of fertile secretions could be linked to her weight and low estrogen levels. Amy reduced her exercise and increased her energy intake (including full-fat dairy products). She conceived naturally after three months and delivered a healthy 7 lb girl at term.

Amy returned to the clinic when her daughter was 18 months old. She had breastfed successfully for six months, but after stopping she remained amenorrhoeic for a further three months. Amy's cycles were now consistently around 21 days with very light bleeds. Her gynaecologist confirmed a normal pelvic scan with normal AFC. He prescribed clomiphene, but Amy was not comfortable with this. Amy's BMI was now 18. She acknowledged her return to intensive exercise, plus a busy job and caring for a toddler. Amy had returned to her old habits and was eating mostly vegetables with hardly any protein and no carbohydrates. Amy decided she could get her BMI up to 20 and then if she did not conceive within three months she would try clomiphene. She conceived on her third cycle with no need for ovulation induction.

Body fat distribution

Body weight and body fat percentage are not the only factors to influence the incidence of normal fertile cycles – the distribution of body fat may also play a part. Women with a more gynaecoid body fat distribution (pear-shape) are more likely to conceive. Consider two different women:

- Woman 1 has a waist:hip ratio of 24:36 inches or 2:3 = 0.66 (< 0.80): the pear.
- Woman 2 has a waist:hip ratio of 30:36 inches or 5:6 = 0.83 (> 0.80): the apple.

In a study of 500 women undergoing intrauterine insemination, the CPR for women with a waist:hip ratio lower than 0.80 was significantly higher than for women with ratios greater than 0.80. [640]

Measurement of waist circumference detects abdominal visceral fat rather than subcutaneous fat. Visceral fat is metabolically active; when increased, it results in increased rates of insulin resistance. Women with a more android body fat distribution (central obesity) are more likely to have increased testosterone, PCOS and insulin resistance (page 210). [23] It has been suggested that self-reported body shape may be a useful proxy measure, in addition to body size, in large-scale surveys because women's perception of body size is consistent with anthropometric measures used to assess obesity and body fat distribution. [576]

NUTRITIONAL HEALTH

Nutrition plays a key role in reproductive health. When trying to conceive, both partners should enjoy a well-balanced diet including protein with each meal and plenty of fruit, vegetables and whole grains, whilst limiting fatty foods and highly refined sugars. Women consuming a diet containing several protein-rich food sources, fruit and whole grains have a reduced risk of preterm delivery. [247]

Increasing numbers of studies demonstrate the impact of diet on sperm quality, ovulatory function and IVF success rates; however, many women planning pregnancy still have an inadequate nutritional intake. More effort needs to be made by health professionals to increase awareness of a healthy diet and lifestyle before and throughout pregnancy. [115]

The importance of preconception nutrition was first recognised following the Dutch famine of 1944–1945. Babies who were born during the famine, but conceived before it began, were slightly lighter than the previous generation, but had no increased risk of congenital or developmental abnormalities. However, babies conceived during the famine had significantly higher rates of low birth weight, perinatal mortality and congenital abnormalities, demonstrating that an inadequate supply of nutrients around the time of conception is more damaging than inadequate nutrition in later pregnancy. A very low calorie intake at conception results in the birth of a normal weight or slightly underweight baby, but there is a significantly higher rate of obesity and type 2 diabetes in adulthood. The offspring's genes had been modified for famine conditions, hence plentiful food results in obesity. [364]

Fetal origins hypothesis

In 1992 Barker, an epidemiologist, proposed the "fetal origins hypothesis". He suggested that chronic illnesses such as coronary heart disease, hypertension, stroke and type 2 diabetes are not always inherited or the result of an unhealthy adult lifestyle but may result from poor nutrition in pregnancy and early infant life. Barker proposed that in poor nutritional conditions fetal development is modified to prepare for survival in a resource-limited environment. [28] The "Barker hypothesis" is now widely accepted as biological fact.

A child's health may be affected by grand-maternal as well as maternal health and lifestyle. A woman's potential for life starts as an immature oocyte within one of her mother's ovaries whilst her mother is still a fetus – hence a woman's potential for life starts within her grandmother's body. Grand-maternal smoking as well as maternal smoking, for example, has been linked to low birth weight and childhood asthma. [295] [355]

Epigenetic effects

A mother's preconception diet can permanently affect the functioning of her child's genes. The primordial germ cells, embryo and fetus are highly susceptible to epigenetic changes influenced by the mother's nutritional status at the time of conception (and by environmental chemicals and possibly severe stress). "Epigenetics" literally means "in addition to changes in the genetic sequence." Epigenetic effects are modifications to DNA that turn genes on and off. This includes any process that alters gene activity without changing the DNA sequence, and leads to modifications that can be transmitted to daughter cells.

Medical Research Council studies in rural Gambia have demonstrated that the dramatic seasonal fluctuations in peri-conceptional nutritional status cause permanent epigenetic effects. Individuals conceived in the rainy season (July to November) when there are plentiful supplies of green leafy vegetables (rich sources of B vitamins and folate) live significantly longer and healthier lives compared with those conceived in the dry season when couscous and rice are staple foods. [605]

Epigenetic changes have consequences for subsequent developmental disorders and disease which may manifest in childhood, throughout life and pass to subsequent generations. [460] [127] The challenge for research is to determine an optimal preconception diet for women and men that would optimise the genetic health of subsequent generations.

Vegetarian vs. non-vegetarian diet and restrained eating

Vegetarians do not eat meat and most do not eat fish. The majority of vegetarians are lacto-vegetarians so include dairy products such as milk, cheese, yogurt and butter. Most vegetarians eat eggs but vegans don't eat any foods from an animal source – just vegetables, grains, nuts and fruits. A restricted diet may be of concern particularly if a woman is underweight or has a low body fat percentage.

One study compared the weight and cycle characteristics of vegetarians with non-vegetarians. All the women had stable BMIs of 18–25 and apparently normal menstrual cycles. They used food and restraint diaries to determine energy intake, and waking temperature to determine their ovulatory status. Vegetarians had lower BMIs and body fat percentages. Average cycle lengths were similar between the two groups, but the vegetarians had longer luteal phase lengths and fewer anovulatory cycles. The women (vegetarian and non-vegetarian) who were most restrained with their eating (i.e. controlled intake to avoid weight gain) showed the highest incidence of ovulatory dysfunction, with shorter luteal phases and fewer ovulatory cycles. [32]

When questioned about body weight, many women who are trying to conceive report that they weighed significantly more during their late teens and early 20s at a time when they were less inhibited with their eating. **Maintaining a tight control over nutritional intake may result in a lower body fat percentage than is optimal for reproductive function.**

Nutritional information

For more information about healthy eating before and during pregnancy, see RCOG guidance on nutrition in pregnancy, [489] the Food Standards Agency website (www.food.gov.uk) and the NHS Choices website (www.nhs.uk). Registered nutritionists are qualified to provide information about food and healthy eating; see The Association for Nutrition website (www.associationfornutrition.org). Nutritionists are *not* qualified to provide information about special diets for medical conditions. Men or women with a chronic medical condition, such as diabetes or coeliac disease, should consult their dietitian about their dietary needs when planning pregnancy; see the Association of UK Dietitians website: www.bda.uk.com.

SEXUAL FUNCTION

The majority of couples who are trying to conceive will have normal sexual functioning and will conceive easily. It has been suggested that negative pressure in the uterus at the time of orgasm may help to suck up sperm, but the link between orgasm and conception is unproven. When sex is satisfying, however, it is likely to increase emotional intimacy – resulting in more frequent sex hence optimising chances of conception. Women should be reassured that loss of seminal fluid after intercourse (flowback) is normal (page 48). There is no scientific evidence that lying flat or lying with the buttocks raised increases the chance of conception but it makes good practical sense to avoid getting up, urinating or washing immediately. Sexual boredom and sexual difficulties are common. In an audit of more than 500 lifestyle questionnaires (average six months trying to conceive), 56% of couples felt that their sex life had been affected – a few reported a positive effect (more sex), but the majority felt that the pressures to conceive had a negative effect, with sex becoming mechanical and less satisfying. [611]

Sexual difficulties

Sexual function can be affected at any stage of the sexual response cycle. The major difference between sexual functioning in men and women is that it is virtually impossible for a man to have intercourse if he is unable to achieve or maintain an erection, whereas it is still physically possible for a woman to have intercourse without being aroused, as demonstrated by the widespread use of vaginal lubricants. As natural conception cannot occur without normal male sexual functioning, this can put a huge pressure on the man and on the relationship. Sexual difficulties may be the cause of fertility delays for some couples, but conversely for others fertility delays may cause sexual difficulties.

Sexual difficulties that may lead to fertility problems

Couples who have difficulty conceiving should be questioned sensitively, but explicitly, about their sexual activity, including the frequency and timing of intercourse, plus the mechanics of intercourse (page 33). Sexual dysfunction may first present as a fertility problem, hence it is vital that this fundamental issue has been addressed prior to starting invasive fertility investigations. Careful questioning must confirm that seminal fluid is being ejaculated into the vagina. Some couples rather naively have anal sex, intercrural sex (between the thighs) or only partial vaginal penetration. Questions about the nature of seminal fluid may reveal that a man has retrograde ejaculation (ejaculates backwards into the bladder). He will feel the sensations of orgasm, but will not release any fluid. Despite the apparently open attitudes to sex, couples still fail to consummate relationships sometimes after many years of embarrassed silence. In the case study of Molly, her entrenched fear about penetration could easily have resulted in non-consummation of the marriage.

CASE STUDY MOLLY, FEAR OF PENETRATION

Molly and Steve had been together for three years and planned to marry within four months. As a committed Catholic, Molly was not yet sexually active. She wanted to learn NFP but planned to start trying to conceive on the honeymoon. Molly kept her charts meticulously but was concerned about "not doing it right". Her anxiety about sex was palpable. She understood very little about her body and had never used tampons. Molly had worried about sex since her mother's disclosure that she had required surgery for a thick hymen before she was able to have sex. Molly had convinced herself that penetration would be impossible. She was offered a gentle internal examination for reassurance but declined, so simple line drawings were used to explain her sexual anatomy.

Molly was given "permission" to use a hand mirror to get to know her genital geography and to take some uninterrupted time to explore her vagina. She learnt about her pelvic floor muscles (page 66) and her ability to contract and relax these powerful muscles using Kegel exercises. She started to feel comfortable inserting first one finger, then two. Her internal exploration helped her to more easily identify secretions and she managed to locate her cervix and recognise its changes. Molly discovered the pleasures of her highly sensitive clitoris. She found that her vaginal walls could expand and lubricate, her hymen felt quite elastic and she could control the degree of digital penetration. She started to use tampons confidently and finally felt in control of her body. Molly was highly receptive to suggestions which increased her understanding of FA, but meanwhile she had become more relaxed about her body and her ability to become sexually aroused and achieve penetration. She was finally able to look forward to her wedding night.

Sexual difficulties resulting from fertility delays The stress of delayed conception, and invasive fertility investigations and treatments, can impact sexual intimacy, creating sexual difficulties for either partner. Intercourse is often avoided because it acts as a reminder of the fertility issues and the inability to achieve what other couples appear to achieve so easily. The added pressure of the public nature and social isolation caused by fertility problems puts further pressure on the relationship.

A man might feel that his partner wants sex only when there is a chance of pregnancy. She may reject him completely at times or avoid "unnecessary" sexual activity, such as oral sex, which would otherwise be an enjoyable part of their lovemaking. The bedroom quickly becomes a battleground. A man may be unable to get an erection or to ejaculate, which can lead to a vicious circle with the fear of failure increasing anxiety and leading to further failure – "performance anxiety".

A study of 439 men with no history of erectile dysfunction found that after six months of timed intercourse, the stress imposed by the thought of obligatory sex caused erectile difficulties in 40% of the men. Many men tried to avoid sex at the fertile time and 10% of the men reported extra-marital affairs. As the number of episodes of timed intercourse increased the number of men with erectile difficulties, avoiding behaviour and extra-marital affairs increased. All 47 men who reported extra-marital affairs experienced erectile difficulties with their spouse. These findings may confirm the link between high cortisol levels and erectile dysfunction. [21]

Facilitating discussion about sex and sexual difficulties

Discussions about sexual activity and intercourse timing form an integral part of FA consultations, whether for planning or avoiding pregnancy. Anxieties about sexual difficulties often arise naturally, but practitioners must be sensitive to clients who find the issues embarrassing. Some women will avoid discussions around sex, sometimes focusing on unimportant details of a chart. Patterns of intercourse may give an indication of possible sexual or relationship difficulties: for example, a woman may not record any acts of intercourse on her chart, or she may only record intercourse sporadically, finding excuses such as tiredness or work stress. This always requires further exploration (page 365 for sexual issues related to avoiding pregnancy). The Female Sexual Function Index (FSFI) can be used as a reliable screening tool particularly in young fertile women. [514] [573] [421]

Identifying the problem area The use of open-ended questions encourages clients to engage in discussion. The following questions may help to elicit useful information:

- How often do you have sex (penis in vagina)?
- Do you ever experience pain during or after intercourse?
- Do you ever experience any bleeding after intercourse?
- Do you use any lubricating gels?
- Do you ever experience any sexual difficulties including lack of desire?
- Do you have any difficulties attaining or maintaining an erection (men)?
- Has anything changed in your sex life since you started trying to conceive?
- Do you struggle to cope with your (or your partner's) fertility problems?

If a problem area is identified, then it is useful to elicit when and how the problem started, whether it is improving or getting worse, whether any other factors help or exacerbate the problem, and whether it is persistent or sporadic in nature or circumstance. The client's own assessment of the cause of the problem may help in exploring how best to deal with the issues and to consider appropriate next steps, including referral within or outside the clinic team. Physical factors must always be excluded before assuming that the problem is purely psychological. See appendix H for further reading and referral to psychosexual-trained doctors and accredited therapists specialising in sexual and relationship issues.

SEX PRE-SELECTION

Many couples are keen to try and influence their baby's sex prior to conception. Interest in sex pre-selection dates back to the ancient Greeks, who believed that male sperm originated from the right testicle and female sperm from the left. In the 18th century French noblemen were reported to have tied up, or even cut off, their left testicle in their quest for an heir. "Son preference" is still common in many parts of the world, but particularly in China and India, where daughter neglect, female infanticide and selective abortion are significant issues.

The sex of the child is determined by whether the egg is fertilised by an X- or Y-chromosome-bearing spermatozoon (page 56). Seminal fluid contains equal numbers of each, with the expected sex ratio at birth being about 105 boys for every 100 girls – hence about 50% of couples will have the sex of their choice by random chance. However, a number of studies have suggested that the sex ratio might vary with the timing of intercourse in relation to ovulation. There are three potential outcomes: a higher ratio of males closer to ovulation, a higher ratio of females closer to ovulation or no difference in the sex ratio.

Higher ratio of males closer to ovulation

Shettles, an American gynaecologist, observed (with phase contrast microscopy) that X- and Y-sperm showed subtle differences in size, motility and resistance to hostile conditions. The larger oval-headed X-bearing sperm were shown to swim more slowly, but live longer and be more resistant to hostile acidic conditions, whilst the smaller, lighter, round-headed, Y-bearing sperm were seen to swim faster but require alkaline conditions for survival. (Evidence from more reliable genotyping techniques suggests that there are no significant morphological differences between mature X and Y sperm.[289][239]) Shettles commented on the imprecision of these factors, but his observations of the physiological differences led him to assert principles to influence the sex of the child:

- To increase the chance of a boy: intercourse should be limited to the time of ovulation with abstinence prior to ovulation during the given cycle. Each act of intercourse should be preceded by an alkaline douche of water and baking soda. Vaginal penetration should be from the rear with deep penetration at the time of male orgasm plus female orgasm to aid sperm penetration – essentially the easier the conditions for conception the greater the chance of a boy.
- To increase the chance of a girl: intercourse should cease 2–3 days before ovulation. Each act of intercourse should be preceded by an acid douche of water and vinegar. Intercourse should take place in a face to face position with shallow vaginal penetration and no female orgasm (Shettles 1970, p. 645 [540]).

Shettles observed 41 couples over a 12-year period. Twenty-two couples were trying for a girl and 19 couples were trying for a boy. Nineteen couples (out of 22) successfully achieved a boy and 16 couples (out of 19) successfully achieved a girl. [540] Shettles results confirmed earlier research by Kleegman which showed that timing a single intrauterine insemination (IUI) in a given cycle close to ovulation resulted in boys in 80% births whereas timing IUI 48 hours before the estimated ovulation resulted in a similar incidence of girls. [331]

A significantly higher proportion of boys from intercourse close to ovulation was similarly reported in a study of nearly 4,000 Jewish women. These women all observed the orthodox ritual of sexual separation until after the mikveh, resuming intercourse within two days of ovulation. The women who resumed intercourse two days after ovulation had a significantly higher proportion of boys. [264]

The Billings the pioneers of the Ovulation Method, strongly advocated Shettles' method. They devised a complex set of rules based on changes in the secretions: essentially, to increase the odds for a boy they asserted that intercourse should be delayed until after peak day whilst to increase the odds for a girl intercourse should be avoided from two days before peak. Sex pre-selection using the Billings Method is still widely promoted as a successful method for choosing the desired sex. [398]

Higher ratio of females closer to ovulation

John France conducted a prospective study in New Zealand which disproved Shettles theory. Thirty-three women used the LH surge, peak day and temperature rise as markers for ovulation. A higher percentage of girls were conceived at the time of ovulation. [185] France conducted a similar prospective study of 91 natural conception cycles. The birth sex ratio favoured boys when intercourse preceded ovulation by two days or longer. France noted that while this association was statistically significant, the number of pregnancies involved was too small to conclude that the relationship was real. [184]

A meta-analysis of six studies, using temperature and secretions, found similar results to France. There was a statistically significant *lower* percentage of male births among conceptions occurring during the most fertile time of the cycle. This study disproved suggestions by Shettles and Billings that intercourse timing around ovulation can be used to pre-select male births. Gray suggested that hormonal levels may be a factor in the sex ratio because ovulation induction (2,608 births) has been shown to result in 46% male births, whilst IVF studies have reported 52% male births. [240]

No association between intercourse timing and sex ratio

Many large, well-conducted studies have failed to find a link between intercourse timing and the sex ratio at birth. The large WHO multi-centre study, which used cervical secretions as a marker for ovulation, reported on the outcome of 140 live births. It showed no significant differences in the sex ratio from varying intervals between the likely act of intercourse leading to conception and the estimated day of ovulation. [619]

The North Carolina Early Pregnancy study, which measured estrogen and progesterone metabolites in urine, found that cycles producing girls and boys (129 live births) had similar patterns of intercourse in relation to ovulation. It concluded that for practical purposes the timing of intercourse in relation to ovulation has no influence on the sex of the baby. [631]

A multi-centre prospective study involving couples using temperature and secretions as markers for ovulation reported on 947 singleton births. There were 101.5 males per 100 females, which was not significantly different from the expected ratio of 105 males per 100 females. There was no significant relationship between the estimated day of conception relative to ovulation, the length of the follicular phase or the planned/unplanned status of the pregnancies. Gray commented that the findings may be affected by the imprecision of the data, but the study suggested that intercourse timing in relation to ovulation cannot be used to influence the sex of the child. [241]

Why the conflicting results?

Contradictory reports on sex pre-selection may be due to poor study design or analysis. Some studies questioned women retrospectively about their intercourse pattern months later (at the time of birth). A very large sample size is needed to detect a difference from the theoretical 50:50 ratio of male:female births. Many studies use subjective indicators of fertility which are less reliable markers of ovulation. Additionally, in the majority of studies, couples had more than one act of intercourse during the fertile time, so it is not possible to determine which intercourse resulted in pregnancy. At least 30 other variables have been suggested which may influence the sex of the baby: for example, rising female birth rate with increasing paternal age, higher male birth rate with increasing socio-economic status and higher incidence of males with increased intercourse frequency. It is possible that stress may play a part. The Oxford Conception Study data showed that of 130 singleton births, women with the highest levels of salivary cortisol had a higher percentage of girls (but this requires further research). [76]

Self-help

Self-help books and Internet forums widely promote a variety of recommendations (mostly based on Shettles method) for sex determination. A number of test kits on the market (with unsubstantiated claims of more than 95% effectiveness) include acid or alkaline vaginal douches, OPKs, thermometers, dietary advice and supplements.

There may be no harm in couples altering their intercourse pattern in an effort to influence the sex of their child, but there have been situations – particularly for women trying to conceive a girl (by avoiding intercourse at their most fertile time) – where significant delays in conception can crucially affect the chances of achieving a healthy pregnancy of either sex. Time delays may be highly detrimental for older women. Couples who would be dissatisfied by a child of the "wrong" sex should be strongly discouraged from attempting to pre-select the sex.

So despite the passion that this subject generates, **there is no reliable scientific evidence to support claims for influencing the sex of the baby by any natural means** – whether through diet, intercourse position or intercourse timing in relation to ovulation. Reliable sex selection techniques are currently possible only using laboratory-based techniques.

Sperm sorting and pre-implantation diagnosis

The two techniques which are permitted in the UK are sperm sorting and pre-implantation genetic diagnosis. Sperm sorting uses flow cytometry with fluorescent dye to separate X- and Y- sperm. Sperm of the appropriate sex are then used for assisted fertility. Sperm sorting is not 100% reliable so is not used in practice in the UK.

Pre-implantation genetic diagnosis (PGD) is the method of choice for sex selection for medical reasons. PGD involves checking the genes and/or chromosomes of embryos created through IVF. An embryo(s) of the appropriate sex is then transferred. UK law allows sex selection only if there is a substantial risk that a sex-linked genetic disease could be passed on to a child. For example, PGD may be used to select female embryos if there is a family history of Duchenne muscular dystrophy or haemophilia, which occur almost exclusively in boys. "Family balancing" for social reasons is not licensed in the UK.

SELF-ASSESSMENT QUESTIONS

Answers are at the end of the chapter.

1 What do NICE Fertility guidelines recommend regarding intercourse timing to optimise chances of conception?
2 Which fertility indicator provides the best marker for timing intercourse to conceive, and why?
3 Describe the role of temperature in pregnancy planning.
4 Define the term "ovarian reserve" and describe the role of ovarian reserve tests as a predictor of fertility potential.
5 What is the fetal origins hypothesis?

WHAT COUPLES NEED TO KNOW WHEN PLANNING PREGNANCY

The following key facts are essential information for couples planning pregnancy:

1. Ensure that the woman has had a blood test in the last five years to confirm that she is immune to rubella (rubella antibody IgG > 10 IU/ml).
2. The woman should start taking 400 mcg folic acid and continue for the first trimester.
3. Discuss any chronic health conditions and prescribed medication (both partners) with your doctor and consider the need for increased folic acid or vitamin D.
4. Eat a healthy, balanced diet to optimise weight, with a multi-vitamin and mineral supplement designed for preconception and pregnancy (for the woman).
5. Aim for intercourse every two to three days to ensure that fresh, healthy sperm are waiting in the tubes prior to ovulation.
6. Ovulation occurs about 14 days before the *next* period starts. The fertile time (about six days) occurs earlier in shorter cycles and later in longer cycles and is most easily recognised by the wetter, transparent, stretchy secretions.
7. A period does not prove ovulation has occurred; similarly, an OPK does not prove the occurrence of ovulation. Waking temperature may confirm the possible occurrence of ovulation, or detect a short luteal phase, but temperature is of no value in timing sex to conceive.
8. It is normal to have the occasional cycle where ovulation does not occur. Anovulatory cycles are more common after stopping hormonal contraception, postpartum and pre-menopausally.
9. Consider any additional stresses and how best to manage this. Identify a relaxation technique or therapy that works for you – consider yoga, mindfulness meditation or acupuncture.
10. If there is no conception after six months of frequent sex across the entire fertile time, seek medical advice.

ANSWERS TO SELF-ASSESSMENT QUESTIONS

1. Vaginal sexual intercourse every two to three days.
2. Cervical secretions. The days when the secretions are wetter, transparent and stretchy provide the best prospective marker and are the best predictor of the chances of conception.
3. A biphasic chart is indicative of ovulation. A luteal phase of less than 10 days may indicate LPD. A monophasic chart is indicative of anovulation. A raised temperature of 20 days or more is indicative of pregnancy.
4. Ovarian reserve describes the quantity of eggs remaining in a woman's ovaries at a certain point in time. Tests for ovarian reserve give an idea of how the reserve compares with other women of similar age, but they cannot predict how long childbearing can safely be delayed. Age is the best predictor of fertility potential. The main use of ovarian reserve tests is to predict ovarian response to stimulation during assisted fertility.
5. The fetal origins hypothesis, originated by Barker, proposes that chronic illnesses such as coronary heart disease, hypertension, stroke and type 2 diabetes are not always inherited or the result of an unhealthy adult lifestyle but may result from poor nutrition in pregnancy and early infant life. Barker suggested that in poor nutritional conditions, fetal development is modified to prepare for survival in a resource-limited environment.

CONCEPTION DELAYS AND ASSISTED FERTILITY

19

The art of medicine consists of keeping the patient amused while nature heals the disease.
(Voltaire, French Philosopher 1694–1778)

About one in seven heterosexual couples in the UK have fertility problems, and most are **subfertile** rather than **infertile**. The term "subfertility" describes any time of reduced fertility resulting in a prolonged time to conception (usually > 1 year), whilst the term "infertility"is reserved for couples who require assisted fertility techniques to achieve a pregnancy. Examples of conditions causing absolute infertility include azoospermia, blockage of both tubes (in male or female), severe uterine abnormalities or premature menopause – in these situations natural conceptions only occur sporadically.

This chapter explores aspects of delayed conception with the emphasis on the information which can be gained from a FA approach. It is not intended to provide comprehensive coverage of infertility, but to give an overview of fertility investigations and treatment, and explore the role of FA in the management of "unexplained" infertility. It also looks at the return of fertility after pregnancy loss. For wider aspects of infertility, assisted conception and recurrent miscarriage see texts such as Balen [23] in appendix H.

TIMES WHEN FERTILITY IS NATURALLY REDUCED

Fertility is naturally suppressed at certain times in a woman's reproductive life: this is a normal physiological response to hormonal changes. Anticipate reduced fertility in:

- postpartum and breastfeeding women;
- women who have suffered miscarriage or pregnancy loss;
- women who are very stressed;
- women whose weight is significantly outside the ideal BMI range;
- women who discontinue hormonal contraception (notably injectable methods); and
- older women.

Reduced fertility as a result of ovulatory dysfunction may be recognised on the chart by a delayed or absent temperature rise, interrupted pattern of secretions, multiple peak, deficient luteal phase or (in severe cases) amenorrhoea. It takes time for a woman's body to re-establish full ovulatory function, but this delay can be hard for women to accept and sometimes equally hard for clinicians.

CAUSES OF FERTILITY PROBLEMS

A delay in conception may be caused by a problem in either or both partners at any stage of the reproductive process. The main causes (and approximate prevalence) are:

- male factors (30%);
- ovulatory disorders (25%);
- tubal damage (20%);
- uterine or peritoneal disorders (10%); and
- unexplained infertility (25%).

Percentages do not add up to 100 as there may be more than one cause. In about 40% of cases disorders are found in both partners. Endometrial factors, gamete or embryo defects, and pelvic conditions such as endometriosis may also play a role. [428] Fertility assessment needs to address this wide range of causes and also encourage discussion around lifestyle factors, intercourse timing and sexual difficulties.

REFERRAL FOR CLINICAL ASSESSMENT

NICE guidelines recommend:

- A woman of reproductive age who has not conceived after one year of unprotected vaginal sexual intercourse, in the absence of any known cause of infertility, should be offered further clinical assessment and investigation along with her partner.
- An earlier referral should be offered for specialist consultation to discuss the options for attempting conception, further assessment and appropriate treatment where:
  - the woman is aged 36 years or over; and
  - there is a known clinical cause of infertility or a history of predisposing factors for infertility. [428]

INVESTIGATION OF FERTILITY PROBLEMS

Figure 19.1 shows the normal progression of fertility tests and investigations. Additional testing may be required for some people with an existing medical condition. Sometimes an investigation may be unnecessary: for example, if a man has a very low sperm count, then IVF with intracytoplasmic sperm injection (ICSI) may be the only option and tubal patency tests may thus be an unnecessary intervention.

Male assessment and semen analysis

The first thing to establish is whether the man has good-quality sperm and whether they have the potential for natural conception. The results of the semen analysis are compared with the WHO reference values (table 19.1). [105] NICE provides guidance on interpreting the results and the timing of repeat tests. [428] Male infertility is a highly specialised area which took a huge leap forward in 1992 when ICSI was first introduced, but the impact of lifestyle factors and oxidative stress are increasingly recognised as affecting sperm health. [356]

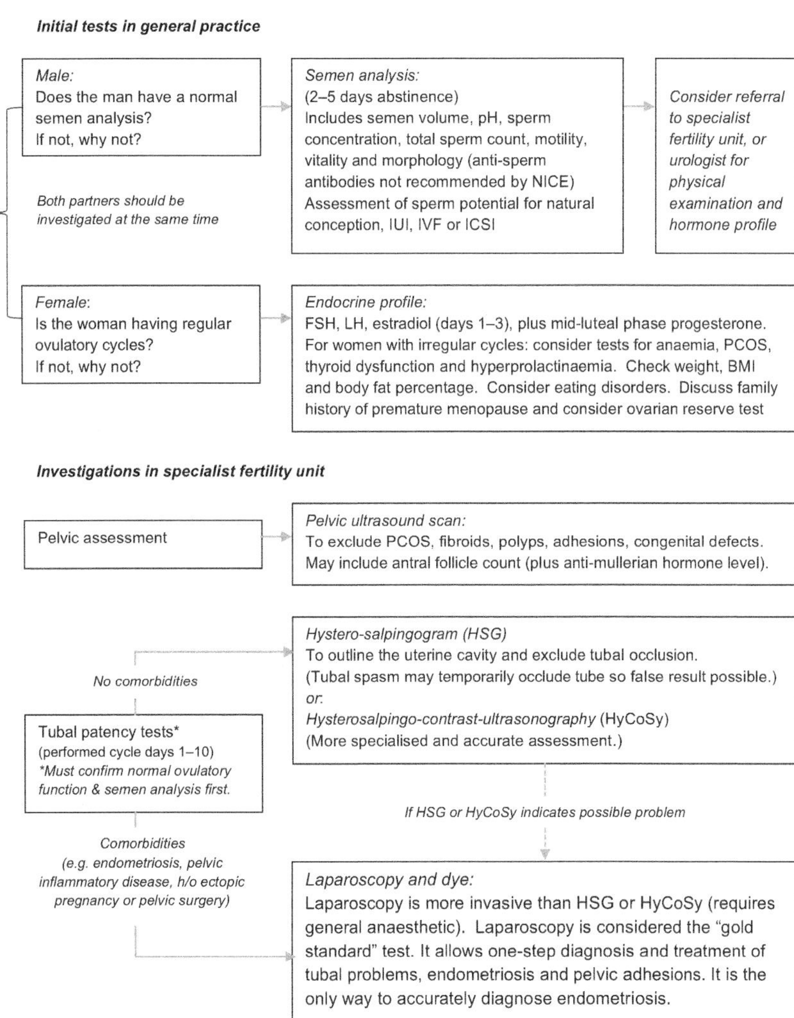

Initial tests in general practice
Male:
Does the man have a normal semen analysis?
If not, why not?
Semen analysis:
(2–5 days abstinence)
Includes semen volume, pH, sperm concentration, total sperm count, motility, vitality and morphology (anti-sperm antibodies not recommended by NICE)
Assessment of sperm potential for natural conception, IUI, IVF or ICSI
Consider referral to specialist fertility unit, or urologist for physical examination and hormone profile
Both partners should be investigated at the same time
Female:
Is the woman having regular ovulatory cycles?
If not, why not?
Endocrine profile:
FSH, LH, estradiol (days 1–3), plus mid-luteal phase progesterone.
For women with irregular cycles: consider tests for anaemia, PCOS, thyroid dysfunction and hyperprolactinaemia. Check weight, BMI and body fat percentage. Consider eating disorders. Discuss family history of premature menopause and consider ovarian reserve test
Investigations in specialist fertility unit
Pelvic assessment
Pelvic ultrasound scan:
To exclude PCOS, fibroids, polyps, adhesions, congenital defects.
May include antral follicle count (plus anti-mullerian hormone level).
Hystero-salpingogram (HSG)
To outline the uterine cavity and exclude tubal occlusion.
(Tubal spasm may temporarily occlude tube so false result possible.)
or:
Hysterosalpingo-contrast-ultrasonography (HyCoSy)
(More specialised and accurate assessment.)
No comorbidities
Tubal patency tests*
(performed cycle days 1–10)
*Must confirm normal ovulatory function & semen analysis first.
If HSG or HyCoSy indicates possible problem
Comorbidities
(e.g. endometriosis, pelvic inflammatory disease, h/o ectopic pregnancy or pelvic surgery)
Laparoscopy and dye:
Laparoscopy is more invasive than HSG or HyCoSy (requires general anaesthetic). Laparoscopy is considered the "gold standard" test. It allows one-step diagnosis and treatment of tubal problems, endometriosis and pelvic adhesions. It is the only way to accurately diagnose endometriosis.

Figure 19.1 Investigation of fertility problems

Progesterone as confirmation of ovulation

The first test for the woman is normally the progesterone assay to confirm ovulation. [428] Progesterone must be measured in the mid-luteal phase. A concentration of more than 30 nmol/l is set as the lower limit associated with ovulation. A level between 16–30 nmol/l indicates a strong possibility of ovulation, but possibly a mistimed test. A level of less than 16 indicates anovulation. It is essential to know the timing of the test in relation to the start of the next period: if there is any doubt, it should be repeated in the next cycle. [23] A raised mid-luteal phase progesterone provides a good indirect marker of ovulation, but does not prove that the follicle ruptured. (Women with LUF syndrome frequently have values higher than 40 nmol/l.) [1] A more comprehensive picture can be gained by using a combination of serial hormonal levels and ultrasound scans to observe follicular growth, ovulation and the development of an adequate corpus luteum. [23]

Table 19.1 WHO reference values for normal semen analysis (adapted from Cooper 2010) [105]

Semen parameter	*Lower reference limit*
Semen volume	≥ 1.5 ml
pH	≥ 7.2
Sperm concentration	≥ 15 million per ml
Total sperm count	≥ 39 million per ejaculate
Total motility	≥ 40%
Progressive motility	≥ 32%
Vitality	≥ 58% live
Morphology	≥ 4% normal forms
White blood cells	< 1 million/mL
Mixed antiglobulin reaction (MAR test) Motile sperm with bound particles (anti-sperm antibodies)	< 50%
Immunobead test; motile sperm with bound beads	< 50%
Additional tests	
Fructose	≥ 13 µmol per ejaculate
Zinc	> 2.4 µmol per ejaculate

Timing progesterone tests

The timing of the progesterone test (loosely referred to as the "Day 21 test") is crucial. It is not easy to time the test to one week before the period is due because cycle lengths can be so variable (figure 3.13 in chapter 3). It is always preferable to use a prospective marker such as the cervical secretions or the LH surge. Suggest the woman aims to time her progesterone test for the following:

- seven days after peak;
- seven days after the urinary LH surge; or
- six days after the temperature rise.

Explain that the results can be interpreted only after the start of the next period to ensure that the test was optimally timed.

Ovarian reserve tests

There are a number of markers for ovarian reserve, including serum FSH, AMH and ultrasound determination of AFC. These are used to predict the likely ovarian response to gonadotrophin stimulation in IVF, but they also give some indication of ovarian age.

FSH As the ovarian reserve diminishes, higher levels of FSH are required to stimulate the follicles and promote the development of a dominant follicle (the pituitary has to "shout louder" to get a response) – hence high levels of FSH indicate diminished ovarian reserve. NICE guidance recommends that FSH levels of 8.9 IU/l or more predict a low response to ovarian stimulation, whilst levels of less than 4 IU/l predict a high response. [428]

AMH Secreted by both late pre-antral and small antral follicles, AMH is a good predictor of ovarian reserve. Women with PCOS have an excess of antral follicles, and individual follicles produce more AMH, hence the concentration is much higher. [349] In older women, with rapidly diminishing ovarian reserve, levels become undetectable approximately five years before the menopause. AMH levels of 5.4 pmol/l or less predict a low response to ovarian stimulation, whilst levels of 25 pmol/l or more predict a high response. [428]

AFC An antral follicle is a resting follicle measuring 2–8 mm in diameter. The number of antral follicles is a good measure of ovarian reserve. An ideal number is 8–10 in each ovary. If there are more than 12, the ovary is polycystic. If the total AFC (i.e. sum from both ovaries) is four or less this indicates a low count and predicts a poor response to ovarian stimulation, with reduced chance of conception. If the total count is more than 16, a high response is anticipated. AMH, together with AFC, allows the clinician to select the most appropriate stimulation protocol for IVF.

Most of the literature about ovarian reserve tests refers specifically to women going through IVF. Some tests are predictive of the number of eggs that could be collected following ovarian stimulation, but they show poor correlation with live-birth rates as they cannot assess egg quality. **Age remains the best predictor of a successful pregnancy, whether through natural or assisted fertility.** [371] [430] [493] [193] [428] [570]

Home tests to assess fertility potential

Many tests which were once only available through the laboratory are now widely available commercially with the advantage of allowing testing in the privacy of the home. This includes home kits and monitors to identify the fertile time (page 172), plus home tests to predict fertility potential. Brezina reviewed some of these tests in 2011, [63] but in this rapidly changing market it is difficult to give up-to-date information. For example: Fertell, which combined a male and female test, was included in the review but is no longer available.

Home semen tests Men frequently find lab-based semen analysis embarrassing and stressful, therefore home tests may be particularly appealing. *SpermCheck Fertility*, an immunodiagnostic test which uses red lines to distinguish between a normal sperm count and a low count, performed well when compared with lab-based WHO-standardised tests. [106] However, a home test gives no indication of other vital semen parameters and provides no additional information about male reproductive health. An abnormal result may encourage a man to undergo a lab-based analysis, but a normal result could be falsely reassuring.

Home tests for ovarian reserve FSH tests (such as *First Response* fertility test) aim to distinguish between a normal and elevated FSH level, but some indicate an abnormal result above 10 IU/l and others as high as 25 IU/l (those claiming to detect menopausal status). A woman whose home test shows a "normal" result may discover that a lab-based test indicates her FSH level is already too high to qualify for IVF. AMH tests are not currently available from the NHS, but they can be done via the Internet. A normal result may be reassuring, but AMH is only part of the picture. An abnormal result showing a low ovarian reserve can be devastating. A personalised service which includes discussion of the results by a health professional provides an opportunity to consider the implications of the result and how best to proceed.

MANAGEMENT OF FERTILITY PROBLEMS

Figure 19.2 shows the treatment options. Some couples may start with a "wait and see" approach or the simplest effective treatment, but others may be advised to proceed straight to IVF with ICSI or even egg (or sperm) donation. NICE guidelines [428] provide clear recommendations

Fertility treatment options
Active expectant management
Education in fertility awareness and lifestyle modifications
Encourage intercourse to coincide with optimal cervical secretions
Observe charts for cyclic abnormalities (temperature may give additional information)
Cycle monitoring with timed intercourse
Serial ultrasound with hormonal assays to monitor follicular development and ovulation
Advise on optimal timing for intercourse based on follicular size (and LH)
Women may continue recording fertility indicators and correlate changes with objective markers
Ovulation induction with timed intercourse
Clomifene citrate (or gonadotrophins) for controlled ovarian hyperstimulation
Advise on optimal timing for intercourse based on follicular size, LH (and cervical secretions)
Intrauterine insemination
Intrauterine insemination (IUI) can be performed during a natural or stimulated cycle
HCG injection is used to trigger ovulation with insemination timed around 36 hours later
Treated sperm (from partner or donor) is inserted through the cervix into the uterine cavity
In vitro fertilisation (IVF) and Intracytoplasmic sperm injection (ICSI)
Ovarian stimulation with gonadotrophins to stimulate multiple follicles followed by egg collection,
sperm collection and preparation (or use of frozen/thawed sperm from partner or donor),
fertilisation with IVF or ICSI, embryo development, transfer and luteal phase support
IVF can be performed in a natural (unstimulated) cycle, but this is not recommended (NICE 2013)
IVF with egg donation
The menstrual cycles of donor and recipient are synchronised
(if recipient is post-menopausal then her uterus is prepared hormonally for transfer)
The donor has her ovaries stimulated to produce multiple eggs (as with IVF)
The eggs are collected and fertilised with recipient partner's (or donor) sperm using IVF or ICSI
The embryo(s) are transferred into the recipient's uterus

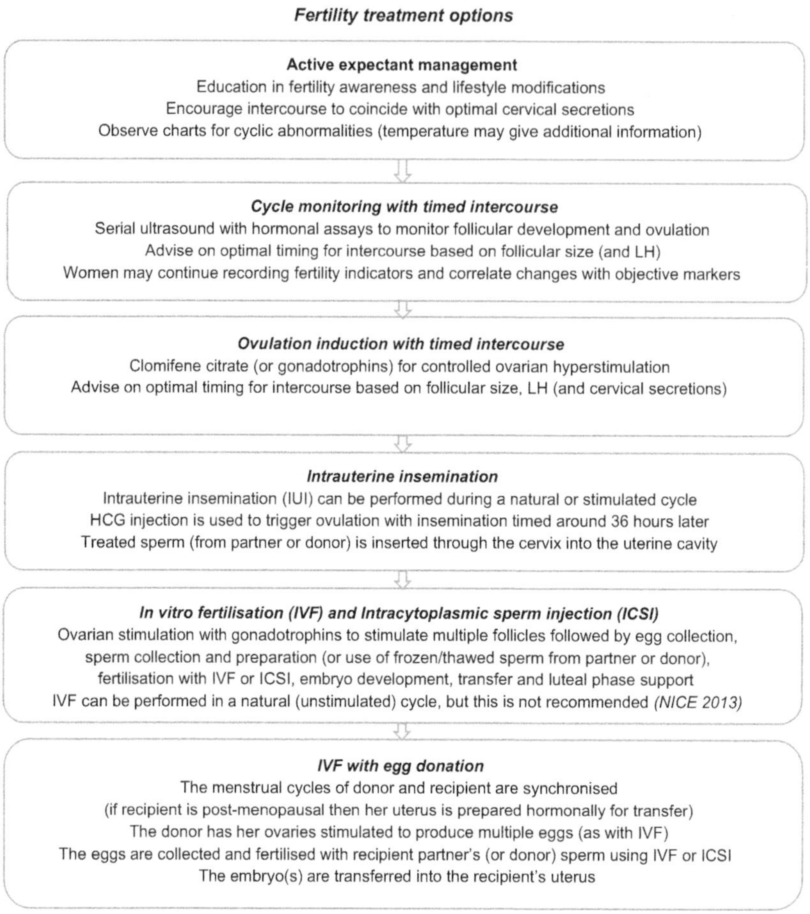

Figure 19.2 Fertility treatment options

on access criteria for IVF on the NHS. Fertility management is a highly specialised area which is outside the scope of this book, but there are some situations where FA may have a role.

Male factor

Women who have an older partner or a partner with sub-optimal sperm may benefit from timing intercourse to coincide with the highest-quality cervical secretions. However, couples with severe male factor problems should not delay and require prompt referral for IVF (possibly with ICSI). [144]

Luteal phase deficiency (LPD)

LPD is a subtle form of ovulatory dysfunction in which ovulation occurs, but the corpus luteum is inadequate, in amount and/or duration, to support implantation and early pregnancy. LPD may be present in short, average or long cycles (page 72). Several different mechanisms may underlie the defect, but the precise mechanism is not understood. LPD occurs in random cycles in women of normal fertility, but it has been linked to subfertility, implantation failure and recurrent miscarriage. LPD is a common concern for women, but its clinical relevance is controversial. It is only of concern if it occurs in most cycles and would therefore impact on chances of conception.

Types of LPD

The BioCycle Study reported on two criteria for LPD:

- Clinical LPD, with a luteal phase length of less than 10 days
- Biochemical LPD, with sub-optimal mid-luteal phase progesterone (< 13 nmol/l)

Both clinical and biochemical LPD were evident amongst women with regular cycles: 9% of cycles showed clinical deficiency, 8% showed biochemical deficiency and 4% met the criteria for both. Both types were associated with lower estradiol levels across the entire cycle. Clinical, but not biochemical, deficiency was associated with lower FSH and LH across the entire cycle. It was proposed that the differences in gonadotrophin levels between the two groups could reflect different underlying causes. [528]

Conditions associated with LPD

LPD is a normal physiological event in specific circumstances. It is described in Brown's continuum as one of the five types of ovarian activity. LPD is associated with stress, irregular cycles, premenstrual spotting, adolescence, postpartum, post-miscarriage, peri-menopause, after hormonal contraception, over- and underweight, eating disorders, excessive exercise and LUF syndrome. LPD is also associated with some pathological conditions including PCOS, thyroid dysfunction (particularly hypothyroidism), hyperprolactinaemia and endometriosis – these conditions should be excluded.

Diagnosis of LPD

There is currently no reliable way to determine luteal function or to know how much impact this has on the prognosis for natural conception. The most commonly used test is serum progesterone (page 343); however, the minimum concentration which defines an adequate luteal phase is not known. As luteal function can vary from cycle to cycle, a random progesterone test has limited value.

Progesterone has some value in predicting the viability of a pregnancy: once pregnancy has become established, hCG stimulates the corpus luteum to produce progesterone. Low progesterone levels in early pregnancy may reflect abnormal hCG stimulation by a non-viable or extra-uterine pregnancy – hence the pregnancy does not fail *because* of low progesterone, the low progesterone reflects a non-viable pregnancy.

Women frequently self-diagnose LPD based on a shortened interval from the time of presumed ovulation to the next period (page 110). Women also express concerns about premenstrual spotting affecting successful implantation (page 207). **If a woman records *three* consecutive cycles with a short luteal phase, further investigation may be warranted.** Premenstrual spotting may be indicative of LPD and requires further assessment. [553]

Treatment of LPD

As the perception of LPD is a progesterone deficiency, women commonly ask about the use of progesterone supplements (pessaries or injections). There is, however, no evidence that this improves pregnancy rates in natural unstimulated cycles. [23] Some women turn to self-help measures, including natural progesterone creams which are rubbed into the skin after ovulation. These are widely promoted to improve luteal function, but there is no evidence of any benefit so their use should be discouraged. The first approach should always be to correct any underlying problems, which in turn optimises the menstrual cycle and the luteal phase.

The development of the corpus luteum is dependent on the preceding phase of follicular growth; similarly, the receptivity of the endometrium depends on estrogen from the developing follicles for proliferation before it can be transformed into a secretory structure. The focus of treatment is therefore normally directed towards the follicular phase. Ovarian stimulation (e.g. with clomiphene citrate) improves follicular growth and development, which subsequently enhances the formation of the corpus luteum, which in turn increases progesterone production.

Self-help measures Women who are restrained in their eating and/or exercise excessively have a higher incidence of LPD and other ovulatory disorders (page 334). A Mediterranean diet, beneficial in terms of cardiovascular disease and diabetes risk, may be less beneficial for optimum fertility: the Mediterranean diet, vegetable protein, fibre and isoflavones have been linked to LPD. Conversely, selenium may have a beneficial effect on luteal function. [9]

Vitex agnus castus (chasteberry) may improve luteal function in women with short luteal phases due to hyperprolactinaemia: 52 women were treated with 20 mg agnus castus (or placebo) daily. After three months, prolactin levels in the treatment group were reduced, luteal phases were normalised and the women showed normal progesterone levels. Two of the women in the treatment group conceived. [404] Vitamin C and other antioxidants may help to prevent oxidative stress and the production of free radicals. Daily supplementation with 750 mg vitamin C significantly increased progesterone levels and pregnancy rates in women with LPD, although there was no significant difference in the miscarriage rate. [276]

Improving cervical secretions

The amount and quality of secretions correlates closely with estrogen levels. Women with low estrogens – for example, older women or those who are underweight – often express concerns about scant, poor-quality secretions. It is important to treat any underlying cause: for example, increasing body fat percentage in an underweight woman (page 331). Subfertile women should be particularly careful to avoid anything that is drying to the vaginal area (e.g. antihistamines) because this may exacerbate the problem (see page 130, table 5.1 and appendix G). Poor-quality secretions are usually related to abnormal follicular development, hence, unless it has been demonstrated that the problem is purely a cervical factor, there is limited value in focusing directly on the improvement of secretions. [81] If cycle monitoring demonstrates abnormal follicular development, then a fertility drug such as clomiphene citrate may be appropriate.

Guaifenesin Expectorant cough mixture is widely promoted on Internet forums to improve cervical secretions. Its main ingredient, guaifenesin, increases respiratory secretions; it may also improve cervical secretions and enhance sperm survival. Forty ovulating women with reduced-quality secretions (and negative post-coital tests) were given 200 mg guaifenesin three times daily from cycle day 5 until the first high temperature. Cervical secretions showed a marked improvement (increased spinnbarkeit and reduced cellularity) in 23 women and slight improvement in seven women; 40% of the participants conceived. In the subgroup of women with cervical problems alone, 80% conceived. [79] *Note:* Cough preparations must be used in their plainest form where the only active ingredient is guaifenesin. Some contain decongestants (e.g. pseudoephedrine) which improve nasal air flow by constricting nasal blood vessels. Decongestants may slow uterine blood flow and have been linked to birth defects, including gastroschisis and ventricular septal defects. [609]

Other self-help remedies There are frequent online discussions about different remedies to improve cervical secretions. Recommendations for measures to increase the volume and liquidity of secretions include a well-balanced diet with increased fluid intake; Vitamin C, an antioxidant (maximum 1,000 mg daily); and evening primrose oil, an essential fatty acid, which has anti-inflammatory properties. Note that evening primrose oil should not be used in the luteal phase or during pregnancy, because it can induce mild uterine contractions. Women may report a difference as a result of lifestyle changes, but the research evidence is lacking.

Short fertile time

Some subfertile couples have a very short fertile time, which significantly reduces their chances of conception. This may be apparent from a reduced number of days with cervical secretions. There may be less than one day between the first normal sperm-mucus test and ovulation (by ultrasound; see page 78). [328] These couples may benefit from education about cervical secretions and more targeted intercourse.

Ovulation disorders, lifestyle change and ovulation induction

Women who are not ovulating may require some form of ovulation induction; however, the first goal is to treat any underlying cause and to optimise health and lifestyle. The most common cause of anovulation is PCOS. Other causes include thyroid disease, hyperprolactinaemia, obesity, rapid weight loss, underweight, eating disorders and excessive exercise (see NICE guidance for WHO classification and treatment of ovulation disorders). [428] Women whose BMI is outside normal limits can improve their chances of regular ovulation, conception and uncomplicated pregnancy by optimising BMI through diet and exercise before proceeding to ovulation induction. **Women who record their fertility indicators whilst implementing lifestyle changes can feel encouraged by positive signs of improved hormone balance:** the temperature may be seen to change from a monophasic pattern through a biphasic pattern with short luteal phase to an adequate luteal phase and hopefully a sustained high temperature confirming pregnancy.

Effect of clomiphene and tamoxifen on secretions

Clomiphene citrate (and tamoxifen), commonly used for ovulation induction, reduce the quantity and quality of secretions, but despite scant poor-quality secretions, given the right conditions, these estrogen antagonists are still effective treatments. [572] [224]

Luteinised unruptured follicle (LUF) syndrome

LUF syndrome describes a condition where the follicle matures but fails to rupture. Despite the failure of ovulation, the action of LH causes the unruptured follicle to undergo luteinisation followed by normal progesterone production and a normal luteal phase. LUF syndrome may be a significant cause of delayed conception. [476] The following facts about LUF are worthy of mention:

- LUF occurs in about 10% of cycles of normal fertile women.
- There is a higher incidence of LUF in subfertile women: it is associated with endometriosis, pelvic adhesions and unexplained infertility.
- LUF can be detected only by serial ultrasound. [86]
- Mid-luteal phase progesterone is typically lower than expected following normal ovulation, but may be at an ovulatory level (page 343).
- Waking temperature may show a normal biphasic curve, but is typically lower than expected following normal ovulation. [527]

- The luteal phase may be of normal duration or shorter; in some cases, it may be longer than anticipated (16 days plus) but pregnancy tests will be negative.
- The following period may be lighter than normal.
- There is an increased incidence of LUF with chronic use of NSAIDs (page 223).
- There is a high incidence of LUF in women treated with clomiphene citrate.

Unexplained infertility

About 25% of couples will be diagnosed with unexplained infertility: routine investigations will have shown a normal semen analysis, normal ovulatory function and patent tubes. Some of these couples may have, as yet, unidentified egg or sperm defects, impaired fertilisation or other subtle causes that may become apparent only during the IVF process. [23]

Some women with unexplained infertility will show classic biphasic charts with a close correlation between fertility indicators, whilst others may observe subtle changes such as premenstrual spotting, short duration of secretions (typical fertile time of less than three days) or a delay between peak day and temperature rise. Peak may occur up to five days before the temperature rise, as in scenario D in figure 10.2 in chapter 10. These subtle changes in the menstrual cycle are not conducive to pregnancy.

NICE guidelines recommend that ovarian stimulation should not be offered to women with unexplained infertility. Clomiphene citrate or unstimulated IUI do not improve live-birth rates. [48] Couples with unexplained infertility who are having regular unprotected intercourse should try to conceive for two years before IVF will be considered. Understandably, many women feel anxious about IVF, but they need to understand that interim steps are unlikely to be effective and may waste valuable fertility time. IVF is a treatment, but it also acts as an investigative process which may give clues about underlying problems. IVF may help to "explain the unexplained".

Expectant management: role of fertility awareness

NICE recognises that where there is no known cause for infertility, expectant management increases the chances of conception. Expectant management is defined as:

> A formal approach that encourages conception through unprotected vaginal intercourse. It involves supportively offering an individual or couple information and advice about the regularity and timing of intercourse and any lifestyle changes which might improve their chances of conceiving. It does not involve active clinical or therapeutic interventions. [428]

However, women who are trying to conceive, express a strong desire to be "doing something". Bhattacharya showed that women with unexplained infertility felt reassured by active treatment and less satisfied by expectant management despite the fact that the treatment did not offer any improvement in live-birth rates. [48]

Gnoth suggested that couples who have a good prognosis (women aged 35 and under, with a normal ovarian reserve, unexplained infertility and trying for less than three years) may still have a reasonable chance of conceiving naturally within the next few cycles, so may benefit from FA education to optimise intercourse timing (page 303). [234] The key indicator for women to observe is the cervical secretions. In addition, both partners should be encouraged to make appropriate lifestyle changes (page 313). **This active expectant management approach helps to optimise conception and avoid mistimed intercourse as a cause of infertility.** Fertility charting has the added benefit of detecting subtle changes in the cycle, which may provide valuable diagnostic information (page 309).

A systematic review evaluated the relationship between cervical secretions and the day-specific pregnancy rate in subfertile couples. It demonstrated that cervical secretions can identify the days with the highest chance of pregnancy. The quality of secretions correlates well with the cycle-specific probability of pregnancy in normal fertile couples but less so in subfertile couples. These results indicated an urgent need for more prospective studies to evaluate the effectiveness of cervical secretions in a subfertile population. [575] Optimising intercourse timing increases the pregnancy rate in couples with unexplained infertility, but it is not known how this natural approach compares with other medicalised approaches such as IUI or IVF. [348] [234] [64]

CONCEPTION DELAYS AFTER PREGNANCY LOSS

The loss of a pregnancy at any stage is a traumatic life event. Each woman's experience will be different, but it can be a devastating time, with approximately 25% of women meeting the criteria for post-traumatic stress disorder one month after pregnancy loss. [155]

Miscarriage

A miscarriage is the loss of a pregnancy before 23 completed weeks, with the majority of miscarriages occurring in the first eight weeks. The most common cause for a single miscarriage is a sporadic chromosomal abnormality, which arises from the egg in about 90% of cases and the sperm in the other 10%. NICE guidelines offer advice on best practice for the diagnosis and initial management of early miscarriage and ectopic pregnancy. [427] Women can be reassured that the method of miscarriage management does not affect subsequent pregnancy rates. [550]

Return of fertility after miscarriage

The first post-miscarriage cycle may be longer than usual. It may be a normal biphasic cycle or show signs of inadequacy. There may be several inadequate cycles before full ovulatory function is restored. The return of ovulation is variable:

- Ovulation returns on *average* 29–50 days post-miscarriage (resulting in pregnancy approximately 9 weeks after a loss).
- Ovulation may return as early as 10 days post-miscarriage (resulting in pregnancy within 4 weeks of a miscarriage). [525]

Time to pregnancy after miscarriage The LIFE study (Longitudinal Investigation of Fertility and the Environment) investigated time to pregnancy in successive attempts to conceive amongst 501 couples experiencing early pregnancy loss. The women (average age 30) used fertility monitors to measure both urinary estrogen and LH in order to optimise intercourse timing. When compared with the first attempt, it took 59% longer to conceive on the second attempt and 43% longer to conceive on the third attempt. It took couples on average one cycle longer to conceive on the third attempt compared with the second; however, for 25% of couples it took three or more cycles longer to conceive in their second attempt. Menstrual diaries showed no difference in intercourse frequency and no difference in the intake of alcohol, smoking or caffeine following the miscarriage. A significantly lower percentage of first cycles following miscarriage were ovulatory when compared with cycles preceding the loss. It was concluded that the longer time to pregnancy may be due to a biological mechanism such as delayed return of ovulation or endometrial changes following miscarriage. [525] **Subfertile couples who conceive naturally but miscarry can be reassured that they have a very good chance of conceiving again**

naturally in the near future and carrying a successful pregnancy. [107] **Following an uncomplicated miscarriage, healthy women can try for another pregnancy whenever they feel ready; however, it could take longer to conceive than expected.** [542]

Information and support for anyone affected by miscarriage, ectopic pregnancy or molar pregnancy is available from Miscarriage Association website (www.miscarriageassociation.org.uk).

Late intrauterine fetal death and stillbirth

A stillbirth is defined as a baby delivered with no signs of life after 23 completed weeks of pregnancy. An intrauterine fetal death refers to a baby with no sign of life in utero. See RCOG guidelines for management, including psychological and social aspects of care. [487]

Returning fertility Women who have suffered a late intrauterine fetal death or stillbirth will start lactating. This can be most distressing for a woman as her breasts physically ache for her baby. Up to one-third of women will experience severe breast pain and may require medical suppression of lactation. As there is no breastfeeding, ovulation may return very quickly. The return of fertility is varied but the following facts are significant:

- Ovulation returns on average around six weeks postpartum.
- Ovulation may occur as early as day 18 with lactation suppression. [487]
- Ovulation precedes the first menstruation in up to 70% of cycles, with the majority of these ovulations determined to be potentially fertile (adequate luteal phase). [303]

Although fertility may return very quickly, late pregnancy loss is highly stressful. Women who wish to use FAMs should follow the postpartum guidelines for women who are not breastfeeding (page 283), anticipating a rapid return to normal fertility but the possibility of delayed fertility with charts showing signs of inadequacy before a return to full ovulatory cycles.

The Stillbirth & Neonatal Death Society website (SANDS, at www.uk-sands.org) offers information and support for anyone who has been affected by the death of a baby before, during or shortly after birth.

Ectopic pregnancy

An ectopic (extra-uterine) pregnancy is a serious condition in which an embryo implants in sites other than the uterine cavity. Over 95% of ectopic pregnancies occur in the Fallopian tube, but rarely the pregnancy may develop in the ovary, cervix or abdominal cavity. In very rare cases an ectopic pregnancy develops simultaneously with an intrauterine pregnancy – a heterotopic pregnancy. A ruptured ectopic is a life-threatening situation, hence the need for early diagnosis: any woman with abdominal pain or vaginal bleeding during early pregnancy should be referred promptly for a trans-vaginal ultrasound scan, progesterone assay and quantitative serum hCG. [108] NICE guidelines offer advice on best practice for the diagnosis and initial management of ectopic pregnancy. [427] Information and support is available from the Ectopic Pregnancy Trust website (www.ectopic.org.uk).

Fertility after ectopic pregnancy

Fertility after an ectopic pregnancy is dependent on whether the affected tube has been spared and the condition of the other tube (in addition to factors such as age). Approximately 60–70% of women who wish to conceive again will have a successful intrauterine pregnancy. The chance of a recurrent ectopic pregnancy is about 10–15%.

A couple are normally advised to wait for three months following an ectopic before trying to conceive again. A woman who has had methotrexate must have serial hCG tests and wait until levels are undetectable before contemplating further pregnancy — this may take up to six months.

Couples should either abstain from intercourse completely or use an effective contraceptive method. Experienced FAM users may, with the support of an experienced practitioner, consider using "life or death rules" (page 228) until it is considered safe to conceive again, but a rapid return to fertility must always be anticipated. Depending on the method of management, a woman may observe a temperature rise within two weeks of treatment. Alternatively, she may have a number of inadequate cycles before resuming full ovulatory function.

Molar pregnancy

A molar pregnancy is an abnormality of the placental tissue in which the chorionic villi become swollen and distended, forming hundreds of fluid-filled vesicles. It is caused by abnormal fertilisation. Molar pregnancy is the most common type of gestational trophoblastic disease (GTD). In a complete molar pregnancy, there is no fetal tissue whilst in a partial mole there is fetal and molar tissue but the fetus is not viable. Molar pregnancy always requires surgical evacuation of the uterus. If molar tissue remains, this can lead to persistent trophoblastic disease and rarely to choriocarcinoma. This requires treatment with methotrexate or other forms of chemotherapy plus prolonged follow-up to monitor declining hCG levels. During this time pregnancy must be strictly avoided. RCOG provides guidance on the management of GTD. [488]

Fertility after molar pregnancy HCG levels should drop back to normal (undetectable) very quickly following surgical evacuation, with a subsequent rapid return to normal fertility. However, if there is any residual molar tissue, hCG levels remain elevated and methotrexate is started. This causes amenorrhoea with fertility returning after three to six months. Some forms of chemotherapy may cause permanent infertility.

Molar pregnancy is highly stressful. A woman has to cope emotionally with the loss of her pregnancy and simultaneously with concerns about cancer and the need for strict pregnancy avoidance. There is no published data related to FA following molar pregnancy. A woman who is recording her fertility indicators might anticipate that, following a straightforward surgical evacuation, the first cycle could be biphasic with an adequate luteal phase; but if additional medical treatment is required, a more gradual return to normal fertility may be anticipated.

Avoiding pregnancy after molar pregnancy It is essential for a woman to use an effective contraceptive method (such as COCs or LARCs) until she is medically advised that it is safe to conceive again. FSRH guidance recommends that women should not rely solely on fertility indicators for prevention of pregnancy when using teratogenic drugs. Clear information should be given regarding the need to abstain from intercourse until the drug has cleared from the system. [215] Some experienced FAM users who cannot cope with total abstinence may be able to use "life or death" rules (page 228) with the support of an experienced practitioner.

Conceiving again after molar pregnancy A woman who has required only surgical evacuation can normally start to conceive again after her hCG levels have been undetectable for six months. If chemotherapy is required, she should wait for one year, ensuring she has adequate supplementation with folic acid for three months preconception. Couples can be reassured that there is no increased risk of complications in further pregnancies, and there is only about 1% risk of another molar pregnancy.

SELF-ASSESSMENT QUESTIONS

Answers are at the end of the chapter.

1 List six different circumstances where fertility may be naturally reduced.
2 What are the five main causes of fertility problems?
3 How can a progesterone test (to confirm ovulation) be optimally timed?
4 LPD may be a normal physiological event, but it may also have a pathological cause. List four possible pathological causes.
5 List the most common cause for a single miscarriage.

PSYCHOLOGICAL AND EMOTIONAL ISSUES

Most people have some kind of mental plan for their future – to find a partner, possibly to marry and to have a family. Having a child may be perceived as a way to cement a relationship, to pass on the family genes, even to give a meaning to life. Anyone facing the fear and uncertainty associated with fertility delays can experience a wide range of emotions including anger, fear, frustration, envy, guilt, negativity, lack of confidence and low self-esteem. Some feel isolated from friends and family. Couples may find it difficult to relate to each other. The pressure may be on to provide a grandchild and intensified if a parent is old or sick, or if there are no other grandchildren. There may be added cultural expectations. Many people discover how much they value their ability to have children only when conception is delayed or following a pregnancy loss.

Fertility counselling Fertility counselling should be available for individuals and couples at all stages: from contemplating whether or not to start a family (or have another child) through investigations and treatment to IVF and beyond. Any couple considering egg, sperm or embryo donation, or planning surrogacy must be offered counselling to help them consider the implications of treatment for themselves and their future child. Fertility counselling may be beneficial following pregnancy loss or when making decisions about stopping treatment and moving on to adoption, fostering or coming to terms with a childless future. For a list of fertility counsellors in the UK, see the British Infertility Counselling Association website (www.bica.net).

A review of the role of fertility counselling highlighted the dangers of neglecting the emotional impact of infertility and viewing it solely in biological or medical terms. It describes the major complementary role of counselling in providing holistic patient-centred care by multidisciplinary staff in fertility clinics. [308] The European Society of Human Reproduction and Embryology (ESHRE) produces guidance for routine psychosocial care for all staff working in fertility clinics and specific guidelines for fertility counsellors (available from the website, www.eshre.eu).

Facing a future without children

One in five women in the UK who were born in the mid-1960s have no children. This figure, which appears to be rising, is almost double that of the previous generation. Many women will be childless by circumstance and not by choice. The rise in childlessness may be explained by a decline in the number of women getting married, greater social acceptability of a child-free lifestyle, delaying having children until it is biologically too late, and the perceived costs and benefits of childbearing vs. work and leisure activities. [441] Support groups such as Gateway Women (http://gateway-women.com) provide friendship and support to help individuals create a meaningful and fulfilling life without children.

ANSWERS TO SELF-ASSESSMENT QUESTIONS

1 Fertility may be naturally reduced postnatally and during breastfeeding, following pregnancy loss, during times of stress, when weight is outside the normal BMI range, after discontinuation of hormonal contraception (notably injectable methods) and in older women.
2 The five main causes of fertility problems are male factors, ovulatory disorders, tubal damage, uterine or peritoneal disorders, and unexplained infertility.
3 The progesterone test should be performed mid-luteal phase. This can be prospectively timed seven days after peak, seven days after the urinary LH surge or six days after the temperature rise. This coincides with day 21 only if the woman has a regular 28-day cycle.
4 Pathological causes of LPD include PCOS, thyroid dysfunction, endometriosis and hyperprolactinaemia.
5 The most common cause for a single miscarriage is a sporadic chromosomal abnormality.Case study planned pregnancy while breastfeeding

PART IV

Teaching fertility awareness

TEACHING FERTILITY AWARENESS

20

Teaching FA is an ongoing educational process rather than a one-off event. Health professionals in primary care services are in a key position to provide essential fertility/reproductive health awareness information to individuals at all stages of reproductive life – this includes information for couples planning pregnancy. Although all professionals should have a working knowledge of the principles of modern FAMs, only those with specialist training should teach these methods to avoid pregnancy.

ESSENTIAL RHA INFORMATION

The essentials of RHA include an understanding of:

- Male and female reproductive anatomy and physiology
- Lifespan of egg and sperm
- Menstrual cycle and its normal variations
- Concepts of the fertile and infertile times in the cycle
- Bodily signs indicating fertility
- Cervical secretions and their role in sperm survival
- Distinction between normal secretions and abnormal vaginal discharge
- Vulnerability of reproductive organs and the damaging effects of STIs
- Safer sex strategies and the protection offered by condoms
- Contraceptive choice, including how the method interrupts fertility, how it fails if not used correctly and how fertility returns after the method is discontinued
- Female age and declining fertility, including the ideal time for having children (and anticipated family size)
- Assisted fertility, including IVF and its limitations with age

Integrating RHA into schools

There is a strong case for integrating RHA into sex and relationships education (SRE) in schools. A review of the literature on adolescent cognitive development, sexual activity, knowledge of fertility and contraceptive risk-taking showed that adolescents have a poor understanding of the basic concepts of ovulation, egg and sperm survival and the menstrual cycle. [516] Roth showed that, as with Luker's risk theory, an adolescent girl's inability to identify her fertile time directly contributes to contraceptive risk-taking behaviour.

Teenagers often believe that they are infertile. Some believe that they are too young to get pregnant, have sex too infrequently or at a time of the cycle when pregnancy is not possible (such as during or just after a period). The added complication here is that a high percentage of early post-menarche cycles will be infertile (anovulatory or short luteal phases), which means that random acts of unprotected sex have a low probability of conception. With increasing age and reproductive maturity, the risks of conception increase and, given time, risk-taking behaviour leads to unintended pregnancy. It is suggested that when young people are educated in FA and can identify the signs of fertility, they are more likely to see themselves as potentially fertile beings with a need to protect themselves from the risk of infection and pregnancy.

Suggested content

Reproductive health awareness sessions in schools should include the essential reproductive health information (as discussed earlier) plus the following topics, delivered at age-appropriate stages across the curriculum:

- Bodily changes associated with puberty
- Why unprotected sex does not always result in pregnancy
- Personal responsibility for sexual activity, including negotiating skills and relationships
- Influence of alcohol and drugs on decision-making and negotiating skills
- Abstinence as a valid choice
- Outercourse (no penetration or exchange of body fluids)
- Information about local contraception and sexual health services
- Privacy and confidentiality
- Pre- and post-course knowledge assessments
- Exploding myths about fertility (e.g. can't get pregnant during a period)
- Evaluation of sessions

In the UK, SRE forms part of personal, social, health and economic education (PSHE). Although a non-statutory subject, staff teaching PSHE require subject-specific training and support in the teaching of these sensitive issues. Groups such as the PSHE Association, Brook (young people's sexual health and well-being charity) and Sex Education Forum provide SRE training and resources for teachers and youth workers. Some schools invite external speakers (or school nurses) to teach RHA/FA particularly in years 9–11 (14–16 years); others are keen to integrate this into staff training. Although some programmes are well-evaluated by students and staff, further research is needed to assess the impact of such interventions in the short and long-term.

TEACHING WOMEN/COUPLES PLANNING PREGNANCY

Women who are planning pregnancy should be taught individually (or preferably as a couple). A single session may be all that is needed with follow-up within three to six months if there is no conception.

The overall aims of preconception sessions are as follows:

- To provide basic FA information to optimise chances of conception
- To encourage optimum preconception health and nutrition
- To identify menstrual irregularities and ensure timely referral for assessment

First session

The first session is ideally scheduled for one hour during which time the practitioner aims to do the following:

- Take medical, obstetric, gynaecological, menstrual and contraceptive history.
- Consider specific preconception health issues, prescribed and bought medication.

- Consider lifestyle factors (e.g. diet, alcohol, smoking, caffeine, weight).
- Confirm immunity to rubella.
- Ensure the woman is taking folic acid (and vitamin D).
- Assess knowledge of menstrual cycle and role of cervical secretions.
- Discuss intercourse frequency and timing.
- Explain that intercourse every two to three days optimises the chance of pregnancy.
- Explain the role of FA to optimise conception.
- Establish past cycle lengths and the potential fertile time.
- Consider use of a simple chart to record cervical secretions and intercourse (appendix C).
- Recording the temperature is not necessary unless there are concerns about ovulatory function.
- Check on the use of OPKs and fertility gadgets.
- Provide handouts to support learning.
- Arrange follow-up appointment as needed.
- Document session on IT system.

Subsequent sessions

Subsequent sessions are ideally scheduled for 30 minutes during which time the practitioner aims to:

- Discuss health and lifestyle modifications.
- Consider intercourse timing and any pressures on the relationship.
- Note any chart irregularities and consider referral for fertility assessment.
- Document session on IT system.

Women who have three consecutive cycles showing a monophasic pattern, short luteal phase, poor quality cervical secretions or more than 2 days premenstrual spotting should be referred for further investigations into ovulatory status.

TEACHING WOMEN/COUPLES AVOIDING PREGNANCY

Health professionals who wish to extend their role to teach FAMs to avoid pregnancy must complete specialist training to become an accredited FA practitioner (see training organisations in appendix H.3)

Fertility awareness practitioner

FA practitioners are usually doctors, nurses or midwives who have achieved professional competence to offer FAMs as part of a comprehensive range of sexual and reproductive health care services. Some organisations (mostly faith-based) train lay users to teach FAMs. It is vital that these teachers have achieve the required level of competence and have adequate support from health professionals.

In order to teach FAMs, practitioners require:

- A thorough knowledge of reproductive physiology
- An in-depth understanding of FAMs for planning or avoiding pregnancy
- Effective communication skills and an ability to teach
- Sensitivity to the intimate nature of observations
- An understanding about relationships and how individuals make decisions

- An appreciation of the difficulties with abstinence and behaviour change
- A non-judgemental, client-focussed approach
- Respect for the client's moral, religious or ethical beliefs
- Respect for client's privacy and confidentiality
- Recognition of limits of expertise with clear referral pathways
- Regular supervision and continuing professional development

Who uses FAMs?

Women find FAMs most appealing because they are natural, do not involve chemicals and are free from side effects. Many perceive FAMs as convenient, easy-to-use, low cost and reliable. Some appreciate learning about their own bodies. The least important aspects (demographically) are religious and moral acceptability. Women's main concerns about FAMs are effectiveness and ease of use. Some perceive self-observation as messy and unnatural; some express concerns about abstinence, interference with spontaneity and whether their partner would accept the method. [558] [197] [403] Modern FAM users vary widely across the age spectrum (although the majority are 25–35 years) and they are of different religions (or non-religious). The majority of users consider two children to be optimum, although Catholic women (often from larger families themselves) may desire three, four or more children. A high proportion of FAM users rely on barrier methods (particularly condoms) during the fertile time. The profile of a typical FAM user in the UK is broadly similar to that of a Persona user: highly educated, in a committed relationship, interested in her own body, and looking for a reliable method without side effects but open to pregnancy at a later stage. [305] It is plausible that more women may be interested in using modern FAMs to avoid pregnancy if health professionals were better informed and the methods were more accessible. [333] [87]

Religious and cultural issues

Pope Paul VI's encyclical *Humanae Vitae* [599] reaffirmed Catholic orthodoxy on the prohibition of contraception. It supported only the use of NFP with abstinence. The encyclical asserted that "each and every marital act must retain its intrinsic relationship to the procreation of human life." This openness to life is very important for some individuals. The issue of contraception for most Catholics is regarded as a matter for personal conscience, with roughly the same percentage (1–2%) of Catholics as non-Catholics using FAMs in the UK. [602] This is similar in most parts of the world, with a study across 15 developing countries finding no obvious link between FAMs and religion. [78] It has been suggested that higher rates of FAMs use are related not to religion, but to their ease of access and local support. [403]

Suitability for use

The majority of couples can use FAMs for avoiding pregnancy, provided consideration is given to the factors which may disturb the cycle and the indicators of fertility. Practitioners must assess a couple's suitability to use FAMs and consider any restrictions on use.

Establish how important it is to avoid pregnancy:

- Consider the impact of pregnancy on the woman and her relationship/family.
- Establish the couple's motivation: to space or limit pregnancy. Are they both in agreement?
- Consider any medical conditions which would make pregnancy a high-risk condition (e.g. epilepsy or cardiovascular disease).

- Consider any prescribed drugs which are contraindicated in pregnancy (e.g. lithium, warfarin and most anti-epileptic drugs). Women using drugs known to have a teratogenic effect should not rely solely on FAMs to avoid pregnancy. Consider a more-effective method, total abstinence or "life or death" rules.

Establish the woman's risk of STI:

- Advise both partners to have a sexual health screen.
- Advise on consistent and correct use of condoms in conjunction with FAMs for anyone at risk of STIs.

Consider factors which could make FAMs more difficult to use:

- Irregular cycles
- Recent use of hormonal contraception
- Postpartum and breastfeeding
- Peri-menopause
- Chronic medical conditions
- Acute illness/infection
- Medication, including bought products
- Lifestyle factors

Contraceptive needs change over reproductive life. Women in committed relationships who are contemplating their first baby, breastfeeding or spacing births may be ideally suited to FAMs, but each woman's situation must be considered on its own merit. [91] [215]

Teaching methods

Ideally both partners should be taught together, whether couples are planning or avoiding pregnancy. This helps to encourage male partner involvement and joint responsibility, which is particularly important in the learning stages. It may not be feasible to see couples together at all sessions. Group teaching can be both effective and cost-effective, but it has limitations. Group sessions, with similar demographic groups, can work well for the presentation of basic FA information but women/couples need access to individual sessions to address personal need.

Face-to-face consultations supported by the use of graphics allow interactive learning. FAM teaching should be a highly participatory process aiming for the couple to become autonomous users. Lack of experienced practitioners may mean that some couples have to travel long distances to clinics. Many services integrate online teaching with email, telephone and Skype support, allowing charts to be sent electronically to an experienced practitioner. There have been no effectiveness studies to validate this approach.

Teaching programmes: avoiding pregnancy

Teaching programmes must be flexible and responsive to client need. A single session is of value, but has its limitations. Most couples require four to six sessions before they can confidently use the method to avoid pregnancy.

The overall aim is to provide the relevant FA information and practical charting skills to enable individuals/couples to confidently use combined-indicator methods to avoid pregnancy.

Setting and equipment

The setting and equipment required for teaching FAMs is minimal. The practitioner will need:

- a comfortable and private room;
- client teaching resources (e.g. laminated sheets);
- thermometers, charts (appendix A) and instructions for use (appendix B); and
- hand-outs or Web-based materials, including FAM guidelines, to support learning.

First session

During the first session (which is ideally one hour) the practitioner should aim to:

- Take medical, obstetric, gynaecological, menstrual and contraceptive history.
- Assess client needs and suitability for use.
- Assess current level of fertility knowledge.
- Teach basic reproductive physiology and changes during the menstrual cycle.
- Teach correct use of thermometer and charting temperatures.
- Teach essentials of observing and charting cervical secretions.
- Establish past cycle lengths and calculation to identify the first fertile day.
- Discuss correct use and typical use failure rates.
- Advise abstinence (or consistent barrier use) during the first cycle.
- Provide guidelines applicable to fertility circumstances.
- Provide handouts to support learning.
- Arrange follow-up appointment (roughly monthly intervals).
- Consider the need for interim telephone or email support.
- Document session on IT system including discussion of effectiveness.

Second and subsequent sessions

On the second and subsequent sessions (which ideally last 30 minutes) the practitioner aims to:

- Ask about experience of charting since last session.
- Review chart noting observing and recording techniques and areas for improvement.
- Explain chart interpretation (if adequate information) and correlation of indicators.
- Use chart summary sheet to support chart interpretation (appendix D).
- Discuss disturbances affecting the chart.
- Reinforce methodology and guidelines.
- Assess woman/couple's skills and confidence in the method.
- Remind of ongoing calculation to identify the first fertile day.
- Discuss option of cervical changes (when woman confident with secretions).
- Discuss relevance of minor indicators.
- Check the intercourse pattern and discuss any risk-taking.
- Consider the impact of abstinence or use of barriers/withdrawal.
- Ensure the method is still appropriate to couple's needs.

Sessions should be interactive and allow time for discussion of difficulties with the method and pressures on the relationship. Most clients will be confident and autonomous in their use of FAMs after about six cycles, but follow-up sessions should be offered at approximately nine months and one year, thereafter offering additional support for experienced users at time of cyclic change or changes in fertility circumstances.

Male involvement Some men are keen to be involved with charting: for example, recording the woman's temperature. Some even wish to plot their own temperatures for a short time, either out of interest or to act as a control for temperature disturbances (see the Gap technique on page 106). Some men like to take responsibility for checking the woman's cervix. In most cases, the woman is the one to assume full responsibility for checking cervical secretions as this is an ongoing assessment over the course of a day.

Managing a client with a difficult chart When faced with a client with a difficult chart, consider the following possibilities:

- Poor teaching or learning: is instruction appropriate to client's educational level and existing knowledge?
- Poor observation or recording: revisit techniques for relevant indicators.
- Disturbances affecting the menstrual cycle or fertility indicators (see table 12.1 in chapter 12).
- Poor adherence: consider motivation, relationship issues and partner dissatisfaction.

An uninterpretable chart should be clearly marked as such. Practitioners must discuss difficult charts with their supervisor, particularly if there is no known reason.

Supporting couples with abstinence and behaviour change FAM consultations must allow time for discussion of sexual activity and difficulties with abstinence or barrier methods because this impacts on effectiveness, user satisfaction and continuity rates. Some practitioners, particularly in faith-based organisations, may feel uncomfortable discussing the use of contraception during the fertile time. Similarly, some couples using FAMs for religious reasons may feel that they should be seen to adhere to the Church's teaching on abstinence, so may be reluctant to be open about their use of barriers or withdrawal (see modification of sexual behaviour on page 229).

Sexual difficulties Couples are encouraged to record all acts of intercourse on the chart. For couples avoiding pregnancy, it is acceptable to limit documentation to the outer limits of the fertile time – this helps to identify any misinterpretation of the rules or risk-taking. If there are few or no recorded acts of intercourse, this warrants further discussion. Lack of interest in sex is commonly reported, [401] but this should always be explored. Couples must feel confident and supported in their use of FAMs if they are to enjoy unrestricted intercourse during the infertile time. The question should always be raised about whether the method suits both partners and whether it may be creating or exacerbating any sexual difficulties (page 336).

Client autonomy Before a couple can be considered independent in their use of FAMs, the woman must be able to confidently identify the limits of her fertile time and apply the appropriate guidelines (see appendix E for autonomy checklist).

Managing client with unintended pregnancy Most practitioners will, at some stage, be confronted by a client with an unintended pregnancy. Although each practitioner is responsible for their own standard of teaching and continuing professional development, they are not responsible for user-related pregnancies. Unintended pregnancies should be discussed with a supervisor and an attempt made to classify the pregnancy (page 241) and consider lessons learnt. Despite the unplanned nature of the pregnancy, many women adjust and happily accept the pregnancy. Couples can learn a lot from an unintended pregnancy and many continue to use FAMs postnatally, provided that they have ongoing support from an experienced practitioner. Conversely users who are self-taught may be distressed by an unintended pregnancy, feel uncertain about where they went wrong and abandon the method, labelling it as unreliable.

FAM TEACHING AND TRAINING

Internationally FAM services comprise a mixture of religious and non-religious organisations with different teaching methodologies. Some teach single-indicator methods whilst others teach combined indicators. Catholic-based organisations are more likely to promote NFP with abstinence (and may teach married couples only), whereas secular organisations are open to all and accept the use of barrier methods/withdrawal. Some FAM services are integrated into health systems, others are faith-based and operate independently, and yet others are operated by sole traders such as complementary therapists as private enterprises. In Europe many established organisations are members of the European Institute for Family Life Education (EIFLE), a non-governmental umbrella organisation which promotes Catholic values.

Teaching and training in the UK

In the UK FAMs are mostly integrated into mainstream NHS services. FertilityUK (a secular service) provides access to a network of accredited practitioners. It also provides multi-disciplinary training for health professionals. The advanced skills course covers the theory and practice of FAMs for planning and avoiding pregnancy. The intensive four-day course is relevant to doctors, nurses and midwives working in general practice, family planning, fertility clinics, and sexual and reproductive health care. Course materials include a course manual, workbook of charts for experiential learning and high-quality laminated client teaching materials. Two modules are held four months apart to allow time for completion of directed study and supervised client teaching. Participants are assessed by a variety of methods, both formative and summative. The course receives Continuing Professional Development credits from the Faculty of Sexual and Reproductive Health Care. For further information, see the FertilityUK website (www.fertilityuk.org).

Appendices

APPENDIX A

Normal fertility chart

Fertility chart

Length of shortest cycle = day: [ ] minus 20 = day: [ ]
(based on past 12 cycle lengths)

Length of this cycle = [ ] days

Temperature taking route: Oral [ ] Vaginal [ ] Rectal [ ] (tick appropriate box)

Time of taking temperature: [ ] a.m.

Name ____________________

Age ____________________

Chart no. ____________________

Comments

Month & Year																																									
Date																																									
Day																																									
°C 37.4																																									37.4
37.3																																									37.3
37.2																																									37.2
37.1																																									37.1
37.0																																									**37.0**
36.9																																									36.9
36.8																																									36.8
36.7																																									36.7
36.6																																									36.6
36.5																																									36.5
36.4																																									36.4
36.3																																									36.3
36.2																																									36.2
36.1																																									36.1
36.0																																									**36.0**
35.9																																									35.9
35.8																																									35.8
35.7																																									35.7
35.6																																									35.6
35.5																																									35.5
Sexual intercourse - circle day of cycle	1	2	3	4	5	6	7	8	9	10	11	12	13	14	15	16	17	18	19	20	21	22	23	24	25	26	27	28	29	30	31	32	33	34	35	36	37	38	39	40	
Cervical Secretions: Wet, slippery, transparent, stretchy																																									
Moist, white, cloudy, sticky																																									
Dry (no secretions seen or felt)																																									
Period																																									
Cervix High, soft, open / Low, firm, closed																																									
Tilted or straight																																									
Fertility test kit or monitor Result																																									
.... Test day																																									

APPENDIX B

Instructions for use

Temperature

1. Use a centigrade liquid-in-glass or digital thermometer and follow the manufacturer's instructions. Most digital thermometers have an audible bleep, a last memory recall feature and a low-battery warning indicator.
2. Take your temperature immediately on waking, before getting out of bed or doing anything. If recording time varies by more than one hour, note this on the chart.
3. Place the bulb of the thermometer under your tongue in contact with the floor of your mouth, close your lips gently and leave until the thermometer produces the audible bleep (takes about one minute). Oral temperatures are usually reliable, but if readings are erratic, your FA practitioner may suggest an internal reading – vaginal or rectal. Make any change in temperature-taking route at the beginning of the cycle.
4. Remove the thermometer, read it and mark the temperature with a dot in the centre of the appropriate square, not on the line. Join the dots to form a continuous graph.
5. If you miss a day, leave a gap on the chart. (Do not join non-consecutive dots)
6. Clean the thermometer with a little cotton wool and cold water.

Cycle length

1. The first day of your period is day 1 of the cycle. Start a new chart on that day.
2. If your period (fresh red bleed) starts during the day, transfer that morning's temperature to a new chart.
3. Record your cycle lengths to estimate the length of your shortest cycle.

Cervical secretions

1. Observe secretions throughout the day and record on the chart in the evening.
2. Observe the sensation (feel), colour (look) and the finger-test (touch).
3. Describe the secretions, using shading in the appropriate box:
   - period, including blood spotting;
   - no secretions seen or felt (dry);
   - moist, white or cloudy, sticky secretions; or
   - wet, slippery, transparent, stretchy secretions.
4. Indicate peak day by extending the shaded area in the column vertically upwards to correlate with the temperature readings. Peak day is the *last* day of highly fertile secretions (last day in top box). Peak day can be recognised only in retrospect (day after peak) when the secretions have changed back to show less fertile characteristics (marked in a lower box).

Cervix (optional)

The infertile cervix is represented by
- a solid black circle showing it to be firm and closed: ●;
- the circle is placed low down, showing it lower in the vagina; and
- a slanted line drawn below shows the tilt (/).

The fertile cervix is represented by
- an open circle showing softening: ◯;
- an inner circle showing that the cervix is more open: ◎;
- the circle is placed higher, showing it higher in the vagina; and
- a vertical line below shows the cervix straight in position (|).

Cyclical symptoms (optional)

- Indicate abdominal pain, breast, or mood changes.

Fertility monitoring devices (optional)

- Indicate test days and results.
- Correlate results with observed fertility indicators.

Sexual Intercourse

- Indicate intercourse by circle around the appropriate day.
- If combining with barrier methods, indicate whether sex is protected or unprotected (e.g. "C" for condom).
- Note any other sexual activity, such as withdrawal method, which could result in pregnancy.

Comments:

Note late nights, alcohol, illness, drugs, travel or stressful times on the appropriate days and/or in the comments box.

For further help, contact FertilityUK at www.fertilityuk.org

Local FA practitioner: ____________________

Tel: ____________________

APPENDIX C

Planning pregnancy chart

Fertility awareness chart: planning pregnancy

Name: ....

Instructions for use:

- o Observe cervical secretions throughout the day. Record on the chart in the evening.
- o The first day of the period (fresh red bleed) is day 1 of the cycle. Start a new chart at the start of each period (4 blank charts below).
- o Record days of period; dry days; moist, white, cloudy, sticky secretions; and days of wetter, slippery, transparent, stretchy secretions.
- o The fertile time starts at the first sign of any secretions and continues for 3 days after peak day (last day of wet, stretchy secretions).
- o Aim for sex at least 2-3 times per week. The days with wetter, transparent, stretchy secretions have the highest chance of pregnancy.

Example chart Sept/Oct

Date	7	8	9	10	11	12	13	14	15	16	17	18	19	20	21	22	23	24	25	26	27	28	29	30	1	2	3													
Day	W	T	F	S	S	M	T	W	T	F	S	S	M	T	W	T	F	S	S	M	T	W	T	F	S	S	M													
								Peak Day →																																
Wet, slippery, transparent, stretchy														1	2	3																								
Moist, white, cloudy, sticky																																								
Dry (no secretions seen or felt)																																								
Period																																								
Day of cycle - circle intercourse	1	2	3	4	5	6	7	8	9	10	11	12	13	14	15	16	17	18	19	20	21	22	23	24	25	26	27	28	29	30	31	32	33	34	35	36	37	38	39	40
											Fertile Time																													

Chart number:

Date																																								
Day																																								
Wet, slippery, transparent, stretchy																																								
Moist, white, cloudy, sticky																																								
Dry (no secretions seen or felt)																																								
Period																																								
Day of cycle - circle intercourse	1	2	3	4	5	6	7	8	9	10	11	12	13	14	15	16	17	18	19	20	21	22	23	24	25	26	27	28	29	30	31	32	33	34	35	36	37	38	39	40

Chart number:

Date																																								
Day																																								
Wet, slippery, transparent, stretchy																																								
Moist, white, cloudy, sticky																																								
Dry (no secretions seen or felt)																																								
Period																																								
Day of cycle - circle intercourse	1	2	3	4	5	6	7	8	9	10	11	12	13	14	15	16	17	18	19	20	21	22	23	24	25	26	27	28	29	30	31	32	33	34	35	36	37	38	39	40

Chart number:

Date																																								
Day																																								
Wet, slippery, transparent, stretchy																																								
Moist, white, cloudy, sticky																																								
Dry (no secretions seen or felt)																																								
Period																																								
Day of cycle - circle intercourse	1	2	3	4	5	6	7	8	9	10	11	12	13	14	15	16	17	18	19	20	21	22	23	24	25	26	27	28	29	30	31	32	33	34	35	36	37	38	39	40

Chart number:

Date																																								
Day																																								
Wet, slippery, transparent, stretchy																																								
Moist, white, cloudy, sticky																																								
Dry (no secretions seen or felt)																																								
Period																																								
Day of cycle - circle intercourse	1	2	3	4	5	6	7	8	9	10	11	12	13	14	15	16	17	18	19	20	21	22	23	24	25	26	27	28	29	30	31	32	33	34	35	36	37	38	39	40

APPENDIX D

Chart summary sheet

Name of client: .... Age: [ ] Chart number: [ ]

You are a new user [ ] You are an experienced user (charting more than 1 year) [ ] (Tick appropriate box)

The length of this menstrual cycle was: [............days]

Your shortest cycle length (S) over the last 12 cycles was: [S = ...days] (if available)

Your peak secretion day (last day of most fertile secretions) was: [Day ....]

Your first high temperature was recorded on : [Day ....]

Your earliest temperature rise (T) (out of the last 12 cycles) was: [Day ....] (if available)

Your first fertile day

Day 6 (new users from cycle 4): [ ] Requires first 3 cycles 26 days or longer

S = [ ] minus 20 = Day: [ ] Requires 12 previous cycle lengths

T = [ ] minus 7 = Day: [ ] Requires 12 previous temperature charts

Your first secretions were on day: [ ]

Your first cervix change was day: [ ] (optional indicator)

So, your first fertile day was day: [ ] your first sign of fertility (whichever comes first) (the lowest number in this section)

Your last fertile day

(Delete as appropriate)

In the 6 low temperatures, you did not have a temperature spike[1] / *or:*

you had a temperature spike on day [ ]

Your 3rd high temperature[2] was day [ ]

Were all 3 high temperatures after peak day? → *Yes. The fertile time has ended*

↓

No. Then, wait for three high temperatures after peak day.

So, your last fertile day was day [ ] **(3 high temperatures after peak day)**

In this cycle, your fertile time started on day .... and ended on day ....

[1] single reading of at least 0.2 deg.C above the one on both sides. One spike can safely be ignored

[2] The third high temperature must be at least 0.2 deg.C. above the six low temperatures.

Summary of guidelines to avoid pregnancy for women of normal fertility

The fertile time starts at the first sign of cervical secretions, the first change in cervix, or the earliest day by calculation (*S minus 20*; *Earliest T. rise minus 7* or *Day Six rule* as appropriate) – whichever comes *first*. The fertile time ends after the third high temperature has been recorded, provided it is a min. 0.2 deg.C above the six low temperatures and they are all after peak day.

APPENDIX E

Autonomy checklist

Date. . . . . *Name. . . . .*

Can the woman / couple confidently:	*Yes*	*No*	*Comments*
Calculate the length of the menstrual cycle?			
Interpret the temperature chart using the *3 over 6 rule?*			
Manage disturbances in temperature including temperature spikes?			
Identify the change from dryness and the start of cervical secretions?			
Identify peak day and correlate this with the temperature rise?			
Identify the changes in the cervix (optional)?			
Apply the *Day 6 rule*?			
Apply the calculation: *S minus 20*?			
Apply the calculation: *earliest temperature rise minus 7*?			
Understand the significance of the minor indicators and their variability?			
Understand factors which affect cycle length, temperature and secretions?			
Apply the guidelines (as appropriate to current circumstances):			
• to achieve pregnancy			
• to avoid pregnancy – to space or limit the family			
• for LAM			
• after stopping hormonal contraception			
• for managing cyclic changes approaching the menopause			
Consider:			
Are both partners in agreement about their family planning intention?			
Does the intercourse pattern indicate any risk-taking behaviour?			
Does abstinence create problems for either partner?			
Are the couple using another family planning method during the fertile time?			
Do the couple understand the effectiveness of FAMs?			
Does the woman understand how and when to access further support?			

APPENDIX F

Body mass index chart

Weight (kg)	Height (ft/in) 5'0	5'0	5'1	5'2	5'3	5'4	5'4	5'5	5'6	5'7	5'7	5'8	5'8	5'9	5'10	5'11	6'0	Weight (st/lbs)
100	43	42	41	40	39	38	37	36	35	35	34	33	32	32	31	30	30	15-10
98	42	41	40	39	38	37	36	36	35	34	33	32	32	31	30	30	29	15-6
96	42	40	39	38	38	37	36	35	34	33	32	32	31	30	30	29	28	15-2
94	41	40	39	38	37	36	35	34	33	33	32	31	30	30	29	28	28	14-11
92	40	39	38	37	36	35	34	33	33	32	31	30	30	29	28	28	27	14-7
90	39	38	37	36	35	34	33	33	32	31	30	30	29	28	28	27	27	14-2
88	38	37	36	35	34	34	33	32	31	30	30	29	28	28	27	27	26	13-12
86	37	36	35	34	34	33	32	31	30	30	29	28	28	27	27	26	25	13-8
84	36	35	35	34	33	32	31	30	30	29	28	28	27	27	26	25	25	13-3
82	35	35	34	33	32	31	30	30	29	28	28	27	26	26	25	25	24	12-13
80	35	34	33	32	31	30	30	29	28	28	27	26	26	25	25	24	24	12-8
78	34	33	32	31	30	30	29	28	28	27	26	26	25	25	24	24	23	12-4
76	33	32	31	30	30	29	28	28	27	26	26	25	25	24	23	23	22	12-0
74	32	31	30	30	29	28	28	27	26	26	25	24	24	23	23	22	22	11-9
72	31	30	30	29	28	27	27	26	26	25	24	24	23	23	22	22	21	11-5
70	30	30	29	28	27	27	26	25	25	24	24	23	23	22	22	21	21	11-0
68	29	29	28	27	27	26	25	25	24	24	23	22	22	21	21	21	20	10-10
66	29	28	27	26	26	25	25	24	23	23	22	22	21	21	20	20	19	10-6
64	28	27	26	26	25	24	24	23	23	22	22	21	21	20	20	19	19	10-1
62	27	26	25	25	24	24	23	22	22	21	21	20	20	20	19	19	18	9-11
60	26	25	25	24	23	23	22	22	21	21	20	20	19	19	19	18	18	9-6
58	25	24	24	23	23	22	22	21	21	20	20	19	19	18	18	18	17	9-2
56	24	24	23	22	22	21	21	20	20	19	19	18	18	18	17	17	17	8-11
54	23	23	22	22	21	21	20	20	19	19	18	18	17	17	17	16	16	8-7
52	23	22	21	21	20	20	19	19	18	18	18	17	17	16	16	16	15	8-3
50	22	21	21	20	20	19	19	18	18	17	17	17	16	16	15	15	15	7-12
48	21	20	20	19	19	18	18	17	17	17	16	16	15	15	15	14	14	7-8
46	20	19	19	18	18	18	17	17	16	16	16	15	15	15	14	14	14	7-3
44	19	19	18	18	17	17	16	16	16	15	15	15	14	14	14	13	13	6-13
42	18	18	17	17	16	16	16	15	15	15	14	14	14	13	13	13	12	6-9
40	17	17	16	16	16	15	15	15	14	14	14	13	13	13	12	12	12	6-4
Height (m)	1.52	1.54	1.56	1.58	1.60	1.62	1.64	1.66	1.68	1.70	1.72	1.74	1.76	1.78	1.80	1.82	1.84	

Grey shaded zone indicates ideal BMI range for fertility

APPENDIX G

Drugs which affect the menstrual cycle

Drug classification	*Usual treatment for*	*Effect on the menstrual cycle and the indicators of fertility*
Analgesics (e.g. paracetamol)	Pain relief	Analgesics are used to provide relief from various forms of pain. – Some analgesics are anti-pyretic, so may cause lower temperatures.
Antibiotics (e.g. ampicillin)	Bacterial infections	Antibiotics are used to kill micro-organisms. Bacterial infections are often accompanied by pyrexia (fever) which may disturb waking temperatures. – May increase or reduce cervical secretions. – May increase susceptibility to candida due to altered vaginal flora. – Persona (fertility monitor) is unsuitable for women on tetracyclines.
Antidepressants and antipsychotics (e.g. SSRIs sertraline and venlafaxine)	Mental health problems	Antidepressants and antipsychotics are widely used in the treatment of mental health conditions. Many psychiatric medications including sedatives, anti-emetics and some selective serotonin reuptake inhibitors (SSRIs) suppress hypothalamic secretion of dopamine. As dopamine is thought to be a prolactin-inhibiting factor, these drugs often cause hyperprolactinaemia. Some drugs affect thyroid function. – May cause disruption to ovulation. – May cause irregular cycles. – May lead to sexual dysfunction. *Note:* Ask women about breast leakage. Check prolactin, full blood count and thyroid function in women who are trying to conceive.
Anti-emetics (e.g. metoclopramide)	Nausea & vomiting Migraine Travel sickness	Anti-emetics are used to treat many forms of nausea and vomiting. – May increase prolactin which can delay or suppress ovulation and result in irregular cycles, short luteal phases or monophasic cycles. – May reduce cervical secretions.
Anti-epileptics (e.g. sodium valproate, carbamazepine, gabapentin)	Prevention of seizures	Anti-epileptics are used in epilepsy as an anticonvulsant. – May cause a variety of different effects on the menstrual cycle. – May cause painful periods, amenorrhoea, reduced secretions and possibly reduced fertility. *Note:* Anti-epileptics cause deficiency in folic acid and vitamin D, so supplements of high dose folic acid and vitamin D may be required during the preconception time. Some of the older anti-epileptic drugs have been linked to an increased risk of congenital abnormalities including neural tube defects, facial defects and congenital heart defects. A preconception medication review is essential.

(*Continued*)

(Continued)

Anti-estrogens (e.g. tamoxifen)	Breast cancer (adjuvant therapy)	An anti-estrogen such as Tamoxifen is a selective estrogen receptor modulator (SERM) which binds to estrogen receptors. In the cells of some tissues (such as the breast) this blocks the action of estrogen, preventing the growth of estrogen-dependent tumours. In other tissues such as the uterus (and bone) SERMs act like weak estrogen and may cause a range of disturbances. – May reduce or suppress cervical secretions. – May cause prolonged or excessive bleeding. – May cause menopausal symptoms with cessation of periods. – May have little effect on the cycle (particularly in younger women). – May continue to have normal biphasic cycles.
Anti-estrogens (in assisted fertility) (e.g. clomiphene or tamoxifen)	Ovulation induction and ovarian stimulation	SERMs such as clomiphene or tamoxifen are also used in different forms of assisted fertility. They are used for ovulation induction as a treatment for anovulation mostly for women with polycystic ovaries (PCOS). They are also used for controlled ovarian hyperstimulation to produce multiple follicles for treatment with intrauterine insemination (IUI) and in-vitro fertilisation (IVF). – May reduce the amount and quality of cervical secretions. – May thin the endometrium (particularly with more than 6 cycles use).
Antifungals (e.g. clotrimazole, fluconazole)	Candida (vaginal thrush)	Antifungal creams, pessaries and tablets kill fungal infections such as Candida. The thick white vaginal discharge of a 'yeast infection' masks normal changes in cervical secretions. – Should help to restore the normal pattern of cervical secretions.
Anti-gonadotrophins (e.g. danazol)	Endometriosis	Anti-gonadotrophins suppress the activity of gonadotrophins (FSH and LH) to treat estrogen-related conditions such as endometriosis. – May cause temporary menopausal symptoms, such as hot flushes. – May prevent ovulation & menstruation so resulting in monophasic cycles or amenorrhoea.
Antihistamines (e.g. chlorphenamine / Piriton)	Allergies including hayfever. Also in some cold and flu preparations	Antihistamines block the action of histamine (which is involved in immune responses and allergies). They dry up respiratory secretions. – May dry cervical secretions, causing persistent dryness or reduced amount and quality secretions particularly with long-term use. – May affect sperm penetration through the cervix so reducing fertility. *Note:* Women who are using cervical secretions as an indicator to avoid pregnancy may not detect early changes in secretions so must have a calendar calculation as a back-up to identify the start of the fertile time.
Antihistamines (for inducing sleep) (e.g. diphenhydramine / Nytol)	Insomnia	Antihistamines have a sedative effect and may be used as a common over-the-counter sleep aid. – May dry up cervical secretions, causing persistent dryness or scant amounts of poor-quality cervical secretions.

Chemotherapy	Many different forms of cancer	Cytotoxic drugs destroy cells and target rapidly dividing cancer cells. Their effect on the menstrual cycle is varied. – May be irregular cycles – shorter or longer cycles with light or heavy periods, anovulatory cycles or amenorrhoea. – May cause damage to the ovaries either immediately or delayed, temporary or permanent with accompanying menopausal symptoms. – May recover full ovarian function and normal fertility after completing treatment, depending on the type of chemotherapy. This is more likely for younger women.
Combined oral contraception	Preventing pregnancy	Combined oral contraceptives (estrogen & progestogen) prevent ovulation, and create a thick mucus plug blocking the cervix. – Most women will feel dry or observe persistent milky secretions. – May be monophasic temperatures. – May notice that all temperatures are at a slightly elevated level. – May induce a mild hyperprolactinaemia with possible galactorrhoea.
Dopamine agonist (bromocriptine)	Raised prolactin & galactorrhoea	A dopamine agonist activates dopamine receptors to reduce pituitary production of prolactin, stop breast leakage and restore normal hormonal balance, ovulation and menstrual function. – Should change monophasic cycles to biphasic cycles with normal length luteal phases. – Should restore normal pattern of cervical secretions.
H2 blockers e.g. cimetidine, ranitidine	Reduce stomach acid e.g. in acid reflux	H2 blockers (histamine H2-receptor antagonists) increase prolactin levels. – May disrupt ovulation – delayed or absent temperature rise. – May affect luteal function – short or inadequate luteal phase. – May reduce libido.
Mucolytics (e.g. guaifenesin)	Coughs expectorant	Mucolytics thin respiratory secretions to make them easier to cough up. – May increase and thin cervical secretions. – May help to improve poor quality secretions, but research is limited.
Non-steroidal anti-inflammatories Cox-2 inhibitors (e.g. ibuprofen, aspirin, mefenamic acid, diclofenac, etoricoxib)	Inflammation and pain including painful periods and inflammatory conditions such as rheumatoid arthritis	Non-steroidal anti-inflammatory drugs (NSAIDs) are used to reduce pain and inflammation; they may also have an antipyretic effect. NSAIDs block the action of prostaglandin – the substances that cause inflammation and pain. Prostaglandins are also involved with regulation of body temperature, melatonin synthesis, sleep and rupture of the ovarian follicle. COX-2 inhibitors are selective NSAIDs with more potent effects on fertility. – May prevent ovulation, yet still show a biphasic temperature curve. – High incidence of luteinised unruptured follicle (LUF) syndrome. – May reduce cervical secretions or cause an interrupted pattern. – May affect fertilisation, tubal function and implantation. *Note:* Women who are trying to conceive should try and restrict their use of NSAIDs. This may be highly significant for women on continuous treatment around ovulation.

(*Continued*)

(Continued)

Progestogen-only contraception	Preventing pregnancy	The main action of progestogen-only methods is to create a thick mucus plug blocking the cervix. Ovulation is generally not affected by progestogen only pills but may be suppressed by longer-acting progestogen-only methods. – May be a biphasic temperature pattern as ovulation is likely to occur with progestogen-only pills. – May be monophasic charts with long-acting reversible contraceptives (LARC) methods (e.g. implanon or depot injections. – May reduce amount and quality of cervical secretions or cause persistent dryness.
Retiniods (Isotretinon – Roaccutane)	Severe (cystic) acne	Retinoids are related to vitamin A and work on the epithelium reducing the production of the skin's natural oils to treat severe acne. They may also have an effect on cervical epithelium. – May dry up cervical secretions. *Note:* Isotretinon carries a high risk of major congenital abnormalities. Women require a highly effective family planning method. If a woman wishes to use FAMs, she should restrict intercourse to the late infertile time for maximum protection against pregnancy (using life or death rules).
Steroids (e.g. cortisone prednisolone)	Rheumatoid arthritis or severe asthma attacks	Corticosteroids are used to treat a large number of allergic and inflammatory conditions. – May inhibit the production of cervical secretions. – May cause irregular cycles, delay or suppress ovulation.
Thyroid replacement (levothyroxine)	Hypothyroidism	Thyroxine replacement improves general health and helps to optimise reproductive function. – May help to re-establish a regular ovulatory cycle with normal length luteal phase. – May re-establish a normal coverline (if temperatures had been lowered overall). – May re-establish an adequate pattern of cervical secretions.

APPENDIX H

Further reading

- *Women's sexual health*. Editor: G. Andrews, Elsevier, 2005.
- *Infertility in practice*. A. Balen, CRC Press, 2014.
- *Human sexuality and its problems*. J. Bancroft, Churchill Livingstone, 2009.
- *The handbook of sexual health in primary care*. Editors: T. Belfield, P. Matthews, C. Moss FPA, 2011.
- *Handbook of contraception and sexual health*. S. Everett, Routledge, 2014.
- *Female fertility and the body fat connection*. R. Frisch, Chicago Press, London, 2002.
- *Contraception: your questions answered*. J. Guillebaud and A. McGregor, Churchill Livingstone, 2012.
- *Llewellyn-Jones fundamentals of obstetrics and gynaecology*. D. Oats and S. Abraham, Mosby Elsevier, 2016.
- *Expecting better*. E. Oster, Orion, London, 2013.
- *Abortion care*. S. Rowlands, Cambridge University Press, 2014.
- *Why zebras don't get ulcers*. R. Sapolsky, Holt, New York, 2004.
- *Fertility and pregnancy: An epidemiological perspective*. A.J. Wilcox, Oxford, 2010.
- Taking charge of your fertility, T. Weschler, Harper Collins, 2016 and companion site www.tcoyf.com (general readership).

PROFESSIONAL ASSOCIATIONS AND RESOURCES

- British Infertility Counselling Association: www.bica.net
- British Fertility Society: www.britishfertilitysociety.org.uk
- British Menopause Society: www.thebms.org.uk
- Brook: www.brook.org.uk
- College of Sexual and Relationship Therapists: www.cosrt.org.uk
- European Society of Human Reproduction and Embryology: www.eshre.eu
- Family Planning Association: www.fpa.org.uk
- Faculty of Sexual and Reproductive Health Care: www.fsrh.org
- FertiSTAT (Fertility Status Awareness Tool): www.fertistat.com
- Global Library of Women's Medicine: www.glowm.com
- Human Fertilisation & Embryology Authority: www.hfea.gov.uk
- Institute of Psychosexual Medicine: www.ipm.org.uk
- International Planned Parenthood Federation: www.ippf.org
- National Preconception Curriculum and Resources Guide: http://beforeandbeyond.org
- PSHE Association: www.pshe-association.org.uk
- Royal College of Obstetricians & Gynaecologists: www.rcog.org.uk
- Sex Education Forum: www.sexeducationforum.org.uk
- UK Teratology Information Service: www.uktis.org
- World Health Organisation: www.who.int/reproductivehealth

PATIENT SUPPORT

- Adoption UK: www.adoptionuk.org
- Beat (beat eating disorders): www.b-eat.co.uk
- Breast Cancer Care: www.breastcancercare.org.uk
- Breast and gynaecological cancers: www.cancerresearchuk.org
- The Daisy Network (premature menopause support): www.daisynetwork.org.uk
- Donor Conception Network: www.dcnetwork.org
- Ectopic Pregnancy Trust: www.ectopic.org.uk
- Endometriosis UK: www.endometriosis-uk.org
- Gateway Women (for women childless by circumstance): http://gateway-women.com
- Infertility Network UK: www.infertilitynetworkuk.com
- Miscarriage Association requires separate bullet miscarriageassociation.org.uk
- SANDS (stillbirth and neonatal death charity): www.uk-sands.org
- Tommy's (information on miscarriage, stillbirth and premature birth): www.tommys.org
- Verity (PCOS support group): www.verity-pcos.org.uk

ORGANISATIONS TEACHING FAMS

- FertilityUK (FA service including network of UK practitioners): www.fertilityuk.org
- European Institute for Family Life Education (European teaching organisations): www.ieef.eu
- Institute for Reproductive Health, Georgetown University (SDM, TDM and LAM for world-wide use): www.irh.org
- IRH standard days method: www.standarddaysmethod.org
- Serena Canada: www.serena.ca
- Australian Council of Natural Family Planning: www.acnfp.com.au
- Natural Fertility New Zealand: www.naturalfertility.co.nz

BIBLIOGRAPHY

[1] Abdulla, U., Diver, M. J., Hipkin, L. J. and Davis, J. C. Plasma progesterone levels as an index of ovulation. *British Journal of Obstetrics and Gynaecology*, 90(6):543–548, Jun 1983.

[2] Abidogun, K. A., Ojengbede, O. A. and Fatukasi, U. I. Prediction and detection of ovulation: An evaluation of the cervical mucus score. *African Journal of Medicine and Medical Sciences*, 22(1):65–69, Mar 1993.

[3] Adams, D. B., Gold, A. R. and Burt, A. D. Rise in female-initiated sexual activity at ovulation and its suppression by oral contraceptives. *New England Journal of Medicine*, 299(21):1145–1150, Nov 1978.

[4] Agarwal, A., Deepinder, F., Cocuzza, M., Short, R.A. and Evenson, D. P. Effect of vaginal lubricants on sperm motility and chromatin integrity: A prospective comparative study. *Fertility and Sterility*, 89(2):375–379, Feb 2008.

[5] Aleandri, V., Spina, V. and Morini, A. The pineal gland and reproduction. *Human Reproduction Update*, 2(3):225–235, 1996.

[6] Anderson, K., Norman, R. J. and Middleton, P. Preconception lifestyle advice for people with subfertility. *Cochrane Database of Systematic Reviews*, (4):CD008189, 2010.

[7] Anderson, L., Lewis, S. E. and McClure, N. The effects of coital lubricants on sperm motility in vitro. *Human Reproduction*, 13(12):3351–3356, Dec 1998.

[8] Andrews, G. *Women's Sexual Health*. Bailliere Tindall, London, 2001.

[9] Andrews, M. A., Schliep, K. C., Wactawski-Wende, J., Stanford, J. B., Zarek, S. M., Radin, R. G., Sjaarda, L. A., Perkins, N. J., Kalwerisky, R. A., Hammoud, A. O. and Mumford, S. L. Dietary factors and luteal phase deficiency in healthy eumenorrheic women. *Human Reproduction*, DOI:10.1093/humrep/dev133, Jun 2015.

[10] Arevalo, M., Sinai, I. and Jennings, V. A fixed formula to define the fertile window of the menstrual cycle as the basis of a simple method of natural family planning. *Contraception*, 60(6):357–360, Dec 1999.

[11] Arevalo, M., Jennings, V., Nikula, M., and Sinai, I. Efficacy of the new TwoDay Method of family planning. *Fertility and Sterility*, 82(4):885–892, Oct 2004.

[12] Arevalo, M., Jennings, V., and Sinai, I. Efficacy of a new method of family planning: The Standard Days Method. *Contraception*, 65(5):333–338, May 2002.

[13] Arevalo, M., Jennings, V., and Sinai, I. Application of simple fertility awareness-based methods of family planning to breastfeeding women. *Fertility and Sterility*, 80(5):1241–1248, Nov 2003.

[14] Arevalo, M., Sinai, I., Olivotti, B., and Bahamondes, L., Implications of cycle length immediately after discontinuation of combined oral contraceptives on use of the Standard Days Method. *International Journal of Gynaecology and Obstetrics*, 111(1):78–81, Oct 2010.

[15] Attarchi, M., Darkhi, H., Khodarahmian, M., Dolati, M., Kashanian, M., Ghaffari, M., Mirzamohammadi, E., and Mohammadi, S. Characteristics of menstrual cycle in shift workers. *Global Journal of Health Sciences*, 5(3):163–172, May 2013.

[16] Backhausen, M. G., Ekstrand, M., Tydén, T., Magnussen, B. K., Shawe, J., Stern, J. and Hegaard, H. K. Pregnancy planning and lifestyle prior to conception and during early pregnancy among Danish women. *European Journal of Contraception and Reproductive Health Care*, 19(1):57–65, Feb 2014.

[17] Baerwald, A. R., Adams, G. P. and Pierson, R. A. A new model for ovarian follicular development during the human menstrual cycle. *Fertility and Sterility*, 80(1):116–122, Jul 2003.

[18] Baerwald, A. R., Adams, G. P. and Pierson, R. A. Ovarian antral folliculogenesis during the human menstrual cycle: A review. *Human Reproduction Update*, 18(1):73–91, Jan 2012.

[19] Bailey, J. and Marshall, J. The relationship of the post-ovulatory phase of the menstrual cycle to total cycle length. *Journal of Biosocial Science*, 2(2):123–132, Apr 1970.

[20] Baird, D. D., McConnaughey, D. R., Weinberg, C. R., Musey, P. I., Collins, D. C., Kesner, J. S., Knecht, E. A., and Wilcox, A. J. Application of a method for estimating day of ovulation using urinary estrogen and progesterone metabolites. *Epidemiology*, 6(5):547–550, Sep 1995.

[21] Bak, C. W., Lyu, S. W., Seok, H. H., Byun, J. S., Lee, J. H., Shim S. H. S. and Yoon, T. K. Erectile dysfunction and extramarital sex induced by timed intercourse: A prospective study of 439 men. *Journal of Andrology*, May 2012.

[22] Baker, R. R. and Bellis, M. A. *Human Sperm Competition*. Chapman & Hall, London, 1994.

[23] Balen, Adam. *Infertility in Practice*, 4th Edition. CRC Press, London, 2014.

[24] Ball, M. A prospective field trial of the "Ovulation Method" of avoiding conception. *European Journal of Obstetrics and Gynecology and Reproductive Biology*, 6(2):63–66, 1976.

[25] Ball, M. Integration of abstinence in NFP. *International Review of Natural Family Planning*, 11(1), 1987.

[26] Barbato, M. and Bertolotti, G. Natural methods for fertility control: A prospective study – first part. *International Journal of Fertility and Sterility*, 33(Suppl):48–51, 1988.

[27] Barbato, M., Pandolfi, A. and Guida, M. A new diagnostic aid for natural family planning. *Advances in Contraception*, 9(4):335–340, Dec 1993.

[28] Barker, D. J. and Martyn, C. N. The maternal and fetal origins of cardiovascular disease. *Journal of Epidemiology and Community Health*, 46(1):8–11, Feb 1992.

[29] Barnes, Broda Otto. *Hypothyroidism: The Unsuspected Illness*. Harper Collins, Toronto, 1976.

[30] Barnhart, K., Mirkin, S., Grubb, G., and Constantine, G. Return to fertility after cessation of a continuous oral contraceptive. *Fertility and Sterility*, 91(5):1654–1656, May 2009.

[31] Barr, S. I, Janelle, K. C. and Prior, J. C. Energy intakes are higher during the luteal phase of ovulatory menstrual cycles. *American Journal of Clinical Nutrition*, 61(1):39–43, Jan 1995.

[32] Barr, S. I., Prior, J. C. and Vigna, Y. M. Restrained eating and ovulatory disturbances: Possible implications for bone health. *American Journal of Clinical Nutrition*, 59(1):92–97, Jan 1994.

[33] Barrett, G., Pendry, E., Peacock, J., Victor, C., Thakar, R. and Manyonda, I. Women's sexual health after childbirth. *British Journal of Obstetrics and Gynaecology*, 107(2):186–195, Feb 2000.

[34] Barrett, J. C. and Marshall, J. The risk of conception on different days of the menstrual cycle. *Population Studies (Cambridge)*, 23(3):455–461, Nov 1969.

[35] Barron, Mary Lee. Light exposure, melatonin secretion, and menstrual cycle parameters: An integrative review. *Biological Research for Nursing*, 9(1):49–69, Jul 2007.

[36] Bath, S. C., Steer, C. D., Golding, J., Emmett, P. and Rayman, M. P. Effect of inadequate iodine status in UK pregnant women on cognitive outcomes in their children: Results from the Avon longitudinal study of parents and children (ALSPAC). *Lancet*, 382(9889):331–337, Jul 2013.

[37] Bauml, K. H. On the relationship between the menstrual cycle and the body weight and food intake of women. *Archives of Psychology (Frankfurt)*, 141(4):237–250, 1989.

[38] Becher, N., Adams Waldorf, K. Hein, M., and Uldbjerg, N. The cervical mucus plug: Structured review of the literature. *Acta Obstetrica Gynecologia Scandinavica*, 88(5):502–513, 2009.

[39] Been, J. V., Nurmatov, U. B., Cox, B., Nawrot, T. S., van Schayck, C. P. and Sheikh, A. Effect of smoke-free legislation on perinatal and child health: A systematic review and meta-analysis. *Lancet*, 383(9928):1549–1560, May 2014.

[40] Behre, H. M., Kuhlage, J., Gassner, C., Sonntag, B., Schem, C., Schneider, H. P. and Nieschlag, E. Prediction of ovulation by urinary hormone measurements with the home use Clearplan fertility monitor: Comparison with transvaginal ultrasound scans and serum hormone measurements. *Human Reproduction*, 15(12):2478–2482, Dec 2000.

[41] Belfield, T., Matthews, P. and Moss, C. *The Handbook of Sexual Health in Primary Care.* FPA, 2011.

[42] Benjamin, F. Basal body temperature recordings in gynaecology and obstetrics. *Journal of Obstetrics and Gynaecology of the British Commonwealth*, 67:177–187, Apr 1960.

[43] Beral, Valerie and Million Women Study Collaborators. Breast cancer and hormone-replacement therapy in the million women study. *Lancet*, 362(9382):419–427, Aug 2003.

[44] Berardono, B., Melani, D., Ranaldi, F., Giachetti, E., and Vanni, P. Is the salivary "ferning" a reliable index of the fertile period? *Acta Europea Fertilitatis*, 24(2):61–65, 1993.

[45] Berglund Scherwitzl, E., Gemzell Danielsson, K., Sellberg, J. A., and Scherwitzl, R. Fertility awareness-based mobile application for contraception. *The European Journal of Contraception and Reproductive Health Care*, DOI: 10.3109/13625187.2016.1154143, 2016.

[46] Bewley, S., Ledger, W. and Nikolaou, D. editors. Reproductive ageing, in *Reproductive Ageing: Chapter 36 Consensus Views Arising from the 56th Study Group*. RCOG Press, London, 2009. 353–356.

[47] Bewley, S., Davies, M., and Braude, P. Which career first? *British Medical Journal*, 331(7517):588–589, Sep 2005.

[48] Bhattacharya, S., Harrild, K., Mollison, J., Wordsworth, S., Tay, C., Harrold, A., McQueen, D., Lyall, H., Johnston, L., Burrage, J., Grossett, S., Walton, H., Lynch, J., Johnstone, A., Kini, S., Raja, A., and Templeton, A. Clomifene citrate or unstimulated intrauterine insemination compared with expectant management for unexplained infertility: Pragmatic randomised controlled trial. *British Medical Journal*, 337:a716, 2008.

[49] Bigelow, J. L., Dunson, D. B. Stanford, J. B. Ecochard, R., Gnoth, C., and Colombo, B. Mucus observations in the fertile window: A better predictor of conception than timing of intercourse. *Human Reproduction*, 19(4):889–892, Apr 2004.

[50] Billings, E., Billings, J., and Caratinich, M. *Atlas of the Ovulation Method*, 2nd Edition. Advocate Press, Melbourne, 1974.

[51] Billings, E. L., Brown, J. B., Billings, J. J., and Burger, H. G. Symptoms and hormonal changes accompanying ovulation. *Lancet*, 1(7745):282–284, Feb 1972.

[52] Billings, John. *The Ovulation Method*. The Advocate Press, Melbourne, 1964.

[53] Blackwell, L. F., Brown, J. B., Vigil, P., Gross, B., Sufi, S., and d'Arcangues, C. Hormonal monitoring of ovarian activity using the ovarian monitor, Part I: Validation of home and laboratory results obtained during ovulatory cycles by comparison with radioimmunoassay. *Steroids*, 68(5):465–476, May 2003.

[54] Blake, D., Smith, D., Bargiacchi, A., France, M. and Gudex, G. Fertility awareness in women attending a fertility clinic. *Australian and New Zealand Journal of Obstetrics and Gynaecology*, 37(3):350–352, Aug 1997.

[55] Bonnar, J. Experience in the use of NFP in the field, in *Genus*. Department of Demographic Sciences, University La Sapienza, Rome, 1998. 119–128.

[56] Bonnar, J., Flynn, A., Freundl, G., Kirkman, R., Royston, R., and Snowden, R. Personal hormone monitoring for contraception. *British Journal of Family Planning*, 24(4):128–134, Jan 1999.

[57] Bonnar, J., Lamprecht, V., and O'Conner, E. Alternatives to vaginal intercourse practiced during the fertile time among calendar method users in Ireland. *Advances in Contraception*, 13(2–3):173–177, 1997.

[58] Borkman, T. and Shivanandan, M. The impact of natural family planning on selected aspects of the couple relationship. *International Review of Natural Family Planning*, 8(1):58–66, 1984.

[59] Bouchard, T., Fehring, R. J. and Schneider, M. Efficacy of a new postpartum transition protocol for avoiding pregnancy. *Journal of the American Board of Family Medicine*, 26(1):35–44, 2013.

[60] British Pregnancy Advisory Service (BPAS). Misconceptions leading to unwanted pregnancies among older women, www.bpas.org (accessed 17.8.16), May 2014.

[61] Braat, D. D., Smeenk, J. J, Manger, A. P., Thomas, C. M., Veersema, S., and J. M. Merkus, J. M. Saliva test as ovulation predictor. *Lancet*, 352(9136):1283–1284, Oct 1998.

[62] Brayer, F. T., Chiazze, Jr, L., and Duffy, B. J. Calendar rhythm and menstrual cycle range. *Fertility and Sterility*, 20(2):279–288, 1969.

[63] Brezina, P. R., Haberl, E. and Wallach, E. At home testing: Optimizing management for the infertility physician. *Fertility and Sterility*, 95(6):1867–1878, May 2011.

[64] Brosens, Ivo and Brosens, Jan. Managing infertility with fertility-awareness methods. *Sexuality, Reproduction & Menopause*, 4(1):13–16, 2006.

[65] Brosens, I., Hernalsteen, P., Devos, A., Cloke, B., and Brosens, J. Self-assessment of the cervical pupil sign as a new fertility-awareness method. *Fertility and Sterility*, 91(3):937–939, Mar 2009.

[66] Brown, J. B., Holmes, J., and Barker, G. Use of the home ovarian monitor in pregnancy avoidance. *American Journal of Obstetrics and Gynecology*, 165(6 Pt 2):2008–2011, Dec 1991.

[67] Brown, James B. Types of ovarian activity in women and their significance: The continuum (a reinterpretation of early findings). *Human Reproduction Update*, 17(2):141–158, 2011.

[68] Brown, S. Controversy persists in the diagnosis of PCOS, in *Focus on Reproduction*, pp. 12–13. ESHRE, www.eshre.eu, January 2014.

[69] Brtnicka, H., Weiss, P., and Zverina, J. Human sexuality during pregnancy and the postpartum period. *Bratisl Lek Listy [Bratislava Medical Journal]*, 110(7):427–431, 2009.

[70] Bryant, M., Truesdale, K. P., and Dye, L. Modest changes in dietary intake across the menstrual cycle: Implications for food intake research. *British Journal of Nutrition*, 96(5):888–894, Nov 2006.

[71] Buffenstein, R., Poppitt, S. D., McDevitt, R. M., and Prentice, A. M. Food intake and the menstrual cycle: A retrospective analysis, with implications for appetite research. *Physiology and Behaviour*, 58(6):1067–1077, Dec 1995.

[72] Bujan, L., Daudin, M., Charlet, J. P., Thonneau, P., and Mieusset, R. Increase in scrotal temperature in car drivers. *Human Reproduction*, 15(6):1355–1357, Jun 2000.

[73] Burger, H. G. Estradiol: The physiological basis of the fertile period. *International Journal of Gynecology and Obstetrics* (supplement), 1:5–9, 1989.

[74] Case, A. M. and Reid, R. L. Effects of the menstrual cycle on medical disorders. *Archives of Internal Medicine*, 158(13):1405–1412, Jul 1998.

[75] Chai, S. and Wild, R. A. Basal body temperature and endometriosis. *Fertility and Sterility*, 54(6):1028–1031, Dec 1990.

[76] Chason, R. J., McLain, A. C., Sundaram, R., Chen, Z., Segars, J. H., Pyper, C., and Buck Louis, G. M. Preconception stress and the secondary sex ratio: A prospective cohort study. *Fertility and Sterility*, 98(4):937–941, Oct 2012.

[77] Chausiaux, O., Hayes, J., Long, C., Morris, S., Williams, G., and Husheer, S. Pregnancy prognosis in infertile couples on the duofertility programme compared with in vitro fertilisation/intracytoplasmic sperm injection. *Touch Briefings*, 92–94, 2011.

[78] Che, Y., Cleland, J. G., and Ali, M. M. Periodic abstinence in developing countries: An assessment of failure rates and consequences. *Contraception*, 69(1):15–21, Jan 2004.

[79] Check, J. H., Adelson, H. G., and Wu, C. H. Improvement of cervical factor with guaifenesin. *Fertility and Sterility*, 37(5):707–708, May 1982.

[80] Check, J. H., Dietterich, C., and Houck, M. A. Ipsilateral versus contralateral ovary selection of dominant follicle in succeeding cycle. *Obstetrics and Gynecology*, 77(2):247–249, Feb 1991.

[81] Check, J. H., Dietterich, C., Lauer, C., and Liss, J. Ovulation-inducing drugs versus specific mucus therapy for cervical factor. *International Journal of Fertility*, 36(2):108–112, 1991.

[82] Chen, L., Malone, K. E., and Li, C. I. Bra wearing not associated with breast cancer risk: A population-based case-control study. *Cancer Epidemiology, Biomarkers and Prevention*, 23(10):2181–2185, Oct 2014.

[83] Chen, Z. E. *Fertility decision-making: A qualitative study in Scotland.* PhD thesis, PhD Sociology, University of Edinburgh, Edinburgh, 2015.

[84] Chiazze, Jr, L., Brayer, F. T., Macisco, Jr, J. J.,Parker, M. P., and Duffy, B. J. The length and variability of the human menstrual cycle. *Journal of the American Medical Association*, 203(6):377–380, Feb 1968.

[85] Chiu, Y. H., Afeiche, M. C., Gaskins, A. J., Williams, P. L., Petrozza, J. C., Tanrikut, C., Hauser, R., and Chavarro, J. E. Fruit and vegetable intake and their pesticide residues in relation to semen quality among men from a fertility clinic. *Human Reproduction*, Mar 2015.

[86] Chizen, D. and Pierson, R. Transvaginal ultrasonography and female infertility. *Global Library Women's Medicine* (www.glowm.com), May 2010. ISSN: 1756–2228.

[87] Choi, J., Chan, S. and Wiebe, E. Natural family planning: Physicians' knowledge, attitudes, and practice. *Journal of Obstetrics and Gynaecology, Canada*, 32(7):673–678, Jul 2010.

[88] Chretien, F. C., Cohen, J., Borg, V., and Psychoyos, A. Human cervical mucus during the menstrual cycle and pregnancy in normal and pathological conditions. *Journal of Reproductive Medicine*, 14(5):192–196, May 1975.

[89] Chrétien, F. C. Cervical mucus: III. physiological roles. *Journal de Gynecologie et Obstetrique Biologie de la Reproduction [Journal of Gynaecology, Obstetrics and Biology of Reproduction] (Paris)*, 6(4):451–488, Jun 1977.

[90] Chrétien, François C. Involvement of the glycoproteic meshwork of cervical mucus in the mechanism of sperm orientation. *Acta Obstetrica Gynecologia Scandinavica*, 82(5):449–461, May 2003.

[91] Clinical Knowledge Summaries [CKS] (National Institute for Health and Care Excellence). Contraception – natural family planning: Scenario: Fertility awareness-based methods, www.cks.nice.org.uk.

[92] Clark, A. M., Ledger, W., Galletly, C., Tomlinson, L., Blaney, F., Wang, X., and Norman, R. J. Weight loss results in significant improvement in pregnancy and ovulation rates in anovulatory obese women. *Human Reproduction*, 10(10):2705–2712, Oct 1995.

[93] Clift, A. F. Observations on certain rheological properties of human cervical secretion. *Proceedings of the Royal Society of Medicine*, 39(1):1–9, Nov 1945.

[94] Clubb, E., Pyper, C. M., and Knight, J. A pilot study on teaching NFP in general practice. In *Current Knowledge and New Strategies for the 1990s: Proceedings of a Conference, Part II, Georgetown University*, Washington, DC. 1989. 130–132.

[95] Cohen, M. R., Stein, Sr, I. F. and Kaye, B. M. Spinnbarkeit: A characteristic of cervical mucus; significance at ovulation time. *Fertility and Sterility*, 3(3):201–209, 1952.

[96] Cole, Laurence A., Ladner, Donald G., and Byrn, Francis W. The normal variabilities of the menstrual cycle. *Fertility and Sterility*, 91(2):522–527, Feb 2009.

[97] Collins, W. P. Hormonal indices of ovulation and the fertile period. *Advances in Contraception*, 1(4):279–294, Dec 1985.

[98] Collins, W. P. The evolution of reference methods to monitor ovulation. *American Journal of Obstetrics and Gynecology*, 165(6 Pt 2):1994–1996, Dec 1991.

[99] Colombo, B. Biometrical research on some parameters of the menstrual cycle. *International Journal of Gynecology and Obstetrics* (supplement), 1:13–18, 1989.

[100] Colombo, B. Evaluation of fertility predictors and comparison of different rules, in *Genus*. Department of Demographic Sciences, University La Sapienza, Rome, 1998. 153–167.

[101] Colombo, B. and Masarotto, G. Daily fecundability: First results from a new data base. *Demographic Research*, 3:39, Sep 2000.

[102] Colombo, B. and Scarpa, B. Calendar methods of fertility regulation: A rule of thumb. *Statistica*, 56(1):3–14, 1996.

[103] Cooney, K. A., Nyirabukeye, T., Labbok, M. H., Hoser, P. H., and Ballard, E. An assessment of the nine-month lactational amenorrhea method (Mama-9) in Rwanda. *Studies in Family Planning*, 27(3):102–171, 1996.

[104] Cooper, K. H. and Abrams, R. M. Attributes of the oral cavity as a site for basal body temperature measurements. *Journal of Obstetric, Gynecologic and Neonatal Nursing*, 13(2):125–129, 1984.

[105] Cooper, T. G., Noonan, E., von Eckardstein, S., Auger, J., Gordon Baker, H. W., Behre, H. M., Haugen, T. B., Kruger, T., Wang, C., Mbizvo, M. T., and Vogelsong, K. M. World Health Organization reference values for human semen characteristics. *Human Reproduction Update*, 16(3):231–245, 2010.

[106] Coppola, M. A., Klotz, K. L., Kim, K. A., Cho, H. Y., Kang, J., Shetty, J., Howards, S. S., Flickinger, C. J., and Herr, J. C. Spermcheck fertility, an immunodiagnostic home test that detects normozoospermia and severe oligozoospermia. *Human Reproduction*, 25(4):853–861, Apr 2010.

[107] Cox, T., van der Steeg, J. W., Steures, P., Hompes, P. G. A., van der Veen, F., Eijkemans, M. J. C., van Leeuwen, J. H., S., Renckens, C., Bossuyt, P. M. M., and Mol, B. W. J. Time to pregnancy after a previous miscarriage in subfertile couples. *Fertility and Sterility*, 94(2):485–488, Jul 2010.

[108] Crochet, J. R., Bastian, L. A., and Chireau, M. V. Does this woman have an ectopic pregnancy? The rational clinical examination systematic review. *Journal of the American Medical Association*, 309(16):1722–1729, Apr 2013.

[109] Cronin, M., Schellschmidt, I. and Dinger, J. Rate of pregnancy after using drospirenone and other progestin-containing oral contraceptives. *Obstetrics and Gynecology*, 114(3):616–622, Sep 2009.

[110] Daly, K. J. and Herold, E. S. Who uses natural family planning? *Canadian Journal of Public Health*, 76(3):207–208, 1985.

[111] Danilenko, K. V., and Samoilova, E.A. Stimulatory effect of morning bright light on reproductive hormones and ovulation: Results of a controlled crossover trial. *Public Library of Science (PLoS) Clinical Trials*, 2(2):e7, 2007.

[112] D'Arbonneau, F., Ansart, S., Le Berre, R., Dueymes, M., Youinou, P. and Pennec, Y. Thyroid dysfunction in Primary Sjogren's Syndrome: A long-term followup study. *Arthritis and Rheumatology*, 49(6):804–809, Dec 2003.

[113] Dauchy, R. T., Xiang, S., Mao, L., Brimer, S., Wren, M. A., Yuan, L., Anbalagan, M., Hauch, A., Frasch, T., Rowan, B. G., Blask, D. E., and Hill, S. M. Circadian and melatonin disruption by exposure to light at night drives intrinsic resistance to tamoxifen therapy in breast cancer. *Cancer Research* (journal), Jul 2014.

[114] Davis, S. R. and Tran, J. Testosterone influences libido and well being in women. *Trends in Endocrinology and Metabolism*, 12(1):33–37, 2001.

[115] de Weerd, S., Steegers, E. A. P., Heinen, M. M., van den Eertwegh, S., Vehof, R. M. E. J., and Steegers-Theunissen, R. P. M. Preconception nutritional intake and lifestyle factors: First results of an explorative study. *European Journal of Obstetrics and Gynecology and Reproductive Biology*, 111(2):167–172, Dec 2003.

[116] DeFelice, Joy. *The Effects of Light on Cervical Mucus Patterns in the Menstrual Cycle: A Clinical Study*. Emergence Publications, Washington, DC, 1979.

[117] DeFranco, E. A., Ehrlich, S., and Muglia, L. J. Influence of interpregnancy interval on birth timing. *British Journal of Obstetrics and Gynaecology*, 121(13):1633–1640, Dec 2014.

[118] Depares, J., Ryder, R. E., Walker, S. M., Scanlon, M. F., and Norman, C. M. Ovarian ultrasonography highlights precision of symptoms of ovulation as markers of ovulation. *British Medical Journal (Clinical Research Edition)*, 292(6535):1562, Jun 1986.

[119] Department of Health, Dublin and WHO. *International Seminar on Natural Family Planning*, Dublin, October 1979.

[120] Devrim, I., Kara, A., Ceyhan, M., Tezer, H., Uludag, A. K., Cengiz, A. B., Yigitkanl, I. and Seccmeer, G. Measurement accuracy of fever by tympanic and axillary thermometry. *Pediatric Emergency Care*, 23(1):16–19, Jan 2007.

[121] Diamond, Jared. *The Rise and Fall of the Third Chimpanzee*. Vintage, London, 1991. 65.

[122] Diaz, S., Cardenas, H., Brandeis, A., Miranda, P., Salvatierra, A. M., and Croxatto, H. B. Relative contributions of anovulation and luteal phase defect to the reduced pregnancy rate of breastfeeding women. *Fertility and Sterility*, 58(3):498–503, Sep 1992.

[123] Diaz, C. A., Seron-Ferre, M., Cardenas, H., Schiappacasse, V., Brandeis, A., and Croxatto, H. B. Circadian variation of basal plasma prolactin, prolactin response to suckling, and length of amenorrhea in nursing women. *Journal of Clinical Endocrinology and Metabolism*, 68(5):946–955, May 1989.

[124] Diaz, S., Aravena, R., Cardenas, H., Casado, M. E., Miranda, P., Schiappacasse, V., and Croxatto, H. B. Contraceptive efficacy of lactational amenorrhea in urban Chilean women. *Contraception*, 43(4):335–352, Apr 1991.

[125] Djerassi, C. Fertility awareness: Jet-age rhythm method? *Science*, 248(4959):1061–1062, Jun 1990.

[126] DOH. Judicial review of emergency contraception, 2002. 257. Available at: http://webarchive.nationalarchives.gov.uk/+/www.dh.gov.uk/en/Publichealth/Healthimprovement/Sexualhealth/Sexualhealthgeneralinformation/DH_4063853, Accessed 18.08.16

[127] Dominguez-Salas, P., Moore, S. E., Baker, M. S., Bergen, A. W., Cox, S. E., Dyer, R. A., Fulford, A. J., Guan, Y., Laritsky, E., Silver, M. J., Swan, G. E., Zeisel, S. H., Innis, S. M., Waterland, R. A., Prentice, A. M., and Hennig, B. J. Maternal nutrition at conception modulates DNA methylation of human metastable epialleles. *Nature Communications*, 5:3746, 2014.

[128] Dorairaj, K. *The Modified Mucus Method of Family Planning*. Indian Social Institute, New Delhi, India, 1980.

[129] Dorairaj, K. Use-effectiveness of fertility awareness among the urban poor. *Social Action*, 34(3):286–306, 1984.

[130] Dorairaj, K. Acceptability of the Modified Mucus Method: Study of the psychosocial factors affecting acceptance. *International Journal of Fertility*, 33(Suppl):78–86, 1988.

[131] Dorairaj, K. The Modified Mucus Method in India. *American Journal of Obstetrics and Gynecology*, 165(6 Pt 2):2066–2067, Dec 1991.

[132] Döring, G. K. Basal temperature measurement for the determination of fertile and infertile days of women. *Deutsche Gesundheitswesen*, 12(14):422–425, Apr 1957.

[133] Döring, G. K. The incidence of anovular cycles in women. *Journal of Reproduction and Fertility*, 6:77–81, 1969.

[134] Drife, J. O. Breast modifications during the menstrual cycle. *International Journal of Gynecology and Obstetrics* (supplement), 1:19–24, 1989.

[135] Duane, M., Contreras, A., Jensen, E. T., and White, A. The performance of fertility awareness-based method apps marketed to avoid pregnancy, *Journal of the American Board of Family Medicine*, 29(4): 508–511, 2016.

[136] Dude, A., Neustadt, A. Martins, S., and Gilliam, M. Use of withdrawal and unintended pregnancy among females 15–24 years of age. *Obstetrics and Gynecology*, 122(3):595–600, Sep 2013.

[137] Dunlop, A. L., Allen, A. S., and Frank, E. Involving the male partner for interpreting the basal body temperature graph. *Obstetrics and Gynecology*, 98(1):133–138, Jul 2001.

[138] Dunlop, A. L., Schultz, R., and Frank, E. Interpretation of the BBT chart: Using the "gap" technique compared to the coverline technique. *Contraception*, 71(3):188–192, Mar 2005.

[139] Dunselman, G. A. J., Vermeulen, N., Becker, C., Calhaz-Jorge, C., D'Hooghe, T., De Bie, B., Heikinheimo, O., Horne, A. W., Kiesel, L., Nap, A., Prentice, A., Saridogan, E., Soriano, D., Nelen, W., European Society of Human Reproduction, and Embryology. Eshre guideline: Management of women with endometriosis. *Human Reproduction*, 29(3):400–412, Mar 2014.

[140] Dunson, D. B., Baird, D. D., Wilcox, A. J., and Weinberg, C. R. Day-specific probabilities of clinical pregnancy based on two studies with imperfect measures of ovulation. *Human Reproduction*, 14(7):1835–1839, Jul 1999.

[141] Dunson, D. B., Sinai, I., and Colombo, B. The relationship between cervical secretions and the daily probabilities of pregnancy: Effectiveness of the twoday algorithm. *Human Reproduction*, 16(11):2278–2282, Nov 2001.

[142] Dunson, D. B., Weinberg, C. R., Baird, D. D., Kesner, J. S., and Wilcox, A. J. Assessing human fertility using several markers of ovulation. *Statistics in Medicine*, 20(6):965–978, Mar 2001.

[143] Dunson, D. B., Baird, D.D., and Colombo, B. Increased infertility with age in men and women. *Obstetrics and Gynecology*, 103(1):51–56, Jan 2004.

[144] Dunson, D. B., Bigelow, J. L., and Colombo, B. Reduced fertilization rates in older men when cervical mucus is suboptimal. *Obstetrics and Gynecology*, 105(4):788–793, Apr 2005.

[145] Dunson, D. B., Colombo, B., and Baird, D. D. Changes with age in the level and duration of fertility in the menstrual cycle. *Human Reproduction*, 17(5):1399–1403, May 2002.

[146] Durai, R. and Ng, P. C. H. Mittelschmerz mimicking appendicitis. *British Journal of Hospital Medicine (London)*, 70(7):419, Jul 2009.

[147] Dye, L. and Blundell, J. E. Menstrual cycle and appetite control: Implications for weight regulation. *Human Reproduction*, 12(6):1142–1151, Jun 1997.

[148] Ecochard, R. and Gougeon, A. Side of ovulation and cycle characteristics in normally fertile women. *Human Reproduction*, 15(4):752–755, Apr 2000.

[149] Ecochard, R., Leiva, R., Bouchard, T., Boehringer, H., Direito, A., Mariani, A., and Fehring, R. Use of urinary pregnanediol 3-glucuronide to confirm ovulation. *Steroids*, 78(10):1035–1040, Oct 2013.

[150] Ecochard, R., Duterque, O., Leiva, R., Bouchard, T. and Vigil, P. Self-identification of the clinical fertile window and the ovulation period. *Fertility and Sterility*, Feb 2015.

[151] Eggert-Kruse, W., Botz, I., Pohl, S., Rohr, G., and Strowitzki, T. Antimicrobial activity of human cervical mucus. *Human Reproduction*, 15(4):778–784, Apr 2000.

[152] Elstein, M. Cervical mucus: Its physiological role and clinical significance. *Advances in Experimental Medicine and Biology*, 144:301–318, 1982.

[153] Elstein, M., Jennings, V.; Spieler, J. *Natural Family Planning and Reproductive Health Awareness: Expanding Options and Improving Health*. New York: Kluwer Academic Publishers, 1997.

[154] Endicott, J., Nee, J., and Harrison, W. Daily record of severity of problems (DRSP): Reliability and validity. *Archives of Women's Mental Health*, 9(1):41–49, Jan 2006.

[155] Engelhard, I. M, van den Hout, M. A., and Arntz, A. Posttraumatic stress disorder after pregnancy loss. *General Hospital Psychiatry*, 23(2):62–66, 2001.

[156] Englander-Golden, P., Chang, H. S., Whitmore, M. R., and Dienstbier, R. A. Female sexual arousal and the menstrual cycle. *Journal of Human Stress*, 6(1):42–48, Mar 1980.

[157] Entwistle, F. M. The evidence and rationale for the UNICEF baby friendly initiative standards, UNICEF UK, 2013.

[158] ESHRE/ASRM. Revised 2003 consensus on diagnostic criteria and long-term health risks related to polycystic ovary syndrome. *Fertility and Sterility*, 81(1):19–25, Jan 2004.

[159] Evans, J. J., Stewart, C. R., and Merrick, A. Y. Oestradiol in saliva during the menstrual cycle. *British Journal of Obstetrics and Gynaecology*, 87(7):624–626, Jul 1980.

[160] Evans-Hoeker, E., Pritchard, D. A., Leann Long, D. L., Herring, A. H., Stanford, J. B., and Steiner, A. Z. Cervical mucus monitoring prevalence and associated fecundability in women trying to conceive. *Fertility and Sterility*, 100(4):1033–1038.e1, Oct 2013.

[161] Everett, Suzanne. *Handbook of Contraception and Sexual Health*. Routledge, London and New York, 2014.

[162] Faundes, A., Lamprecht, V., Osis, M. J., and Lopes, B. C. Simplifying NFP: Preliminary report of a pilot study of the "collar" method in Brazil. *Advances in Contraception*, 13(2–3):167–171, 1997.

[163] Faundes, A., Segal, S. J., Adejuwon, C. A., Brache, V., Leon, P., and Alvarez-Sanchez, F. The menstrual cycle in women using an intrauterine device. *Fertility and Sterility*, 34(5):427–430, Nov 1980.

[164] Fehring, R., and Schneider, H. P. Comparison of abstinence and coital frequency between two natural methods of family planning. *Journal of Midwifery and Women's Health*, 528–532, DOI: 10/1111/jmwh.12216, 2014.

[165] Fehring, R. J., Hanson, L., and Stanford, J. B. Nurse-midwives' knowledge and promotion of lactational amenorrhea and other natural family planning methods for child spacing. *Journal of Midwifery and Women's Health*, 46(2):68–73, 2001.

[166] Fehring, Richard J. Accuracy of the peak day of cervical mucus as a biological marker of fertility. *Contraception*, 66(4):231–235, Oct 2002.

[167] Fehring, R. J., Schneider, M. and Barron, M. L. Efficacy of the Marquette method of natural family planning. *MCN: The American Journal of Maternal/Child Nursing*, 33(6):348–354, 2008.

[168] Fehring, R. J., Schneider, M., Barron, M. L., and Pruszynski, J. Influence of motivation on the efficacy of natural family planning. *MCN: The American Journal of Maternal/Child Nursing*, 38(6):352–358, 2013.

[169] Fehring, R. J., Schneider, M., Raviele, K., and Barron, M. L. Efficacy of cervical mucus observations plus electronic hormonal fertility monitoring as a method of natural family planning. *Journal of Obstetric Gynecologic and Neonatal Nursing*, 36(2):152–160, 2007.

[170] Fehring, R. J., Schneider, M., Raviele, K., Rodriguez, D., and Pruszynski, J. Randomized comparison of two Internet-supported fertility-awareness-based methods of family planning. *Contraception*, 88(1):24–30, Jul 2013.

[171] Fenster, L., Waller, K., Chen, J., Hubbard, A. E., Windham, G. C., Elkin, E., and Swan, S. Psychological stress in the workplace and menstrual function. *American Journal of Epidemiology*, 149(2):127–134, Jan 1999.

[172] Ferin, J. Determination de la periode sterile premenstruelle par la courbe thermique (determination of the premenstrual sterile period by the temperature curve). *Bruxelles Medical*, 27:2786–2793, 1947.

[173] Ferin, M. Clinical review 105: Stress and the reproductive cycle. *Journal of Clinical Endocrinology and Metabolism*, 84(6):1768–1774, Jun 1999.

[174] Ferreira-Poblete, A. The probability of conception on different days of the cycle with respect to ovulation: An overview. *Advances in Contraception*, 13(2–3):83–95, 1997.

[175] Ferrell, R. J., Simon, J. A., Pincus, S. M., Rodriguez, G., O'Connor, K. A., Holman, D. J., and Weinstein, M. The length of peri-menopausal menstrual cycles increases later and to a greater degree than previously reported. *Fertility and Sterility*, 86(3):619–624, Sep 2006.

[176] Ferris, D. G., Nyirjesy, P., Sobel, J. D., Soper, D., Pavletic, A., and Litaker, M. S. Over-the-counter antifungal drug misuse associated with patient- diagnosed vulvovaginal candidiasis. *Obstetrics and Gynecology*, 99(3):419–425, Mar 2002.

[177] Flynn, A. M., Docker, M., Brown, J. B., and Kennedy, K. I. Ultrasonographic patterns of ovarian activity during breastfeeding. *American Journal of Obstetrics and Gynecology*, 165(6 Pt 2):2027–2031, Dec 1991.

[178] Flynn, A. M., Docker, M., Morris, R., et al. The reliability of women's subjective assessment of the fertile period, relative to urinary gonadotrophins and follicular ultrasonic measurements during the menstrual cycle. In *conference proceedings from XIth World Congress on Fertility and Sterility*, Dublin, June 1983 (edited by John Bonnar), 3–11.

[179] Flynn, A. M., James, P., Collins, W. P., and Royston, P. Symptothermal and hormonal markers of potential fertility in climacteric women. *American Journal of Obstetrics and Gynecology*, 165(6 Pt 2):1987–1989, Dec 1991.

[180] Fordney-Settlage, D. A review of cervical mucus and sperm interactions in humans. *International Journal of Fertility*, 26(3):161–169, 1981.

[181] Formuso, C., Stracquadanio, M., and Ciotta, L. Myo-inositol vs. d-chiro inositol in pcos treatment. *Minerva Ginecologica*, 67(4):321–325, Aug 2015.

[182] Family Planning Association and National Opinion Polls; FAP survey results, In brief (newsletter), 2, Spring 2007.

[183] Family Planning Association, Conceivable, In brief (newsletter), 1, Spring 2010.

[184] France, J. T., Graham, F. M., Gosling, L., Hair, P., and Knox, B. S. Characteristics of natural conceptual cycles occurring in a prospective study of sex preselection: Fertility awareness symptoms, hormone levels, sperm survival, and pregnancy outcome. *International Journal of Fertility*, 37(4):244–255, 1992.

[185] France, J. T., Graham, F. M., Gosling, L., and Hair, P. I. A prospective study of the preselection of the sex of offspring by timing intercourse relative to ovulation. *Fertility and Sterility*, 41(6):894–900, Jun 1984.

[186] France, M., France, J., and Townend, K. Natural family planning in New Zealand: A study of continuation rates and characteristics of users. *Advances in Contraception*, 13(2–3):191–198, 1997.

[187] France, M. M. A study of the lactational amenorrhoea method of family planning in New Zealand women. *New Zealand Medical Journal*, 109(1022):189–191, May 1996.

[188] Frank-Herrmann, P., Freundl, G., Gnoth, C. H., et al. Natural family planning with and without barrier method use in the fertile phase: Efficacy in relation to sexual behaviour: A German prospective long-term study. *Advances in Contraception*, 13:179–189, 1997.

[189] Frank-Herrmann, P., Heil, J., Gnoth, C., Toledo, E., Baur, S., Pyper, C., Jenetzky, E., Strowitzki, T., and Freundl, G. The effectiveness of a fertility awareness based method to avoid pregnancy in relation to a couple's sexual behaviour during the fertile time: A prospective longitudinal study. *Human Reproduction*, 22(5):1310–1319, May 2007.

[190] Frank-Herrmann, P., Gnoth, C., Baur, S., Strowitzki, T., and Freundl, G. Determination of the fertile window: Reproductive competence of women – European cycle databases. *Gynecological Endocrinology*, 20(6):305–312, Jun 2005.

[191] Fraser, I. S., Critchley, H. O. D., Broder, M., and Munro, M. G. The Figo recommendations on terminologies and definitions for normal and abnormal uterine bleeding. *Seminars in Reproductive Medicine*, 29(5):383–390, Sep 2011.

[192] Freely, M., and Pyper, C. *Pandora's Clock*. Cedar, London, 1994.

[193] Freeman, E. W., Sammel, M. D., Lin, H. Boorman, D. W., and Gracia, C. R. Contribution of the rate of change of antimullerian hormone in estimating time to menopause for late reproductive-age women. *Fertility and Sterility*, 98(5):1254–1259, Aug 2012.

[194] Freundl, G. Present stage of knowledge of reproductive biology concerning natural family planning, in *Genus*, Vol. 54, Number 3–4. Universita degli Studi di Roma La Sapienza, Rome, 1998. 57–74.

[195] Freundl, G. European multicenter study of natural family planning (1985–1995): efficacy and drop-out; *Advances in Contraception*, 15: 69–83, 1999.

[196] Freundl, G., Bremme, M., Frank-Herrmann, P., Baur, S., Godehardt, E., and Sottong, U. The cue fertility monitor compared to ultrasound and lh peak measurements for fertile time ovulation detection. *Advances in Contraception*, 12(2):111–121, Jun 1996.

[197] Freundl, G., Frank, P., Bauer, S., and Döring, G. Demographic study on the family planning behaviour of the German population: The importance of natural methods. *International Journal of Fertility*, 33(Suppl):54–58, 1988.

[198] Freundl, G., Frank-Hermann, P., and Gnoth, C. Rhythm and devices. In *Paper Presented at the 4th Congress of the European Society of Contraception*, Barcelona, June 12–15. 1996.

[199] Freundl, G., Frank-Herrmann, P., and Bremme, M. Results of an efficacy-finding study (EFS) with the computer-thermometer cyclotest 2 plus containing 207 cycles. *Advances in Contraception*, 14(4):201–207, Dec 1998.

[200] Freundl, G., Frank-Herrmann, P., Brown, S., and Blackwell, L. A new method to detect significant basal body temperature changes during a woman's menstrual cycle. *European Journal of Contraception and Reproductive Health Care*, 1–9, Aug 2014.

[201] Freundl, G., Frank-Herrmann, P., and Gnoth, C. Cycle monitors and devices in natural family planning. *Journal of Reproductive Medicine and Endocrinology*, 7:1–9 (early online), DOI: 10.3109/13625187.2014.948612, 2010.

[202] Freundl, G., Frank-Herrmann, P., Godehardt, E., Klemm, R., and Bachhofer, M. Retrospective clinical trial of contraceptive effectiveness of the electronic fertility indicator Ladycomp/Babycomp. *Advances in Contraception*, 14(2):97–108, Jun 1998.

[203] Freundl, G., Godehardt, E., Kern, P. A., Frank-Herrmann, P., Koubenec, H. J., and Gnoth, C. Estimated maximum failure rates of cycle monitors using daily conception probabilities in the menstrual cycle. *Human Reproduction*, 18(12):2628–2633, Dec 2003.

[204] Freundl, G., Sivin, I., and Batar, I. State-of-the-art of non-hormonal methods of contraception: Iv. natural family planning. *Human Reproduction*, 15(2):113–123, Apr 2010.

[205] Frisch, R. E. Body fat, menarche, fitness and fertility. *Human Reproduction*, 2(6):521–533, Aug 1987.

[206] Frisch, R. E. Fatness and fertility. *Sci Am*, 258(3):88–95, Mar 1988.

[207] Frisch, R. E. *Female Fertility and the Body Fat Connection*. Chicago Press, Chicago and London, 2002.

[208] Faculty of Sexual and Reproductive Healthcare (FSRH). Postnatal sexual and reproductive health, FSRH Clinical Guidance, 2009.

[209] Faculty of Sexual and Reproductive Healthcare (FSRH). UK medical eligibility criteria for contraceptive use (UKMEC 2009), FSRH, RCOG, 2009.

[210] Faculty of Sexual and Reproductive Healthcare (FSRH) Contraception for women aged over 40 years, FSRH Clinical Guidance, 2010.

[211] Faculty of Sexual and Reproductive Healthcare (FSRH). Emergency contraception, FSRH Clinical Guidance, 2011.

[212] Faculty of Sexual and Reproductive Healthcare (FSRH). Progestogen-only implants, FSRH Clinical Guidance, 2014.

[213] Faculty of Sexual and Reproductive Healthcare (FSRH). Progestogen-only injectable contraception, FSRH Clinical Guidance, 2014.

[214] Faculty of Sexual and Reproductive Healthcare (FSRH). Barrier methods for contraception and STI prevention, FSRH Clinical Guidance, 2015.

[215] Faculty of Sexual and Reproductive Healthcare (FSRH). Fertility awareness methods, FSRH Clinical Guidance, 2015.

[216] Faculty of Sexual and Reproductive Healthcare (FSRH). Intrauterine contraception, FSRH Clinical Guidance, 2015.

[217] Faculty of Sexual and Reproductive Healthcare (FSRH). Progestogen-only pills, FSRH Clinical Guidance, 2015.

[218] Fukuda, M., Fukuda, K., Yding Andersen, C., and Byskov, A. G. Does anovulation induced by oral contraceptives favor pregnancy during the following two menstrual cycles? *Fertility and Sterility*, 73(4):742–747, Apr 2000.

[219] Gadow, E. C., Jennings, V. H., López-Camelo, J. S., Paz, J. E., da Graça Dutra, M., Leguizamón, G., Simpson, J. L., Queenan, J. T., and Castilla, E. E. Knowledge of likely time of ovulation and contraceptive use in unintended pregnancies. *Advances in Contraception*, 15(2):109–118, 1999.

[220] Gall, H., Glowania, H. J., and Fischer, M. Circadian rhythm of testosterone level in plasma: I. physiologic 24-hour oscillations of the testosterone level in plasma. *Andrologia*, 11(4):287–292, 1979.

[221] Gallagher, J. Mobile phone effect on fertility – "research needed", Available from www.bbc.co.uk/news/health-27767981, June 2014.

[222] Galletly, C., Clark, A., Tomlinson, L., and Blaney, F. Improved pregnancy rates for obese, infertile women following a group treatment program: An open pilot study. *General Hospital Psychiatry*, 18(3):192–195, May 1996.

[223] Gangestad, S. W., and Thornhill, R. Human oestrus. *Proceedings of the Royal Society of Biological Sciences*, 275(1638):991–1000, May 2008.

[224] Gelety, T. J., and Buyalos, R. P. The effect of clomiphene citrate and menopausal gonadotropins on cervical mucus in ovulatory cycles. *Fertility and Sterility*, 60(3):471–476, Sep 1993.

[225] Germano, E., and Jennings, V. New approaches to fertility awareness based methods: Incorporating the standard days and two day methods into practice. *Journal of Midwifery and Women's Health*, 51(6):471–477, 2006.

[226] Gioti, A., Wigby, S., Wertheim, B., Schuster, E., Martinez, P., Pennington, C. J., Partridge, L., and Chapman, T. Sex peptide of drosophila melanogaster males is a global regulator of reproductive processes in females. *Proceedings of the Royal Society of Biological Sciences*, 279(1746):4423–4432, Sep 2012.

[227] Girotto, S., Del Zotti, F., Baruchello, M., Gottardi, G., Valente, M., Battaggia, A., Rosa, B., Fedrizzi, P., Campanella, M., Zumerle, M., and Bressan, F. The behavior of Italian family physicians regarding the health problems of women and, in particular, family planning (both contraception and NFP). *Advances in Contraception*, 13(2–3):283–293, 1997.

[228] Glasier, A., and McNeilly, A. S. Physiology of lactation. *Balliere's Clinical Endocrinology and Metabolism*, 4(2):379–395, Jun 1990.

[229] Glasier, A., McNeilly, A. S., and Howie, P. W. Hormonal background of lactational infertility. *International Journal of Fertility*, 33(Suppl):32–34, 1988.

[230] Gnoth, C., Frank-Herrmann, P., Bremme, M., Freundl, G., and Godehardt, E. How do self-observed cycle symptoms correlate with ovulation? *Zentralblatt für Gynäkologie*, 118(12):650–654, 1996.

[231] Gnoth, C., Frank-Herrmann, P., Freundl, G., Kunert, J., and Godehardt, E. Sexual behavior of natural family planning users in Germany and its changes over time. *Advances in Contraception*, 11(2):173–185, Jun 1995.

[232] Gnoth, C., Frank-Herrmann, P., Schmoll, A., Godehardt, E., and Freundl, G. Cycle characteristics after discontinuation of oral contraceptives. *Gynecological Endocrinology*, 16(4):307–317, Aug 2002.

[233] Gnoth, C., Godehardt, D., Godehardt, E., Frank-Herrmann, P., and Freundl, G. Time to pregnancy: Results of the German prospective study and impact on the management of infertility. *Human Reproduction*, 18(9):1959–1966, Sep 2003.

[234] Gnoth, C., Frank-Herrmann, P., and Freundl, G. Opinion: Natural family planning and the management of infertility. *Archives of Gynecology and Obstetrics*, 267(2):67–71, Dec 2002.

[235] Goldstein, I., and Rothstein, L. *The Potent Male*. Regenesis Cycle Publishing, Norwalk, CT, 1995.

[236] Gorrindo, T., Lu, Y., Pincus, S., Riley, A., Simon, J. A., Singer, B. H., and Weinstein, M. Lifelong menstrual histories are typically erratic and trending: A taxonomy. *Menopause*, 14(1):74–88, 2007.

[237] Gould, J. E., Overstreet, J. W., and Hanson, F. W. Assessment of human sperm function after recovery from the female reproductive tract. *Biology of Reproduction*, 31(5):888–894, Dec 1984.

[238] Gracia, C. R., Sammel, M. D., Freeman, E. W., Lin, H., Langan, E., Kapoor, S. and Nelson, D. B. Defining menopause status: Creation of a new definition to identify the early changes of the menopausal transition. *Menopause*, 12(2):128–135, Mar 2005.

[239] Grant, V. J. Entrenched misinformation about x and y sperm. *British Medical Journal*, 332(7546):916, Apr 2006.

[240] Gray, R. H. Natural family planning and sex selection: Fact or fiction? *American Journal of Obstetrics and Gynecology*, 165(6 Pt 2):1982–1984, Dec 1991.

[241] Gray, R. H., Simpson, J. L., Bitto, A. C., Queenan, J. T., Li, C., Kambic, R. T., Perez, A., Mena, P., Barbato, M., Stevenson, W., and Jennings, V. Sex ratio associated with timing of insemination and length of the follicular phase in planned and unplanned pregnancies during use of natural family planning. *Human Reproduction*, 13(5):1397–1400, May 1998.

[242] Gray, R. H., Simpson, J. L., Kambic, R. T., Queenan, J. T., Mena, P., Perez, A., and Barbato, M. Timing of conception and the risk of spontaneous abortion among pregnancies occurring during the use of natural family planning. *American Journal of Obstetrics and Gynecology*, 172(5):1567–1572, May 1995.

[243] Gray, S. J. Comparison of effects of breast-feeding practices on birth-spacing in three societies: Nomadic Turkana, Gainj, and Quechua. *Journal of Biosocial Science*, 26(1):69–90, Jan 1994.

[244] Greenberg, J. A., Bell, S. J., and Van Ausdal, W. Omega-3 fatty acid supplementation during pregnancy. *Reviews in Obstetrics and Gynecology*, 1(4):162–169, 2008.

[245] Greenstein, D., Jeffcote, N., Ilsley, D., and Kester, R. C. The menstrual cycle and Raynaud's phenomenon. *Angiology*, 47(5):427–436, May 1996.

[246] Gribble, J. N., Lundgren, R. I., Velasquez, C. and Anastasi, E. E. Being strategic about contraceptive introduction: The experience of the standard days method. *Contraception*, 77(3):147–154, Mar 2008.

[247] Grieger, J. A., Grzeskowiak, L. E., and Clifton, V. L. Preconception dietary patterns in human pregnancies are associated with preterm delivery. *Journal of Nutrition*, 144(7):1075–1080, Jul 2014.

[248] Grimes, D. A., Gallo, M. F., Grigorieva, V., Nanda, K., and Schulz, K. F. Fertility awareness-based methods for contraception. *Cochrane Database of Systematic Reviews* (4):CD004860, 2004.

[249] Grimes, D. A., Lopez, L. M., Raymond, E. G., Halpern, V,, Nanda, K., and Schulz, K. F. Spermicide used alone for contraception. *Cochrane Database of Systematic Reviews*, 12:CD005218, 2013.

[250] Gross, B. A., and Eastman, C. J. Prolactin and the return of ovulation in breastfeeding women. *Journal of Biosocial Science* (supplement), 9:25–42, 1985.

[251] Gross, B. A., Burger, H, and W. H. O. Task Force on Methods for the Natural Regulation of Fertility. Breastfeeding patterns and return to fertility in Australian women. *Australian and New Zealand Journal of Obstetrics and Gynaecology*, 42(2):148–154, May 2002.

[252] Grundy, A., Richardson, H., Burstyn, I. Lohrisch, C., SenGupta, S. K., Lai, A. S., Lee, D. Spinelli, J. J., and Aronson, K. J. Increased risk of breast cancer associated with long-term shift work in Canada. *Occupational and Environmental Medicine*, 70(12):831–838, Dec 2013.

[253] Gude, Dilip. Thyroid and its indispensability in fertility. *Journal of Human Reproductive Sciences*, 4(1):59–60, Jan 2011.

[254] Gudgeon, K., Leader, L., and Howard, B. Evaluation of the accuracy of the home ovulation detection kit, Clearplan, at predicting ovulation. *Medical Journal of Australia*, 152(7):344, 346, 349, Apr 1990.

[255] Guida, M., Tommaselli, G. A., Palomba, S., Pellicano, M., Moccia, G., Di Carlo, C., and Nappi, C. Efficacy of methods for determining ovulation in a natural family planning program. *Fertility and Sterility*, 72(5):900–904, Nov 1999.

[256] Guillebaud, J., and MacGregor, A. Aspects of human fertility and fertility awareness, in *Contraception: Your Questions Answered*. Churchill Livingstone, Edinburgh, 2013. 19–39.

[257] Dik, J., Habbema, F., Eijkemans, Marinus J. C., Leridon, Henri, and Te Velde, Egbert R. Realizing a desired family size: When should couples start? *Human Reproduction*, 30(9):2215–2221, Sep 2015.

[258] Hahn, S., Janssen, O. E., Tan, S., Pleger, K., Mann, K., Schedlowski, M., , Kimmig, R., Benson, S., Balamitsa, E., and Elsenbruch, S. Clinical and psychological correlates of quality-of-life in polycystic ovary syndrome. *European Journal of Endocrinology*, 153(6):853–860, Dec 2005.

[259] Hale, G. E., Manconi, F., Luscombe, G., and Fraser, I. S. Quantitative measurements of menstrual blood loss in ovulatory and anovulatory cycles in middle- and late-reproductive age and the menopausal transition. *Obstetrics and Gynecology*, 115(2 Pt 1):249–256, Feb 2010.

[260] Hampton, K. D., Mazza, D., and Newton, J. M. Fertility-awareness knowledge, attitudes, and practices of women seeking fertility assistance. *Journal of Advanced Nursing*, 65(5):1076–1084, May 2013.

[261] Hanan, A. J. A., and Taee, A. L. The value of cervical score in predicting ovulation in natural and stimulated cycles. *Medical Journal of Babylon*, 5(1):63–67, 2008.

[262] Hann, L. E., Hall, D. A., Black, E. B., and Ferrucci, J. T., Jr. Mittelschmerz: Sonographic demonstration. *Journal of the American Medical Association*, 241(25):2731–2732, Jun 1979.

[263] Hansen, L. K., Becher, N., Bastholm, S., Glavind, J., Ramsing, Mette, Kim, C. J., Romero, R., Jensen, J. S., and Uldbjerg, N. The cervical mucus plug inhibits, but does not block, the passage of ascending bacteria from the vagina during pregnancy. *Acta Obstetrica et Gynecologica Scandinavica*, 93(1):102–108, Jan 2014.

[264] Harlap, S. Gender of infants conceived on different days of the menstrual cycle. *New England Journal of Medicine*, 300(26):1445–1448, Jun 1979.

[265] Harlow, S. D., and Matanoski, G. M. The association between weight, physical activity, and stress and variation in the length of the menstrual cycle. *American Journal of Epidemiology*, 133(1):38–49, Jan 1991.

[266] Harlow, S. D., Gass, M., Hall, J. E., Lobo, R., Maki, P., Rebar, R. W., Sherman, S., Sluss, P. M., de Villiers, T. J., and S. T. R. A. W 10 Collaborative Group. Executive summary of the stages of reproductive aging workshop + 10: Addressing the unfinished agenda of staging reproductive aging. *Fertility and Sterility*, 97(4):843–851, Apr 2012.

[267] Harper, C. Contraception and the perimenopause. *British Journal of Sexual Medicine*, 12–14, Sept/Oct 1995.

[268] Hartman, C. G. *Science and the Safe Period*. Williams and Wilkins, Baltimore, 1962.

[269] Harvey, A. T., Hitchcock, C. L., and Prior, J. C. Ovulation disturbances and mood across the menstrual cycles of healthy women. *Journal of Psychosomatic Obstetrics and Gynaecology*, 30(4):207–214, Dec 2009.

[270] Hassan, M. A. M., and Killick, S. R. Is previous use of hormonal contraception associated with a detrimental effect on subsequent fecundity? *Human Reproduction*, 19(2):344–351, Feb 2004.

[271] Hassan, M. A. M., and Killick, S. R. Negative lifestyle is associated with a significant reduction in fecundity. *Fertility and Sterility*, 81(2):384–392, Feb 2004.

[272] Hatch, M. C., Figa-Talamanca, I., and Salerno, S. Work stress and menstrual patterns among American and Italian nurses. *Scandinavian Journal of Work, Environment and Health*, 25(2):144–150, Apr 1999.

[273] Heffner, L., and Schust, D. *The Reproductive System at a Glance*. Number 40. Blackwell Publishing, Malden, MA, 2006.

[274] Heitmann, R. J., Langan, K. L., Huang, R. R., Chow, G. E., and Burney, R. O. Premenstrual spotting of 2 days or more is strongly associated with histologically confirmed endometriosis in women with infertility. *American Journal of Obstetrics and Gynecology*, 211(4):358.e1–358.e6, Oct 2014.

[275] Henderson, B. J., and Whissell, C. Changes in women's emotions as a function of emotion valence, self-determined category of premenstrual distress, and day in the menstrual cycle. *Psychological Reports*, 80(3 Pt 2):1272–1274, Jun 1997.

[276] Henmi, H., Endo, T., Kitajima, Y., Manase, K., Hata, H., and Kudo, R., Effects of ascorbic acid supplementation on serum progesterone levels in patients with a luteal phase defect. *Fertility and Sterility*, 80(2):459–461, Aug 2003.

[277] Henry, L. Some data on natural fertility. *Eugen Q*, 8:81–91, Jun 1961.

[278] HFEA. *Human Fertilization and Embryology Act*. Her Majesty's Stationery Office, London, 1990.

[279] Hight-Laukaran, V., Labbok, M. H., Peterson, A. E., Fletcher, V., von Hertzen, H., and Van Look, P. F. Multicenter study of the lactational amenorrhea method: should read: II. Acceptability, utility, and policy implications. *Contraception*, 55(6):337–346, Jun 1997.

[280] Hilgers, T. W. *The Medical and Surgical Practice of NaProTechnology*. Pope Paul VI Institute Press, Omaha, NE, 2004.

[281] Hilgers, T. W., Abraham, G. E., and Cavanagh, D. Natural family planning: I. the peak symptom and estimated time of ovulation. *Obstetrics and Gynecology*, 52(5):575–582, Nov 1978.

[282] Hilgers, T. W., Daly, K. D., Prebil, A. M., and Hilgers, S. K. Natural family planning iii: Intermenstrual symptoms and estimated time of ovulation. *Obstetrics and Gynecology*, 58(2):152–155, Aug 1981.

[283] Hilgers, T. W., Daly, K. D., Prebil, A. M., and Hilgers, S. K. Cumulative pregnancy rates in patients with apparently normal fertility and fertility-focused intercourse. *Journal of Reproductive Medicine*, 37(10):864–866, Oct 1992.

[284] Hilgers, T. W., and Stanford, J. B. Creighton model naproeducation technology for avoiding pregnancy: Use effectiveness. *Journal of Reproductive Medicine*, 43(6):495–502, Jun 1998.

[285] Hjollund, N. H., Jensen, T. K., Bonde, J. P., Henriksen, T. B., Andersson, A. M., Kolstad, H. A., Ernst, E., Giwercman, A., Skakkebaek, N. E., and Olsen, J. Distress and reduced fertility: A follow-up study of first-pregnancy planners. *Fertility and Sterility*, 72(1):47–53, Jul 1999.

[286] HMSO. *Abortion Act 1967*. Her Majesty's Stationery Office, London, 1967.

[287] Hoekstra, C., Zhao, Z. Z., Lambalk, C. B., Willemsen, G., Martin, N. G., Boomsma, D. I., and Montgomery, G., W. Dizygotic twinning. *Human Reproduction Update*, 14(1):37–47, 2008.

[288] Holt, J. G. H. *Marriage and Periodic Abstinence*, 2nd Edition (1st Edition 1937). Longmans, London, 1960.

[289] Hossain, A. M., Barik, S., and Panduang, M. K. Lack of significant morphological differences between human x and y spermatozoa and their precursor cells (spermatids) exposed to different prehybridization treatments. *Journal of Andrology*, 22(1):119–123, 2001.

[290] Howard, C. R., Howard, F. M., Lanphear, B., deBlieck, E. A., Eberly, S., and Lawrence, R. A. The effects of early pacifier use on breastfeeding duration. *Pediatrics*, 103(3):E33, Mar 1999.

[291] Howie, P. W., McNeilly, A. S., Houston, M. J., Cook, A., and Boyle, H. Effect of supplementary food on suckling patterns and ovarian activity during lactation. *British Medical Journal (Clinical Research Edition)*, 283(6294):757–759, Sep 1981.

[292] Howie, P. W., McNeilly, A. S., Houston, M. J., Cook, A., and Boyle, H. Fertility after childbirth: Post-partum ovulation and menstruation in bottle and breast feeding mothers. *Clinical Endocrinology (Oxford)*, 17(4):323–332, Oct 1982.

[293] HSCIC. Infant feeding survey UK – 2010, Available from www.hscic.gov.uk/catalogue/pub08694 (accessed 31.12.15), 2010.

[294] Hull, M. G., Glazener, C. M., Kelly, N. J., Conway, D. I., Foster, P. A., Hinton, R. A., Coulson, C., Lambert, P. A., Watt, E. M., and Desai, K. M. Population study of causes, treatment, and outcome of infertility. *British Medical Journal (Clinical Research Edition)*, 291(6510):1693–1697, Dec 1985.

[295] Hypponen, E. Smith, G. D., and Power, C. Effects of grandmothers' smoking in pregnancy on birth weight: Intergenerational cohort study. *British Medical Journal*, 327(7420):898, Oct 2003.

[296] Ingram, J., Hunt, L., Woolridge, M., and Greenwood, R. The association of progesterone, infant formula use and pacifier use with the return of menstruation in breastfeeding women: A prospective cohort study. *European Journal of Obstetrics and Gynecology and Reproductive Biology*, 114(2):197–202, Jun 2004.

[297] Inoue, H., Ono, J., Masuda, W., Tomohiro, I., Yokata, M., and Inenga, K. Rheological properties of human saliva and salivary mucins. *Journal of Oral Biosciences*, 50(2):134–141, 2008.

[298] Insler, V., Melmed, I., Eichenbrenner, H., Serr, D. M., and Lunenfeld, B. The cervical score: A simple semi-quantitative method for monitoring of the menstrual cycle. *International Journal of Gynaecology and Obstetrics*, 10(223), 1972.

[299] International Planned Parenthood Federation (IPPF). Periodic abstinence, in *Family Planning Handbook for Health Professionals*, p. 105. IPPF Medical Publications, London, 1997.

[300] Institute for Reproductive Health, Georgetown University. *Glossary of Natural Family Planning Terms*, Second edition. Washington, DC, 1993.

[301] Institute for Reproductive Health (IRH). Fertility awareness across the life course: A comprehensive literature review, FAM Project, Institute for Reproductive Health at Georgetown University, Available from www.irh.org, 2013.

[302] Institute for Reproductive Health (IRH). Process for integrating the standard days method into services: Essential steps, Institute for Reproductive Health, Georgetown University, Washington, DC, 2013.

[303] Jackson, E., and Glasier, A., Return of ovulation and menses in postpartum nonlactating women: A systematic review. *Obstetrics and Gynecology*, 117(3):657–662, Mar 2011.

[304] Jahnke, R., Larkey, L., Rogers, C., Etnier, J., and Lin, F., A comprehensive review of health benefits of qigong and tai chi. *American Journal of Health Promotion*, 24(6):e1–e25, 2010.

[305] Janssen, C. J., and van Lunsen, R. H. Profile and opinions of the female persona user in the Netherlands. *European Journal of Contraception and Reproductive Health Care*, 5(2):141–146, Jun 2000.

[306] Jennings, V., and Landy, H. Explaining ovulation awareness-based family planning methods. *Contemporary Ob/Gyn*, 51(7):48–54, Jul 2006.

[307] Johnston, J. A., Roberts, D. B., and Spencer, R. B. A survey evaluation of the efficacy and efficiency of natural family planning services and methods in Australia: Report of a research project, St. Vincent's Hospital, Darlinghurst, NSW, 1978.

[308] Jolly, J. and McCrystal, P. The role of counselling in the management of patients with infertility. *The Obstetrician & Gynaecologist*, 17(2):83–89, Apr 2015.

[309] Jones, E., Dimmock, P. W., and Spencer, S. A. A randomised controlled trial to compare methods of milk expression after preterm delivery. *Archives of Disease in Childhood, Fetal and Neonatal Edition*, 85(2):F91–F95, Sep 2001.

[310] Jones, E., and Spencer, S. A., Optimizing the provision of human milk for preterm infants. *Archives of Disease in Childhood, Fetal and Neonatal Edition*, 92(4):F236–F238, Jul 2007.

[311] Jones, G., Carlton, J., Weddell, S., Johnson, S., and Ledger, W. L. Women's experiences of ovulation testing: A qualitative analysis. *Reproductive Health*, 12(1):116, 2015.

[312] Kakuno, Y., Amino, N., Kanoh, M., Kawai, M., Fujiwara, M., Kimura, M., Kamitani, A., Saya, K., Shakuta, R., Nitta, S., Hayashida, Y., Kudo, T., Kubota, S., and Miyauchi, A. Menstrual disturbances in various thyroid diseases. *Endocrine Journal*, 57(12):1017–1022, 2010.

[313] Kalo-Klein, A., and Witkin, S. S. Candida albicans: Cellular immune system interactions during different stages of the menstrual cycle. *American Journal of Obstetrics and Gynecology*, 161(5):1132–1136, Nov 1989.

[314] Kambic, R. The effectiveness of natural family planning methods for birth spacing: A comprehensive review, in *Human Fertility Regulation: Demographic and Statistical Aspects*. Edizioni Libreria Cortina, Verona, 1999. 63–90.

[315] Kambic, R. T. Natural family planning use-effectiveness and continuation. *American Journal of Obstetrics and Gynecology*, 165(6 Pt 2):2046–2048, Dec 1991.

[316] Kambic, R. T., and Lamprecht, V. Calendar rhythm efficacy: A review. *Advances in Contraception*, 12(2):123–128, Jun 1996.

[317] Katz, D. F. Human cervical mucus: Research update. *American Journal of Obstetrics and Gynecology*, 165(6 Pt 2):1984–1986, Dec 1991.

[318] Katz, D. F., Slade, D. A., and Nakajima, S. T. Analysis of pre-ovulatory changes in cervical mucus hydration and sperm penetrability. *Advances in Contraception*, 13(2–3):143–151, 1997.

[319] Kazi, A., Kennedy, K. I., Visness, C. M., and Khan, T. Effectiveness of the lactational amenorrhea method in Pakistan. *Fertility and Sterility*, 64(4):717–723, Oct 1995.

[320] Keefe, E. A practical open-scale thermometer for timing human ovulation. *New York State Journal of Medicine*, 49(21):2554–2555, Nov 1949.

[321] Keefe, E. F. Self-observation of the cervix to distinguish days of possible fertility. *Bulletin of the Sloane Hospital for Women in Columbia*, 8(4):129–136, Dec 1962.

[322] Keefe, E., Cephalad shift of the cervix uteri: Sign of the fertile time in women. *International Review of Natural Family Planning*, 1:55–60, 1977.

[323] Kegel, A. H. The nonsurgical treatment of genital relaxation; use of the perineometer as an aid in restoring anatomic and functional structure. *Annals of Western Medicine and Surgery*, 2(5):213–216, May 1948.

[324] Kennedy, K. I., Gross, B. A., Parenteau-Carreau, S., Flynn, A. M., Brown, J. B., and Visness, C. M. Breastfeeding and the symptothermal method. *Studies in Family Planning*, 26(2):107–115, 1995.

[325] Kennedy, K. I., Labbok, M. H., and Van Look, P. F. Consensus statement: Lactational amenorrhea method for family planning. *International Journal of Gynaecology and Obstetrics*, 54(1):55–57, Jul 1996.

[326] Kennedy, K. I., Parenteau-Carreau, S., Flynn, A., Gross, B., Brown, J. B., and Visness, C. The natural family planning – lactational amenorrhea method interface: Observations from a prospective study of breastfeeding users of natural family planning. *American Journal of Obstetrics and Gynecology*, 165(6 Pt 2):2020–2026, Dec 1991.

[327] Kennedy, K. I. Consensus statement: Breastfeeding as a family planning method. *Lancet*, 2(8621):1204–1205, Nov 1988.

[328] Keulers, M. J., Hamilton, C. J. C. M., Franx, A., Evers, J. L. H., and Bots, R. S. G. M. The length of the fertile window is associated with the chance of spontaneously conceiving

an ongoing pregnancy in subfertile couples. *Human Reproduction*, 22(6):1652–1656, Jun 2007.

[329] Killick, S. R., Leary, C., Trussell, J., and Guthrie, K. A. Sperm content of pre-ejaculatory fluid. *Human Fertility (Cambridge)*, 14(1):48–52, Mar 2011.

[330] Klaus, H., Goebel, J. M., Muraski, B., Egizio, M. T., Weitzel, D., Taylor, R. S., Fagan, M. U., Ek, K., and Hobday, K. Use-effectiveness and client satisfaction in six centers teaching the billings Ovulation Method. *Contraception*, 19(6):613–629, Jun 1979.

[331] Kleegman, S. J. Can sex be predetermined by the physician? *Excerpta Medica No. 109*, 1966.

[332] Knaus, H. On the time of women's ability to conceive during the intermenstrual period. *Munchener Medizinische Wochenschrift/12. Juli 1929*: PMID: 347273 [Article in German].

[333] Knight, J., and Pyper, C. Integrating fertility awareness into family planning consultations. *Contraceptive Education Bulletin*, 5, Spring 1999.

[334] Knight, J., and Pyper, C. Postnatal contraception what are the choices? *Nurse Practitioner*, 5:23–25, 2002.

[335] Kong, A., Frigge, M. L., Masson, G., Besenbacher, S., Sulem, P., Magnusson, G., et al. Rate of de novo mutations and the importance of father's age to disease risk. *Nature*, 488(7412):471–475, Aug 2012.

[336] Kramer, M. S., and Kakuma, R. Optimal duration of exclusive breastfeeding. *Cochrane Database of Systematic Reviews*, 8:CD003517, 2012.

[337] Krohn, P. L. Intermenstrual pain (the mittelschmerz) and the time of ovulation. *British Medical Journal*, 803–805, May 1949.

[338] Kutteh, W. H., Chao, C. H., Ritter, J. O., and Byrd, W. Vaginal lubricants for the infertile couple: Effect on sperm activity. *International Journal of Fertility and Menopausal Studies*, 41(4):400–404, 1996.

[339] Köhler, G., and Lober, R. Endometriosis and basal temperature. *Zentralblatt für Gynäkologie*, 110(7):419–422, 1988.

[340] La Marca, A., Grisendi, V., and Griesinger, G. How much does AMH really vary in normal women? *International Journal of Endocrinology*, 2013:959487, 2013.

[341] Labbok, M. Breastfeeding, fertility and family planning. *Global Library of Women's Medicine* (ISSN: 1756–2228), DOI 10.3843/GLOWM.10397, 2008.

[342] Labbok, M., Cooney, K., and Coly, S. *Guidelines: Breastfeeding, Family Planning and the lactational amenorrhoea method (LAM)*. Institute for Reproductive Health, Georgetown University, Washington, DC, 1994.

[343] Labbok, M. H., Hight-Laukaran, V., Peterson, A. E., Fletcher, V., von Hertzen, H., and Van Look, P. F. Multicenter study of the lactational amenorrhea method: I. efficacy, duration, and implications for clinical application. *Contraception*, 55(6):327–336, Jun 1997.

[344] Labyak, S., Lava, S., Turek, F., and Zee, P. Effects of shiftwork on sleep and menstrual function in nurses. *Healthcare for Women International*, 23(6–7):703–714, 2002.

[345] Lamprecht, V., and Trussell, J. Natural family planning effectiveness: Evaluating published reports. *Advances in Contraception*, 13(2–3):155–165, 1997.

[346] Lamprecht, V. M., and Grummer-Strawn, L. Development of new formulas to identify the fertile time of the menstrual cycle. *Contraception*, 54(6):339–343, Dec 1996.

[347] Latz, L., and Reiner, C. Natural conception control. *Journal of the American Medical Association*, 105(16):1241–1246, 1935.

[348] Leader, L. R., Russell, T., and Stenning, B. The use of Clearplan home ovulation detection kits in unexplained and male factor infertility. *Australia and New Zealand Journal of Obstetrics and Gynaecology*, 32(2):158–160, May 1992.

[349] Ledger, W.L. Measurement of antimullerian hormone: Not as straightforward as it seems. *Fertility and Sterility*, 101(2):339, Feb 2014.

[350] Lee, S., Kim, J., Jang, B., Hur, S., Jung, U., Kil, K., et al. Fluctuation of peripheral blood t, b, and nk cells during a menstrual cycle of normal healthy women. *Journal of Immunology*, 185(1):756–762, Jul 2010.

[351] Leiva, R., Burhan, U., Kyrillos, E., Fehring, R., McLaren, R., Dalzell, C., and Tanguay, E., Use of ovulation predictor kits as adjuncts when using fertility awareness methods (fams): A pilot study. *Journal of the American Board of Family Medicine*, 27(3):427–429, 2014.

[352] Lenton, E. A., Landgren, B. M., and Sexton, L. Normal variation in the length of the luteal phase of the menstrual cycle: Identification of the short luteal phase. *British Journal of Obstetrics and Gynaecology*, 91(7):685–689, Jul 1984.

[353] Leridon, H. Can assisted reproduction technology compensate for the natural decline in fertility with age? A model assessment. *Human Reproduction*, 19(7):1548–1553, Jul 2004.

[354] Levy, A. Interpreting raised serum prolactin results. *British Medical Journal*, 348:g3207, 2014.

[355] Li, Y., Langholz, B., Salam, M. T., and Gilliland, F. D. Maternal and grandmaternal smoking patterns are associated with early childhood asthma. *Chest*, 127(4):1232–1241, Apr 2005.

[356] Lipshultz, L. I. *Infertility in the Male*. Cambridge University Press, Cambridge, 2009.

[357] Llarena, N. C., Estevez, S. L., Tucker, S. L., and Jeruss, J. S. Impact of fertility concerns on tamoxifen initiation and persistence. *Journal of the National Cancer Institute*, 107(10), Epub2015/08/27, Oct 2015.

[358] Lockwood, G. Infertility and early pregnancy loss, in *Women's Health*. Oxford University Press, Oxford, 1998. 256.

[359] Lopez, L. M., Steiner, M., Grimes, D. A., Hilgenberg, D. and Schulz, K. F. Strategies for communicating contraceptive effectiveness. *Cochrane Database of Systematic Reviews*, 4:CD006964, 2013.

[360] Louis, G. M., Lum, K. J., Sundaram, R., Chen, Z., Kim, S., Lynch, C. D., Schisterman, E. F., and Pyper, C., Stress reduces conception probabilities across the fertile window: Evidence in support of relaxation. *Fertility and Sterility*, 95(7):2184–2189, Jun 2011.

[361] Lousse, J-C., and Donnez, J., Laparoscopic observation of spontaneous human ovulation. *Fertility and Sterility*, 90(3):833–834, Sep 2008.

[362] Lucas, N., Rosario, R., and Shelling, A., New Zealand university students' knowledge of fertility decline in women via natural pregnancy and assisted reproductive technologies. *Human Fertility (Cambridge)*, epub (early online), 1–7, Feb 2015.

[363] Luker, K. *Taking Chances: Abortion and the Decision Not to Contracept*. University of California Press, Berkeley, 1975.

[364] Lumey, L. H., Ravelli, A. C., Wiessing, L. G., Koppe, J. G., Treffers, P. E., and Stein, Z. A. The Dutch famine birth cohort study: Design, validation of exposure, and selected characteristics of subjects after 43 years follow-up. *Paediatric Perinatal Epidemiology*, 7(4):354–367, Oct 1993.

[365] Lundgren, R. I., Karra, M. V., and Yam, E. A. The role of the standard days method in modern family planning services in developing countries. *European Journal of Contraception and Reproductive Health Care*, 17(4):254–259, Aug 2012.

[366] Lundsberg, L. S., Pal, L., Gariepy, A. M., Xu, X., Chu, M. C., and Illuzzi, J. L. Knowledge, attitudes, and practices regarding conception and fertility: A population-based survey among reproductive-age united states women. *Fertility and Sterility*, 101(3):767–774.e2, Mar 2014.

[367] Lynch, C. D., Sundaram, R., Maisog, J. M., Sweeney, A. M., and Louis, G. M. Buck. Preconception stress increases the risk of infertility: Results from a couple-based prospective cohort study – the life study. *Human Reproduction*, 29(5):1067–1075, May 2014.

[368] Lynch, C. D., Jackson, L. W., and Buck Louis, G. M., Estimation of the day-specific probabilities of conception: Current state of the knowledge and the relevance for epidemiological research. *Paediatric Perinatal Epidemiology l*, 20(Suppl 1):3–12, Nov 2006.

[369] Lynch, C. D., Sundaram, R., Buck Louis, G. M. Lum, K., and Pyper, C., Are increased levels of self-reported psychosocial stress, anxiety, and depression associated with fecundity? *Fertility and Sterility*, 82(2):453–458, Aug 2012.

[370] Lyons, R. A., Saridogan, E., and Djahanbakhch, O. The reproductive significance of human fallopian tube cilia. *Human ReproductionUpdate*, 12(4):363–372, 2006.

[371] Maheshwari, A., Bhattacharya, S., and Johnson, N. P. Predicting fertility. *Human Fertility (Cambridge)*, 11(2):109–117, Jun 2008.

[372] Mansfield, P. K., Carey, M., Anderson, A., Barsom, S. H., and Koch, P. B., Staging the menopausal transition: Data from the Tremin Research Program on Women's Health. *Women's Health Issues*, 14(6):220–226, 2004.

[373] Mansour, D., Gemzell-Danielsson, K., Inki, P., and Jensen, J. T. Fertility after discontinuation of contraception: A comprehensive review of the literature. *Contraception*, 84(5):465–477, Nov 2011.

[374] Mansour, D., Inki, P., and Gemzell-Danielsson, K., Efficacy of contraceptive methods: A review of the literature. *European Journal of Contraception and Reproductive Health Care*, 15(1):4–16, Feb 2010.

[375] Marinakis, G., and Nikolaou, D., What is the role of assisted reproduction technology in the management of age-related infertility? *Human Fertility (Cambridge)*, 14(1):8–15, Mar 2011.

[376] Marinho, A. O., Sallam, H. N., Goessens, L., Collins, W. P., and Campbell, S. Ovulation side and occurrence of mittelschmerz in spontaneous and induced ovarian cycles. *British Medical Journal (Clinical Research Edition)*, 284(6316):632, Feb 1982.

[377] Marshall, J. Thermal changes in the normal menstrual cycle. *British Medical Journal*, 1:102–104, Jan 12 1963.

[378] Marshall, J. Predicting length of menstrual cycle. *Lancet*, 1(7379):263–5, Jan 30 1965.

[379] Marshall, J. A statistical analysis of the time of conception in relation to the temperature in 5013 cycles. In *United Nations: Dept. of Economic and Social Affairs: Proceedings of the World Population Conference, Belgrade, 30 August-10 September 1965: Vol. 2. Selected Papers and Summaries: Fertility, Family Planning, Mortality*. New York, UN, 1967. 294–296. (E/CONF.41/3).

[380] Marshall, J. A field trial of the Basal-Body-Temperature Method of regulating births. *Lancet*, 2(7558):8–10, Jul 1968.

[381] Marshall, J. Cervical-mucus and Basal Body-Temperature Method of regulating births: Field trial. *Lancet*, 2(7980):282–283, Aug 1976.

[382] Marshall, J. A prospective trial of the muco-thermal method of natural family planning. *International Review of NFP*, 10(2):139–143, 1985.

[383] Marshall, J. *Love One Another: Psychological Aspects of Natural Family Planning*. Sheed and Ward, New York, 1996.

[384] Marshall, J., and Rowe, B. Psychologic aspects of the Basal Body Temperature Method of regulating births. *Fertility and Sterility*, 21(1):14–19, Jan 1970.

[385] Marshall, John. *The Infertile Period – Principles and Practice*. Darton, Longman and Todd, London, 1963.

[386] Marshall, M., and Aumack Yee, K. *Reproductive Health Awareness: A Wellness, Selfcare Approach*. Centre for Development and Population Activities, Washington, DC, 2003.

[387] Martinez, A. R., van Hooff, M. H., Schoute, E., van der Meer, M., Broekmans, F. J., and Hompes, P. G. The reliability, acceptability and applications of basal body temperature (BBT) records in the diagnosis and treatment of infertility. *European Journal of Obstetrics, Gynecology and Reproductive Biology*, 47(2):121–127, Nov 1992.

[388] Martinez, A. R., Zinaman, M. J., Jennings, V. H., and Lamprecht, V. M. Prediction and detection of the fertile period: The markers. *International Journal of Fertility and Menopausal Studies*, 40(3):139–155, 1995.

[389] Marx, V. *The Semen Book*. Free Associate Books, London, 2001.

[390] Masters, W. H., and Johnson, V. E. The sexual response cycle of the human female: Iii. the clitoris: Anatomic and clinical consideration. *Western Journal of Surgery, Obstetrics and Gynecology*, 70:248–257, 1962.

[391] Masters, W. H., and Johnson, V. E. The sexual response of the human male: I. gross anatomic considerations. *Western Journal of Surgery, Obstetrics and Gynecology*, 71:85–95, 1963.

[392] Matsumoto, S., Nogami, Y., and Ohkuri, S. Statistical studies on menstruation: A criticism on the definition of normal menstruation. *Gunma Journal of Medical Sciences*, 11:294–318, 1962a.

[393] May, K. Monitoring reproductive hormones to detect the fertile period: Development of persona – the first home use system. *Advances in Contraception*, 13(2–3):139–141, 1997.

[394] McCarthy, J. J., and Rockette, H. E. A comparison of methods to interpret the basal body temperature graph. *Fertility and Sterility*, 39(5):640–646, May 1983.

[395] McGovern, P. G., Myers, E. R., Silva, S., Coutifaris, C., Carson, S. A., Legro, R. S., Schlaff, W. D., Carr, B. R., Steinkampf, M. P., Giudice, L. C., Leppert, P. C., Diamond, M. P., and N. I. C. H. D. National Cooperative Reproductive Medicine Network. Absence of secretory endometrium after false-positive home urine luteinizing hormone testing. *Fertility and Sterility*, 82(5):1273–1277, Nov 2004.

[396] McNeilly, A. S. Lactational control of reproduction. *Reproduction, Fertility and Development*, 13(7–8):583–590, 2001.

[397] McNeilly, A. S., Glasier, A. F., Howie, P. W., Houston, M. J., Cook, A., and Boyle, H. Fertility after childbirth: Pregnancy associated with breast feeding. *Clinical Endocrinology (Oxford)*, 19(2):167–173, Aug 1983.

[398] McSweeney, L. Successful sex pre-selection using natural family planning. *African Journal of Reproductive Health*, 15(1):79–84, Mar 2011.

[399] Medina, J. E., Cifuentes, A., Abernathy, J. R., Spieler, J. M., and Wade, M. E. Comparative evaluation of two methods of natural family planning in Columbia. *American Journal of Obstetrics and Gynecology*, 138(8):1142–1147, Dec 1980.

[400] Menarguez, M., Pastor, L. M., and Odeblad, E. Morphological characterization of different human cervical mucus types using light and scanning electron microscopy. *Human Reproduction*, 18(9):1782–1789, Sep 2003.

[401] Mercer, C. H., Tanton, C., Prah, P., Erens, B.. Sonnenberg, P., Clifton, S., et al. Changes in sexual attitudes and lifestyles in Britain through the life course and over time: Findings from the national surveys of sexual attitudes and lifestyles (NATSAL). *Lancet*, 382(9907):1781–1794, Nov 2013.

[402] Micu, M. C., Micu, R., and Ostensen, M., Luteinized unruptured follicle syndrome increased by inactive disease and selective cyclooxygenase 2 inhibitors in women with inflammatory arthropathies. *Arthritis Care and Research (Hoboken)*, 63(9):1334–1338, Sep 2011.

[403] Mikolajczyk, R. T., Stanford, J. B., and Rauchfuss, M. Factors influencing the choice to use modern natural family planning. *Contraception*, 67(4):253–258, Apr 2003.

[404] Milewicz, A., Gejdel, E., Sworen, H., Sienkiewicz, K., Jedrzejak, J., Teucher, T., and Schmitz, H. Vitex agnus castus extract in the treatment of luteal phase defects due to latent hyperprolactinemia: Results of a randomized placebo-controlled doubleblind study. *Arzneimittelforschung*, 43(7):752–756, Jul 1993.

[405] Miller, G., Tybur, J., and Jordan, B. Ovulatory cycle effects on tip earnings by lap dancers: Economic evidence for human oestrus? *Evolution & Human Behavior*, 28(6), 2007.

[406] Ming, L., Xiaoling, P., Yan, L., Lili, W., Qi, W., Xiyong, Y., Boyao, W., and Ning, H. Purification of antimicrobial factors from human cervical mucus. *Human Reproduction*, 22(7):1810–1815, Jul 2007.

[407] Miolo, L., Colombo, B., and Marshall, J. A database for biometric research on changes in basal body temperature in the menstrual cycle. *Statistica, Anno*, 53(4):563–572, 1993.

[408] Moghissi, K. S. Prediction and detection of ovulation. *Fertility and Sterility*, 34(2):89–98, Aug 1980.

[409] Moghissi, K. S., Puscheck, E. E., and Kahn, S., Documentation of ovulation. *Global Library of Women's Medicine*, DOI 10.3843/GLOWM.10325, 2008.

[410] Moghissi, K. S., Syner, F. N., and Evans, T. N. A composite picture of the menstrual cycle. *American Journal of Obstetrics and Gynecology*, 114(3):405–418, Oct 1972.

[411] Moglia, M. L., Nguyen, H. V., Chyjek, K., Chen, K. T., and Castano, P. M. Evaluation of Smartphone menstrual cycle tracking applications using an adapted APPLICATIONS scoring system. *Obstetrics and Gynecology*, 127(6), 1153–1160, 2016.

[412] Moore, E. R., Anderson, G. C., Bergman, N., and Dowswell, T. Early skin-to-skin contact for mothers and their healthy newborn infants. *Cochrane Database of Systematic Reviews*, 5:CD003519, 2012.

[413] Moran, L. J., Ko, H., Misso, M., Marsh, K., Noakes, M., Talbot, M., et al. Dietary composition in the treatment of polycystic ovary syndrome: A systematic review to inform evidence-based guidelines. *Journal of the Academy of Nutrition and Dietetics*, 113(4):520–545, Apr 2013.

[414] Morris, N., Underwood, L., and Easterling, W., Jr. Temporal relationship between basal body temperature nadir and luteinizing hormone surge in normal women. *Fertility and Sterility*, 27(7):780–783, Jul 1976.

[415] Mu, Q., and Fehring, R. J., Efficacy of achieving pregnancy with fertility-focused intercourse. *MCN: American Journal of Maternal/Child Nursing*, 39(1):35–40, 2014.

[416] Mucharski, Jan. *History of the Biologic Control of Human Fertility*. Married Life Information, Oak Ridge, NJ, 1982.

[417] Munro, M. G., Critchley, H. O. D., and Fraser, I. S. The Figo systems for nomenclature and classification of causes of abnormal uterine bleeding in the reproductive years: Who needs them? *American Journal of Obstetrics and Gynecology*, 207(4):259–265, Oct 2012.

[418] Murphy, J., and Laux, J. *The Rhythm Way to Family Happiness; a Lifetime Reference for the Use of the rhythm method: A Practical Manual for Application of the Medical Findings of Dr. K. Ogino and Dr. H. Knaus*. Staple Press, London, 1959.

[419] Murphy, P. J., Myers, B. L., and Badia, P. Nonsteroidal anti-inflammatory drugs alter body temperature and suppress melatonin in humans. *Physiology and Behaviour*, 59(1):133–139, Jan 1996.

[420] Münster, K., Schmidt, L., and Helm, P. Length and variation in the menstrual cycle – a cross-sectional study from a Danish county. *British Journal of Obstetrics and Gynaecology*, 99(5):422–429, May 1992.

[421] Nappi, R. E., Albani, F., Vaccaro, P., Gardella, B., Salonia, A., Chiovato, L., Spinillo, A., and Polatti, F. Use of the Italian translation of the female sexual function index (FSFI) in routine gynecological practice. *Gynecological Endocrinology*, 24(4):214–219, Apr 2008.

[422] Nassaralla, C. L., Stanford, J. B., Daly, K. D., Schneider, M., Schliep, K. C., and Fehring, R. J. Characteristics of the menstrual cycle after discontinuation of oral contraceptives. *Journal of Women's Health (Larchmt)*, 20(2):169–177, Feb 2011.

[423] United Nations. World contraceptive use 2012, UN, Department of Economic and Social Affairs, Population Division, 2012.

[424] Navarretta, V. Sexual behavior and natural family planning teaching experiences. *International Journal of Gynecology and Obstetrics* (supplement), 1:157–160, 1989.

[425] Nepomnaschy, P. A., Welch, K., McConnell, D., Strassmann, B. I., and England, B. G., Stress and female reproductive function: A study of daily variations in cortisol, gonadotrophins, and gonadal steroids in a rural Mayan population. *American Journal of Human Biology*, 16(5):523–532, 2004.

[426] National Institute for Health and Clinical Excellence (NICE). Heavy menstrual bleeding, clinical guideline 44, Available from www.nice.org.uk/guidance/cg44, January 2007.
[427] National Institute for Health and Clinical Excellence (NICE). Ectopic pregnancy and miscarriage, clinical guideline 154, Available from www.nice.org.uk/guidance/cg154, December 2012.
[428] National Institute for Health and Clinical Excellence (NICE). Fertility: Assessment and treatment for people with fertility problems, clinical guideline 156, Available from www.nice.org.uk/guidance/cg156, February 2013.
[429] National Institute for Health and Clinical Excellence (NICE). Menopause: Diagnosis and management, clinical guideline NG 23, Available from www.nice.org.uk/guidance/ng23, November 2015.
[430] Nikolaou, Dimitrios. How old are your eggs? *Current Opinion in Obstetrics and Gynecology*, 20(6):540–544, Dec 2008.
[431] Norman, R. J., Noakes, M., Wu, R., Davies, M. J., Moran, L., and Wang, J. X. Improving reproductive performance in overweight/obese women with effective weight management. *Human ReproductionUpdate*, 10(3):267–280, 2004.
[432] Norman, R. J., and Wu, R., The potential danger of cox-2 inhibitors. *Fertility and Sterility*, 81(3):493–494, Mar 2004.
[433] Oats, J., and Abraham, S. *Llewellyn-Jones Fundamentals of Obstetrics and Gynaecology*, 10th Edition. Elsevier, Amsterdam, 2016.
[434] Odeblad, E. The functional structure of human cervical mucus. *Acta Obstetrica et Gynecologica Scandinavica*, 47:57–79, 1968.
[435] Odeblad, E. The biophysical properties of the cervico-vaginal secretions. *International Review of Natural Family Planning*, 7(1):1–56, Spring 1983.
[436] Odeblad, E. Cervical mucus and their functions. *Journal of the Irish College of Physicians and Surgeons*, 26(1):27–32, 1997.
[437] European Society of Human Reproduction and Embryology (ESHRE) Amsterdam. Greening, D., daily sex helps reduce sperm DNA damage and improve fertility. In *Science Daily, 1 July 2009*, Available from www.sciencedaily.com/re-leases/2009/06/090630075311.htm, 2009.
[438] Diaz, A., Laufer, M. R., and Breech, L. L. American Academy of Pediatrics Committee on Adolescence, American College of Obstetricians, Gynecologists Committee on Adolescent Health Care. Menstruation in girls and adolescents: Using the menstrual cycle as a vital sign. *Pediatrics*, 118(5):2245–2250, Nov 2006.
[439] O'Herlihy, C., Robinson, H. P., and de Crespigny, L. J. Mittelschmerz is a preovulatory symptom. *British Medical Journal*, 280:986, Apr 1980.
[440] International Conference on Population and Development. Cairo conference maps out "path to a better reality". *ICPD 94* Newsletter Number 19, Sept 1994.
[441] Office for National (ONS). Cohort fertility, 2012: Statistical bulletin, 2012.
[442] Paes, B. F., Vermeulen, K., Brohet, R. M., van der Ploeg, T., and de Winter, J. P. Accuracy of tympanic and infrared skin thermometers in children. *Archives of Disease in Childhood*, 95(12):974–978, Dec 2010.
[443] Paffoni, A., Ferrari, S., Vigano, P., Pagliardini, L., Papaleo, E., Candiani, M., Tirelli, A., Fedele, L., and Somigliana, E. Vitamin D deficiency and infertility: Insights from in vitro fertilization cycles. *Journal of Clinical Endocrinology and Metabolism*, 99(11):2372–2376, Nov 2014.
[444] Pallone, S. R., and Bergus, G. R. Fertility awareness-based methods: Another option for family planning. *Journal of the American Board of Family Medicine*, 22(2):147–157, 2009.
[445] Panzetta, S. Breastfeeding as contraception, Patient information leaflet for Camden Primary Care Trust, May 2010.
[446] Panzetta, S., Lactational amenorrhoea method contraception: Improving knowledge. *Community Practitioner*, 84(10):35–37, Oct 2011.

[447] Panzetta, S., and Shawe, J., Lactational amenorrhoea method: The evidence is there, why aren't we using it? *Journal of Family Planning and Reproductive Health Care*, 39(2):136–138, Apr 2013.

[448] Papaioannou, S., Delkos, D., and Pardey, J. Vaginal core body temperature assessment identifies pre-ovulatory body temperature rise and detects ovulation in advance of ultrasound folliculometry. In *European Society for Human Reproduction and Endocrinology 30th Annual Conference: Poster Presepresent*, Munich, 2014.

[449] Papaioannou, S., Aslam, M., Al Watter, B.H., Milnes, R.C., and Knowles, T.G. Ovulation assessment by vaginal temperature analysis (the ovusense advanced fertility monitoring system) in comparison to oral temperature measurement. *Fertility and Sterility*, 98(3):S160, 2012.

[450] Parenteau-Carreau, S. The return of fertility in breastfeeding women. *International Review of Natural Family Planning*, 8(1):34–43, 1984.

[451] Parenteau-Carreau, S., and Infante-Rivard, C. Self-palpation to assess cervical changes in relation to mucus and temperature. *International Journal of Fertility*, 33(Suppl):10–16, 1988.

[452] Planned Parenthood. Withdrawal method, Available from www.plannedparenthood.org/health-info/birth-control/withdrawal-pull-out-method (accessed 30.7.14).

[453] Parry, B. L., Berga, S. L., Mostofi, N., Klauber, M. R., and Resnick, A. Plasma melatonin circadian rhythms during the menstrual cycle and after light therapy in premenstrual dysphoric disorder and normal control subjects. *Journal of Biological Rhythms*, 12(1):47–64, Feb 1997.

[454] Pasquali, R., Gambineri, A., and Pagotto, U. The impact of obesity on reproduction in women with polycystic ovary syndrome. *British Journal of Obstetrics and Gynaecology*, 113(10):1148–1159, Oct 2006.

[455] Pastor, Zlatko. Female ejaculation orgasm vs. coital incontinence: A systematic review. *Journal of Sexual Medicine*, 10(7):1682–1691, Jul 2013.

[456] Peccatori, F. A., Azim, H. A., Jr, Orecchia, R., Hoekstra, H. J., Pavlidis, N., Kesic, V., Pentheroudakis, G., and E. S. M. O. Guidelines Working Group. Cancer, pregnancy and fertility: Esmo clinical practice guidelines for diagnosis, treatment and followup. *Annals of Oncology*, 24(Suppl 6):vi160–vi170, Oct 2013.

[457] Pehlivanoglu, B., Balkanci, Z. D., Ridvanagaoglu, A. Y., Durmazlar, N., Ozturk, G., Erbas, D., and Okur, H. Impact of stress, gender and menstrual cycle on immune system: Possible role of nitric oxide. *Archives of Physiology and Biochemistry*, 109(4):383–387, Oct 2001.

[458] Penev, Plamen D. Association between sleep and morning testosterone levels in older men. *Sleep*, 30(4):427–432, Apr 2007.

[459] Penketh, R. J., Taylor, L. M., and Shah, S. Bladder fever: Rare complication of the "safe period" method of contraception. *British Medical Journal (Clinical Research Edition)*, 285(6336):171–172, Jul 17 1982.

[460] Perera, F., and Herbstman, J., Prenatal environmental exposures, epigenetics, and disease. *Reproductive Toxicology*, 31(3):363–373, Apr 2011.

[461] Perez, A., Labbok, M. H., and Queenan, J. T. Clinical study of the lactational amenorrhoea method for family planning. *Lancet*, 339(8799):968–970, Apr 1992.

[462] Perez, A., Vela, P., Masnick, G. S., and Potter, R. G. First ovulation after childbirth: The effect of breast-feeding. *American Journal of Obstetrics and Gynecology*, 114(8):1041–1047, Dec 1972.

[463] Perez, A., Zabala, A., Larrain, A., Widmer, S., Nunez, M., and Baranda, B. The clinical efficiency of the Ovulation Method (Billings). *Revista Chilena de Obstetricia y Ginecologia*, 48:97–102, 1983.

[464] Petersen, M. H., and Hauge, H. N. Can training improve the results with infrared tympanic thermometers? *Acta Anaesthesiologica Scandinavica*, 41(8):1066–1070, Sep 1997.

[465] Peterson, A. E., Perez-Escamilla, R., Labbok, M. H., Hight, V., von Hertzen, H., and Van Look, P. Multicenter study of the lactational amenorrhea method iii: Effectiveness, duration, and satisfaction with reduced client-provider contact. *Contraception*, 62(5):221–230, Nov 2000.

[466] Peterson, B. D., Pirritano, M., Tucker, L., and Lampic, C., Fertility awareness and parenting attitudes among American male and female undergraduate university students. *Human Reproduction*, 27(5):1375–1382, May 2012.

[467] Phillips, O., and Simpson, J. Contraception and congenital malformations. *Global Library of Women's Medicine*, DOI: 10.3843/glowm.10398, 2008.

[468] Pinkerton, J. V., Guico-Pabia, C. J., and Taylor, H. S. Menstrual cycle-related exacerbation of disease. *American Journal of Obstetrics and Gynecology*, 202(3):221–231, Mar 2010.

[469] Porucznik, C. A., Cox, K. J., Schliep, K. C., and Stanford, J. B. Pilot test and validation of the peak day method of prospective determination of ovulation against a handheld urine hormone monitor. *BioMed Central (BMC) Women's Health*, 14:4, 2014.

[470] Potts, M., and Short, R. *Ever Since Adam and Eve, the Evolution of Human Sexuality*. Cambridge: Cambridge University Press, 1999.

[471] Prasad, A., Mumford, S. L., Buck Louis, G. M., Ahrens, K. A., Sjaarda, L. A., Schliep, K. C., et al. Sexual activity, endogenous reproductive hormones and ovulation in premenopausal women. *Hormones and Behavior*, 66(2):330–338, Jul 2014.

[472] Pyper, C. Reproductive health awareness, an important dimension to be integrated into existing programmes. *Advances in Contraception*, 13:331–338, 1997.

[473] Pyper, C., and Knight, J. Fertility awareness methods of family planning: The physiological background, methodology and effectiveness of fertility awareness methods. *The Journal of Family Planning and Reproductive Health Care*, 27(2):103–110, 2001.

[474] Pyper, C., and Knight, J. Fertility awareness methods of family planning for achieving or avoiding pregnancy, in *The Global Library of Women's Medicine*, DOI: 10.3843/GLOWM.10384, 2008.

[475] Pyper, C. M. Fertility awareness and natural family planning. *European Journal of Contraception and Reproductive Health Care*, 2(2):131–146, Jun 1997.

[476] Qublan, H., Amarin, Z., Nawasreh, M., Diab, F., Malkawi, S., Al-Ahmad, N., and Balawneh, M. Luteinized unruptured follicle syndrome: Incidence and recurrence rate in infertile women with unexplained infertility undergoing intrauterine insemination. *Human Reproduction*, 21(8):2110–2113, Aug 2006.

[477] Rabinerson, D., and Horowitz, E. G-spot and female ejaculation: Fiction or reality? *Harefuah*, 146(2):145–7, 163, Feb 2007.

[478] Radwan, H., Mussaiger, A. O., and Hachem, F., Breast-feeding and lactational amenorrhea in the United Arab Emirates. *Journal of Pediatric Nursing*, 24(1):62–68, Feb 2009.

[479] Ramsay, D. T., Kent, J. C., Hartmann, R. A., and Hartmann, P. E. Anatomy of the lactating human breast redefined with ultrasound imaging. *Journal of Anatomy*, 206(6):525–534, Jun 2005.

[480] Rapkin, A. J., and Akopians, A. L. Pathophysiology of premenstrual syndrome and premenstrual dysphoric disorder. *Menopause International*, 18(2):52–59, Jun 2012.

[481] Rasmussen, K. M., and Geraghty, S. R. The quiet revolution: Breast-feeding transformed with the use of breast pumps. *American Journal of Public Health*, 101(8):1356–1359, Aug 2011.

[482] Ratto, M. H., Leduc, Y. A., Valderrama, X. P., van Straaten, K. E., Delbaere, L. T. J., Pierson, R. A., and Adams, G. P., The nerve of ovulation-inducing factor in semen. *Proceedings of the National Academy of Sciences of the USA*, 109(37):15042–15047, Aug 2012.

[483] Royal College of Obstetricians and Gynaecologists (RCOG). Exercise in pregnancy, 2006.

[484] RCOG. Management of premenstrual syndrome, 2007.

[485] RCOG. Clinical governance advice no. 7: Presenting information on risk, 2008.
[486] RCOG. Alternatives to HRT for the management of symptoms of the menopause, 2010.
[487] RCOG. Late intrauterine fetal death and stillbirth, 2010.
[488] RCOG. The management of gestational trophoblastic disease: Green-top guideline no. 38, 2010.
[489] RCOG. Nutrition in pregnancy: Scientific impact paper no. 18, 2010.
[490] RCOG. The care of women requesting induced abortion: Evidence-based clinical guideline number 7, 2011.
[491] RCOG. Management of women with mental health issues during pregnancy and the postnatal period, 2011.
[492] RCOG. Pregnancy and breast cancer, Green-top Guideline No. 12, 2011.
[493] RCOG. Reproductive ageing. *Scientific Advisory Committee Opinion Paper 24 January 2011*, 1–5, 2011.
[494] RCOG. Women's health care: A proposal for change: 4.1 life course approach, RCOG Expert Advisory Group, 2011.
[495] RCOG. Bacterial sepsis following pregnancy: Green-top guideline no. 64b, 2012.
[496] RCOG. Air travel and pregnancy: Scientific impact paper no. 1, 2013.
[497] RCOG. Chemical exposure during pregnancy: Dealing with potential, but unproven, risks to child health, scientific impact paper no 37, RCOG, 2013.
[498] RCOG. Long-term consequences of polycystic ovary syndrome, 2014.
[499] RCOG. Alcohol and pregnancy, 2015.
[500] RCOG. Best practice in postpartum family planning, 2015.
[501] Reilly, T. The menstrual cycle and human performance: An overview. *Biological Rhythm Research*, 31(1):2000.
[502] Reiss, Herbert, editor. *Reproductive Medicine from A-Z*. Oxford University Press, Oxford, 1998.
[503] Rice, F. J., Lanctot, C. A., and Garcia-Devesa, C. Effectiveness of the symptothermal method of natural family planning: An international study. *International Journal of Fertility*, 26(3):222–230, 1981.
[504] Robinson, J. E., Wakelin, M., and Ellis, J. E. Increased pregnancy rate with use of the Clearblue Easy fertility monitor. *Fertility and Sterility*, 87(2):329–334, Feb 2007.
[505] Roetzer, J. Supplemented basal body temperature and regulation of conception. *Archiv für Gynäkologie*, 206(2):195–214, 1968.
[506] Roetzer, J. Sympto-thermal Method and family planning. *Acta Medica Romana*, 16(30):339–348, 1978.
[507] Roetzer, J. *Family Planning the Natural Way: A Complete Guide to the Symptothermal Method*. Fleming H. Revell Co., Old Tappan, NJ, 1981.
[508] Rogow, D., and Horowitz, S. Withdrawal: A review of the literature and an agenda for research. *Studies in Family Planning*, 26(3):140–153, 1995.
[509] Roland, M. The fern test: A critical analysis. *Obstetrics and Gynecology*, 11(1):30–34, Jan 1958.
[510] Rollason, J. C.B., Outtrim, J. G., and Mathur, R. S. A pilot study comparing the Duofertility(®) monitor with ultrasound in infertile women. *International Journal of Women's Health*, 6:657–662, 2014.
[511] Romans, S., Clarkson, R., Einstein, G., Petrovic, M., and Stewart, D. Mood and the menstrual cycle: A review of prospective data studies. *Gender Medicine*, 9(5):361–384, Oct 2012.
[512] Ronda, E., García, A. M., Sánchez-Paya, J., and Moen, B. E. Menstrual disorders and subfertility in Spanish hairdressers. *European Journal of Obstetrics, Gynecology and Reproductive Biology*, 147(1):61–64, Nov 2009.
[513] Roos, J., Johnson, S., Weddell, S., Godehardt, E., Schiffner, J., Freundl, G., and Gnoth, C. Monitoring the menstrual cycle: Comparison of urinary and serum reproductive hormones

referenced to true ovulation. *European Journal of Contraception and Reproductive Health Care*, 20(6):438–50, May 2015.

[514] Rosen, R., Brown, C., Heiman, J., Leiblum, S., Meston, C., Shabsigh, R., Ferguson, D., and D'Agostino, R., Jr. The female sexual function index (FSFI): A multidimensional self-report instrument for the assessment of female sexual function. *Journal of Sex and Marital Therapy*, 26(2):191–208, 2000.

[515] Rossouw, J. E., Anderson, G. L., Prentice, R. L., LaCroix, A. Z., Kooperberg, C., Stefanick, M. L., et al. Risks and benefits of estrogen plus progestin in healthy postmenopausal women: Principal results from the women's health initiative randomized controlled trial. *Journal of the American Medical Association*, 288(3):321–333, Jul 2002.

[516] Roth, B. Fertility awareness as a component of sexuality education: Preliminary research findings with adolescents. *Nurse Practitioner*, 18(3):40, 43, 47–408 passim, Mar 1993.

[517] Rowlands, S., editor. *Abortion Care*. Cambridge University Press, Cambridge, 2014.

[518] Royston, J. P. Basal body temperature, ovulation and the risk of conception, with special reference to the lifetimes of sperm and egg. *Biometrics*, 38(2):397–406, Jun 1982.

[519] Royston, J. P., and Abrams, R. M. The choice between rectum and mouth as sites for basal body temperature measurements. *British Journal of Family Planning*, 7:110–111, 1982.

[520] Royston, J. P., Abrams, R. M., Higgins, M. P., and Flynn, A. M. The adjustment of basal body temperature measurements to allow for time of waking. *British Journal of Obstetrics and Gynecology*, 87(12):1123–1127, Dec 1980.

[521] Sandhu, R. S., Wong, T. H., Kling, C. A., and Chohan, K. R. In-vitro effects of coital lubricants and synthetic and natural oils on sperm motility. *Fertility and Sterility*, 101(4):941–944, Jan 2014.

[522] Santoro, N., Crawford, S. L., Lasley, W. L., Luborsky, J. L., Matthews, K. A., McConnell, D., Randolph, J. F., Jr, Gold, E. B., Greendale, G. A., Korenman, S. G., Powell, L., Sowers, M. F., and Weiss, G. Factors related to declining luteal function in women during the menopausal transition. *Journal of Clinical Endocrinology and Metabolism*, 93(5):1711–1721, May 2008.

[523] Sapolsky, Robert M. *Why Zebras Don't Get Ulcers*. Holt, New York, 2004.

[524] Sapra, K. J., Kim, S., Eisenberg, M. L., Chen, Z., and Louis, G. M. Buck. Male underwear and semen quality in a population-based preconception cohort. *Fertility and Sterility*, 104(3, supplement):e45, 2015.

[525] Sapra, K. J., McLain, A. C., Maisog, J. M., Sundaram, R., and Louis, G. M. Buck. Successive time to pregnancy among women experiencing pregnancy loss. *Human Reproduction*, Aug 2014.

[526] Scarpa, B., and Dunson, D. B. Bayesian methods for searching for optimal rules for timing intercourse to achieve pregnancy. *Statistics in Medicine*, 26(9):1920–1936, Apr 2007.

[527] Scarpellini, F., Curto, C., and Scarpellini, L. LUF syndrome biological diagnosis by basal body temperature graph. *Acta Europea Fertiliatis*, 24(3):113–115, 1993.

[528] Schliep, K. C., Mumford, S. L., Hammoud, A. O., Stanford, J. B., Kissell, K. A., Sjaarda, L. A., et al. Luteal phase deficiency in regularly menstruating women: Prevalence and overlap in identification based on clinical and biochemical diagnostic criteria. *Journal of Endocrinology and Metabolism*, 99(6):E1007–E1014, Jun 2014.

[529] Schmid, Thomas E., Eskenazi, Brenda, Marchetti, Francesco, Young, Suzanne, Weldon, Rosana H., Baumgartner, Adolf, Anderson, Diana, and Wyrobek, Andrew J. Micronutrients intake is associated with improved sperm DNA quality in older men. *Fertility and Sterility*, Aug 2012.

[530] Schreiber, C. A., Sober, S., Ratcliffe, S., and Creinin, M. D. Ovulation resumption after medical abortion with mifepristone and misoprostol. *Contraception*, 84(3):230–233, Sep 2011.

[531] Schreiber, S., Minute, M., Tornese, G., Giorgi, R., Duranti, M., Ronfani, L., and Barbi, E. Galinstan thermometer is more accurate than digital for the measurement of body temperature in children. *Paediatric Emergency Care*, 29(2):197–199, Feb 2013.

[532] Schwartz, D., Macdonald, P. D., and Heuchel, V. Fecundability, coital frequency and the viability of ova. *Population Studies (Cambridge)*, 34(2):397–400, Jul 1980.

[533] Schwartz, D., and Mayaux, M. J. Female fecundity as a function of age: Results of artificial insemination in 2193 nulliparous women with azoospermic husbands: Federation cecos. *New England Journal of Medicine*, 306(7):404–406, Feb 1982.

[534] Seshadri, S., Oakeshott, P., Nelson-Piercy, C., and Chappell, L. C. Prepregnancy care. *British Medical Journal*, 344:e3467, 2012.

[535] Severino, S. K., Wagner, D. R., Moline, M. L., Hurt, S. W., Pollak, C. P., and Zendell, S. High nocturnal body temperature in premenstrual syndrome and late luteal phase dysphoric disorder. *American Journal of Psychiatry*, 148(10):1329–1335, Oct 1991.

[536] Shamim, N., Usala, S. J., Biggs, W. C., and McKenna, G. B. The elasticity of cervical-vaginal secretions is abnormal in polycystic ovary syndrome: Case report of five PCOS women. *Indian Journal of Endocrinology and Metabolism*, 16(6):1019–1021, Nov 2012.

[537] Sharma, R., Biedenharn, K. R., Fedor, J. M., and Agarwal, A., Lifestyle factors and reproductive health: Taking control of your fertility. *Reproductive Biology and Endocrinology*, 11:66, 2013.

[538] Shawe, J., Mann, S., and Stephenson, J., The move to integrated contraception and sexual health services: Have we forgotten family "planning"? *Journal of Family Planning and Reproductive Health Care*, 35(4):250–253, Oct 2009.

[539] Sherman, B. M., Chapler, F. K., Crickard, K., and Wycoff, D. Endocrine consequences of continuous antiestrogen therapy with tamoxifen in premenopausal women. *Journal of Clinical Investigation*, 64(2):398–404, Aug 1979.

[540] Shettles, L. B. Factors influencing sex ratios. *International Journal of Gynecology and Obstetrics*, 8(5):643–647, 1970.

[541] Sheynkin, Y., Jung, M.l, Yoo, P., Schulsinger, D., and Komaroff, E. Increase in scrotal temperature in laptop computer users. *Human Reproduction*, 20(2):452–455, Feb 2005.

[542] Sholapurkar, S. L. Is there an ideal interpregnancy interval after a live birth, miscarriage or other adverse pregnancy outcomes? *Journal of Obstetrics and Gynaecology*, 30(2):107–110, Feb 2010.

[543] Short, R. V., Lewis, P. R., Renfree, M. B., and Shaw, G. Contraceptive effects of extended lactational amenorrhoea: Beyond the Bellagio consensus. *Lancet*, 337(8743):715–717, Mar 1991.

[544] Sinai, I., Jennings, V., and Arévalo, M. The twoday algorithm: A new algorithm to identify the fertile time of the menstrual cycle. *Contraception*, 60(2):65–70, Aug 1999.

[545] Sinai, I., and Arévalo, M. It's all in the timing: Coital frequency and fertility awareness-based methods of family planning. *Journal of Biosocial Sciences*, 38(6):763–777, Nov 2006.

[546] Sinai, I., and Cachan, J. A bridge for postpartum women to standard days method®: Ii. efficacy study. *Contraception*, 86(1):16–21, Jul 2012.

[547] Sinai, I., Lundgren, R., Arévalo, M., and Jennings, V. Fertility awareness-based methods of family planning: Predictors of correct use. *International Family Planning Perspectives*, 32(2):94–100, Jun 2006.

[548] Sinding, C., Kemper, E., Spornraft-Ragaller, P., and Hummel, T. Decreased perception of bourgeonal may be linked to male idiopathic infertility. *Chemical Senses Journal*, 38(5):439–445, Jun 2013.

[549] Singer, D., Mann, E., Hunter, M. S., Pitkin, J., and Panay, N. The silent grief: Psychosocial aspects of premature ovarian failure. *Climacteric*, 14(4):428–437, Aug 2011.

[550] Smith, L. F. P., Ewings, P. D., and Quinlan, C., Incidence of pregnancy after expectant, medical, or surgical management of spontaneous first trimester miscarriage: Long term follow-up of miscarriage treatment (MIST) randomised controlled trial. *British Medical Journal*, 339:b3827, 2009.

[551] Snick, H. K., Snick, T. S., Evers, J. L., and Collins, J. A. The spontaneous pregnancy prognosis in untreated subfertile couples: The Walcheren primary care study. *Human Reproduction*, 12(7):1582–1588, Jul 1997.
[552] Snick, H. K. A. Should spontaneous or timed intercourse guide couples trying to conceive? *Human Reproduction*, 20(10):2976–2979, Oct 2005.
[553] Sonntag, B., and Ludwig, M., An integrated view on the luteal phase: Diagnosis and treatment in subfertility. *Clinical Endocrinology (Oxford)*, 77(4):500–507, Oct 2012.
[554] Soules, M. R., Sherman, S., Parrott, E., Rebar, R., Santoro, N., Utian, W., and Woods, N. Executive summary: Stages of reproductive aging workshop (straw). *Fertility and Sterility*, 76(5):874–878, Nov 2001.
[555] Spehr, M., Gisselmann, G., Poplawski, A., Riffell, J. A., Wetzel, C. H., Zimmer, R. K., and Hatt, H. Identification of a testicular odorant receptor mediating human sperm chemotaxis. *Science*, 299(5615):2054–2058, Mar 2003.
[556] Spence, J. E. Anovulation and monophasic cycles. *Annals of the New York Academy of Sciences*, 816:173–176, Jun 1997.
[557] Spieler, J., and Collins, W. Potential fertility – defining the window of opportunity. *Journal of International Medical Research*, 29(Suppl 1):3A–13A, 2001.
[558] Stanford, J. B., Lemaire, J. C., and Thurman, P. B. Women's interest in natural family planning. *Journal of Family Practice*, 46(1):65–71, Jan 1998.
[559] Stanford, J. B., Thurman, P. B., and Lemaire, J. C. Physicians' knowledge and practices regarding natural family planning. *Obstetrics and Gynecology*, 94(5 Pt 1):672–678, Nov 1999.
[560] Stanford, J.B. Revisiting the fertile window. *Fertility and Sterility*, Mar 2015.
[561] Stanford, J. B., Smith, K. R., and Dunson, D. B. Vulvar mucus observations and the probability of pregnancy. *Obstetrics and Gynecology*, 101(6):1285–1293, Jun 2003.
[562] Stanford, J. B., Smith, K. R., and Varner, M. W. Impact of instruction in the Creighton model fertility care system on time to pregnancy in couples of proven fecundity: Results of a randomised trial. *Paediatric Perinatal Epidemiology*, 28(5):391–399, Sep 2014.
[563] Stanford, J. B., White, G. L., and Hatasaka, H. Timing intercourse to achieve pregnancy: Current evidence. *Obstetrics and Gynecology*, 100(6):1333–1341, Dec 2002.
[564] Steiner, A. Z., Long, D. L., Tanner, C., and Herring, A. H. Effect of vaginal lubricants on natural fertility. *Obstetrics and Gynecology*, 120(1):44–51, 2012.
[565] Stern, J., Larsson, M., Kristiansson, P., and Tyden, T. Introducing reproductive life plan-based information in contraceptive counselling: An rct. *Human Reproduction*, 28(9):2450–2461, Sep 2013.
[566] Stirling, A., and Glasier, A. Estimating the efficacy of emergency contraception – how reliable are the data? *Contraception*, 66(1):19–22, Jul 2002.
[567] Stoddard, A., and Eisenberg, D. L. Controversies in family planning: Timing of ovulation after abortion and the conundrum of postabortion intrauterine device insertion. *Contraception*, 84(2):119–121, Aug 2011.
[568] Suarez, S. S., and Pacey, A. A. Sperm transport in the female reproductive tract. *Human ReproductionUpdate*, 12(1):23–37, 2006.
[569] Summa, K. C., Vitaterna, M. H., and Turek, F. W. Environmental perturbation of the circadian clock disrupts pregnancy in the mouse. *PLoS ONE*, 7(5):e37668, DOI:10.1371/journal.pone.0037668, 2012.
[570] Tal, R., Tal, O., Seifer, B. J., and Seifer, D. B. Antimullerian hormone as predictor of implantation and clinical pregnancy after assisted conception: A systematic review and meta-analysis. *Fertility and Sterility*, 103(1):119–130.e3, Jan 2015.
[571] Taranissi, M., and El-Toukhy, T. Immunotherapy for IVF implantation failure: Just in case, or just in time, in *How to Improve Your ART Success Rates: An Evidence-Based Review of Adjuncts to IVF*. Cambridge University Press, Cambridge, 2011. 204–206.

[572] Tepper, R., Lunenfeld, B., Shalev, J., Ovadia, J., and Blankstein, J. The effect of clomiphene citrate and tamoxifen on the cervical mucus. *Acta Obstetrica et Gynecologica Scandinavica*, 67(4):311–314, 1988.

[573] ter Kuile, M. M., Brauer, M., and Laan, E. The female sexual function index (FSFI) and the female sexual distress scale (FSDS): Psychometric properties within a dutch population. *Journal of Sexual and Marital Therapy*, 32(4):289–304, 2006.

[574] Thapa, S., Wonga, M. V., Lampe, P. G., Pietojo, H., and Soejoenoes, A. Efficacy of three variations of periodic abstinence for family planning in Indonesia. *Studies in Family Planning*, 21(6):327–334, 1990.

[575] Thijssen, A., Meier, A., Panis, K., and Ombelet, W. "fertility awareness-based methods" and subfertility: A systematic review. *Facts, Views and Visions in ObGyn*, 6(3):113–123, 2014.

[576] Thoma, M. E., Hediger, M. L., Sundaram, R., Stanford, J. B., Peterson, C. M., Croughan, M. S., et al. Comparing apples and pears: Women's perceptions of their body size and shape. *Journal of Women's Health (Larchmont)*, 21(10):1074–1081, Oct 2012.

[577] Thyma, Paul. *The Double Check Method of Family Planning*. Marriage Life Information, Fall River, MA, 1977.

[578] Tietze, C. Statistical contributions to the study of human fertility. *Fertility and Sterility*, 7(1):88–95, 1956.

[579] Tietze, C., Poliakoff, S. R., and Rock, J. The clinical effectiveness of the rhythm method of contraception. *Fertility and Sterility*, 2(5):444–450, 1951.

[580] Tiplady, S., Jones, G., Campbell, M., Johnson, S., and Ledger, W. Home ovulation tests and stress in women trying to conceive: A randomized controlled trial. *Human Reproduction*, 28(1):138–151, Jan 2013.

[581] Tommaselli, G. A., Guida, M., Palomba, S., Barbato, M., and Nappi, C. Using complete breastfeeding and lactational amenorrhoea as birth spacing methods. *Contraception*, 61(4):253–257, Apr 2000.

[582] Toth, M. J., Tchernof, A., Sites, C. K., and Poehlman, E. T. Menopause-related changes in body fat distribution. *Annals of the New York Academy of Sciences*, 904:502–506, May 2000.

[583] Treloar, A. E., Boynton, R. E., Behn, B. G., and Brown, B. W. Variation of the human menstrual cycle through reproductive life. *International Journal of Fertility*, 12(1 Pt 2):77–126, 1967.

[584] Trussell, J. Statistical flaws in evidence for the Frisch hypothesis that fatness triggers menarche. *Human Biology*, 52(4):711–720, Dec 1980.

[585] Trussell, J. Measuring the contraceptive efficacy of persona. *Contraception*, 63(2):77–79, Feb 2001.

[586] Trussell, J. Contraceptive efficacy, in *Contraceptive Technology*, edited by Hatcher, R., 20th Revised Edition. Ardent Media, New York, 2011. 779–863.

[587] Trussell, J. and Grummer-Strawn, L. Contraceptive failure of the Ovulation Method of periodic abstinence. *International Family Planning Perspectives*, 16(1):5–15, 1990.

[588] Trussell, J., and Grummer-Strawn, L. Further analysis of contraceptive failure of the Ovulation Method. *American Journal of Obstetrics and Gynecology*, 165(6 Pt 2):2054–2059, Dec 1991.

[589] Trussell, James. Contraceptive failure in the United States. *Contraception*, 83(5):397–404, May 2011.

[590] Tulandi, T., Plouffe, L., Jr, and McInnes, R. A. Effect of saliva on sperm motility and activity. *Fertility and Sterility*, 38(6):721–723, Dec 1982.

[591] Tyden, T., Svanberg, A. S., Karlstrom, P., Lihoff, L., and Lampic, C., Female university students' attitudes to future motherhood and their understanding about fertility. *European Journal of Contraception and Reproductive Health Care*, 11(3):181–189, Sep 2006.

[592] Unfer, V., Carlomagno, G., Dante, G., and Facchinetti, F. Effects of myo-inositol in women with pcos: A systematic review of randomized controlled trials. *Gynecological Endocrinology*, 28(7):509–515, Jul 2012.

[593] United States Agency for International Development (USAID). Costing the standard days method, DHS occasional paper no. 6, 2013.

[594] Utting, D., and Bewley, S. Family planning and age-related reproductive risk. *The Obstetrician & Gynaecologist*, 13:5–41, 2011.

[595] Valdes, V., Labbok, M. H., Pugin, E., and Perez, A. The efficacy of the lactational amenorrhea method (LAM) among working women. *Contraception*, 62(5):217–219, Nov 2000.

[596] Van der Wijden, C., and Manion, C. Lactational amenorrhea for family planning. *Cochrane Database of Systematic Reviews* (10):CD001329, DOI: 10.1002/14651858.CD001329.pub2, 2008.

[597] Vande Vusse, L., Hanson, L., Fehring, R. J., Newman, A., and Fox, J., Couples' views of the effects of natural family planning on marital dynamics. *Journal of Nursing Scholarship*, 35(2):171–176, 2003.

[598] Vargas, J., Crausaz, M., Senn, A., and Germond, M., Sperm toxicity of "nonspermicidal" lubricant and ultrasound gels used in reproductive medicine. *Fertility and Sterility*, 95(2):835–836, Feb 2011.

[599] Pope Paul VI. Humanae vitae: Encyclical of Pope Paul VI on the regulation of birth, Available from www.papalencyclicals.net/Paul06/p6humana.htm, 1968.

[600] Vigil, P., Cortes, M. E., Ziga, A., Riquelme, J., and Ceric, F. Scanning electron and light microscopy study of the cervical mucus in women with polycystic ovary syndrome. *J Electron Microsc (Tokyo)*, 58(1):21–27, Jan 2009.

[601] Vollman, R. F. *The Menstrual Cycle: Major Problems in Obstetrics and Gynecology*, Vol. 7. Saunders, Philadelphia, 1977.

[602] VonFragstein, M., Flynn, A., and Royston, P. Analysis of a representative sample of natural family planning users in England and Wales, 1984–1985. *International Journal of Fertility*, 33(Suppl):70–77, 1988.

[603] Wade, M. E., McCarthy, P., Braunstein, G. D., Abernathy, J. R., Suchindran, C. M., Harris, G. S., Danzer, H. C., and Uricchio, W. A. A randomized prospective study of the use-effectiveness of two methods of natural family planning. *American Journal of Obstetrics and Gynecology*, 141(4):368–376, Oct 1981.

[604] Walker, A. E. *The Menstrual Cycle*. London: Routledge, 1997.

[605] Waterland, R. A., Kellermayer, R., Laritsky, E., Rayco-Solon, P., Harris, R. A., Travisano, M., et al. Season of conception in rural Gambia affects dna methylation at putative human metastable epialleles. *PLoS Genetics*, 6(12):e1001252, 2010.

[606] Watson, C. J., Grando, D., Garland, S. M., Myers, S., Fairley, C. K., and Pirotta, M., Premenstrual vaginal colonization of candida and symptoms of vaginitis. *Journal of Medical Microbiology*, 61(Pt 11):1580–1583, Nov 2012.

[607] Weissmann, M. C., Foliaki, L., Billings, E. L., and Billings, J. J. A trial of the Ovulation Method of family planning in Tonga. *Lancet*, 2(7781):813–816, Oct 1972.

[608] Wentz, A. C. Premenstrual spotting: Its association with endometriosis but not luteal phase inadequacy. *Fertility and Sterility*, 33(6):605–607, Jun 1980.

[609] Werler, M. M. Teratogen update: Pseudoephedrine. *Birth Defects Research Part A Clinical and Molecular Teratology*, 76(6):445–452, Jun 2006.

[610] Weschler, T. *Taking Charge of Your Fertility*. London: Vermillion, 2003.

[611] West, Z., and Knight, J. Ticking all the boxes: A unique fertility questionnaire to assess preconception health and lifestyle factors in a midwife-led integrated care clinic. In *Abstracts of the 22nd Annual Meeting of the European Society of Human Reproduction and Endocrinology*, Prague, Czech Republic, 18–21 June 2006.

[612] White, C. P., Hitchcock, C. L., Vigna, Y. M., and Prior, J. C. Fluid retention over the menstrual cycle: 1-year data from the prospective ovulation cohort. *Obstetrics and GynecologyInternational*, 2011:138451, 2011.

[613] World Health Organisation (WHO). Biology of fertility control by periodic abstinence: Report of a who scientific group. *World Health Organisation Technical Report Series*, 360:5–20, 1967.

[614] WHO. Temporal relationships between ovulation and defined changes in the concentration of plasma estradiol-17 beta, luteinizing hormone, follicle-stimulating hormone, and progesterone: I. probit analysis: World health organization, task force on methods for the determination of the fertile period, special programme of research, development and research training in human reproduction. *American Journal of Obstetrics and Gynecology*, 138(4):383–390, Oct 1980.

[615] WHO. A prospective multi-centre trial of the Ovulation Method of natural family planning: I. the teaching phase. *Fertility and Sterility*, 36(2):152–158, Aug 1981.

[616] WHO. A prospective multi-centre trial of the Ovulation Method of natural family planning: II. the effectiveness phase. *Fertility and Sterility*, 36(5):591–598, Nov 1981.

[617] WHO. A prospective multi-centre trial of the Ovulation Method of natural family planning: III. characteristics of the menstrual cycle and of the fertile phase. *Fertility and Sterility*, 40(6):773–778, Dec 1983.

[618] WHO. Temporal relationships between indices of the fertile period. *Fertility and Sterility*, 39(5):647–655, May 1983.

[619] WHO. A prospective multi-centre study of the Ovulation Method of natural family planning: IV. the outcome of pregnancy: *Fertility and Sterility*, 41(4):593–598, Apr 1984.

[620] WHO. Fertility Awareness Methods – health for all 2000. In *Report on a WHO Workshop*, Poland, 1986.

[621] WHO. A prospective multicenter trial of the Ovulation Method of natural family planning: V. psychosexual aspects: *Fertility and Sterility*, 47(5):765–772, May 1987.

[622] WHO. The world health organization multinational study of breast-feeding and lactational amenorrhea: III. pregnancy during breast-feeding: WHO task force on methods for the natural regulation of fertility. *Fertility and Sterility*, 72(3):431–440, Sep 1999.

[623] WHO. The World Health Organization multinational study of breast-feeding and lactational amenorrhea: IV. postpartum bleeding and lochia in breast-feeding women: WHO task force on methods for the natural regulation of fertility. *Fertility and Sterility*, 72(3):441–447, Sep 1999.

[624] WHO. The optimal duration of exclusive breast-feeding: Report of an expert consultation, Geneva, Switzerland, 28–30 March 2001, Department of Nutrition for Health and Development, Available from www.who.int/nut.

[625] Wiegratz, I., Mittmann, K., Dietrich, H., Zimmermann, T., and Kuhl, H. Fertility after discontinuation of treatment with an oral contraceptive containing 30 microg of ethinyl estradiol and 2 mg of dienogest. *Fertility and Sterility*, 85(6):1812–1819, Jun 2006.

[626] Wilcox, A. J. *Fertility and Pregnancy: An Epidemiological Perspective*. Oxford University Press, Oxford, 2010.

[627] Wilcox, A. J., Baird, D. D., and Weinberg, C. R. Time of implantation of the conceptus and loss of pregnancy. *New England Journal of Medicine*, 340(23):1796–1799, Jun 1999.

[628] Wilcox, A. J., Baird, Donna Day, Dunson, David B., McConnaughey, D. Robert, Kesner, James S., and Weinberg, Clarice R. On the frequency of intercourse around ovulation: Evidence for biological influences. *Human Reproduction*, 19(7):1539–1543, Jul 2004.

[629] Wilcox, A. J., Dunson, D., and Baird, D. D. The timing of the "fertile window" in the menstrual cycle: Day specific estimates from a prospective study. *British Medical Journal*, 321(7271):1259–1262, Nov 2000.

[630] Wilcox, A. J., Dunson, D. B., Weinberg, C. R., Trussell, J., and Baird, D. D. Likelihood of conception with a single act of intercourse: Providing benchmark rates for assessment of post-coital contraceptives. *Contraception*, 63(4):211–215, Apr 2001.

[631] Wilcox, A. J., Weinberg, C. R., and Baird, D. D. Timing of sexual intercourse in relation to ovulation: Effects on the probability of conception, survival of the pregnancy, and sex of the baby. *New England Journal of Medicine*, 333(23):1517–1521, Dec 1995.

[632] Wilcox, A. J., Weinberg, C. R., and Baird, D. D. Post-ovulatory ageing of the human oocyte and embryo failure. *Human Reproduction*, 13(2):394–397, Feb 1998.

[633] Wimpissinger, F., Springer, C., and Stackl, W. International online survey: Female ejaculation has a positive impact on women's and their partners' sexual lives. *British Journal of Urology International*, 112(2):E177–E185, Jul 2013.

[634] Wise, L. A., Hatch, E. E., Stanford, J., McKinnon, C. J., Wesselink, A., and Rothman, K. J. A randomised trial of web-based fertility-tracking software and fecundability. *Fertility and Sterility*, 104(3,supplement): e113, 2015.

[635] Wojcieszek, A. M., and Thompson, R. Conceiving of change: A brief intervention increases young adults' knowledge of fertility and the effectiveness of in vitro fertilization. *Fertility and Sterility*, 100(2):523–529, Aug 2013.

[636] WHO. Family planning/contraception, www.who.int/mediacentre/factsheets/fs351/en/.

[637] Wyndham, N., Gabriela, P., Figueira, M., and Patrizio, P. A persistent misperception: Assisted reproductive technology can reverse the "aged biological clock". *Fertility and Sterility*, 97(5):1044–1047, Mar 2012.

[638] Xiao, E., Xia-Zhang, L., and Ferin, M. Inadequate luteal function is the initial clinical cyclic defect in a 12-day stress model that includes a psychogenic component in the rhesus monkey. *Journal of Endocrinology and Metabolism*, 87(5):2232–2237, May 2002.

[639] Yairi-Oron, Y., Rabinson, J., and Orvieto, R. A simplified approach to religious infertility. *Fertility and Sterility*, 86(6):1771–1772, Dec 2006.

[640] Zaadstra, B. M., Seidell, J. C., Van Noord, P. A., te Velde, E. R., Habbema, J. D., Vrieswijk, B., and Karbaat, J. Fat and female fecundity: Prospective study of effect of body fat distribution on conception rates. *British Medical Journal*, 306(6876):484–487, Feb 1993.

[641] Zachariah, M., Fleming, R., and Acharya, U., Management of obese women in assisted conception units: A UK survey. *Human Fertility (Cambridge)*, 9(2):101–105, Jun 2006.

[642] Zimecki, M., The lunar cycle: Effects on human and animal behavior and physiology. *Postepy Higieny I Medycyny Doswiadczalnej (Online)*, 60:1–7, 2006.

[643] Zinaman, M., and Stevenson, W. Efficacy of the symptothermal method of natural family planning in lactating women after the return of menses. *American Journal of Obstetrics and Gynecology*, 165(6 Pt 2):2037–2039, Dec 1991.

[644] Zinaman, M. J., Hughes, V., Queenan, J. T., Labbok, M. H., and Albertson, B. Acute prolactin and oxytocin responses and milk yield to infant suckling and artificial methods of expression in lactating women. *Pediatrics*, 89(3):437–440, Mar 1992.

[645] Zinaman, M., Johnson, S., Ellis, J., and Ledger, W. Accuracy of perception of ovulation day in women trying to conceive. *Current Medical Research and Opinion*, 28(5):749–754, May 2012.

[646] Zukerman, Z., Weiss, D. B., and Orvieto, R. Does preejaculatory penile secretion originating from Cowper's gland contain sperm? *Journal of Assisted Reproduction and Genetics*, 20(4):157–159, Apr 2003.

INDEX

Page numbers in italic format indicate figures and tables.

T - #1039 - 101024 - C0 - 246/174/24 - PB - 9781138790100 - Matt Lamination